METHODS IN MOLECULAR BIOLOGY

Series Editor
John M. Walker
School of Life and Medical Sciences
University of Hertfordshire
Hatfield, Hertfordshire, AL10 9AB, UK

For further volumes:
http://www.springer.com/series/7651

Computational Drug Discovery and Design

Edited by

Mohini Gore

Department of Basic and Applied Sciences, Dayananda Sagar University, Bangalore, KA, India

Umesh B. Jagtap

Department of Biotechnology, Shivaji University, Kolhapur, MH, India;
Department of Botany, Government Vidarbha Institute of Science and Humanities, Amaravati, MH, India

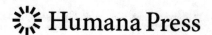 Humana Press

Editors
Mohini Gore
Department of Basic and Applied
Sciences
Dayananda Sagar University
Bangalore, KA, India

Umesh B. Jagtap
Department of Biotechnology
Shivaji University
Kolhapur, MH, India

Department of Botany
Government Vidarbha Institute of Science
and Humanities
Amaravati, MH, India

ISSN 1064-3745   ISSN 1940-6029   (electronic)
Methods in Molecular Biology
ISBN 978-1-4939-9276-8   ISBN 978-1-4939-7756-7   (eBook)
https://doi.org/10.1007/978-1-4939-7756-7

Printed on acid-free paper

This Humana Press imprint is published by the registered company Springer Science+Business Media, LLC part of
Springer Nature.
The registered company address is: 233 Spring Street, New York, NY 10013, U.S.A.

Preface

Computer-aided drug design is an indispensable approach for accelerating and economizing the costly and time-consuming process of drug discovery and development. In the recent years, there has been a spurt in the protein and ligand structure data. This has led to a surge in the number of databases and bioinformatics tools to manage and process the available data. Optimal application of the vast array of available computational tools is crucial for the discovery and design of novel drugs.

The aim of this volume on *Computational Drug Discovery and Design* is to provide methods and techniques for identification of drug target, binding sites prediction, high-throughput virtual screening, lead discovery and optimization, and prediction of pharmacokinetic properties using computer-based methodologies. This volume includes an overview of the possible techniques of the available computational tools, developing prediction models for drug target prediction and de novo design of ligands. Structure-based drug designing, fragment-based drug designing, molecular docking, and scoring functions for assessing protein-ligand docking protocols have been outlined with practical examples. Phylogenetic analysis for protein functional site prediction has been described. Virtual screening and microarray studies for identification of potential compounds for drug discovery have been described using examples. The use of molecular dynamics simulation for virtual ligand screening, studying the protein-ligand interaction, estimating ligand binding free energy, and calculating the thermodynamic properties of bound water has been presented with stepwise protocols. In silico screening of pharmacokinetic and toxicity properties of potential drugs has been demonstrated. The currently available algorithms and software for protein-protein docking have been discussed with latest examples. Protocols for quantitative structure-activity relationship have been described. Computational approaches for the prediction of protein dynamics and protein aggregation have been presented with relevant protocols. The important methods of enhanced molecular dynamics have been analyzed with the help of practical procedure description. In silico analysis for inclusion of solvent in docking studies has been described with detailed methodology. We have also included a chapter on data analytics protocol, which is useful to summarize independent studies on drug designing.

There is abundant literature available on bioinformatics. However, there is very limited literature which will provide a step-by-step approach to utilize the various bioinformatics tools. In this volume, we present a stepwise description of the protocols for the use of bioinformatics tools in drug discovery and design. This volume will assist graduate and postgraduate students, researchers, and scholars working in the fields of drug discovery and design, pharmacology, bioinformatics, chemoinformatics, computational biology, medicinal chemistry, molecular biology, and systems biology to effectively utilize computational methodologies in the discovery and design of novel drugs.

We would like to express our heartfelt gratitude to the series editor John Walker for his valuable advice and support during every stage of development of this book. We thank all the authors who contributed to this book in a timely manner and shared their practical knowledge by providing stepwise methodology for the utilization of bioinformatics tools for drug discovery and design. We hope that this volume will be helpful to both novice in the field of bioinformatics and scientists actively engaged in drug discovery research.

Bangalore, KA, India   *Mohini Gore*
Kolhapur, MH, India   *Umesh B. Jagtap*

Contents

Contributors

AMR H. A. ABDALLAH • *Department of Medicinal Chemistry and Molecular Pharmacology, College of Pharmacy, Purdue University, West Lafayette, IN, USA*

SAMIA ACI-SÈCHE • *Institut de Chimie Organique et Analytique (ICOA), UMR7311 CNRS-Université d'Orléans, Université d'Orléans, Orléans Cedex 2, France*

MATTEO ALDEGHI • *Structural Bioinformatics and Computational Biochemistry, Department of Biochemistry, University of Oxford, Oxford, UK; Department of Theoretical and Computational Biophysics, Max Planck Institute for Biophysical Chemistry, Göttingen, Germany*

ADRIANO D. ANDRICOPULO • *Laboratório de Química Medicinal e Computacional, Centro de Pesquisa e Inovação em Biodiversidade e Fármacos, Instituto de Física de São Carlos, Universidade de São Paulo (USP), São Carlos, SP, Brazil*

DAVID B. ASCHER • *Department of Biochemistry and Molecular Biology, University of Melbourne, Parkville, VIC, Australia; Department of Biochemistry, University of Cambridge, Cambridge, UK*

HEVAL ATAS • *Department of Health Informatics, Graduate School of Informatics, METU, Ankara, Turkey; Cancer Systems Biology Laboratory (CanSyL), METU, Ankara, Turkey*

KHALED BARAKAT • *Faculty of Pharmacy and Pharmaceutical Sciences, University of Alberta, Edmonton, AB, Canada*

DAMIAN BARTUZI • *Department of Synthesis and Chemical Technology of Pharmaceutical Substances with Computer Modelling Lab, Medical University of Lublin, Lublin, Poland*

SHAHERIN BASITH • *National Leading Research Laboratory (NLRL) of Molecular Modeling & Drug Design, College of Pharmacy and Graduate School of Pharmaceutical Sciences, Ewha Womans University, Seoul, Republic of Korea*

PHILIP C. BIGGIN • *Structural Bioinformatics and Computational Biochemistry, Department of Biochemistry, University of Oxford, Oxford, UK*

JOSEPH P. BLUCK • *Structural Bioinformatics and Computational Biochemistry, Department of Biochemistry, University of Oxford, Oxford, UK*

PASCAL BONNET • *Institut de Chimie Organique et Analytique (ICOA), UMR7311 CNRS-Université d'Orléans, Université d'Orléans, Orléans Cedex 2, France*

ABDENNOUR BRAKA • *Institut de Chimie Organique et Analytique (ICOA), UMR7311 CNRS-Université d'Orléans, Université d'Orléans, Orléans Cedex 2, France; Centre de Biophysique Moléculaire (CBM), CNRS, UPR 4301, Orléans Cedex 2, France*

YANG CAO • *Center of Growth, Metabolism and Aging, Key Lab of Bio-Resources and Eco-Environment of Ministry of Education, College of Life Sciences, Sichuan University, Chengdu, People's Republic of China*

ISHWAR CHANDRA • *Computer Aided Drug Design and Molecular Modelling Lab, Department of Bioinformatics, Alagappa University, Karaikudi, Tamil Nadu, India*

RADHA CHAUBE • *Department of Zoology, Institute of Science, Banaras Hindu University, Varanasi, Uttar Pradesh, India*

SUN CHOI • *National Leading Research Laboratory (NLRL) of Molecular Modeling & Drug Design, College of Pharmacy and Graduate School of Pharmaceutical Sciences, Ewha Womans University, Seoul, Republic of Korea*

BENJAMIN P. COSSINS • *Computer-Aided Drug Design and Structural Biology, UCB Pharma, Slough, UK*

GEORGES CZAPLICKI • *Institute of Pharmacology and Structural Biology, UMR 5089, University of Toulouse III, Toulouse, France*

WENTAO DAI • *Shanghai Center for Bioinformation Technology, Shanghai, People's Republic of China*

JULIEN DIHARCE • *Institut de Chimie Organique et Analytique (ICOA), UMR 7311 CNRS-Université d'Orléans, Université d'Orléans, Orléans Cedex 2, France*

TUNCA DOĞAN • *Department of Health Informatics, Graduate School of Informatics, METU, Ankara, Turkey; Cancer Systems Biology Laboratory (CanSyL), METU, Ankara, Turkey; European Molecular Biology Laboratory, European Bioinformatics Institute (EMBL-EBI), Cambridge, UK*

TIANHUA FENG • *Faculty of Pharmacy and Pharmaceutical Sciences, University of Alberta, Edmonton, AB, Canada*

LEONARDO G. FERREIRA • *Laboratório de Química Medicinal e Computacional, Centro de Pesquisa e Inovação em Biodiversidade e Fármacos, Instituto de Física de São Carlos, Universidade de São Paulo (USP), São Carlos, SP, Brazil*

FRANCIS GAUDREAULT • *National Research Council Canada, Ottawa, Canada*

JODI A. HADDEN • *Department of Chemistry and Biochemistry, University of Delaware, Newark, DE, USA*

MAR HUERTAS • *Department of Fisheries and Wildlife, Michigan State University, East Lansing, MI, USA; Department of Biology, Texas State University, San Marcos, TX, USA*

AGNIESZKA A. KACZOR • *Department of Synthesis and Chemical Technology of Pharmaceutical Substances with Computer Modelling Lab, Medical University of Lublin, Lublin, Poland; School of Pharmacy, University of Eastern Finland, Kuopio, Finland*

LISA M. KAMINSKAS • *School of Biomedical Sciences, University of Queensland, St. Lucia, QLD, Australia*

SHASHANK P. KATIYAR • *Department of Biochemical Engineering and Biotechnology, DBT-AIST International Laboratory for Advanced Biomedicine (DAILAB), Indian Institute of Technology Delhi, New Delhi, India*

DAISUKE KIHARA • *Department of Biological Science, Purdue University, West Lafayette, IN, USA; Department of Computer Science, Purdue University, West Lafayette, IN, USA*

LESLIE A. KUHN • *Department of Biochemistry and Molecular Biology, Michigan State University, East Lansing, MI, USA; Department of Fisheries and Wildlife, Michigan State University, East Lansing, MI, USA; Department of Computer Science and Engineering, Michigan State University, East Lansing, MI, USA*

ANJANI KUMARI • *Department of Biochemical Engineering and Biotechnology, DBT-AIST International Laboratory for Advanced Biomedicine (DAILAB), Indian Institute of Technology Delhi, New Delhi, India*

PRIYANKA KUMARI • *Department of Biotechnology, Delhi Technological University, Delhi, India*

ALASTAIR D. G. LAWSON • *Computer-Aided Drug Design and Structural Biology, UCB Pharma, Slough, UK*

YOONJI LEE • *National Leading Research Laboratory (NLRL) of Molecular Modeling & Drug Design, College of Pharmacy and Graduate School of Pharmaceutical Sciences, Ewha Womans University, Seoul, Republic of Korea*

SIU-WAI LEUNG • *State Key Laboratory of Quality Research in Chinese Medicine, Institute of Chinese Medical Sciences, University of Macau, Macao, China; School of Informatics, University of Edinburgh, Edinburgh, UK*

WEIMING LI • *Department of Fisheries and Wildlife, Michigan State University, East Lansing, MI, USA*

MARKUS A. LILL • *Department of Medicinal Chemistry and Molecular Pharmacology, College of Pharmacy, Purdue University, West Lafayette, IN, USA*

VIDHI MALIK • *Department of Biochemical Engineering and Biotechnology, DBT-AIST International Laboratory for Advanced Biomedicine (DAILAB), Indian Institute of Technology Delhi, New Delhi, India*

DARIUSZ MATOSIUK • *Department of Synthesis and Chemical Technology of Pharmaceutical Substances with Computer Modelling Lab, Medical University of Lublin, Lublin, Poland*

LAURENT MAVEYRAUD • *Institute of Pharmacology and Structural Biology, UMR 5089, University of Toulouse III, Toulouse, France*

GRÉGORY MENCHON • *Laboratory of Biomolecular Research, Paul Scherrer Institute, Villigen PSI, Switzerland*

ZHICHAO MIAO • *European Molecular Biology Laboratory, European Bioinformatics Institute, Cambridge, UK; Wellcome Trust Sanger Institute, Cambridge, UK*

LOUIS-PHILIPPE MORENCY • *Department of Pharmacology and Physiology, Faculty of Medicine, Université de Montréal, Montréal, QC, Canada*

RAFAEL NAJMANOVICH • *Department of Pharmacology and Physiology, Faculty of Medicine, Université de Montréal, Montréal, QC, Canada*

ABHIGYAN NATH • *Department of Zoology, Institute of Science, Banaras Hindu University, Varanasi, Uttar Pradesh, India*

UMESH PANWAR • *Computer Aided Drug Design and Molecular Modelling Lab, Department of Bioinformatics, Alagappa University, Karaikudi, Tamil Nadu, India*

SAMUEL PEÑA-DÍAZ • *Institut de Biotecnologia i Biomedicina, Universitat Autònoma de Barcelona, Bellaterra, Spain; Departament de Bioquímica i Biologia Molecular, Universitat Autònoma de Barcelona, Bellaterra, Spain*

JUAN R. PERILLA • *Department of Chemistry and Biochemistry, University of Delaware, Newark, DE, USA*

DOUGLAS E. V. PIRES • *Centro de Pesquisas René Rachou, FIOCRUZ, Belo Horizonte, Brazil*

JORDI PUJOLS • *Institut de Biotecnologia i Biomedicina, Universitat Autònoma de Barcelona, Bellaterra, Spain; Departament de Bioquímica i Biologia Molecular, Universitat Autònoma de Barcelona, Bellaterra, Spain*

SEBASTIAN RASCHKA • *Department of Biochemistry and Molecular Biology, Michigan State University, East Lansing, MI, USA*

SERGEY A. SAMSONOV • *Laboratory of Molecular Modeling, Department of Theoretical Chemistry, Faculty of Chemistry, University of Gdańsk, Gdansk, Poland*

RICARDO N. DOS SANTOS • *Departamento de Físico-Química, Universidade Estadual de Campinas (UNICAMP), Campinas, SP, Brazil*

ANNE M. SCOTT • *Department of Fisheries and Wildlife, Michigan State University, East Lansing, MI, USA*

JANA SELENT • *GPCR Drug Discovery Group, Research Programme on Biomedical Informatics (GRIB), Universitat Pompeu Fabra (UPF)-Hospital del Mar Medical Research Institute (IMIM), Parc de Recerca Biomèdica de Barcelona (PRBB), Barcelona, Spain*

JIYE SHI • *Computer-Aided Drug Design and Structural Biology, UCB Pharma, Slough, UK*

WOONG-HEE SHIN • *Department of Biological Science, Purdue University, West Lafayette, IN, USA*

KAMYA SINGH • *Department of Biochemical Engineering and Biotechnology, DBT-AIST International Laboratory for Advanced Biomedicine (DAILAB), Indian Institute of Technology Delhi, New Delhi, India*

SANJEEV KUMAR SINGH • *Computer Aided Drug Design and Molecular Modelling Lab, Department of Bioinformatics, Alagappa University, Karaikudi, Tamil Nadu, India*

TOMASZ MACIEJ STĘPNIEWSKI • *GPCR Drug Discovery Group, Research Programme on Biomedical Informatics (GRIB), Universitat Pompeu Fabra (UPF)-Hospital del Mar Medical Research Institute (IMIM), Parc de Recerca Biomèdica de Barcelona (PRBB), Barcelona, Spain*

DURAI SUNDAR • *Department of Biochemical Engineering and Biotechnology, DBT-AIST International Laboratory for Advanced Biomedicine (DAILAB), Indian Institute of Technology Delhi, New Delhi, India*

VENKATESAN SURYANARAYANAN • *Computer Aided Drug Design and Molecular Modelling Lab, Department of Bioinformatics, Alagappa University, Karaikudi, Tamil Nadu, India*

ALAN TALEVI • *Laboratorio de Investigación y Desarrollo de Bioactivos (LIDeB), Faculty of Exact Sciences, National University of La Plata (UNLP), Buenos Aires, Argentina; Argentinean National Council of Scientific and Technical Research (CONICET), Buenos Aires, Argentina*

NURCAN TUNCBAG • *Department of Health Informatics, Graduate School of Informatics, METU, Ankara, Turkey; Cancer Systems Biology Laboratory (CanSyL), METU, Ankara, Turkey*

SALVADOR VENTURA • *Institut de Biotecnologia i Biomedicina, Universitat Autònoma de Barcelona, Bellaterra, Spain; Departament de Bioquímica i Biologia Molecular, Universitat Autònoma de Barcelona, Bellaterra, Spain*

YING YANG • *Department of Medicinal Chemistry and Molecular Pharmacology, College of Pharmacy, Purdue University, West Lafayette, IN, USA*

SZE CHUNG YUEN • *State Key Laboratory of Quality Research in Chinese Medicine, Institute of Chinese Medical Sciences, University of Macau, Macao, China*

HONGMEI ZHU • *State Key Laboratory of Quality Research in Chinese Medicine, Institute of Chinese Medical Sciences, University of Macau, Macao, China*

SONIA ZIADA • *Institut de Chimie Organique et Analytique (ICOA), UMR7311 CNRS-Université d'Orléans, Université d'Orléans, Orléans Cedex 2, France*

Chapter 1

Computer-Aided Drug Design: An Overview

Alan Talevi

Abstract

The term drug design describes the search of novel compounds with biological activity, on a systematic basis. In its most common form, it involves modification of a known active scaffold or linking known active scaffolds, although de novo drug design (i.e., from scratch) is also possible. Though highly interrelated, identification of active scaffolds should be conceptually separated from drug design. Traditionally, the drug design process has focused on the molecular determinants of the interactions between the drug and its known or intended molecular target. Nevertheless, current drug design also takes into consideration other relevant processes than influence drug efficacy and safety (e.g., bioavailability, metabolic stability, interaction with antitargets).

This chapter provides an overview on possible approaches to identify active scaffolds (including in silico approximations to approach that task) and computational methods to guide the subsequent optimization process. It also discusses in which situations each of the overviewed techniques is more appropriate.

Key words ADMET, Anti-target, Computer-aided drug design, Ligand-based approaches, Molecular optimization, Pharmacophore, QSAR, Structure-based approaches, Target-based approaches, Virtual screening

1 Introduction

The term drug design describes the search of novel compounds with biological activity, on a systematic, rational basis. Basically, it relies on experimental information of the intended molecular target or a similar biomolecule (direct drug design) and/or known binders of such target (indirect drug design). Lately, however, the idea of using direct or indirect structural information on relevant anti-targets has gained increasing attention to improve ligand selectivity and reduce off-target interactions, leading to enhanced safety and even improved pharmacokinetic profile [1–4]. In other words, modern drug design not only relies on available molecular information on the proposed molecular targets but also on the information on antitargets.

In its most common form, drug design involves modification of a known active scaffold (molecular optimization) or linking known

Mohini Gore and Umesh B. Jagtap (eds.), *Computational Drug Discovery and Design*, Methods in Molecular Biology, vol. 1762, https://doi.org/10.1007/978-1-4939-7756-7_1, © Springer Science+Business Media, LLC, part of Springer Nature 2018

active scaffolds, although de novo drug design (i.e., from scratch) is of course also possible (e.g., fragment growing approximations). In any case, a starting point or seed is required to build up or optimize the active compound. Computer-aided methods have gained a prominent role in both stages of modern drug discovery: searching for starting points and making rational decisions regarding which chemical modifications are more convenient to introduce to them.

Whereas in silico or virtual screening (VS) (i.e., using computational methods to explore vast collections of chemicals and identify novel active scaffolds) represents a rational way of finding starting points to implement a drug design campaign, it should be conceptually separated from drug design. Drug design is intrinsically and unequivocally related to finding *molecular novelty*, that is, novel chemical entities. Novelty is the key, underlying drug design. In contrast, in silico screening, which can be and usually is coupled with drug design, typically explores the known chemical universe in search of new active motifs. The novelty in virtual screening is not in the chemistry of the emerging hits, but in uncovering an unknown, hidden association between known chemicals and a given biological activity. There are, however, many alternatives to in silico screening to discover such association.

Besides its rationality, an attractive aspect of computer-aided drug design is its accessibility. The technology gap between high- and low-income countries is smaller for computer-aided drug discovery than for any other process or approach in the drug discovery cycle. This is in part because many computational resources and applications have been made publicly available, and many computational tools used in the field run fairly smoothly in any modern personal computer.

It should be emphasized, though, that several constrains operate on the process of drug design. First, synthetic feasibility of the designed compounds should not be neglected [5]. A proposed compound might not be synthetically attainable due to universal technical reasons (lack of a given synthetic route) or to local limitations (e.g., lack of access to required technology and/or reactants, expensive synthesis). Equally important is the fact that drug discovery is a challenging multiobjective problem, where numerous pharmaceutically relevant objectives should be simultaneously addressed [6], a problem further complicated by the fact that, occasionally, some of those objectives might be conflicting, resulting in very complex solution spaces. For example, it is in general accepted that higher selectivity leads to safer medications; however, efficacious treatments for complex disorders might require multi-target therapeutic agents which, by definition, are not exquisitely selective [7]. On the other hand, as implicit in the famous Lipinski's rule of five and similar rules of thumb [8], a certain degree of aqueous solubility is often pursued to assure absorption, but an excessive solubility could be detrimental to absorption and

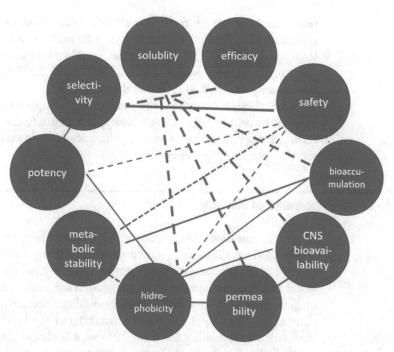

Fig. 1 A complex, conflicting interplay is observed between pharmaceutically relevant properties that are taken into consideration when facing a drug design project. An inverse, possibly conflicting relationship between two properties is indicated by a dashed line. Oppositely, a direct, favorable relationship is shown with a continuous line

biodistribution. Introduction of lipophilic substituents into adequate positions of a ligand often translates into a gain in potency [8], and certain degree of lipophilicity is also desirable in central nervous system medications to achieve brain bioavailability [9]. However, high lipophilicity conspires against both drug dissolution [10] and metabolic stability [11]. The key word in drug design seems to be balance, which explains why multiobjective optimization methods have gained such popularity in the field in the past years [6, 12].

A scheme illustrating the complex interplay between some pharmaceutically important drug properties is shown in Fig. 1. Naturally, the scheme is an oversimplification. The nature of the relationship between two properties might not be linear and many counterexamples to the illustrated relationships can be found, e.g., while it is accepted that lipophilicity has a positive impact on cell permeability, excessively high lipophilic drugs might become sequestered inside the cell, with little improvement on permeability across biological barriers (prominently, endothelial and epithelial tissues) [13], thus determining a parabolic relationship between lipophilicity and permeability. In general, hit identification is potency-driven, preferring ligands with affinities in the nM range. Whereas potent ligands are undoubtedly pursued in some cases (e.g., to treat anti-infectious diseases), the most potent ligand might not be the first choice if trying to restore sensitive physiologic systems (e.g., the brain or the heart) to its normal functioning, since highly potent ligands will tend to impair normal functioning and produce intolerable side effects.

This chapter overviews the computational approaches that can be used to find novel active chemotypes and guide the subsequent molecular optimization. General principles of rational drug design are also tangentially visited.

2   Where to Start—The Value of Novelty

A critical question when conceiving a drug discovery project is where to start. Obviously, any target-driven drug discovery project today starts by choosing one (single-target agents) or more (tailored multitarget agents) drug targets. What makes a good drug target? First, it must be disease-modifying. Second, it must be druggable, that is, it should be modulated by binding a small molecule or, according to some authors, a biologic [14, 15]. If no ligand is known to bind the potential target, druggability prediction can be performed, which generally involves examining the target surface for binding sites, or checking the existence of similar proteins which have already proven to be druggable [16–18]. Other desirable features include assayability, differential expression throughout the body and a favorable intellectual property situation (no competitors focused working on the same target!) [14].

Second, if we exclude entirely de novo approximations, where forcefully one should begin from a model of the molecular target, any other approach requires a starting (and hopefully novel) active scaffold (ligand) into which chemical modifications are introduced.

Leaving aside serendipitous discoveries (which are of course useful but unsystematic), hints on potential active scaffolds of natural origin can be found in traditional medicine. Alternatively, one might resort to information on the natural ligand of an intended molecular target to start a drug design project.

At this point, it is worth emphasizing that chemical structural novelty is a key factor in the pharmaceutical sector. Novelty is a fundamental requisite to obtain intellectual property rights on an invention (and thus exclusivity). And although recently drug repurposing (finding new medical uses to already known drugs) has raised considerable interest within the health community, it also faces nontrivial intellectual property, regulatory, and commercial challenges [19, 20]. Accordingly, the search of novel active chemotypes remains a priority within the pharmaceutical industry due to their intellectual property potential.

High-throughput screening (HTS) methods are among the most frequent approaches to explore the vast universe of known chemicals in search of novel active scaffolds. It is the modern version of the traditional trial-and-error, "exhaustive" screening. The rationality of HTS lies in the integration of automation and miniaturization to the screening process, which results in efficient exploration of the chemical space [21]. Moreover, the approach has been greatly improved by the design of target-focused libraries [22] and the recognition of privileged scaffolds [23] (molecular frameworks/building blocks that are present in many biologically active ligands against a diverse array of targets). However, it should be mentioned that HTS requires very expensive technological platforms which are not frequently found in the academic sector or low- and middle-income countries.

In contrast, VS requires considerably more accessible technology, with many resources being completely publicly available, from specialized software to online chemical repositories. The term VS refers to the application of a diversity of computational approaches to rank digital chemical collections or libraries in order to establish which compounds are more likely to obtain favorable results when experimentally tested through in vitro and/or animal models. They have been conceived to minimize the volume of experimental testing and optimize the results, thus being advantageous in terms of cost-efficiency, bioethics, and environmental impact.

VS approaches can be essentially classified in two categories: structure-based (or direct or target-based) and ligand-based (or indirect) approximations.

Molecular docking is prominently used for structure-based VS. Starting from an experimental structure of the target (or, at worst, a homolog from other species or another protein belonging to the same family, i.e., comparative or homology modeling), the binding event is simulated and a scoring function is used to predict, for the most likely binding poses, the free energy difference due to the binding of the screened compounds to the target. While rigid (computationally undemanding) or more accurate, flexible (computationally demanding) approximations are possible, docking can be considered a computationally demanding VS approach in comparison with ligand-based methods. A search/sampling algorithm is used to generate a diversity of ligand-binding orientations (rigid-body approximations) or ligand binding orientations and conformations (flexible approximations). A major obstacle for the implementation of structure-based VS approaches comes from the fact that the structures of many validated drug targets have not yet been solved experimentally. Another caveat of docking relates to the empirical nature of scoring functions, which in general, depending on the type of scoring function, include a variable degree of parameterization. This limits the reliability of the method, plagued by a high incidence of false positives [24]. Since the scoring functions are parameterized/trained against a number of experimentally determined binding affinities or experimental structures, the performance of the docking approach tends to be highly system-dependent and scores are, at best, weakly predictive of affinities [25]. Results are sometimes improved when different scoring functions are combined into a consensus score [25]. A persistent problem of the scoring function is the elusive entropic contribution to free-energy [24, 26] which is ignored in many cases or very approximately estimated in others. The reader should remember that, upon the binding event, the ligand will lose translational, rotational, and conformational freedom, whereas the target will mostly lose conformational freedom. The contributions of desolvation and water molecules mediating ligand–protein interactions (which also impact the initial and final entropy of the system) should not be neglected either [27, 28], but often are. Free energy simulations, which employ molecular dynamics or Monte Carlo simulations, provide a much more rigorous solution to binding free-energy estimation [24, 29, 30]. The emergence of low cost parallel computing is starting to relegate docking to the role of a prescreening tool, in favor of molecular dynamics-based VS [24, 29]. *See* Fig. 2 for a caption of a ligand–protein interaction simulation.

Ligand-based approximations may be applied whenever a model of the target structure is not available or to complement structure-based approximations. Concisely, ligand-based screening methods can be classified into similarity searches, machine learning approaches (prominently, supervised machine learning used in the frame of the Quantitive Structure–Activity Relationhip—QSAR—theory) and superposition approximations [31–33]. These techniques differ in a number of factors, from their requisites to their active enrichment or scaffold hopping.

Similarity search employs molecular fingerprints obtained from 2D or 3D molecular representations, comparing database compounds with one or more reference molecules in a pairwise manner. Remarkably, only one reference molecule (e.g., the physiologic ligand of a target protein) is required to implement a similarity-based VS campaign. Similarity searches are frequently the only option to explore the chemical universe for active compounds when lacking experimental knowledge on the target or related proteins, or when the number of known ligands is too small and impedes using supervised machine learning approaches.

Supervised machine learning approaches operate by building models from example inputs to make data-driven predictions on the database compounds. Machine learning approximations require several learning or calibration examples. The general model development protocol involves dataset compilation and curation (*see* **Note 1**); splitting the dataset into representative training (calibration) and test (validation) sets (whenever the size of the database allows it) (*see* **Note 2**); choosing which molecular descriptors

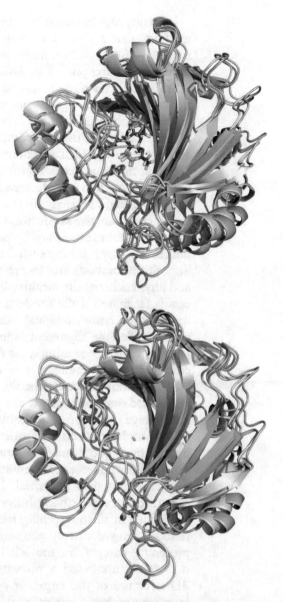

Fig. 2 Snapshots from a molecular dynamics simulation of the interaction between anticonvulsant sulfamides and carbonic anhydrase. Note the significant conformational changes induced by the ligand binding event

should be included into the model (*see* **Note 3**); weighing the contribution of such descriptors to the modeled activity; validating the model internally and externally and; checking the applicability domain of the model whenever a prediction is made [34]. Molecular diversity of the training samples is critical for VS applications of supervised machine learning: the molecular diversity of the calibration examples is directly correlated with a wide applicability domain of the resulting model.

Finally, superposition techniques are conformation-dependent methods that analyze how well a compound superposes onto a reference compound or, more frequently, how well they fit a fuzzy model (pharmacophore) in which functional groups are stripped off their exact chemical nature to become generic chemical properties relevant for the ligand–target interaction (hydrophobic points, H-bond donor, H-bond acceptors, charged groups, etc.). The pharmacophore is thus a geometric, 3D arrangement of generic, abstract features which are essential for the drug–target recognition event. Some approaches that have been used for pharmacophore generation can also include negative features (features that conspire against biological activity) in the model. In contrast with docking, which considers the key features required for drug–target interaction in a direct manner, superposition techniques do the same in an indirect way, by inferring such features from known ligands. Superimposition methods are, by far, the most visual, easy to interpret and physicochemically intuitive ligand-based approaches. The process is facilitated if the modeler counts on an active rigid analog with limited conformational freedom. Usually, though, one may resort to flexible alignment (superimposition) of a set of flexible ligands, either generating a set of low energy conformations and considering each conformer of each ligand in turn or exploring conformational space on the fly, i.e., the conformational search is performed simultaneously to the pattern identification stage (alignment stage) [35, 36]. It should be noted that, when applying pharmacophore-based VS, orientation sampling is probably as important as conformational sampling, since chemical diversity is expected in the screened chemical library and defining an orientation criteria is thus nontrivial. It should also be mentioned that structure-based pharmacophores are also possible [37].

Which in silico screening method should be chosen to start a rational drug discovery project? Of course, as indicated in the preceding paragraphs, the selection is restricted by the available data (structure-based approaches require experimentally solved 3D structure of the target or similar target; supervised machine learning requires a minimum of calibration samples, and so on.). But even if the technical requirements to implement any approach were met…is there a single approach that universally, consistently outperforms the remaining ones? Is there a method of first choice?

As a rule, the more complex approximations (structure-based approaches and, then, pharmacophore superposition) are the most advantageous in terms of scaffold hopping (they retrieve more molecular diverse hits), while simpler approaches are computationally more efficient while simultaneously achieving good active enrichment metrics [38]. Furthermore, structure-based approaches and pharmacophores explain, in an explicit or implicit way, respectively, the molecular basis of ligand–target interaction. They are visual and easily interpretable, two points which are not covered

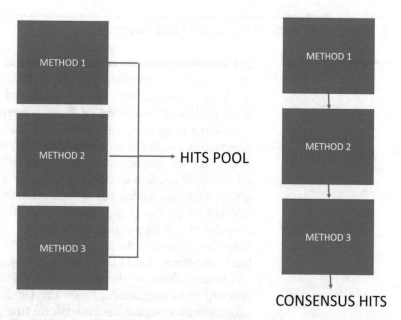

Fig. 3 While in parallel VS hybrid methods result in combination of complementary sets of hits (thus retrieving more chemical diversity), serial hybrid methods tend to produce more robust, consensus hit sets

by other approximations. These advantages should not be underestimated. Not only are they important from an epistemological perspective (they provide results and explanations), they also provide a visual support to their predictions and visual support is extremely important to communicate results to nonspecialized audiences (e.g., scientific collaborators from other fields, investors). Having said so, one should have in mind that the efficacy of a given technique is highly dependent on the chosen molecular target. Regarding VS approaches, a gold standard has not been found yet, a fact that explains the need of rigorous in silico validation before moving to VS and subsequent wet experiments. Some validation approaches are briefly discussed (*see* **Note 4**).

Frequently, different techniques are complementary in nature [39] and the simplest methods have surprisingly good outcomes in some cases. This allows the definition of hybrid protocols combining simple and complex approximations either serially or in parallel [40] (Fig. 3); serial combined approaches tend to provide robust solutions.

A final and important step to prune the hits emerging from systematic screening involves filtering out promiscuous compounds, unspecific inhibitors and reactive compounds, such as PAINS and REOS filters [41, 42].

3 The Actual Design: Hit to Lead and Beyond

Let us assume that one or more hits have emerged from systematic (wet or in silico) screening (or, maybe, that a starting active scaffold has been obtained from natural ligands of the intended target or from traditional medicine or from a serendipitous observation). The actual drug design process starts here, and involves introducing changes to the active scaffold in order to optimize the interaction with the target thus gaining potency, and/or to provide selectivity in relation to nontargeted similar proteins (e.g., nontargeted isoforms). Today, the optimization of other pharmaceutically relevant properties (e.g., chemical and biological stability) is also considered. Hits emerging from VS are usually active in the μM range (or, at best, in the high nM range) [43, 44]. A similar scenario has been observed in HTS campaigns [45]. Molecular optimization will usually decrease the dissociation (affinity) constant in about two orders of magnitude. From the 1990s onward, however, the pharmaceutical sector has understood that potency is not the only property to take into consideration, a realization that was expressed in the adoption of the "fail early, fail cheap" philosophy with the inclusion of in silico in vitro absorption, distribution, metabolism, excretion, and toxicity (ADMET) filters in the early stages of drug discovery [46, 47] and the emergent interest in low affinity ligands within certain therapeutic categories [48]. Classical optimization strategies include extension, ring variations, ring expansion or contraction, bioisosteric replacement and rigidification. In the case of (complex) active compounds of natural origin, simplification is also explored.

With the exception of similarity methods, which are of no use for optimization purposes, all the other approaches described in Subheading 2 of the chapter can be used to guide optimization. If the structure of the intended target has been solved, docking and structure-based pharmacophores are the first choices to guide optimization. They are the only methods that allow exploring, in a rational manner and without the need of trial and error learning, interactions with regions of the target that have not been exploited with previously known ligands. Among ligand-based approximations, pharmacophore superposition is the friendliest approach to molecular optimization. However, the QSAR approach is also suitable for design purposes, guiding the substitutions made onto the active scaffold; moreover, the *inverse QSAR* approach (in which, from molecular descriptors, new molecules having the desired activity could be "recovered") are also suitable for design of de novo molecules [49–51]. It should be noted that, while classification models are useful for VS campaigns, since they can compensate model errors related to data compiled from different laboratories, outlier compounds and mislabeled data points [34], when the

QSAR model is meant for optimization purposes regression modeling can be particularly useful, since the training dataset is usually synthesized inhouse and experimentally tested in the same laboratory. Furthermore, whereas VS applications require chemically diverse datasets, QSAR models used in optimization campaigns would typically display a narrower applicability domain, since they are obtained from a set of compounds with a common scaffold which has been modified to explore the surrounding chemical space.

4 In Silico ADMET Filters and Antitargets

From the 1990s onward, the search of more potent derivatives of an active scaffold has been balanced with early detection of potential bioavailability and toxicity issues. As a result, in silico and in vitro ADME filters are now fully integrated in the early stages of drug discovery and development. Such strategy has resulted in an impressive reduction of project termination rates related to ADME issues [46, 47] though pharmacokinetics and bioavailability still represent a significant cause for attrition at Phase I clinical trials [52–54]. Toxicology failures (both at preclinical and clinical stage) represent one of the key challenges still facing the pharmaceutical industry [52–54].

The earliest ADME filters involved simple rules of thumb derived from distribution analysis of physicochemical properties of drugs having or lacking a desired behavior. Lipinski's rule of five at Pfizer pioneered this kind of analysis [8], which was later followed by other similar rules related to the prediction of drug bioavailability, such as Veber's [55]. This trend was also explored in relation to toxicity, e.g., the "3/75" rule [56]. Later, however, arguments have been raised against rigid implementations of these kinds of rules [57], and the possible advantages of moving beyond the "rule of five" chemical space for difficult targets have been emphasized [58, 59], as well as notable systematic exceptions to this rule (e.g., natural products) [59, 60]. Lipinski himself, when first reporting his famous rule, recognized that acceptable drug absorption depended on the triad "potency–permeability–solubility", and that his computational alert did not factor in drug potency (a point of his analysis that is often overlooked) [8]; he also recognized the potential contribution of drug formulation to oral bioavailability, a contribution that can be addressed today through in silico tools [61].

It has been suggested that control of physicochemical properties is unlikely to have a significant effect on attrition rates; moreover, if a safety issue results from the primary drug target mechanism or from specific off-target interactions (e.g., hERG channel blockade), it is unlikely that physicochemical properties would be predictive of toxicity [52]. A similar point could be made regarding prediction of bioavailability issues linked to specific interactions with enzymes (e.g., CYP450 enzymes) or transporters (e.g., ABC efflux transporters). In these cases, using previously discussed computational tools (docking, pharmacophores, QSAR models) in connection with the antitarget concept could be more advantageous.

The use of more complex (yet simple) multiparameter algorithms that address the interplay of physicochemical properties could also prove rewarding [12].

5   Final Remarks

We have presented an overview of the most relevant methods used in computer-aided drug design. While human beings (and scientist in particular) are naturally inclined to a way of thinking based on pattern recognition and identification of generalities, successful drug design comprises such a complex interplay between a number of objectives (e.g., efficacy, safety, and desired physicochemical properties) that the drug designer should beware oversimplification and dogmatic principles, which may lead not only to bad decisions, but also to loss of opportunities and novelty.

As the name itself suggests, drug design per se resembles an attentive artisan craftwork. The screening stages and the application of ADMET-related computational alerts, in contrast, involve more automated decisions, compatible with the idea of efficient exploration and fast pruning of a vast chemical universe. Fast pruning usually leads, however, to an over reduced chemical space. Flexible decision rules should be preferred over rigid ones, since they expand the borders of the more frequently explored regions of the chemical universe.

The decision to stop a drug candidate for toxicological or pharmacokinetic reasons involves complex and subtle judgements that should take into consideration cost–benefit analysis and available options to compensate the predicted difficulties (e.g, formulation alternatives, targeted-drug carriers). It is advised to be careful with excessive automation, to favor critical case-by-case decision-making as much as possible and to consider difficulties in a multidisciplinary way, including contributions of different professionals involved in the drug discovery cycle at each stage of the drug project.

6   Notes

1. Compiling and curating a dataset is one of the most important steps in supervised machine learning. The dataset will be used to infer the model and to validate it. The inferred model will

only be as good as the biological or biochemical data from which it is derived: the unknown noise in the training data is one of the factors that influence the generalization error. It is accepted that biochemical data (e.g., dissociation constants) are cleaner than biological data. The activities of all the training instances should be of comparable quality. Ideally, they should have been measured in the same laboratory under the same conditions, so that variability in the measured biological or biochemical activity only (or mostly) reflects treatment variability. This requirement is often accomplished when building models for optimization purposes from a series of inhouse synthesized compounds, but rarely met when building models for VS purposes (in this case, the need of a large and diverse training set frequently leads to compile experimental data from different laboratories).

Data distribution should be studied in order to avoid poorly populated regions within the studied chemical space as well as highly populated narrow intervals: extrapolation is forbidden but intrapolation in regions which are poorly populated by training examples is also risky. The dependent variable should span at least two or three orders of magnitude, from the least to the most active compound, and it should be (if possible) uniformly distributed across the range of activity (rarely achieved). The inclusion of leverage points (outliers, i.e., data exceptions represented by extreme values in the descriptor or response space which is not due to measurement or labelling errors) is discouraged.

Conscientiously curate the dataset: read data sources carefully and remove training examples extracted from inadequate or dubious experimental protocols. There are currently several databases that compile experimental data for small molecules (e.g., ChEMBL); such resources are manually curated from primary scientific literature. ChEMBL developers flag activity values that are outside a range typical for a given activity type, possibly missing data and suspected or confirmed author errors. Classification models can be used to alleviate the influence of data heterogeneity; they are useful for VS applications but less practical for models intended for optimization purposes.

Not only experimental data but also chemical structures should be curated. Do not underestimate the importance of this step: it is quite common that medicinal chemistry papers and chemical databases include structural mistakes. Remove those data points that are usually not handled by conventional cheminfomatic techniques: inorganic and some organometallic compounds, counterions, salts and mixtures (there exist molecular descriptors, however, that can be used to characterize ionic species if the dataset molecules are charged at the biologically relevant pH and it is thus suspected that molecular charge can influence drug–target interactions). Duplicates should also be removed to avoid exaggerated incidence of a single compound on the model. Some chemical functions and moieties that can be represented in multiple ways should be standardized: aromatic rings, nitro groups, etc. Tautomeric groups should also be curated. Many of the previous steps can be performed in an automated manner by specialized software applications (e.g., ChemAxon's Standardizer). It is advisable, though, to manually verify a random subset of the resulting curated molecular structures to ensure everything has gone well. Also note that some software applications used for molecular descriptor calculation impose restrictions to the molecular representations that can be input (e.g., explicit or implicit hydrogens, and aromatic rings).

2. Once the dataset has been compiled, it is typically split into a training set (to calibrate the model) and an independent test set (which will be used to estimate the model's predictive ability). Partitioning the dataset is not a trivial task. Often, training and test sets are obtained through random sampling or activity range algorithms. These approaches are especially appropriate when training and test sets are comparable in size, but better results are expected with more rational partitioning procedures such as sphere exclusion algorithms when test sets are small in comparison with the corresponding training sets. This is the typical situation: only 10–20% of the dataset is usually reserved for the test set. If active and inactive compounds are included in the training set, it is preferred that both categories are balanced in order to avoid bias toward the prediction of the overrepresented category.

3. Molecular descriptors are numerical variables that reflect chemical information encoded within a symbolic representation of a chemical compound. There is an extensive diversity of descriptors available to reflect different aspects of a molecule, from simple functional group counts to time-demanding quantum descriptors. Two fundamental aspects can be considered at this stage. First, the throughput speed associated to different kinds of descriptors. Second, the interpretability of each type of descriptor. If the models are intended to be used to screen large collections of chemicals, the selected molecular descriptors should ideally be easy to compute. If the model is expected to describe structure–activity relationships of a reduced number of chemically similar compounds, more computationally demanding descriptors could be afforded.

If 3D descriptors are considered, an interesting question is what conformation should be used to compute the correspondent descriptor values. An ideal solution to account for the conformation dependency would be to determine the bound (also called bioactive) conformation and the conformational energy. Defining the bound conformation is a difficult and time-consuming task. Bound conformations of ligands can be obtained experimentally by NMR or X-ray crystallography, but the number of ligands which have not been cocrystallized with the target protein greatly exceeds the number that have. Crystal structures also have limitations, from data acquisition and data refinement errors to the potential inadequacy of crystal structures to represent the conformational ensemble in solution. Precious clues on the active conformation can be obtained when rigid ligands with restricted conformational freedom are available. When no clues on the bioactive conformation can be inferred from experimental data or rigid ligands, the modeler has no alternative but to sample the potential energy surface of the ligands; a number of methods (all of them computationally demanding) are available for such purpose, including systematic search, stochastic approaches, and molecular dynamics. Very frequently very rough approximations are performed in this stage, from using the presumed global energy minimum or a local energy minimum (which is not representative of the bioactive conformation) to energy minimization procedures in vacuum that neglect solvent effects. Note that the strain energy is characteristically below 10 kcal/mol, but there are exceptions.

In most applications, a subset of descriptors will be chosen from a relatively large pool of descriptors. There is a diversity of methods to proceed with descriptor selection (genetic algorithms, stepwise approaches, replacement method, and many others). What number of descriptors should be allowed into the model? In our experience, at least 10 training compounds per independent variable is a good choice to control the generalization error, avoiding overfitting. Some authors propose that, for noisy data, an optimal trade-off between approximation and estimation errors is achieved if the number of parameters in the model is around the cubic root of the number of training examples (this is the most conservative approach that we have so far heard). In any case, overfitting can be retrospectively controlled with adequate validation protocols.

4. With the sole exception of similarity searches, which are not subjected to in silico validation (direct experimental validation of the predictions is performed) all the other described approaches (structure-based approximations, machine learning and pharmacophores) should be validated in silico, although how the validation process is executed depends on each technique. In the case of docking, for instance, the most frequent validation criteria include a method's ability to reproduce the

correct bound conformation of a ligand–protein complex (*redocking*), its ability to assign better scores to high affinity ligands than to decoys (the Directory of Useful Decoys is a practical resource to obtain such decoys) and the ability to produce scores that show some correlation with the measured affinities of known ligands.

Regarding validation of supervised machine learning techniques, it can be classified in internal and external validation. In the internal validation approaches, the training set itself is used to assess the model stability and predictive power; in external validation, a holdout sample absolutely independent from the training set is used to test the predictive ability. Though there is a diversity of techniques used for internal validation purposes, the most frequent are cross-validation and Y-randomization. In cross-validation, different proportions of training examples are iteratively held out from the training set used for model development; the model is thus regenerated without the removed examples and the regenerated model is applied to predict the dependent variable for the held out compound/s. The process is repeated at least until every training compound has been removed from the training set once. When only one compound is held out in each cross-validation round, we will speak of leave-one-out cross validation. If larger subsets of training samples are removed in each round, we will speak of leave-group-out, multifold cross-validation, leave-many-out cross-validation, or leave-some-out cross-validation. Obviously, the more compounds removed per cycle, the more challenging the cross-validation test. Cross-validation in general and leave-one-out cross-validation in particular tend to be overoptimistic. Y-randomization involves scrambling the value of the experimental/observed dependent across the training instances, thus abolishing the relationship between the response and the molecular structure. Since the response is now randomly assigned to the training cases, poor statistical parameters are expected to be found if the model is regenerated from the scrambled data.

With regard to external validation, i.e., using an independent test set to establish the model predictive power, it has been regarded as the most rigorous validation step, although some conditions should be met for the results to be reliable: the test sample should be representative of the training sample; at least 20 hold out examples are advised when the test set is randomly chosen from the dataset, and, if possible, at least 50. Some authors suggest that only internal validation is advised for small (<50 examples) datasets. In that case not only valuable and scarce training cases would be lost if resorting to external validation, but the reduced test set will give dubious results. In that scenario, leave-group-out using folds comprising 30% of the training set has provided robust results across several small datasets.

Acknowledgments

The author thanks CONICET and University of La Plata, where he holds permanent positions.

References

1. Klabunde T, Everts A (2005) GPCR antitarget modeling: pharmacophore models for biogenic amine binding GPCRs to avoid GPCR-mediated side effects. Chembiochem 6:876–889

2. Raschi E, Vasina V, Poluzzi E, De Ponti F (2008) The hERG K+ channel: target and antitarget strategies in drug development. Pharmacol Res 57:181–195

3. Crivori P (2008) Computational models for P-glycoprotein substrates and inhibitors. In: Vaz RJ, Klabunde T (eds) Anti-targets: prediction and prevention of drug side effects. Wiley-VCH, Weinheim

4. Zamora I (2008) Site of metabolism predictions: facts and experiences. In: Vaz RJ, Klabunde T (eds) Anti-targets: prediction and prevention of drug side effects. Wiley-VCH, Weinheim

5. Hartenfeller M, Schneider G (2011) De novo drug design. Methods Mol Biol 672:299–323

6. Nicolaou CA, Brown N (2013) Multi-objective optimization methods in drug design. Drug Discov Today Technol 10:e427–e435

7. Talevi A (2016) Tailored multi-target agents. Applications and design considerations. Curr Pharm Des 22:3164–3170

8. Lipinski CA, Lombardo F, Dominy BW, Feeney PJ (1997) Experimental and computational approaches to estimate solubility and permeability in drug discovery and development settings. Adv Drug Deliv Rev 23:3–25

9. Pajouhesh H, Lenz GR (2005) Medicinal chemical properties of successful central nervous system drugs. NeuroRx 2:542–553

10. Gupta S, Kesarla R, Omri A (2013) Formulation strategies to improve the bioavailability of poorly absorbed drugs with special emphasis on self-emulsifying systems. ISRN Pharm 2013(848043)

11. Miller DC, Klute W, Calabrese A, Brown AD (2009) Optimising metabolic stability in lipophilic chemical space: the identification of a metabolic stable pyrazolopyrimidine CRF-1 receptor antagonist. Bioorg Med Chem Lett 19:6144–6147

12. Wager TT, Hou X, Verhoest PR, Villalobos A (2010) Moving beyond rules: the development of a central nervous system multiparameter optimization (CNS MPO) approach to enable alignment of druglike properties. ACS Chem Neurosci 1:435–449

13. He X (2009) Integration of physical, chemical, mechanical and biopharmaceutical properties in solid dosage oral form development. In: Qiu Y, Chen Y, Zhang GGZ, Liu L, Porter WR (eds) Developing solid dosage oral forms: pharmaceutical theory and practice, 1st edn. Academic press, Burlington

14. Gashaw I, Ellinghaus P, Sommer A, Asadullah K (2011) What makes a good drug target. Drug Discov Today 16:1037–1043

15. Knowles J, Gromo G (2003) Target selection in drug discovery. Nat Rev Drug Discov 2:63–69

16. Schmidtke P, Barril X (2010) Understanding and predicting druggability. A high-throughput method for detection of drug binding sites. J Med Chem 53:5858–5867

17. Yuan Y, Pei J, Lai L (2013) Binding site detection and druggability prediction of protein targets for structure-based drug design. Curr Pharm Des 19:2326–2333

18. Barril X (2013) Druggability predictions: methods, limitations and applications. WIREs Comput Mol Sci 3:327–338

19. Smith RB (2011) Repositioned drugs: integrating intellectual property and regulatory strategies. Drug Discov Today Ther Strateg 8:131–137

20. Novac N (2013) Challenges and opportunities of drug repositioning. Trends Pharmacol Sci 34:267–272

21. Szymanski P, Markowicz M, Mikiciuk-Olasik E (2012) Adaptation of high-throughput screening in drug discovery - toxicological screening. Int J Mol Sci 13:427–452

22. Harris CJ, Hill RD, Sheppard DW, Slater MJ, Stouten PF (2011) The design and application of target-focused compound libraries. Comb Chem High Throughput Screen 14:521–531

23. Welsch ME, Snyder SA, Stockwell BR (2010) Privileged scaffolds for library design and drug discovery. Curr Opin Chem Biol 14:347–361

24. Procacci P (2016) Reformulating the entropic contribution of molecular docking scoring functions. J Comput Chem 37:1819–1827

25. Gilson MK, Zhou HX (2007) Calculation of protein-ligand binding affinities. Annu Rev Biophys Biomol Struct 36:21–42

26. Bello M, Martínez-Archundia M, Correa-Basurto J (2013) Automated docking for novel drug discovery. Expert Opin Drug Discov 8:821–834

27. Bodnarchuck MS (2016) Water, water, everywhere… It's time to stop and think. Drug Discov Today 21:1139–1146

28. Mysinger MM, Schoichet BK (2010) Rapid context-dependent ligand desolvation in molecular docking. J Chem Inf Model 50:1561–1573

29. Ge H, Wang Y, Li C et al (2013) Molecular dynamics-based virtual screening: accelerating the drug discovery process by high-performance computing. J Chem Inf Model 53:2757–2764

30. Wang L, Wu Y, Deng Y et al (2015) Accurate and reliable prediction of relative ligand binding potency in prospective drug discovery by way of a modern free-energy calculation protocol and force field. J Am Chem Soc 137:2695–2703

31. Lavechia A (2015) Machine-learning approaches in drug discovery: methods and applications. Drug Discov Today 20:318–331

32. Lemmen C, Zimmermann M, Lengauer T (2002) Multiple molecular superpositioning as an effective tool for virtual database screening. In: Klebe G (ed) Virtual screening: an alternative or complement to high-throughput screening? 1st edn. Kluwer Academic Publishers, Marburg

33. Kristensen TG, Nielsen J, Pedersen CNS (2013) Methods for similarity-based virtual screening. Comput Struct Biotechnol J 5: e201302009

34. Talevi A, Bruno-Blanch LE (2016) Virtual screening applications in the search of novel antiepileptic drug candidates. In: Talevi A, Rocha L (eds) Antiepileptic drug discovery. Novel Approaches. Humana Press, New York

35. Schneidman-Duhovny D, Dror O, Inbar Y, Nussinov R, Wolfson HJ (2008) Deterministic pharmacophore detection via multiple flexible alignment of drug-like molecules. J Comput Biol 15:737–754

36. Cottrell SJ, Gillet VJ, Taylor R, Wilton DJ (2004) Generation of multiple pharmacophore hypothesis using multiobjective optimization techniques. J Comput Aided Mol Des 18:665–682

37. Pirhadi S, Shiri F, Ghasemi JB (2013) Methods and applications of structure based pharmacophores in drug discovery. Curr Top Med Chem 13:1036–1047

38. Zhang Q, Muegge I (2006) Scaffold hopping through virtual screening using 2D and 3D similarity descriptors: ranking, voting, and consensus scoring. J Med Chem 9:1536–1548

39. Krüger DM, Evers A (2010) Comparison of structure- and ligand-based virtual screening protocols considering hit list complementarity and enrichment factors. ChemMedChem 5:148–158

40. Talevi A, Gavernet L, Bruno-Blanch LE (2009) Combined virtual screening strategies. Curr Comput Aided Drug Des 5:23–37

41. Pouliot M, Jeanmart S (2016) Pan assay interference compounds (PAINS) and other promiscuous compounds in antifungal research. J Med Chem 59:497–503

42. Walters WP, Stahl MT, Murcko MA (1998) Virtual screening – an overview. Drug Discov Today 3:160–178

43. Zhu T, Cao S, Su PC, Patel R, Shah D, Chokshi HB, Szukala R, Johnson ME, Hevener KE (2013) Hit identification and optimization in virtual screening: practical recommendations based upon a critical literature analysis. J Med Chem 56:6560–6572

44. Ripphausen P, Nisius B, Pletason L, Bajorath J (2010) Quo vadis, virtual screening? A comprehensive survey of prospective applications. J Med Chem 53:8461–8467

45. Neetoo-Isseliee Z, MacKenzie AE, Southern C, Jerman J, McIver EG, Harries N, Taylor DL, Milligan G (2013) High-throughput identification and characterization of novel, species-selective GPR35 agonists. J Pharmacol Exp Ther 344:568–578

46. Kola I, Landis J (2004) Can the pharmaceutical industry reduce attrition rates? Nature Rev Drug Discov 3:711–716

47. Schuster D, Laggner C, Langer T (2005) Why drugs fail – a study on side effects in new chemical entities. Curr Pharm Des 11:3545–3559

48. Talevi A (2016) Computatonal approaches for innovative antiepileptic drug discovery. Expert Opin Drug Discov 11:1001–1016

49. Brown N, Lewis RA (2006) Exploiting QSAR methods in lead optimization. Curr Opin Drug Discov Devel 9:419–424

50. Wong WWL, Burkowski FJ (2009) A constructive approach for discovering new drug leads: using a kernel methodology for the inverse-QSAR problem. J Cheminform 1:4

51. Miyako T, Kaneko H, Funatsu K (2016) Inverse QSPR/QSAR analysis for chemical structure generation (from y to x). J Chem Inf Model 56:286–299

52. Waring MJ, Arrowsmith J, Leach AR et al (2015) An analysis of the attrition of drug candidates from four major pharmaceutical companies. Nat Rev Drug Discov 14:475–486

53. Cook D, Brown D, Alexander R, March R, Morgan P, Satterthwaite G, Pangalos MN (2014) Lessons learned from the fate of Astra-Zeneca's drug pipeline: a five-dimensional framework. Nat Rev Drug Discov 13:419–431

54. Roberts RA, Kavanagh SL, Mellor HR, Pollard CE, Robinson S, Platz SJ (2014) Reducing attrition in drug development: smart loading preclinical safety assessment. Drug Discov Today 19:341–347

55. Veber DF, Johnson SR, Cheng HY, Smith BR, Ward KW, Kopple KD (2002) Molecular properties that influence the oral bioavailability of drug candidates. J Med Chem 45:2615–2623

56. Price DA, Blagg J, Jones L, Greene N, Wager T (2009) Physicochemical drug properties associated with in vivo toxicological outcomes: a review. Expert Opin Drug Metab Toxicol 5:921–931

57. Sutherland JJ, Raymond JW, Stevens JL, Baker TK, Watson DE (2012) Relating molecular properties and in vitro assay results to in vivo drug disposition and toxicity outcomes. J Med Chem 55:6455–6466

58. Doak BC, Zheng J, Dobritzsch D, Kihlberg J (2016) How beyond rule of 5 drugs and clinical candidates bind to their targets. J Med Chem 59:2312–2327

59. Doak BC, Over B, Giordanetto F, Kihlberg J (2014) Oral druggable space beyond the rule of 5: insights from drugs and clinical candidates. Chem Biol 21:1115–1142

60. Lipinski CA (2016) Rule of five in 2015 and beyond: target and ligand structural limitations, ligand chemistry structure and drug discovery project decisions. Adv Drug Deliv Rev 101:34–41

61. Bergström CAS, Charman WN, Porter CJH (2016) Computational prediction of formulation strategies for beyond-rule-of-5 compounds. Adv Drug Deliv Rev 101:6–21

Chapter 2

Prediction of Human Drug Targets and Their Interactions Using Machine Learning Methods: Current and Future Perspectives

Abhigyan Nath, Priyanka Kumari, and Radha Chaube

Abstract

Identification of drug targets and drug target interactions are important steps in the drug-discovery pipeline. Successful computational prediction methods can reduce the cost and time demanded by the experimental methods. Knowledge of putative drug targets and their interactions can be very useful for drug repurposing. Supervised machine learning methods have been very useful in drug target prediction and in prediction of drug target interactions. Here, we describe the details for developing prediction models using supervised learning techniques for human drug target prediction and their interactions.

Key words Drug target identification, Drug target interaction, Feature selection, Machine learning

1 Introduction

One of the salient steps in the drug-discovery pipeline is the identification of drug targets or druggable proteins. Druggable proteins can be defined as those proteins which can be regulated by interaction with a drug and whose interaction can be exploited to produce a therapeutic effect. Majority of druggable targets belongs to the G-protein coupled receptors, ion-channels, and kinases [1]. Traditionally microarrays [2] including both nucleic acid microarrays [3] and protein microarrays [4, 5] are used for identification and validation of drug targets. Also one of the alternative suitable methods is high throughput NMR-based screening for drug target interaction [6]. Expression profiling, biochemical and cell based assays, and cell and model organism based genetics which involves perturbation of gene function are the three major methods for drug target discovery [7]. Novel drug targets can be identified broadly under three major levels—physiological, mechanistic, and genetic levels [8].

Mohini Gore and Umesh B. Jagtap (eds.), *Computational Drug Discovery and Design*, Methods in Molecular Biology, vol. 1762, https://doi.org/10.1007/978-1-4939-7756-7_2, © Springer Science+Business Media, LLC, part of Springer Nature 2018

Experimental methods for drug target identification and drug–target interaction are costly and time consuming. A computational predictor at the human proteome level will be of great importance for the pharmaceutical industry. Computational methods can also expedite the process of drug target identification by reducing the time consumed in the experimental methods.

The three important challenges that are being tackled in the drug-discovery pipeline are the drug target identification/prediction, drug–target interaction prediction, and prediction of drug binding residues. Accurate and most significant prediction methods can facilitate in reducing the target search space. The prediction of drug–target interaction is a challenging task as it presents a situation of many to many mapping (i.e., a single drug can interact with many targets and vice versa). Furthermore, the prediction of drug binding residues is also an inevitable job in target identification study. Availability of very limited number of target structures in repositories directs most of the studies to adopt sequence feature extraction based prediction [9–11], however a structure based analysis of druggable pockets using physicochemical properties have also been reported [12]. A similar druggable microenvironment analysis resulted in the development of DrugFEATURE [13]. There are only few validated and well-proven drug target prediction methods available. Further reliable improvements and innovative methods can be used to increase the prediction rate in drug target discovery. Discovery of a large number of putative drug targets and their interactions with known drugs are still a basic need of medicinal sciences for curing life-threatening diseases. Computational methods can reduce the cost and time which is involved in drug target identification. The promiscuity of drug–target interactions makes it difficult to develop machine learning based classification models. Prediction of new drug targets and drug target interactions can open new doors for drug discovery and drug repurposing for a given disease. The drug targets and their interactions may facilitate the understanding of drug action at molecular level and increase the success rate of drug discovery. The major steps for prediction of drug targets and their interactions are shown in Figs. 1 and 2, respectively.

2 Materials

2.1 Machine Learning Platforms

For the development of machine learning models, there are many open source platforms like WEKA [14], KNIME [15], RapidMiner [16], H_2O [17], and Scikit-learn [18]. WEKA, KNIME, RapidMiner, and Scikit-learn provide a plethora of data preprocessing, classification, and clustering algorithms, while H_2O is mostly dedicated to deep learning neural networks. H_2O can be implemented in both R and python. Graphical User Interface (GUI) facility is

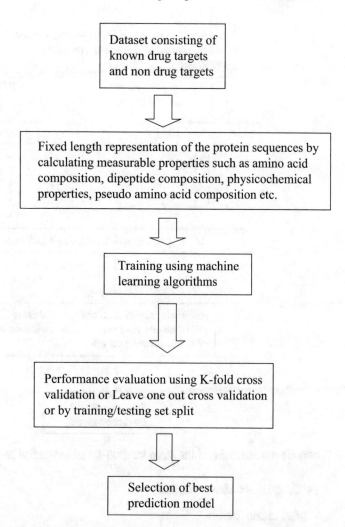

Fig. 1 Schematic representation of the steps for drug target prediction

available in WKEA, KNIME, and Rapidminer which makes it easy to experiment with a large number data processing and machine learning algorithms.

One of the common formats consisting of feature values for a group of instances, which is almost supported by all the above-mentioned machine-learning platforms, is the Attribute-Relation File Format (ARFF). The ARFF file consists of header and data part. The header part consists of title, name of the relation, a list of attributes (features) with their types and the data part consists of the values of the calculated features with the class information for each instance. In Fig. 3 we have presented dummy ARFF file consisting of features for two classes—drug targets and nontargets with four features (Molecular weight, mean hydrophobicity, aromatic amino acid composition, and charged amino acid composition).

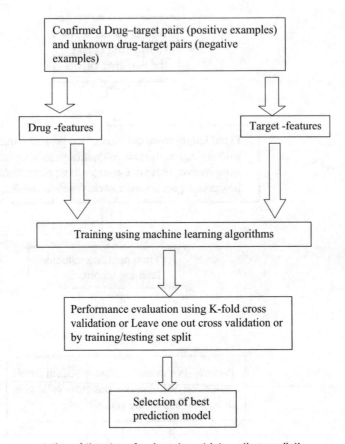

Fig. 2 Schematic representation of the steps for drug–target interaction prediction

```
% 1. Title: Drug Target

@RELATION Class

@ATTRIBUTE Mol Weight               NUMERIC
@ATTRIBUTE Mean Hydrophobicity      NUMERIC
@ATTRIBUTE Aromatic AA Composition  NUMERIC
@ATTRIBUTE Charged AA Composition   NUMERIC
@ATTRIBUTE class        {Class-drug target, Class-non target}

@DATA
    5.1,3.5,1.4,0.2, Class- drug target
    4.9,3.0,1.4,0.2, Class- drug target
    4.7,3.2,1.3,0.2, Class- drug target
    4.6,3.1,1.5,0.2, Class- drug target
    5.0,3.6,1.4,0.2, Class- drug target
    5.4,3.9,1.7,0.4, Class- non target
    4.6,3.4,1.4,0.3, Class- non target
    5.0,3.4,1.5,0.2, Class- non target
    4.4,2.9,1.4,0.2, Class- non target
    4.9,3.1,1.5,0.1, Class- non target
```

Fig. 3 The structure of an ARFF file

2.2 Databases for Creating the Dataset

A number of databases are now available consisting of specialized information about drug and their targets. For example DrugBank [19] consists of information about drug–target relationships; likewise Matador [20] also consists of direct and indirect drug–target relationships. Similarly SuperTarget [20] and Therapeutic Target Database (TTD) [21] also have high quality information about drug–target relationships. Along with the drug–target relationship data, Integrity [22] provides associated disease information also. Potential Drug Target Database (PDTD) [23] augments the information of drug–target relationship with structural data of the target while BindingDB [24] is one of the major databases consisting of experimentally derived protein–ligand binding affinities.

2.3 Tools and Servers for the Calculation of Features

A number of stand-alone programs and web servers are available which can be used to generate a variety of features of protein targets and non targets. PROFEAT [25, 26] is one of the oldest web servers capable of calculating structural and physicochemical properties from proteins sequences. PseAAC-builder [27] which is a stand-alone program and PseAAC [28] a web server are dedicated to the generation of various modes of pseudo amino acid composition [29]. Pse-in-One [30] which is a web server providing services for the calculation of pseudo components for proteins as well as nucleic acids. Complimentary to other programs ProtDcal [31] can also be used for generating a number of numerical descriptors from protein sequences as well as from 3D structures. Apart from the above mentioned stand-alone programs and web servers, propy [32] and protr [33], a python and an R package respectively may be implemented for the calculation of a large number of attributes as per the need of the problem. Various types of molecular descriptors of molecular compounds can also be easily computed using web servers like PaDEL [34], MODEL [35], and Mold2 [36]. These calculated features can be used as features in developing prediction models for drug–target interactions.

3 Methods

3.1 Dataset Creation

For any supervised learning algorithm there should be a labeled dataset, i.e., data instances along with their classes. The foremost requirement for training a supervised learning algorithm is the availability of a benchmark dataset having proper representation of the various classes (in case of binary classification—positive and negative classes), but seldom it is so. A dataset is said to be imbalanced when the number of data points (instances/examples) belonging to a particular class overwhelms the number of data points of the other class. In the case of human drug target prediction the number of instances belonging to the drug target is less as compared to the non targets. In such cases the machine learning algorithms have difficulty in learning the concepts of the minority class (drug targets) as compared to the majority class (nondrug targets) (*see* **Note 1**). The generated classifier behaves like a majority class classifier. For handling the imbalance data problem two types of approaches can be applied (1) intrinsic approaches (2) extrinsic approach. The intrinsic approaches involves the adaption in machine learning algorithms for handling the class imbalance, while extrinsic approaches are algorithm independent and involves changes in the dataset to handle class imbalance, a popular example is SMOTE [37] and its variants. Known drug targets are considered as the positive class while proteins which are not confirmed as targets are considered as non drug targets (negative class). Likewise confirmed/ known drug–target pairs are considered positive examples and unknown drug–target pairs are considered as negative examples.

3.2 Feature Engineering

The machine learning algorithm requires a fixed length representation of the protein sequences. Many packages and web servers are now available which can be used to calculate the various measurable properties from the protein sequences. In [9] authors have calculated amino acid composition, dipeptide composition, and amino acid property group to discriminate between human drug targets and non targets. Apart from simple sequence features, sophisticated features like pseudo amino acid composition can also be calculated with the help of various programs as mentioned in Subheading 2.

3.3 Feature Selection

Certain learning algorithms may perform worse, when learning concepts to discriminate between classes form high dimensional data, this situation is known as the "curse of dimensionality." The aim of feature selection algorithms is to select a minimum set of features while achieving maximum classification accuracy (*see* **Note 2**). Using a reduced feature set provides many advantages as reduced training time, model simplification, and reduction in overfitting. Feature selection can be stated as:Given a set of predicted/calculated features (attributes) F and a target variable (class) "C." Find minimum of set f achieving maximum classification of C. In majority of cases feature selection improves the performance of classification algorithm.

There are basically two main approaches for feature selection (1) Wrapper approach (2) Filter approach. In wrapper approach, one keeps adding features using a certain classifier until no further improvement can be achieved (forward search) or one can start with the full feature set and keeps on removing one feature at a time until no further improvement is recorded. Alternatively one can use both adding and removing features in two phases. Filter methods are independent of classifier but uses association of features with the target class for feature selection [38].

3.4 Performance Evaluation

Various threshold dependent and threshold independent performance evaluation metrics can be used for judging the performance of the machine learning algorithms (*see* **Note 3**).

Sensitivity: This can be defined as % of correctly predicted drug targets.

$$\text{Sensitivity} = \frac{TP}{(TP + FN)} \times 100 \tag{1}$$

Specificity: This can be defined as % of correctly predicted nondrug targets.

$$\text{Specificity} = \frac{TN}{(TN + FP)} \times 100 \tag{2}$$

Accuracy: This can be defined as the % of correctly predicted drug targets and nondrug targets.

$$\text{Accuracy} = \frac{TP + TN}{(TP + FP + TN + FN)} \times 100 \tag{3}$$

Matthews Correlation Coefficient (MCC): For binary classification problems it's a useful performance evaluation metric. Its values ranges from −1 to +1 (worse to best).

$$\text{MCC} = \frac{(TP \times TN) - (FP \times FN)}{\sqrt{(TP + FN)(TP + FP)(TN + FP)(TN + FN)}} \tag{4}$$

Youden's index: This performance evaluation metric gives an indication about the model's ability to avoid failures. Higher values are better.

$$\Upsilon = \text{Sensitivity} - (1 - \text{Specificity}) \tag{5}$$

Area under the Curve (AUC): The area under the receiver operation characteristic curves know as AUC and can be used to summarize the ROC by a single numerical quantity. Its values ranges from 0 to 1 and is threshold independent [39].

g -means: This is the geometric mean of sensitivity and specificity

$$g - \text{means} = \sqrt{\text{Sensitivty} \times \text{Specificity}} \tag{6}$$

3.5 Conclusion and Future Perspective

Machine learning methods have advantage over sequence alignment based methods as they can take into account of the hidden similarities between features for generating successful prediction models. Sequence feature generation step should account to cover as much as possible of chemical and genomic space. Protein–protein interaction data notably from databases like STRING [40], BioGRID [41] and Human Protein Reference Databases(HPRD)

[42], subcellular location, knowledge of functional domains, gene expression profiles can be incorporated as useful features. A variety of network properties (like betweenness and connectivity) can also be calculated which can be used as features along with other sequence and structure based features. Integrating different types of attributes/features should result in more accurate predictors. Most of the machine learning techniques are black-box prediction methods which does not allow to interpret the relationship between attributes used in developing the classification methods, rule based prediction methods can compensate for this shortcoming. It is imperative to accurately develop computational methods for predicting drug targets which is one of the preliminary stages of drug development pipelines which will facilitate to reap benefits in the later stages of the pipeline.

The human drug target space is enormous and a prediction system which can sensitively predict drug targets is needed. Machine learning methods can augment wet lab methods. With the advent of big data technologies, the vast chemical and genomic space could be mined more successfully and efficiently. As development in the field of machine learning continues to grow, the future of prediction of drug targets and their interaction is promising.

4 Notes

1. The human drug target classification presents a case of imbalance data problem where the number of human drug targets is far less than the nondrug targets. Using an algorithm which can take into account data imbalance will be more suitable, alternatively datasets can be balanced using SMOTE and its variants.

2. In some cases it is useful to standardize/normalize the features for better learning for certain machine learning algorithms.

3. There are two major ways to evaluate the performance of machine learning algorithms: K fold cross-validation and training/testing set split based evaluation. The two common versions of cross-validation are the tenfold cross-validation and fivefold cross-validation. Leave one out cross-validation (LOOCV) is a special case of K fold cross-validation where K = n (total number of samples in the dataset). In K fold cross-validation, the dataset is broken into K subsets, then each subset is used once as a testing set while the remaining (K-1) subsets are used for building the prediction model. In LOOCV each sample is kept once for testing while the model is built upon the rest of the samples. If the data is plentiful, then both tenfold cross-validation and train/test split methods of evaluation should be used.

Acknowledgment

Partial support from UGC-CAS to RC is acknowledged.

References

1. Wang S, Sim TB, Kim YS, Chang YT (2004) Tools for target identification and validation. Curr Opin Chem Biol 8:371–377

2. Howbrook DN, van der Valk AM, O'Shaughnessy MC, Sarker DK, Baker SC, Lloyd AW (2003) Developments in microarray technologies. Drug Discov Today 8:642–651

3. Vernell R, Helin K, Müller H (2003) Identification of target genes of the p16INK4A-pRB-E2F pathway. J Biol Chem 278:46124–46137

4. Mitchell P (2002) A perspective on protein microarrays. Nat Biotechnol 20:225–229

5. Cutler P (2003) Protein arrays: the current state-of-the-art. Proteomics 3:3–18

6. Sem DS, Yu L, Coutts SM, Jack R (2001) Object-oriented approach to drug design enabled by NMR SOLVE: first real-time structural tool for characterizing protein–ligand interactions. J Cell Biochem 84:99–105

7. Jackson PD, Harrington JJ (2005) High-throughput target discovery using cell-based genetics. Drug Discov Today 10:53–60

8. Lindsay MA (2005) Finding new drug targets in the 21st century. Drug Discov Today 10:1683–1687

9. Kumari P, Nath A, Chaube R (2015) Identification of human drug targets using machine-learning algorithms. Comput Biol Med 56:175–181

10. Han LY, Zheng CJ, Xie B, Jia J, Ma XH, Zhu F et al (2007) Support vector machines approach for predicting druggable proteins: recent progress in its exploration and investigation of its usefulness. Drug Discov Today 12:304–313

11. Li Q, Lai L (2007) Prediction of potential drug targets based on simple sequence properties. BMC Bioinformatics 8:353

12. Perola E, Herman L, Weiss J (2012) Development of a rule-based method for the assessment of protein Druggability. J Chem Inf Model 52:1027–1038

13. Liu T, Altman RB (2014) Identifying Druggable targets by protein microenvironments matching: application to transcription factors. CPT Pharmacometrics Syst Pharmacol 3:e93

14. Hall M, Frank E, Holmes G, Pfahringer B, Reutemann P, Witten IH (2009) The WEKA data mining software: an update. SIGKDD Explor Newsl 11:10–18

15. Berthold MR, Cebron N, Dill F, Gabriel TR et al (2009) KNIME - the Konstanz information miner: version 2.0 and beyond. SIGKDD Explor Newsl 11:26–31

16. Hofmann M, Klinkenberg R (eds) (2013) RapidMiner: data mining use cases and business analytics applications. Chapman & Hall/CRC, Boca Raton, FL

17. Cook D (2016) Practical machine learning with H2O: powerful, scalable techniques for deep learning and AI. O'Reilly Media, Boston

18. Pedregosa F, Varoquaux G, Gramfort A, Michel V et al (2011) Scikit-learn: machine learning in python. J Mach Learn Res 12:2825–2830

19. Wishart DS, Knox C, Guo AC, Shrivastava S, Hassanali M, Stothard P et al (2006) DrugBank: a comprehensive resource for in silico drug discovery and exploration. Nucleic Acids Res 34:D668–D672

20. Günther S, Kuhn M, Dunkel M, Campillos M, Senger C, Petsalaki E et al (2008) SuperTarget and matador: resources for exploring drug-target relationships. Nucleic Acids Res 36:D919–D922

21. Chen X, Ji ZL, Chen YZ (2002) TTD: therapeutic target database. Nucleic Acids Res 30:412–415

22. Emig D, Ivliev A, Pustovalova O, Lancashire L, Bureeva S, Nikolsky Y et al (2013) Drug target prediction and repositioning using an integrated network-based approach. PLoS One 8:e60618

23. Gao Z, Li H, Zhang H, Liu X, Kang L, Luo X et al (2008) PDTD: a web-accessible protein database for drug target identification. BMC Bioinformatics 9:104

24. Liu T, Lin Y, Wen X, Jorissen RN, Gilson MK (2007) BindingDB: a web-accessible database of experimentally determined protein–ligand binding affinities. Nucleic Acids Res 35:D198–D201

25. Li ZR, Lin HH, Han LY, Jiang L, Chen X, Chen YZ (2006) PROFEAT: a web server for computing structural and physicochemical features of proteins and peptides from amino acid sequence. Nucleic Acids Res 34:W32–W37

26. Rao HB, Zhu F, Yang GB, Li ZR, Chen YZ (2011) Update of PROFEAT: a web server for

computing structural and physicochemical features of proteins and peptides from amino acid sequence. Nucleic Acids Res 39:W385–W390

27. Du P, Wang X, Xu C, Gao Y (2012) PseAAC-builder: a cross-platform stand-alone program for generating various special Chou's pseudo-amino acid compositions. Anal Biochem 425:117–119

28. Shen HB, Chou KC (2008) PseAAC: a flexible web server for generating various kinds of protein pseudo amino acid composition. Anal Biochem 373:386–388

29. Chou KC (2001) Prediction of protein cellular attributes using pseudo-amino acid composition. Proteins 43:246–255

30. Liu B, Liu F, Wang X, Chen J, Fang L, Chou KC (2015) Pse-in-one: a web server for generating various modes of pseudo components of DNA, RNA, and protein sequences. Nucleic Acids Res 43:W65–W71

31. Ruiz-Blanco YB, Paz W, Green J, Marrero-Ponce Y (2015) ProtDCal: a program to compute general-purpose-numerical descriptors for sequences and 3D-structures of proteins. BMC Bioinformatics 16:162

32. Cao DS, Xu QS, Liang YZ (2013) Propy: a tool to generate various modes of Chou's PseAAC. Bioinformatics 29:960–962

33. Xiao N, Cao DS, Zhu MF, Xu QS (2015) Protr/ProtrWeb: R package and web server for generating various numerical representation schemes of protein sequences. Bioinformatics 31:1857–1859

34. Yap CW (2011) PaDEL-descriptor: an open source software to calculate molecular descriptors and fingerprints. J Comput Chem 32:1466–1474

35. Li ZR, Han LY, Xue Y, Yap CW, Li H, Jiang L (2007) MODEL—molecular descriptor lab: a web-based server for computing structural and physicochemical features of compounds. Biotechnol Bioeng 97:389–396

36. Hong H, Xie Q, Ge W, Qian F, Fang H, Shi L (2008) Mold2, molecular descriptors from 2D structures for Chemoinformatics and Toxicoinformatics. J Chem Inf Comput Sci 48:1337–1344

37. Chawla NV, Bowyer KW, Hall LO, Kegelmeyer WP (2002) SMOTE: synthetic minority oversampling technique. J Artif Intell Res 16:321–357

38. Witten IH, Frank E, Hall MA (eds) (2011) Data mining: practical machine learning tools and techniques. Morgan Kaufmann Publishers Inc., San Francisco

39. Bradley AP (1997) The use of the area under the ROC curve in the evaluation of machine learning algorithms. Pattern Recogn 30:1145–1159

40. Szklarczyk D, Franceschini A, Wyder S, Forslund K, Heller D, Huerta-Cepas J et al (2015) STRING v10: protein–protein interaction networks, integrated over the tree of life. Nucleic Acids Res 43:D447–D452

41. Chatr-aryamontri A, Oughtred R, Boucher L, Rust J, Chang C, Kolas NK et al (2017) The BioGRID interaction database: 2017 update. Nucleic Acids Res 45:D369–D379

42. Keshava Prasad TS, Goel R, Kandasamy K, Keerthikumar S, Kumar S, Mathivanan S et al (2009) Human protein reference database--2009 update. Nucleic Acids Res 37:D767–D772

Chapter 3

Practices in Molecular Docking and Structure-Based Virtual Screening

Ricardo N. dos Santos, Leonardo G. Ferreira, and Adriano D. Andricopulo

Abstract

Drug discovery has evolved significantly over the past two decades. Progress in key areas such as molecular and structural biology has contributed to the elucidation of the three-dimensional structure and function of a wide range of biological molecules of therapeutic interest. In this context, the integration of experimental techniques, such as X-ray crystallography, and computational methods, such as molecular docking, has promoted the emergence of several areas in drug discovery, such as structure-based drug design (SBDD). SBDD strategies have been broadly used to identify, predict and optimize the activity of small molecules toward a molecular target and have contributed to major scientific breakthroughs in pharmaceutical R&D. This chapter outlines molecular docking and structure-based virtual screening (SBVS) protocols used to predict the interaction of small molecules with the phosphatidylinositol-bisphosphate-kinase PI3Kδ, which is a molecular target for hematological diseases. A detailed description of the molecular docking and SBVS procedures and an evaluation of the results are provided.

Key words Autodock vina, Drug discovery, Molecular modeling, Structure-based drug design, X-ray crystallography

1 Introduction

Modern drug research and development (R&D) relies on the discovery of low-molecular weight compounds that interact with disease-related biological macromolecules (known as receptors or molecular targets) in a selective way. Although the number of molecular targets that can be modulated by pharmacological agents is estimated in approximately 10,000 gene products, only 4% of these macromolecules are being investigated in drug discovery programs [1]. In view of the potential that this unexplored space represents, understanding the fundamentals that drive ligand–receptor interactions is of critical importance to drug R&D [2]. In this context, structure-based drug design (SBDD), that is, the use of structural information of molecular targets to improve aspects related to ligand binding, is a core approach in the pharmaceutical industry [3].

Mohini Gore and Umesh B. Jagtap (eds.), *Computational Drug Discovery and Design*, Methods in Molecular Biology, vol. 1762, https://doi.org/10.1007/978-1-4939-7756-7_3, © Springer Science+Business Media, LLC, part of Springer Nature 2018

Over the past two decades, advances in SBDD have been fostered by the integration of spectroscopic methods, such as X-ray crystallography, and in silico techniques, such as molecular dynamics, homology modeling and molecular docking [4]. The synergistic use of these methodologies, particularly in the preclinical phase of the R&D process, has enabled the determination of the 3D structures of many biological macromolecules along with the accurate characterization of their binding site features, such as steric and electrostatic properties. This valuable knowledge has been the key to the understanding of ligand–receptor molecular recognition phenomena [5]. By integrating these data with up-to-date technologies in pharmaceutical R&D, SBDD has successfully supported the development of pioneering therapies for highly complex and prevalent conditions [6].

The use of SBDD strategies enables the conception of ligands with specific steric and electrostatic properties that will effectively interact with a target pharmacological receptor [4, 5]. SBDD consists of a cyclic process that begins with the resolution of the 3D structure of the molecular target. Next, molecular modeling investigations are performed to find putative ligands. Subsequently, promising compounds are commercially purchased or synthesized, followed by experimental evaluation of potency, affinity, and selectivity against the investigated receptor. Once active molecules are identified, the 3D structure of the ligand–receptor complex is determined, enabling the identification of the intermolecular interactions that drive the molecular recognition process. Additionally, determining the structure of the ligand–receptor complex enables the construction of relationships between biological activity and structural features [7]. Finally, taking into account these studies, molecular optimization efforts are conducted to improve the ligand properties, mainly those related to affinity, selectivity, and efficiency.

1.1 Molecular Docking

Molecular docking is a broadly used SBDD technique. This technique is applied to predict the most likely 3D conformations of small-molecule ligands within target binding sites and to provide quantitative projections of the energy variations involved in the intermolecular recognition event [8]. In addition, these quantitative estimations of the binding energetics provide rankings for the docked compounds, which is a useful parameter for selecting ligands for experimental profiling. Molecular docking can be divided into two distinct steps: exploration of the ligand conformational space within the binding cavity and estimation of the binding energy for each predicted conformation [9, 10].

1.1.1 Conformational Search

To explore the conformational space, molecular docking programs modify the structural parameters of the ligands, such as dihedral angles and translational and rotational degrees of freedom. Two strategies are usually employed by conformational search algorithms: (1) systematic and (2) stochastic search methods [11]. Systematic search strategies entail small changes in the structural parameters that alter the ligand conformation in a gradual fashion [10]. By exploring the energy landscape of the conformational space, the algorithm converges to a conformation that corresponds to the minimum energy solution. Systematic search algorithms are effective in probing the conformational space; however, a local minimum conformation can be provided instead of the global minimum conformation. This shortcoming can be solved by executing several searches simultaneously starting from a broad range of different conformations. In addition, as systematic search methods explore all combinations of the structural parameters, the number of possible combinations grows exponentially with the degrees of freedom of the ligand, leading to the so-called combinatorial explosion. Docking packages such as FRED and DOCK address this issue using incremental construction algorithms, which gradually build the ligand structure into the binding site [12, 13]. Incremental algorithms break down the ligand structure in several fragments and then add each part sequentially in complementary regions of the binding site until the whole structure has been reconstructed. The conformational search step is performed individually for the added fragments, decreasing the degrees of freedom to be probed and avoiding combinatorial explosion.

In contrast, stochastic methods explore the energy landscape by randomly changing the ligand structural parameters [14]. Stochastic algorithms generate sets of diverse solutions, exploring a broad range of the conformational space. This approach is useful for avoiding confining the conformations at local minima, thus increasing the likelihood of generating global minimum solutions [10, 14]. Genetic algorithms (GAs), one of the most successful applications of stochastic search strategies, are implemented in widely used programs such as AutoDock and GOLD [15, 16]. Genetic algorithms apply the principles of natural selection by encoding the initial conformation of the ligand in a vector termed the chromosome. Taking this chromosome as a starting point, the algorithm generates an ensemble of conformations covering a wide range of the conformational space. Next, the chromosomes with the lowest energy values are selected as starting points for the generation of the next ensemble of conformations. By repeating the GA routine several times, the mean energy of the population is diminished by transferring favorable structural features from one generation of chromosomes to another, decreasing the energy landscape to be probed [10, 16].

1.1.2 Estimation of the Binding Energy

In addition to predicting the binding conformation of ligands, molecular docking algorithms apply scoring functions to evaluate the binding energy of the proposed solutions [17]. The energy variation that occurs during the formation of the ligand–receptor complex is measured by the binding constant (K_d) and Gibbs free energy (ΔG_L) [18]. Scoring functions estimate these parameters using three types of algorithms: (1) force-field-based, (2) empirical, and (3) knowledge-based functions [19]. Those methods based on force fields calculate the binding energy by summing bonded (bond stretching, angle bending, and dihedral variation) and nonbonded contributions (electrostatic and van der Waals interactions). Force-field-based methods use ab initio calculations and the equations of classical mechanics to estimate the contribution of each of these terms to the total binding energy. Empirical scoring functions use training sets consisting of protein–ligand complexes with known binding affinities to generate statistical models. The terms used in the derivation of the models consist of hydrogen-bonding, ionic and non-polar interactions, as well as desolvation effects and entropic contributions [20]. The accuracy of empirical scoring functions depends directly on the quality of the data used to generate the model. The other approach, knowledge-based scoring functions, uses data from known ligand–receptor complexes to calculate pairwise energy potentials and generate a general equation [21]. These potentials are constructed by taking into account the frequency with which two different atoms are found to interact in a series of ligand–receptor complexes. The different types of interactions are classified and weighted according to their occurrence to generate the final scoring function, which is a sum of these individual interactions. In short, current molecular docking programs predict the conformation of a small molecule within the target binding site with reasonable accuracy, as confirmed by comparing complexes predicted by different algorithms with their respective X-ray structures. The major limitation is the lack of a suitable function to estimate desolvation contributions, entropic effects, and protein flexibility with reasonable accuracy [22, 23].

1.2 Virtual Screening

Virtual screening is the use of fast and cost-effective computational methods to identify potentially active molecules from virtual databases [24]. Exploring virtual compound collections is one of the most widespread strategies in drug discovery, and several pharmacological agents can trace their origins to virtual screening efforts [2, 6]. Strategies that rely on docking compounds from libraries against a given molecular target are termed structure-based virtual screening (SBVS) and are the focus of this chapter [24]. In addition to the prediction of likely binding conformations, SBVS offers a convenient method of ranking the docked molecules using scoring functions. This classification criterion can be used solely or in combination with other procedures for selecting promising molecules for experimental profiling.

SBVS strategies usually rely on the following procedures: (1) molecular target selection and preparation, (2) compound database selection, (3) molecular docking, and (4) analysis of results. Careful analyses of the available information concerning the structure and function of the investigated molecular target along with its known ligands are highly recommended when devising an SBVS workflow [25]. Once the molecular target structure is selected, it undergoes important procedures aimed at preparing it for molecular docking. Usually, these procedures consist of adding hydrogen atoms (*see* **Note 1**), eliminating noncrystallographic water molecules, assigning partial charges and specifying protonation states for the amino acid residues [26].

The next critical step is the selection of the set of compounds that will be used in the molecular docking studies. Usually, freely available virtual databases that encompass a wide chemical diversity are used [27]. In general, these compound repositories are interactive interfaces that allow for the application of chemical filters to search and select focused subsets representing a specific chemical space. Molecules in these databases are stored as line notations (e.g., SMILES, SMARTS, or InChI files), which are automatically converted into 3D structures with appropriate ionization states, partial charges, and stereochemistry once downloaded [13, 27].

The next phase consists of docking the selected compounds into the target binding site. The conformational search routine probes the energy landscape of each compound, and those compounds ranked as promising hits are selected for post-docking analysis, the next stage of this process. This procedure involves visualizing the predicted ligand–receptor complexes and enables the examination of critical features, such as binding conformations and intermolecular interactions. The analysis of these elements is useful for deciding on which of the top-scoring compounds have to be prioritized for experimental studies [8, 10, 24]. Another important aspect that can be evaluated by visualizing the structures is whether the docking solutions for known ligands match crystallographic conformations. This step is important for assessing whether the docking simulations can reproduce experimental data.

Considering the above-discussed principles, it is clear that outlining robust molecular docking and SBVS campaigns is not a straightforward task. Given the success achieved by these approaches and the variety of programs, algorithms, and resources available, a wide diversity of strategies can be employed. Next, we will provide a detailed workflow that will introduce to the reader the basic tasks for conducting a molecular docking and SBVS effort.

2   Materials

In this section, we will describe the computational tools that are required to generate the molecular target and database inputs, develop the molecular docking simulations and visualize the results. In general, this step-by-step guide assumes that the readers will develop their molecular docking and SBVS studies on a Unix-like computer operating system (e.g., any version of Linux Ubuntu or Mac OS X or later).

2.1   Initial Data

2.1.1   Molecular Target 3D Structures

Selecting a suitable 3D conformation of the molecular target, i.e., the spatial coordinates that define the relative position of each atom within the structure, is a critical step in performing a molecular docking study. One of the most commonly used sources of 3D structural data for biological macromolecules, the Protein Data Bank (PDB), incorporates structures determined by biophysical methods such as X-ray crystallography, NMR spectroscopy, and cryo-electron microscopy. PDB is freely accessible at http://www.rcsb.org/ and will be used in this chapter to obtain the 3D structure of the molecular target [28].

2.1.2   Small-Molecule Database

The other required component for a molecular docking effort is the 3D structure of the small molecules to be evaluated. The structure of these compounds can be obtained from distinct sources. Several virtual compound databases are freely available, and the selection of these collections depends on the goals of each drug discovery project. For example, focused databases enclosing a specific chemical space are available for specific classes of proteins. Other collections concentrate on specific sources of compounds, for example, the NuBBE database compiles various natural products from organisms that are native to Brazil (http://nubbe.iq.unesp.br/portal/nubbedb.html) [29]. On the other hand, when no information is available about known active ligands or when the investigated target is known for interacting with different chemical classes, general libraries containing widely diverse chemotypes can be used. This type of collection generally contains hundreds of thousands (or millions) of entries [30, 31]. Some examples of these general and large repositories are the ChemSpider (http://www.chemspider.com/) and ZINC (http://zinc.docking.org/) databases [32, 33].

2.2   Computational Tools

In this section, we will introduce all programs that will be used in this tutorial. Currently, there are numerous software programs and tools available for use in each stage of the molecular docking procedure. The tools enumerated here are well-established and freely accessible programs (*see* **Note2**).

2.2.1 *AutoDock Vina*   AutoDock Vina, one of the most cited molecular docking software programs, combines an efficient stochastic conformational search algorithm and accurate and well-rated force-field-based and empirical scoring functions [34]. The combination of its efficacy and suitability for parallelization results in a low computational cost making this program an attractive option for performing SBVS studies against large compound libraries. Executable files and theoretical details about AutoDock Vina and its installation and use can be accessed at http://vina.scripps.edu.

2.2.2 *BKChem*   In addition to chemical databases, novel molecules can be drawn from scratch using chemical drawing suites. Frequently, a series of molecules known to be active against an investigated molecular target are used as references to design novel compounds. BKChem is an open-source chemical drawing program that provides a user-friendly interface for generating 2D structures that can be used as an initial sketch to build 3D conformations. The program is able to assign important features such as specific protonation states and chirality and can be accessed at http://bkchem.zirael.org [35].

2.2.3 *Open Babel*   This toolbox is an open and collaborative resource broadly used to interpret and interconvert a variety of chemical file extensions [36]. Extremely convenient for converting chemical formats that are not compatible with distinct programs, this platform allows for a smooth and straightforward workflow along the molecular docking process. Open Babel includes other useful functionalities such as filtering and searching routines, as well as generation of 3D coordinates and prediction of protonation states. This resource is available at http://openbabel.org.

2.2.4 *UCSF Chimera*   UCSF Chimera is a molecular modeling software for visualization and analysis of a wide range of data related to biomolecular systems [37]. This software is able to handle 3D structures of macromolecules and small-molecule ligands, density maps, sequence alignments, molecular docking results, conformational ensembles, and molecular dynamics trajectories. This resource is also suitable for generating high-quality illustrations and animations for scientific purposes. UCSF Chimera can be downloaded at http://www.cgl.ucsf.edu/chimera.

3   Methods

To perform the molecular docking protocol described herein, phosphatidylinositol-4,5-bisphosphate 3-kinase (PI3Kδ) was selected [38–40]. PI3Ks play a key role in the regulation of several signaling pathways related to fundamental cellular processes such as differentiation, proliferation, metabolism, motility, and cell growth. These kinases catalyze the conversion of phosphatidylino-sitol 4,5-bisphosphate (PIP$_2$) to phosphatidylinositol 3,4,5-trisphosphate (PIP$_3$), which activates downstream intracellular signaling cascades. PI3Kδ belongs to class I PI3Ks and is predominantly expressed in leukocytes; therefore, it represents a potential target for the treatment of hematological diseases.

Idelalisib (Zydelig®, Gilead Sciences) is an inhibitor of PI3Kδ that was recently approved by the FDA for the treatment of chronic lymphocytic leukemia and indolent non-Hodgkin's lymphomas [41–44]. This chapter uses the idelalisib-PI3Kδ complex to run the molecular docking protocol (*see* Note 3). First, we will predict the binding mode of idelalisib to PI3Kδ. Next, we will use the same system to run an SBVS against a large compound database. This part of the chapter is intended to familiarize the reader with elementary tasks concerning chemical library acquisition, SBVS running, and analysis of results.

3.1 Characterization of the Macromolecular Target

The X-ray structure of the PI3K δ-idelalisib complex can be downloaded by entering the code *4XE0* in the search box of the PDB interface (http://www.rcsb.org/) (*see* Note 3). Each PDB entry contains information on experimental details, related literature, the biological relevance of the macromolecule, and statistical indicators on the quality of the 3D model. Accordingly, on the first page of the *4XE0* entry, the Structure Summary tab (Macromolecules section) shows that this macromolecular structure is formed by a polypeptide chain composed of 939 amino acid residues. The Small Molecules section provides information about the presence of low-molecular weight compounds as elements of the crystallographic complex. In this section, idelalisib is identified by its structure and IUPAC name. This inhibitor is distinguished within the crystallographic structure by the code *40L*.

Important points that should be noted when selecting a 3D molecular model are the statistical parameters that indicate the quality of the structure. Despite the existence of many other indicators, the resolution of the X-ray structure is the key parameter that measures the overall quality of the model. In a simple definition, the crystallographic resolution expresses how well detailed the electron density map is that was used to specify the coordinates of each atom in the 3D structure. Lower values mean a higher resolution and, consequently, higher accuracy in the assignment of the atom coordinates. While structures with resolution under 1.5 Å are particularly suited for molecular docking, lower-resolution models (~3 Å) can be used as long as we keep in mind that uncertainty in atom coordinates always increases with the value of the resolution [45].

Returning to the Structure Summary tab and looking at the Experimental Data and Validation section, we observe that although *4XE0* has the acceptable value 2.43 Å, it is not a high-resolution X-ray structure. Nevertheless, this crystallographic model is able to provide good molecular docking results as will be demonstrated in the next sections [46, 47].

3.2 Single-Ligand Docking

3.2.1 Generating the Ligand

Now that we have an overall view of the system to be studied, we can generate the input files to perform the molecular docking analysis. First, open a text terminal (also known as the console) in your OS, and use the following commands to generate a working folder named *Docking*:

```
mkdir Docking
```

Next, move to this folder by typing:

```
cd Docking
```

Then generate a new 3D structure of the ligand idelalisib (distinct from the crystallographic one) to use an equitable input conformation for the docking analysis. Instead of directly drawing the 3D structure of the ligand using a molecular editor, a safer protocol is to sketch a 2D structure and then use this file to automatically generate the 3D representation. This approach is useful for handling compounds with large or intricate structures that contain charged groups and asymmetric carbons, such as those commonly found in natural products. In these cases, drawing 3D structures from scratch can become a significant source of error. Looking at the structure of idelalisib (Fig. 1a), we can use BKChem to reproduce it in a 2D format. Open BKChem by typing *bkchem* on the terminal. After drawing the full structure (with the correct chirality), the generated data should be saved in *mol* extension by selecting *File → Export → Molfile* and should be named *ligand.mol* in the *Docking* directory. Finally, type the following command to convert the idelalisib 2D structure into a *pdb* 3D model with optimized geometry using Open Babel:

```
obabel -imol ligand.mol -h -opdb -O ligand.pdb --gen3d
-minimize
```

The generated 3D structure of the compound will be observed in the UCSF Chimera environment. To do this, open chimera through the installation icon, go to *File → Open*, and select the file *ligand.pdb*. Another way to open the file in Chimera is to type the following in the terminal:

```
chimera ligand.pdb
```

3.2.2 Generating the Receptor

Now, we will use the crystallographic structure of PI3Kδ to generate the input file for the receptor. In the Chimera interface, load the

A   B

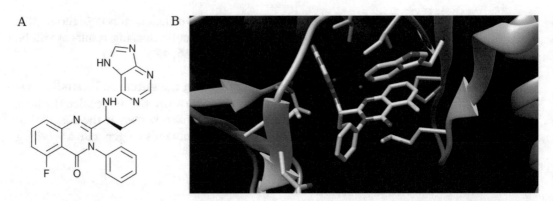

Fig. 1 (a) Molecular structure of idelalisib. (b) View of the PI3Kδ enzyme (PDB ID: *4XE0*)—idelalisib complex. The protein backbone is in cartoon representation. The ligand and residues in the binding site are depicted as sticks. Water molecules are illustrated as spheres

PI3Kδ structure by going to *File → Fetch by ID*. In the newly opened window, select *PDB*, type *4XE0* in the adjacent blank form, and press the *Fetch* button, which will load the PI3Kδ structure. By pressing the left button of the mouse and moving the cursor over the window, we can rotate the protein, observe its secondary and tertiary structures, and examine the binding mode of idelalisib (*40L*). Next, use the ligand coordinates to delimitate the target binding site for the molecular docking simulations (*see* **Note 3**). To do this, go to *Select → Residue → 40L*, and zoom in to it by selecting *Actions → Focus*. This step will generate the image shown in Fig. 1b. Using the mouse to rotate the structure, identify the sole asymmetrical carbon of idelalisib. Select this atom by pressing Ctrl and the left mouse button. Find its coordinates by going to *Favorites → Command Line* and typing the following line in the new *Command* field at the bottom of the Chimera interface:

```
getcrd selection
```

This action will generate a new line in the status bar (lower area of the window). The status bar contains the description of the selected atom followed by its X, Y, Z Cartesian coordinates. Record these numbers in a footnote; they will be used to define the center of the binding site. If selecting the asymmetrical carbon atom is difficult, replace *selection* in the above command by *::40L@C19* to obtain the same result. Finally, remove the crystallographic ligand from the binding site by going to *Select → Residue → 40L* and *Actions → Atoms/Bonds → delete*.

The binding site of PI3Kδ does not contain unusual residue types or electronic states; however, these odd configurations can occur in some crystallographic structures. It is advisable to always verify the presence of uncommon representations and fix them whenever required. This verification can be performed using the

Dock Prep tool available in Chimera, which can be accessed by selecting *Tools → Structure Editing → Dock Prep*. Leaving enabled all options except for *Delete solvent, Delete non-complexes ions* and *Add charges* is the recommended setting. After choosing these settings, a second window will allow the parameterization of the protonation states. This option is useful when the system has multiple protonation possibilities for the binding site residues. In this case, we will keep the default protonation states. Select *OK* on the current window, and when the next option becomes available, save the generated receptor structure in the working directory as *receptor.mol2*.

3.2.3 Running the Molecular Docking Simulation

Having prepared the ligand and receptor input files, we will dock idelalisib into the binding cavity of PI3Kδ. Using Chimera, open the 3D structure of idelalisib (*ligand.pdb*) and go to *Tools → Surface/Binding Analysis → AutoDock Vina*. A new window will pop up with several options describing the parameters that will be used for docking (Fig. 2a). In the *Output file* section, enter a name for the file that will record the final docking results (e.g., *run1*) in the previously created *Docking* folder, and click on *Set Output Location*. In the *Receptor* and *Ligand* options, choose the receptor and ligand to be used (these are *4XE0* and *ligand.pdb*, respectively). Over the blank fields in the *Receptor search* area, enter the X, Y, Z coordinates recorded in Subheading 3.2.2 in the *Center* item (Fig. 2a). The next field, named *Size*, defines the length in Å of each side of the box that will delimitate the binding site. The optimal value for this parameter changes according to the volume and geometry of the binding site of the system under study. In general, this parameter should include all residues that could engage in intermolecular interactions with the ligand; however, it should not be excessively large because that could cause staggering of the conformational search. A reasonable value to be selected in our case is 15 for all axes.

After filling the parameters for the binding site, a wire-frame box showing the selected binding site region will appear (Fig. 2a). Next, we should consider the parameters for receptor and ligand handling. First, the option *Add hydrogens in Chimera* should be ignored, as we already set up protonation states during receptor preparation. Furthermore, because Autodock Vina considers hydrogen atoms bound exclusively to polar atoms to compute the molecular interactions, enable *Merge charges and remove non-polar atoms* and *Merge charges and remove lone pairs* in both Receptor and Ligand options. Because we do not have chains with non-standard residues, settings to *Ignore chains of non-standard residues* and *Ignore all non-standard residues* have no effect and should be ignored. In addition, we should consider the presence of the two

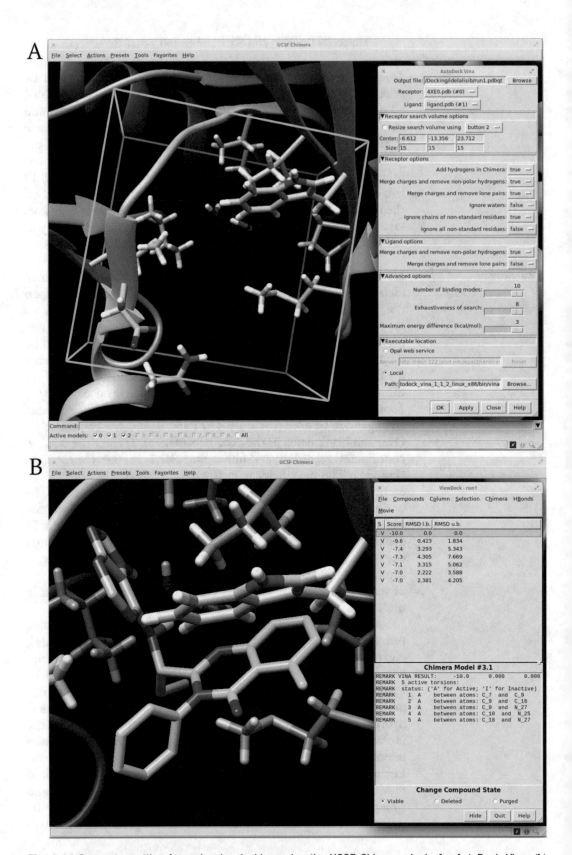

Fig. 2 (a) Parameter setting for molecular docking using the UCSF Chimera plugin for AutoDock Vina. (b) Predicted conformations for idelalisib in the PI3Kδ binding site. The protein backbone is in cartoon representation. The ligand, water and residues in the binding site are depicted as sticks

crystallographic water molecules in the binding site of PI3Kδ by setting the option *Ignore waters* to false.

Finally, the section *Advanced options* is used to specify output parameters, such as the maximum number of binding modes generated for each docking analysis, the extension of the conformational search procedures and the energy gap between the accepted solutions. In general, setting higher values increases the probability of finding likely solutions; however, it also increases computational time. Therefore, we should always consider the available computational resources and the desired duration of the simulation to set those parameters appropriately. Because we are dealing with only one compound with low structural complexity, we can use the maximum allowed values.

The Chimera interface to AutoDock Vina allows the molecular docking to be run locally or to use a remote web server. Because you downloaded Vina (http://vina.scripps.edu/download.html) on your machine, use the *local* option at the *Executable* section, and select the Vina program location using the *Browse* option. Finally, run the molecular docking simulation by clicking *OK*. This procedure will generate the *running* message in the status bar.

3.2.4 Visualizing Results

After running the molecular docking procedure, the ViewDock window containing the scores of the predicted binding solutions will open (Fig. 2b). Each 3D conformation can be observed by clicking on the corresponding score. Each value corresponds to the predicted binding energy, in kcal/mol, calculated by the AutoDock Vina scoring function. Therefore, the more negative the value, the higher the probability of the ligand–receptor interaction occurring in experimental tests. Additionally, the hydrogen bonds for each of the predicted ligand–receptor complexes can be observed in the ViewDock window by selecting the following option: *HBonds* → *Add Count to Entire Receptor*. In the new window, enable *Label H-bond with distance* and *Relax H-bond constraints*, change the parameter *Line width* to 10, and select *inter-model* in the section *Find these bonds* on the right. Leave all the remaining options disabled, and click *OK*. Next, to explicitly display the atoms of the receptor binding site, go to *Actions* → *Atoms/Bonds* → *show* and then to *Actions* → *Ribbon* → *hide* on the main menu of Chimera.

At this point, we should see a colorful line displaying the ligand–receptor hydrogen bonds (Fig. 3a). If your simulation led to the correct prediction, you should observe a distinct interaction between the backbone valine 628 amino group and the ligand N3 nitrogen of the 7H–purine ring (Fig. 3a). Explore the other predicted conformations, and look for the interactions in each complex.

Having identified all the predicted conformations, we can compare these solutions with the crystallographic binding mode of

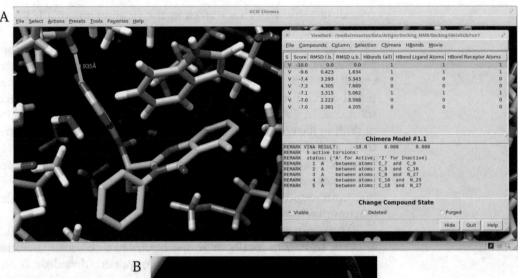

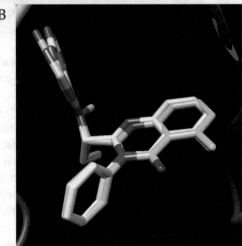

Fig. 3 (**a**) Analysis of the hydrogen bond interactions for a predicted PI3Kδ-idelalisib complex. (**b**) Comparison of the best docking solution (lowest energy) with the crystallographic conformation of idelalisib. The RMSD between the predicted and experimental models is 0.374 Å. The protein backbone is in cartoon representation. The ligand, water and residues in the binding site are depicted as sticks

idelalisib (*see* **Note 3**). To do this, open the original PI3Kδ structure in Chimera by going to *File → Fetch by ID* and writing its PDB code (*4XE0*) at the blank field. If all steps were performed correctly, the top-scoring conformation should be very similar to the crystallographic one (root mean square deviation, RMSD = 0.374 Å), as shown in Fig. 3b.

4 Virtual Screening

In this section, we will use multiple ligands in the molecular docking simulation to perform an SBVS protocol. Several compound libraries covering a wide range of structural and physicochemical features are available on the web. In this example, we will use the NuBBE database to predict likely ligands for PI3Kδ.

4.1 Obtaining the Compound Library

The front page of the NuBBE database (http://nubbe.iq.unesp. br/portal/nubbedb.html) shows a form that allows the user to search compounds based on specific characteristics (e.g., substructure, physicochemical properties, and source). First, we will select a subset of compounds to be screened from the database. Leaving all fields in the form blank, select *Isolated from a microorganism* in the source section, and click on *Search compound(s)* located at the bottom of the page. This procedure will generate a list of entries, each one containing a set of information, such as the accession code, structure and chemical class. Download the file containing all the 3D molecular structures of this selected group of compounds by clicking on the *mol2* link in the results section. Extract and copy the generated *mol2* files to a new folder named VS inside your working *Docking* directory. Next, open a terminal in this folder.

4.2 Running the Virtual Screening

The Chimera-Autodock Vina interface supports docking studies using a single molecule at a time. To perform the SBVS with the dataset containing multiple molecules downloaded from NuBBE, we need to run Autodock Vina independently. First, generate a configuration file for the docking parameters by creating a text file using any editor (e.g., gedit) and copying the following data inside:

```
center_x = -6.612
center_y = -13.356
center_z = 23.712
size_x = 15.00
size_y = 15.00
size_z = 15.00
energy_range = 3
exhaustiveness = 8
num_modes = 1
```

Note that these parameters are the same as those inserted in the Chimera interface while running the molecular docking analyses (Fig. 2a); however, only one conformation for each molecule (*num_modes = 1*) will be generated in this SBVS protocol. Save this new file as *conf.txt* in the current folder (VS). Next, use the following script to automate the docking procedure for all molecules. To do this, create another text file, and copy the following data inside:

```
#! /bin/bash
mkdir results
for i in *.mol2; do
a="${i%.*}"
obabel -imol2 $i -opdbqt -O $a.pdbqt
 vina --config conf.txt --receptor ../*.receptor.pdbqt --
ligand $a.pdbqt --out results/$a.docked.pdbqt
done
rm *.pdbqt
cat results/*.docked.pdbqt > all.docked.pdbqt
```

Save this new file as vs.*sh* in the VS folder in which the compound dataset and the file *conf.txt* are located. Finally, run the screening by executing the above-generated script with the following command:

```
bash vs.sh
```

The calculations should take several minutes. At the end of the process, the Auto Dock Vina algorithm will create a folder named *results* containing the docked conformation for each molecule evaluated. In addition, this algorithm will generate a single file containing all docking results concatenated in a file named *all.docked.pdbqt*. To analyze these results, go to Chimera, and open the receptor structure saved in the *Docking* folder. To do this, go to *File* → *Open*, and choose the file *receptor.mol2*. To visualize the SBVS results using Chimera's ViewDock tool, go to *Tools* → *Surface/ Binding Analysis* → *ViewDock*, and open the concatenated file *all. docked.pdbqt*. Similar to the visual analyses performed for idelalisib, a table with all predicted conformations and their energy values allows the selection and exploration of each docking solution. The *Hbonds* tool can be used again to identify the hydrogen bonds formed in each ligand–receptor complex.

5   Further Considerations

Despite the capabilities of molecular docking in predicting the conformation of a ligand in the target binding site, the calculated interaction energy should not be considered a reliable estimation of ligand–receptor affinity. Once docking programs use simple physical models that do not consider nonclassical phenomena (entropic, desolvation, and quantic effects), their estimations of binding energies are rarely accurate. However, because the accuracy of this measure is equal for all molecules in an SBVS study, the relative energy ranking among conformations is valid and useful for distinguishing ligands with a high probability of binding to the target in experimental tests.

Another fundamental aspect that should be considered when searching for potential candidates for experimental evaluation is the physicochemical profile of each molecule. SBDD does not consider pharmacokinetics aspects; therefore, estimation of properties such as the partition coefficient ($\log P$) and polar surface area (PSA) can be used as a preliminary filter to remove compounds that are likely to show permeability and solubility problems and, consequently, poor pharmacokinetic profiles. Several computational tools are freely available and should be used to estimate the physicochemical properties of dataset molecules before performing an SBVS study [48–50].

Another important aspect that should be considered is the presence of crystallographic water molecules in the target binding site. In some cases, these molecules are tightly bound to the molecular target, requiring for their displacement the formation of at least equally favorable ligand–receptor interactions. However, their displacement is not required, as they can mediate specific ligand–receptor interactions, becoming a component of the binding site themselves, which is the case for PI3Kδ. For crystallographic structures with high resolution, an interesting strategy is to perform docking studies considering both situations—with and without crystallographic water molecules. It should be noted that multiple water molecules in the binding site can substantially increase the complexity of the SBVS workflow since different combinations of these molecules can be considered [51, 52].

6   Notes

1. In the protocol described in this chapter, the final structures generated by the molecular docking program present implicit non-polar hydrogen atoms. This result does not affect the overall interpretation of the molecular interactions; however, it is useful to recover all-atom 3D structures for use as inputs in further computational studies (e.g., molecular dynamics simulations). Full 3D structures in PDB format can be generated from the final docking solutions by typing the following command in Open Babel:

```
obabel -ipdbqt molecule.pdbqt -h -opdb -O molecule.pdb
```

2. The software applications described in this workflow are all free-of-charge and present detailed documentation on their installation and use. Most of these applications are accessible through package repositories for widely used UNIX-based distributions and can be installed by typing a single command in the terminal window. This is the case for BKChem, Open-Babel, and AutoDock Vina. To verify the availability of the Open Babel program in a Debian-based OS (e.g., Ubuntu), enter the following command in the terminal:

```
apt-cache search openbabel
```

Once the package is downloaded into the OS repository, it can be installed by typing:

```
sudo apt-get install openbabel
```

Similarly, the same conveniences are available for Mac and non-Debian-based Linux through MacPorts and yum tools, respectively.

3. As a validation step for the methodology presented herein, it is suggested to always try to reproduce crystallographic conformations whenever they are available. In the absence of a crystallographic binding conformation, one molecule from the compound collection selected for the SBVS can be chosen for a preliminary molecular docking run. This approach is useful for generating the receptor input and providing an initial view of the structural peculiarities of the system under investigation.

Acknowledgments

We gratefully acknowledge financial support from the State of Sao Paulo Research Foundation (FAPESP, Fundação de Amparo à Pesquisa do Estado de São Paulo), grants 2015/13667-9, 2013/25658-9, and 2013/07600-3.

References

1. Jin L, Wang W, Fang G (2014) Targeting protein-protein interaction by small molecules. Annu Rev Pharmacol Toxicol 54:435–456

2. Blaney J (2012) A very short history of structure-based design: how did we get here and where do we need to go? J Comput Aided Mol Des 26:13–14

3. Kinch MS, Hoyer DA (2015) History of drug development in four acts. Drug Discov Today 20:1163–1168

4. Kalyaanamoorthy S, Chen YP (2011) Structure-based drug design to augment hit discovery. Drug Discov Today 16:831–839

5. Honarparvar B, Govender T, Maguire GE et al (2014) Integrated approach to structure-based enzymatic drug design: molecular modeling, spectroscopy, and experimental bioactivity. Chem Rev 114:493–537

6. Eder J, Sedrani R, Wiesmann C (2014) The discovery of first-in-class drugs: origins and evolution. Nat Rev Drug Discov 13:577–587

7. Shoichet BK, Kobilka BK (2012) Structure-based drug screening for G-protein-coupled receptors. Trends Pharmacol Sci 33:268–272

8. Meng XY, Zhang HX, Mezei M, Cui M (2011) Molecular docking: a powerful approach for structure-based drug discovery. Curr Comput Aided Drug Des 7:146–157

9. Kitchen DB, Decornez H, Furr JR et al (2004) Docking and scoring in virtual screening for drug discovery: methods and applications. Nat Rev Drug Discov 3:935–949

10. Ferreira LG, dos Santos RN, Oliva G et al (2015) Molecular docking and structure-based drug design strategies. Molecules 20:13384–13421

11. Yuriev E, Agostino M, Ramsland PA (2011) Challenges and advances in computational docking: 2009 in review. J Mol Recognit 24:149–164

12. McGann M (2012) FRED and HYBRID docking performance on standardized datasets. J Comput Aided Mol Des 26:897–906

13. Ewing TJ, Makino S, Skillman AG, Kuntz ID (2001) DOCK 4.0: search strategies for automated molecular docking of flexible molecule databases. J Comput Aided Mol Des 15:411–428

14. Gorelik B, Goldblum A (2008) High quality binding modes in docking ligands to proteins. Proteins 71:1373–1386

15. Morris GM, Goodsell DS, Huey R, Olson AJ (1996) Distributed automated docking of flexible ligands to proteins: parallel applications of AutoDock 2.4. J Comput Aided Mol Des 10:293–304

16. Jones G, Willett P, Glen RC, Leach AR, Taylor R (1997) Development and validation of a genetic algorithm for flexible docking. J Mol Biol 267:727–748

17. Santos RN, Andricopulo AD (2013) Physics and its interfaces with medicinal chemistry and drug design. Braz J Phys 43:268–280

18. Foloppe N, Hubbard R (2006) Towards predictive ligand design with free-energy based computational methods? Curr Med Chem 13:3583–3608

19. Huang SY, Grinter SZ, Zou X (2010) Scoring functions and their evaluation methods for protein–ligand docking: recent advances and future directions. Phys Chem Chem Phys 12:12899–12908

20. Murray C, Auton TR, Eldridge MD (1998) Empirical scoring functions. II. The testing of an empirical scoring function for the prediction of ligand-receptor binding affinities and the use of Bayesian regression to improve the quality of the model. J Comput Aided Mol Des 12:503–519

21. Huang SY, Zou X (2006) An iterative knowledge-based scoring function to predict protein–ligand interactions: I. Derivation of interaction potentials. J Comput Chem 27:1866–1875

22. Mysinger MM, Shoichet BK (2010) Rapid context-dependent ligand desolvation in molecular docking. J Chem Inf Model 50:1561–1573

23. Ruvinsky AM (2007) Role of binding entropy in the refinement of protein–ligand docking predictions: analysis based on the use of 11 scoring functions. J Comput Chem 28:1364–1372

24. Lionta E, Spyrou G, Vassilatis DK, Cournia Z (2014) Structure-based virtual screening for drug discovery: principles, applications and recent advances. Curr Top Med Chem 14:1923–1938

25. Scior T, Bender A, Tresadern G, Medina-Franco JL, Martínez-Mayorga K, Langer T, Cuanalo-Contreras K, Agrafiotis DK (2012) Recognizing pitfalls in virtual screening: a critical review. J Chem Inf Model 52:867–881

26. Jain AN, Nicholls A (2008) Recommendations for evaluation of computational methods. J Comput Aided Mol Des 22:133–139

27. Moura Barbosa AJ, Del Rio A (2012) Freely accessible databases of commercial compounds for high- throughput virtual screenings. Curr Top Med Chem 12:866–877

28. Rose PW, Prlić A, Ali A et al (2017) The RCSB protein data bank: integrative view of protein, gene and 3D structural information. Nucleic Acids Res 45:D271–D281

29. Valli M, dos Santos RN, Figueira LD et al (2013) Development of a natural products database from the biodiversity of Brazil. J Nat Prod 76:439–444

30. Williams AJ (2008) Public chemical compound databases. Curr Opin Drug Discov Devel 11:393–404

31. Nicola G, Liu T, Gilson MK (2012) Public domain databases for medicinal chemistry. J Med Chem 55:6987–7002

32. Williams A, Tkachenko V (2014) The Royal Society of Chemistry and the delivery of chemistry data repositories for the community. J Comput Aided Mol Des 28:1023–1030

33. Irwin JJ, Sterling T, Mysinger MM et al (2012) ZINC: a free tool to discover chemistry for biology. J Chem Inf Model 52:1757–1768

34. Trott O, Olson AJ (2010) AutoDock Vina: improving the speed and accuracy of docking with a new scoring function, efficient optimization and multithreading. J Comput Chem 31:455–461

35. Pirhadib S, Sunseria J, Koes DR (2016) Open source molecular modeling. J Mol Graph Model 69:127–143

36. O'Boyle NM, Banck M, James CA et al (2011) Open babel: an open chemical toolbox. J Cheminform 3:33

37. Pettersen EF, Goddard TD, Huang CC et al (2004) UCSF chimera: a visualization system for exploratory research and analysis. J Comput Chem 25:1605–1612

38. Knight ZA, Gonzalez B, Feldman ME et al (2006) A pharmacological map of the PI3-K family defines a role for p110alpha in insulin signaling. Cell 125:733–747

39. Wu P, Liu T, Hu Y (2009) PI3K inhibitors for cancer therapy: what has been achieved so far? Curr Med Chem 16:916–930

40. Brana I, Siu LL (2012) Clinical development of phosphatidylinositol 3-kinase inhibitors for cancer treatment. BMC Med 10:161

41. Wu M, Akinleye A, Zhu X (2013) Novel agents for chronic lymphocytic leukemia. J Hematol Oncol 6:36

42. Graf SA, Gopal AK (2016) Idelalisib for the treatment of non-Hodgkin lymphoma. Expert Opin Pharmacother 17:265–274

43. Greenwell BI, Flowers CR, Blum KA et al (2017) Clinical use of PI3K inhibitors in B-cell lymphoid malignancies: today and tomorrow. Expert Rev Anticancer Ther 17 (3):271–279. https://doi.org/10.1080/14737140.2017.1285702

44. Somoza JR, Koditek D, Villaseñor AG et al (2015) Structural, biochemical, and biophysical characterization of idelalisib binding to phosphoinositide 3-kinase δ. J Biol Chem 290:8439–8446

45. Davis AM, Teague SJ, Kleywegt GJ (2003) Application and limitations of X-ray crystallographic data in structure-based ligand and drug design. Angew Chem Int Ed Engl 42:2718–2736

46. Sastry GM, Adzhigirey M, Day T (2013) Protein and ligand preparation: parameters, protocols, and influence on virtual screening enrichments. J Comput Aided Mol Des 27:221–234

47. Blundell TL, Jhoti H, Abell C (2002) High-throughput crystallography for lead discovery in drug design. Nat Rev Drug Discov 1:45–54

48. Moda TL, Torres LG, Carrara AE et al (2008) PK/DB: database for pharmacokinetic properties and predictive in silico ADME models. Bioinformatics 24:2270–2271

49. Clark DE (2005) Computational prediction of ADMET properties: recent developments and future challenges. In: Dixon DA (ed) Annual reports in computational chemistry, vol 1. Elsevier, Amsterdam, pp 133–151

50. Waterbeemd H, Gifford E (2003) ADMET in silico modelling: towards prediction paradise? Nat Rev Drug Discov 2:192–204

51. Roberts BC, Mancera RL (2008) Ligand–protein docking with water molecules. J Chem Inf Model 48:397–408

52. Kirchmair J, Spitzer GM, Liedl KR (2011) Consideration of water and solvation effects in virtual screening. In: Sotriffer C (ed) Virtual screening: principles, challenges, and practical guidelines. Wiley-VCH Verlag, Weinheim

Chapter 4

Phylogenetic and Other Conservation-Based Approaches to Predict Protein Functional Sites

Heval Atas, Nurcan Tuncbag, and Tunca Doğan

Abstract

Proteins use their functional regions to exploit various activities, including binding to other proteins, nucleic acids, or drugs. Functional sites of the proteins have a tendency to be more conserved than the rest of the protein surface. Therefore, detection of the conserved residues using phylogenetic analysis is a general approach to predict functionally critical residues. In this chapter, we describe some of the available methods to predict functional sites and demonstrate a complete pipeline with tool alternatives at several steps. We explain the standard procedure and all intermediate stages including homology detection with BLAST search, multiple sequence alignment (MSA) and the construction of a phylogenetic tree for a given query sequence. Additionally, we demonstrate the prediction results of these methods on a case study. Finally, we discuss the possible challenges and bottlenecks throughout the pipeline. Our step-by-step description about the functional site prediction could be a helpful resource for the researchers interested in finding protein functional sites, to be used in drug discovery research.

Key words Drug discovery, Evolutionary conservation, Functional site, Multiple sequence alignment, Phylogenetic analysis, Predictive approaches

1 Introduction

Proteins do not act in isolation, rather they interact with other molecules such as proteins, nucleic acids and small molecules through their functional sites. Therefore, identification of the functional sites is crucial to determine the function and activity of proteins in a cell, which eventually helps in site-specific drug design to inhibit pathological effect of the disease-related protein interactions. The Universal Protein Resource (UniProt) is a knowledgebase that provides comprehensive protein sequence and annotations, including functions [1]. The majority of the published information about the properties of proteins are organized and recorded in UniProt protein pages. These annotations cover both the experimentally known information and the results of some major computational (i.e., predictive) approaches. Functional sites

Mohini Gore and Umesh B. Jagtap (eds.), *Computational Drug Discovery and Design*, Methods in Molecular Biology, vol. 1762, https://doi.org/10.1007/978-1-4939-7756-7_4, © Springer Science+Business Media, LLC, part of Springer Nature 2018

on proteins can be determined by experimental approaches; however, it is challenging to identify those sites for all proteins due to practical issues and high costs associated with experimental procedures. Therefore, computational approaches have emerged for the prediction of the functional sites (extensively reviewed in [2]). Most of the frequently used computational approaches depend on the information that functional sites are evolutionarily more conserved than the rest of the protein surface. However, there are also other sequence and structure based features that can be used to distinguish functional sites such as the secondary structure information, solvent accessibility and structural conservation [3, 4]. Given that the protein structure is more conserved than the sequence, structural comparison can recover more distant relationships across proteins. In previous studies, a large scale comparison has been applied to all known protein binding sites and shown that although global structures of some protein complexes are different their binding regions are structurally similar [2, 5, 6]. Sequence conservation has been also used in combination with geometric features of functional sites for prediction to improve the performance [7].

Determination of the conserved regions in a protein sequence to predict functional residues starts with the multiple sequence alignment (MSA) of the query protein sequence and its homologs [4]. MSA reveals highly conserved positions on the input sequences. Some methods first construct a phylogenetic tree on the basis of the MSA results, instead of analyzing sequence conservation directly from the MSA [8]. A phylogenetic tree represents the evolutionary relationships between protein sequences, which provides subfamily-specific mutations of protein families [9]. The evolutionary trace (ET) method has been developed as the first implementation of this idea, which does not use only identical residues but also consider amino acid similarities [10]. As a kind of more improved version of ET method, ConSurf also generates phylogenetic trees of homologous sequences using the neighbor-joining algorithm based on the MSA results and computes position-specific conservation scores for each amino acid in the sequence. Also, it retrieves structural information of proteins from PDB if available [11, 12]. INTREPID, another functional site prediction method, performs phylogenetic tree analysis in combination with a Jensen–Shannon divergence based positional conservation score [4]. INTREPID has been extensively compared to ET and ConSurf methods in predicting functional residues [13]. The latest release of ET method as a database and web server is called Universal Evolutionary Trace (UET) [14].

Apart from these methods, there are also machine learning-based approaches such as PROFisis that identifies residues at protein–protein interaction (PPI) interfaces. This method uses PPI information obtained from experimentally known 3D structures; however, it does not require 3D structure of the query protein for the analysis. Instead, it uses predicted structural features of the sequence, combined with the evolutionary information [15].

There is one more approach worth mentioning regarding the prediction of functional sites, which is the coevolution-based approach. At the residue level, coevolution simply refers to the correlated changes across proteins that are important for the maintenance of the protein structure, function, and stability [16]. These approaches also use MSA of a protein family to search coevolved amino acids [17–19]. Among them, CoeViz provides a web server to analyze coevolved residues in a protein [20].

In this chapter, we describe a procedure to predict functional sites of proteins using phylogenetic analysis. We detail all steps starting from searching for homologous sequences of the query protein to performing MSA and finally predicting functionally important residues with alternative selection of tools at different steps (*see* Subheading 2). We discuss how to determine parameters or options of each external tool (BLAST, Clustal Omega, etc.) and what challenges might be experienced at different stages of the functional site prediction procedure.

2   Methods

The procedure below describes a path that can be followed for evaluating *a protein* in terms of identifying its functional sites with alternative solutions. We illustrate the whole pipeline in Fig. 1 as a flowchart where the input is the query protein sequence and the output is the active site information. We need to note that the methods reviewed in this chapter are predictive approaches; therefore, they may have false positives and false negatives besides the true positives. Also, the results of the predictive methods may not highly overlap with each other in some cases, due to the employment of different approaches.

A given protein sequence (P_Q) can be computationally annotated in terms of active/functional sites (i.e., the main focus of this chapter), highly conserved functional regions (e.g., domains and motifs) and sequence-wide generic annotations (e.g., protein families, subcellular locations, biological processes). Below, we describe the methods for functional site annotation:

2.1   Sequence Homology Search (BLAST)

Search the homologs of P_Q using the UniProt BLAST tool (http://www.uniprot.org/blast/) by entering P_Q in FASTA format in the sequence window and clicking run BLAST button. The parameters of BLAST tool are explained in **Note 1**. The algorithm scans the entire target database to find similar sequences to P_Q and display the results (i.e., homologous protein sequences in the target database) ranked by similarities. The homologous sequences with the

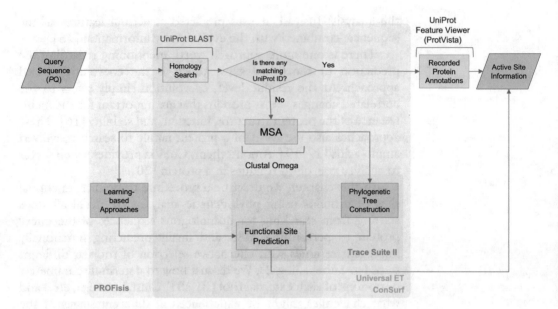

Fig. 1 The general flowchart to perform phylogenetic analysis to predict protein functional sites. The input is a query sequence and the output is the active site information which are represented with parallelograms. The processes and decisions involved in each approach is highlighted with a rectangular shade. Universal ET and ConSurf are highlighted in light green, Trace Suite II in orange, and PROFisis in light blue. The common processes and decisions across all these methods are shown in the intersection of the shaded rectangles

highest similarity values will be valuable for our purpose in the result page. According to the observed similarity values:

(a) If the identity value between the first homolog(s) in the results list and P_Q is 100% and the protein lengths are the same, the user can directly check the UniProt page of this protein (by clicking on the UniProt accession number of the corresponding protein) to observe the experimental and computational annotations, since P_Q and the resulting homolog will possess the exact same functional properties. If the highest ranked homolog is a UniProtKB/Swiss-Prot database protein (marked by yellow document symbol at the "status" column in the BLAST results table), the functional information in UniProt will be richer and more reliable, since the protein entries in UniProtKB/Swiss-Prot are reviewed with manual curation. At this point, the user is advised to continue from Subheading 2.2.

(b) If the identity value is between 90 and 100% (together with a very similar protein length), it will still be sufficient to transfer generic whole-sequence and region based annotations from the resulting protein to the query protein. The user can investigate the UniProt protein page of the homologous protein(s) for the generic functional annotations. However, active sites may differ between the query and resulting sequences; as a result, transferring site specific annotations will not be possible. The user is advised to continue from Subheading 2.3 following a quick investigation in UniProt protein page of the similar resulting protein, as described in Subheading 2.2.

(c) If the identity value is below 90%, it is still possible to transfer the generic functions but not the site-specific ones; as a result, following the procedure from Subheading 2.3 is advised.

2.2 Recorded Protein Annotation (UniProt)

In a UniProt protein page (e.g., human Mast/stem cell growth factor receptor KIT protein -UniProt id: P10721- at http://www. uniprot.org/uniprot/P10721), sequence properties and annotations are grouped under distinct titles (function, taxonomy, pathology, PTMs, expression, interaction, structure, family and domain, sequence, etc.). The left pane shows these titles for easy navigation on the main part of the page. The sources of functional information in UniProt are explained in **Note 2**.

Under the heading "Function," various types of functional information are listed. First of all, a paragraph made up of curated free-text is given. This is a summary of relevant literature publications, references of which are given at the end of the paragraph. Second, region and site specific information (e.g., catalytic, metal, active, and binding sites) is listed in tables, together with the respective positions of the corresponding regions/sites on the sequence. Third, the annotated functions in terms of the Gene Ontology (GO) system is given for the three main GO categories: molecular function, biological process and the cellular component. Clicking a functional GO term in this list opens up the details of the corresponding functional term in the QuickGO web-service. QuickGO is both a database and an easy to use browser for protein GO annotations [21]. Furthermore, clicking "Complete GO annotation..." button in the UniProt protein page will take the user to the dedicated protein GO annotation page in QuickGO (e.g., QuickGO page of the human KIT protein: http://www.ebi.ac. uk/QuickGO/GProtein?ac=P10721).

Under "Family & domains" section, subheading "Phylogenomic databases" displays the clickable links to the corresponding pages in different phylogeny resources (eggNOG, GeneTree, OMA, OrthoDB, etc.). Another subheading "Family and domain databases" shows the information and links for the domains that the corresponding proteins are known to—or predicted to—contain, in various resources (InterPro, Pfam, SUPFAM, Gene3D, etc.). Each domain/family entry in these databases is displayed with a functional description and site-specific information (if possible).

Near the top of the left pane there is the "feature viewer" button and clicking on it will display the ProtVista tool to visualize all of the annotated features of the protein (e.g., human KIT protein at

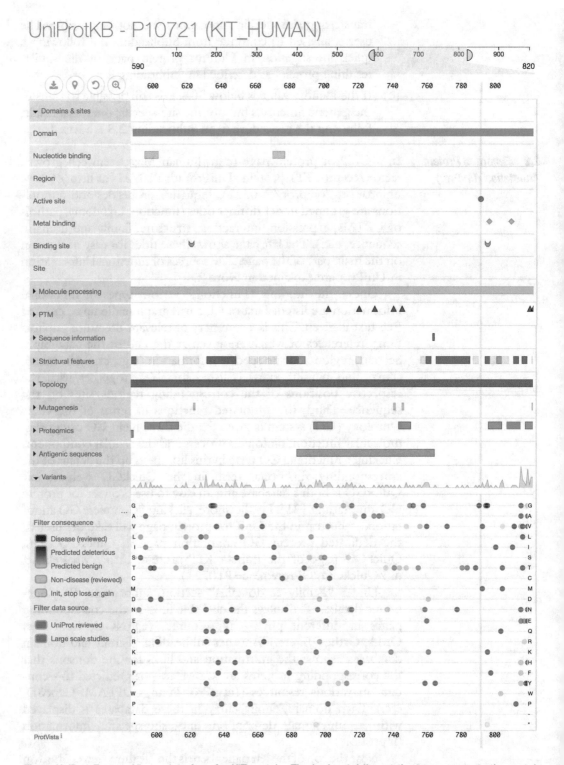

Fig. 2 UniProt Feature Viewer interface for KIT protein. The horizontal line at the top represents the protein sequence with markings at each hundredth residue. The gray area and the half-circles at each side of it indicates the area zoomed in. The user can change the size and position of the zoomed-in area by dragging the

http://www.uniprot.org/uniprot/P10721#showFeaturesViewer).
In this mode, the features are grouped under certain blocks (e.g.,
"Domain & sites"), which corresponds to the sections in the main
UniProt protein pages. Clicking on the titles of these blocks will
reveal a more detailed view with subheadings. A snapshot from
"feature viewer" for human KIT protein is shown in Fig. 2.

(a) Clicking on "Domains & sites" will show functional domains,
regions and motifs; along with residue specific features. The
viewer displays the position of a feature on the protein
sequence by placing boxes/nodes at different positions along
the horizontal axis. Clicking on a box will reveal a new table,
showing the properties of that feature.

(b) Clicking on "Mutagenesis" will show the site specific mutation information. This title will only be visible if there is
mutation information for that protein in the literature that is
recorded in UniProt. When any mutation locating box is
clicked, the opened table will display the description, mutation
states and the evidence containing the relevant literature
publications.

(c) Finally, clicking "Variants" will show detailed site-specific variation information, obtained from the literature and from
other biological data resources. Position indicating circles are
colored according to the quality of the variation (i.e., disease,

---

Fig. 2 (continued) half-circles at each direction. At the top left, there are buttons for downloading the
displayed information in different formats, highlighting a selected region on the sequence, resetting the
view to the default and for zooming-in and out. Each horizontal block on the tool interface displays a specific
type of protein feature. Each block is a drop down menu that displays the sub-features upon clicking on the
name of the main feature (e.g., clicking on "Domains & sites" block reveals domain, region, active site, metal
binding, binding site, etc.). In order to indicate the exact position of a feature on the sequence, a colored node
is placed at the corresponding position on the horizontal axis. The color, shape, and width of the node/box is
respective to the type and the length of the feature (i.e., site-based features span only one residue; however,
region-based features such as domains may span hundreds of residues). For example, there is an active site
at the 792nd position of the KIT protein sequence. Clicking on the node of a feature will display two properties:
(1) a yellow vertical line will highlight that position along all of the feature blocks (e.g., the line shown in the
figure), which enables the observation of the correspondence between different types of features on the
sequence, and (2) a table displaying the details of the corresponding feature annotation such as the
description, the source of information and etc. At the bottom of the feature viewer, information about variants
is shown. The detailed view of variants block displays 20 different amino acids on the vertical axis, which
indicates the substituted amino acid at a specific position in the corresponding protein. The circular nodes that
indicate variations are colored according to the known or predicted effect of the variation (e.g., red for known
disease causing variants, different shades of blue for predicted deleterious effects, green for known
nondisease association, and yellow for initiation, stop loss or gain). For example, for the human KIT protein,
it has been recorded that a recorded variant has a glycine instead of an aspartic acid at the 52nd position. The
source of this information is the COSMIC database, the tissue of this sample is the large-intestine and the
effect of this variation was predicted to be mostly benign

nondisease, deleterious/benign). Clicking on the circles will again reveal a table displaying the description of the effect, variation states, the source database where the information is obtained from (e.g., COSMIC) and the associated disease with clickable links to the corresponding disease databases (e.g., OMIM). When any feature defining node/box is clicked, the column corresponding to the location of the feature on the sequence is highlighted all the way on the vertical axis. This enables the user to observe if a recorded variation is corresponding to an active site, or a structural unit on the protein.

It is possible to observe all of the recorded features of a protein in one place using UniProt protein pages and its visualizer the feature viewer tool. Both the information curated from the literature and the information imported from other biological resources are extensively referenced. So that, the user can check the source data repository or publication for a more detailed investigation. When taxonomic information (i.e., organism) matches between P_Q and the observed protein (along with conditions that the observed protein is 100% identical to P_Q and their sequence lengths are the same), all of the recorded features (including variants and mutagenesis) are applied to P_Q as well, since they are basically the same protein.

This way, the known active site information has been observed for P_Q; however, for some of the proteins this information is incomplete. In this case, the user is advised to continue from Subheading 2.3 to complement the observed sequence features with predictions.

2.3 Multiple Sequence Alignment (Clustal Omega)

In order to uncover the potential active/critical sites in P_Q, a conservation-based approach, multiple sequence alignment (MSA), will be performed. To perform MSA for P_Q, select the similar sequences (i.e., BLAST hits) by checking the boxes at the first column of the UniProt BLAST results. However, sequences that are 100% identical to the query protein are often lead to overestimation of critically important residues. Due to this reason, these sequences will be left out. Once the sequences are selected (including P_Q) click Align button to start the MSA using the integrated Clustal Omega program. It is also possible to run MSA in UniProt by entering the sequences manually on the Align interface (http://www.uniprot.org/align/) or using Clustal Omega tool interface (http://www.ebi.ac.uk/Tools/msa/clustalo/), where the user is able to change the parameters of the tool (*see* **Note 3**).

The resulting page display the output MSA with site-specific conservation information for each position in the alignment with symbols: "*", ":", ".", and "", indicating that all residues at the corresponding position are: identical (i.e., fully conserved), conservation between different amino acid groups of highly similar properties, conservation between different amino acid groups of low similarity and no similarity, respectively.

Various sequence feature options are given (active site, domain, helix, chain, etc.) at the left pane and checking the corresponding boxes enable displaying these features on the aligned sequences with distinct colors. It is possible to easily observe the site specific information on the aligned sequences and to infer the properties of P_Q by observing if the same amino acid presents in the feature carrying column on the output MSA. Clustal Omega tool generates a guide tree from the output of the MSA, which is useful to observe the inferred evolutionary relationship between the aligned sequences.

As mentioned above the MSA parameters can be adjusted when the procedure is run using the Clustal Omega interface (http://www.ebi.ac.uk/Tools/msa/clustalo/). FASTA formatted sequences of to be aligned proteins can be copy-pasted to the sequence window. The results page is similar to the UniProt Align tool interface. It is possible to download the phylogenetic tree, which is constructed using the resulting MSA.

As a result of MSA, the functional positions can be inferred on P_Q. In the case of no (or limited) functional region/site information due to either low conservation or the lack of region/site specific annotation for the aligned sequences, it may still possible to identify potential active sites on the sequences using MSA outputs *via* evolutionary tracing methods or by trying alternative approaches, explained starting from Subheading 2.4.

2.4 Evolutionary Trace (TraceSuite II)

Search functionally important sites via TraceSuite II web server (http://mordred.bioc.cam.ac.uk/~jiye/evoltrace/evoltrace.html) either by uploading or by copy-pasting the MSA output. It is optional to enter PDB id(s) belong to the protein structure of P_Q, if this information is available. If so, place P_Q at the top of the alignment and change its FASTA header to ">PDBid", where PDBid should be replaced with the actual 4 digit PDB structure entry identifier of the protein. If there is no PDB annotation for P_Q but there is a BLAST resulting protein that satisfy the conditions explained in Subheading 2.1, **item a**, then its PDB id can also be used here. When provided, the structural information will help determining the functional residues according to their location (i.e., as either at the core or on the surface of the proteins).

After hitting the start trace button, the algorithm displays the results page following the run. In this page, there are two types of output: (1) a partitioned phylogenetic tree, and (2) the evolutionary trace demonstrating the inferred active sites on the partitions of aligned sequences, where the buried residues are highlighted. It is also possible to display the evolutionary trace mapped to each structure (only available if the structural information is given at the input level), for each partition with highlighted buried/exposed residues (see **Note 4**). Clicking the given PDB id at the bottom of the results page will reveal the evolutionary trace mappings for different partitions on the corresponding structure. Residue positions in the output needs to be checked to match with the positions in the query sequence P_Q (see **Note 5**). However, it is easier to follow the positions of the annotated residues on the structures. At the "evolutionary trace mapped to each structure" page, clicking on "Molscript input file" will display the list of buried/exposed residues with their respective positions on the structure. One important note here is that, the annotated residue positions on the structure and the query sequence usually does not match since the crystal structures are only available for some parts of protein sequences. It is possible to observe the position of a residue on the crystallized structure (as opposed to the position on the whole protein sequence), using the PDB service (e.g., residues position information for the crystal structure of KIT protein: https://www.rcsb.org/pdb/explore/remediatedSequence.do?structureId=1T46).

Partitions illustrated in the output are referred from the constructed phylogenetic tree on which each partition is labelled with a vertical line. Prediction is more stringent in the first partition, as there are more classes of homologs compared to the second partition. From the first partition to the last partition, more residues are labelled as important. In TraceSuite II, residues vary among distant homologs (homologs across the classes obtained from the partitioning) rank better than the residues vary among close homologs (homologs within the same class) in the phylogenetic tree. At the evolutionary trace output on the main results page, the buried residues are marked according the tenth partition, which is the main interest.

Up to this point, we have demonstrated a workflow to infer functional sites on a query sequence. Below, the alternative ways to obtain similar information using all-in-one tools, are explained.

2.5 All-in-One Web Servers for Functional Site Prediction

(a) **Universal Evolutionary Trace (ET)**

Universal ET tool works with the same principle as TraceSuite II; however, it either takes an amino acid sequence in FASTA format, a UniProt accession, a PDB identifier or a PDB structure file as an input, and calculates the functionally important residues following a methodology similar to the one described above. Universal ET stores the precomputed evolutionary traces for UniProt protein records and PDB structure records; as a result, when queried with accessions/ids the system is able to display the precomputed results without any computation, which accelerates the analysis. Entering protein structure information at the input level

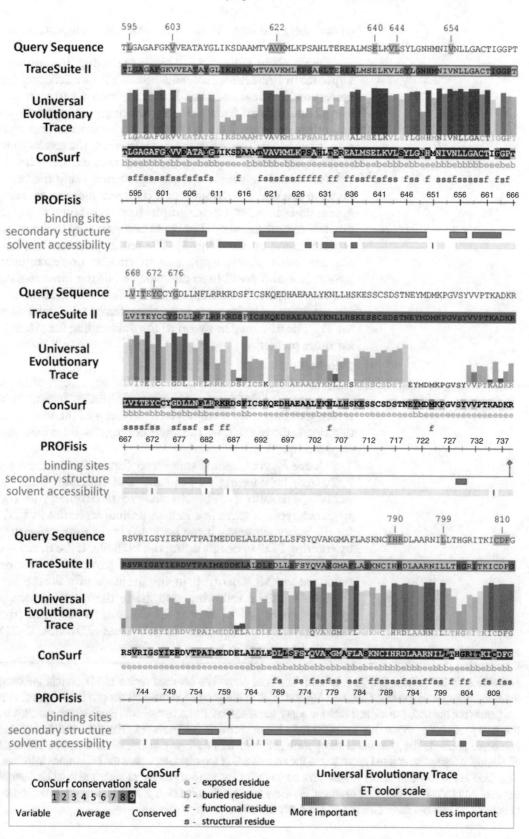

(if available) will improve the functional importance inference in most cases.

Search P_Q in Universal ET by first selecting "Amino acid sequence in FASTA format" and entering its sequence to the corresponding field and click Run trace button (http://mam moth.bcm.tmc.edu/uet/). A progress page will be displayed and refreshed every 10 s, which includes information on each step of the procedure. After the run is finished, the results page displays the query sequence in a way that each residue is colored according the functional importance, using the color range in the visible light spectrum (i.e., red: more important, green: mid-range, and blue/purple: less important). It is also possible to visualize the ET ranks as histograms by clicking the corresponding button (Fig. 3). The results page also displays the generated phylogenetic tree in circular or rectangular layout. It is also possible to download all of the intermediate and resulting files in a compressed file. Here, the residues that are predicted to be important are the inferred functional sites for P_Q. The user may move on to the Subheading 2.5, **item b** for more predictions.

(b) **ConSurf**

The second alternative method, ConSurf, accepts either a sequence or an MSA or a phylogenetic tree as input. As a result, ConSurf can be employed at any step of the workflow described above. Below, the methodology is described for sequence queries.

Query P_Q via ConSurf web server (http://consurf.tau.ac. il/2016/) by entering its sequence and selecting "Amino-Acids" (it is also possible to analyze nucleotides) as the sequence type. If there is a known protein structure in PDB for the query sequence, it can be added in the next step either by entering PDB id or uploading the PDB file. If the query is a protein sequence without a known 3D structure, it can be predicted via MODELLER in the presence of a license key (optional). In the following step, paste the query sequence into the box in FASTA format for ConSurf to run MSA (the sequence will be extracted directly from PDB file if 3D

Fig. 3 Human KIT protein and its predicted functional sites. The selected region of KIT protein involving imatinib binding sites (residues between 594 and 812) is represented in three blocks and the results of four computational methods are aligned with the query sequence, on the horizontal axis. Blue colored residues on the query sequence shows the experimentally known imatinib binding sites. The predicted buried and conserved positions (i.e., functional sites) are highlighted with light gray in TraceSuite II output. Universal ET outputs a histogram colored according to the importance of the residues, where the importance increases from blue to red. ConSurf colors residues based on their conservation scores, as well. It also labels buried/exposed and functional/structural residues. PROFisis displays the predicted protein binding sites, secondary structures and solvent accessibilities on the query sequence

structure information is added). When the method is ran without structural information, the underlying algorithm that complete the prediction task is ConSeq [22]. For this example, use default parameters for homolog search. It is possible to enter a job title and an e-mail address to get the link of the results (optional). The number of homologous sequences is a limitation for the Consurf run (*see* **Note 6**). Clicking "Submit" button will start the analysis, which can take from minutes to a few hours according to the query.

Submitting the job will open the job status page that shows running parameters, run process, and running messages. When the job is completed, the results page will include links for the final prediction results, input sequence data, the MSA, phylogenetic tree, and additional links for high resolution figures including the protein structure. In the output, the first option displays the conserved sites/regions, colored on the sequence according to the conservation scores. In ConSurf a conservation scale from 1 to 9 was employed (with distinct colors), where 1 represents the least and 9 represents the most conserved residues. Additionally, ConSurf predicts if the residues are buried or exposed to the solvent. Predictions for functional residues (conserved and exposed) and structural residues (conserved and buried) are also labelled with different colors below the sequence (*see* **Note 4**). It is important to note that the sequence based output is provided only when the structural information is not included at the input level. If the structure information is added in the first place, the conservation predictions are shown as marked on the 3D structure. Furthermore, ConSurf produces a phylogenetic tree using the MSA output. It is possible to download the whole output as a zip file.

(c) **Machine learning based approach (PROFisis)**

Run the program for P_Q via the PredictProtein (https://www.predictprotein.org/) service, which normally requires registration (*see* **Note 7**). Enter the query amino acid sequence and hit the PredictProtein button. When the results are generated, it will be displayed automatically on the screen. In the output, predicted binding sites for protein interactions, secondary structure, solvent accessibility, transmembrane helices, disordered and flexible region, disulfide bridges, subcellular localization, gene ontology terms of proteins, and effect of point mutations are shown. Results can be displayed separately by clicking relevant part from the left panel or all-in-one by clicking the "Dashboard." In the figure, place the cursor over the interested region to observe the annotation details including the annotated residues, sequence length, type of the prediction and its evidence, for the selected region. It is also possible to view the results in html or xml format by clicking the corresponding boxes on the upper right-hand corner and to export the graphical output to an image. Results can be reached any time from "My Predictions" button after logging in to the system.

There are also stand alone tools such as INTREPID that can be used by downloading and installing their packages, instead of doing interactive analysis *via* web servers. Users having advanced knowledge in scripting may refer to these tools and run them on their local computers.

3 Case Study: Human KIT Protein and Its Predicted Functional Sites

As an example, human KIT protein (UniProt accession: P10721) is chosen to illustrate the functional site prediction procedure using the defined work-flow (including TraceSuite II), Consurf, Universal Evolutionary Trace and PROFisis. KIT protein, which is a kinase inhibitor, has a crystal structure in a bound state with imatinib (i.e., an anticancer drug) in PDB (id: 1t46). Using this structure and KIT's sequence, we aimed to find the residues in contact with the drug molecule (i.e., functional sites). The residues having contact with imatinib are experimentally known; however, we have only used this information in order to compare the prediction results with the known sites.

At the beginning of the analysis we have obtained the sequence of the KIT protein from the UniProt database and assumed that this is an unknown sequence. Then, we searched for the homologs of our query using KIT protein's sequence via UniProt BLAST tool with default parameters. The top ranked result of the BLAST analysis was naturally the actual KIT protein record in UniProt. After that, the homologous sequences found at the BLAST analysis (except the hits with 100% identity to the query and the fragment sequences) are analyzed with MSA using the Align tool in UniProt. The output MSA was investigated manually by highlighting the known functional sites on the aligned sequences. Following MSA analysis, fasta formatted output MSA was given to TraceSuite II together with the structural information (by changing the FASTA header of the query sequence to ">1t46" in the MSA output). The results of TraceSuite II (i.e., the evolutionary trace mapped on sequences and on the given structure, and the constructed phylogenetic tree) have been investigated. Finally, human KIT protein was analyzed with ConSurf, Universal Evolutionary Trace, and PROFisis, by directly entering its sequence to the corresponding web-services. In ConSurf analysis, the structural information was not given at the input.

We used the original graphical output of each web server to prepare Fig. 3. In this figure, the first row displays the query sequence with highlighted experimentally known drug binding sites. This is followed in successive rows by the results of the functional site prediction methods explained in this chapter (i.e., Tracesuite II, Universal ET, ConSurf, and PROFisis). In Fig. 3, we only illustrated the residues between the positions 594 and 812 (in three blocks), since imatinib is known to bind to the residues in this region. TraceSuite II gives the output on the residues of the given structure by highlighting buried and conserved residues in light gray. If the exposed and conserved residues are of interest, they can be browsed at the resulting evolutionary trace, which was mapped to the given structure. Universal Evolutionary Trace method provided a histogram that was colored according to the importance of each residue. ConSurf was used in the sequence input mode (ConSeq tool) and provided conservation scores along with exposed vs. buried and functional vs. structural residue predictions. For PROFisis, binding sites, secondary structures, and solvent accessibilities are shown at different rows.

As shown in Fig. 3, all methods recover most of the imatinib interacting binding sites located on KIT protein, except PROFisis. As observed, most of the methods gave high scores to the residues around the actual binding sites, as well. There can be two possible reasons behind this: (1) the residues at the proximity of binding sites may also play roles in binding; as a result, they are conserved, and (2) the predictive approaches often consider the properties of the neighbors of the corresponding residue while calculating conservation/importance, which results in a smoothed scoring curve. Apart from that, the tested methods also predicted a few additional residues on the sequence, which may be targets for other molecules, located in the core region or just false positive hits.

4   Notes

1. The parameters of BLAST are as follows: The first option is the target database. In this menu, BLAST search database can be selected as either UniProtKB (as a whole or divided to taxonomic nodes, or including only reviewed sequences in UniPRotKB/Swiss-Prot) or UniRef (i.e., sequence clusters at different similarity levels, which is useful for eliminating redundant sequences) or UniParc (i.e., sequence archive is the largest set possible including the deleted sequences as well, not advised to be used unless for specific objectives). The second parameter option is the E-value threshold, which is a threshold statistical measure indicating the number of returned matches. E-values lower than 0.1 are generally accepted as significantly similar hits. It is also possible to select a higher E-value to enlarge the

size of results, while less significant hits can be discarded by unchecking their boxes, before the MSA procedure. The third option is the selection of the similarity matrix. A similarity matrix assigns scores to each amino acid pair combination, proportional to the probability of observing the corresponding substitution in the nature. BLOSUM62 is the generally accepted matrix to detect weak similarities between protein sequences. BLOSUM80 performs better in finding highly similar proteins and BLOSUM45 is a better choice to detect highly distant sequences. Auto option can be selected in order for the algorithm to decide for the best matrix for the query sequence. The fourth parameter option is for filtering low complexity regions in proteins, to avoid false matches specific to those regions. If the query protein is known to include low complexity regions, this filter can be selected to obtain more specific results. The fifth option is for switching the allowance of gaps, where the default selection is "yes." The last option is for limiting the number of returned hits. Usually, 250 hits or less is sufficient to build a MSA.

2. The sources of protein annotations in UniProt include: (1) - in-house manual curation, (2) in-house automated predictions, and (3) imports from external resources. This way, UniProt aims to provide comprehensive information on the properties of proteins. However, included data does not cover the results of most of the external predictive approaches available in the literature. Due to this reason, it is natural to observe differences between the information in UniProt and the results of a prediction method (e.g., functional site information obtained from different resources in our case study). UniProt aims to incorporate only the most reliable annotations backed up by strong evidence; as a result, a predictive approach may provide relatively higher coverage on a query protein, where a portion of its predictions can also be false positives. Nevertheless, predicted information obtained from other resources can be evaluated along with UniProt annotations. For example, predicted active residues can be compared to mutagenesis and variation information provided in UniProt protein pages, which can be utilized to infer disease relations and for drug targeting.

3. The parameters of Clustal Omega are as follows: The first option is the selection of the input data as protein, DNA or RNA. The second one is the output format, which can be selected among Clustal, Pearson, MSF, PHYLIP and etc. "More options" button will reveal the parameters about the tool such as the number of iterations at different steps of the algorithm (e.g., sequence alignment and tree generation). Higher number of iterations will refine the results with the cost of longer computation times. Usually the default values

will provide a good balance between results' quality and run times.

One important point about running MSA procedure is the similarity between input sequences, which should neither be too high nor too low. Results of a BLAST search may constitute a good list for a MSA; nevertheless, 100% identical sequences to the BLAST query should be removed from the list. However, this operation cannot remove the sequences among the BLAST results that are identical to each other (i.e., not identical to the BLAST query sequence). To solve this problem, BLAST operation can be carried out using UniRef90 instead of UniProtKB, as the target database. This way, the results will include only one sequence from each 90% similarity cluster. Afterward, MSA can be run with these BLAST results with default parameters. This alternative operation is especially recommended when BLAST returns many highly identical sequences when ran against UniProtKB database.

4. In addition to conservation predictions, both Consurf and TraceSuite II label residues based on whether they are buried or exposed. However, this information does not tell about if the buried residue is located on the protein surface or in the core region. Functional site residues are located in the surface of the protein and have tendency to be buried. Residues that are important for the stability of the protein are located in the core region. To discriminate if the residue is located in the core or in the surface region, 3D structure information is necessary and the accessible surface area calculations need to be performed. The sequence based version of ConSurf titled: "ConSeq" aims to obtain a distinction between structural and functional residues (apart from exposed vs. buried) using neural networks; however, the performance of this type of prediction was reported to be relatively low [22].

5. Residue numbers in the output of TraceSuite II is labelled according to the partitioned MSA results, which may not represent the correct residue positions of the query protein. In this case, user needs to traceback and relabel the residue numbers accordingly.

6. One limitation of Consurf is that it does not run for less than 50 homologous sequences.

7. It is possible to run the PROFisis tool without registering and logging in using this link: https://ppopen.informatik.tu-muenchen.de/. However, in this mode it is not possible to store the results of the analysis. In some cases PROFisis inaccurately displays the positions of the predicted binding sites on the graphical results, it is advised to check the precise positions of the predicted sites either from the text based output or by dragging the mouse cursor over the binding site representing diamond shaped nodes on the graphical output.

Acknowledgements

H.A. acknowledges TUBITAK 2211 Doctoral Fellowship Program. N.T. thanks to the TUBITAK Career Development Program (Project no: 117E192). T.D. acknowledges TUBITAK BIDEB 2218 Program.

References

1. The UniProt Consortium (2017) UniProt: the universal protein knowledgebase. Nucleic Acids Res 45:D158–D169. https://doi.org/10.1093/nar/gkw1152

2. Keskin O, Tuncbag N, Gursoy A (2016) Predicting protein-protein interactions from the molecular to the proteome level. Chem Rev 116:4884–4909. https://doi.org/10.1021/acs.chemrev.5b00683

3. Pazos F, Bang J-W (2006) Computational prediction of functionally important regions in proteins. Curr Bioinforma 1:15–23. https://doi.org/10.2174/157489306775330633

4. Capra JA, Singh M (2007) Predicting functionally important residues from sequence conservation. Bioinformatics 23:1875–1882. https://doi.org/10.1093/bioinformatics/btm270

5. Keskin O, Tsai C-J, Wolfson H, Nussinov R (2004) A new, structurally nonredundant, diverse data set of protein-protein interfaces and its implications. Protein Sci 13:1043–1055. https://doi.org/10.1110/ps.03484604

6. Tuncbag N, Gursoy A, Guney E et al (2008) Architectures and functional coverage of protein–protein interfaces. J Mol Biol 381:785–802. https://doi.org/10.1016/j.jmb.2008.04.071

7. Bray T, Chan P, Bougouffa S et al (2009) SitesIdentify: a protein functional site prediction tool. BMC Bioinformatics 10:379. https://doi.org/10.1186/1471-2105-10-379

8. Kc DB, Livesay DR (2011) Topology improves phylogenetic motif functional site predictions. IEEE/ACM Trans Comput Biol Bioinform 8:226–233. https://doi.org/10.1109/TCBB.2009.60

9. Pazos F, Valencia A (2001) Similarity of phylogenetic trees as indicator of protein-protein interaction. Protein Eng 14:609–614. https://doi.org/10.1093/protein/14.9.609

10. Lichtarge O, Bourne HR, Cohen FE (1996) An evolutionary trace method defines binding surfaces common to protein families. J Mol Biol 257:342–358. https://doi.org/10.1006/jmbi.1996.0167

11. Landau M, Mayrose I, Rosenberg Y et al (2005) ConSurf 2005: the projection of evolutionary conservation scores of residues on protein structures. Nucleic Acids Res 33:W299–W302. https://doi.org/10.1093/nar/gki370

12. Ashkenazy H, Abadi S, Martz E et al (2016) ConSurf 2016: an improved methodology to estimate and visualize evolutionary conservation in macromolecules. Nucleic Acids Res 44:W344–W350. https://doi.org/10.1093/nar/gkw408

13. Sankararaman S, Sjölander K (2008) INTREPID--INformation-theoretic TREe traversal for protein functional site IDentification. Bioinformatics 24:2445–2452. https://doi.org/10.1093/bioinformatics/btn474

14. Lua RC, Wilson SJ, Konecki DM et al (2016) UET: a database of evolutionarily-predicted functional determinants of protein sequences that cluster as functional sites in protein structures. Nucleic Acids Res 44:D308–D312. https://doi.org/10.1093/nar/gkv1279

15. Ofran Y, Rost B (2007) ISIS: interaction sites identified from sequence. Bioinformatics 23:e13–e16. https://doi.org/10.1093/bioinformatics/btl303

16. de Juan D, Pazos F, Valencia A (2013) Emerging methods in protein co-evolution. Nat Rev Genet 14:249–261. https://doi.org/10.1038/nrg3414

17. Hopf TA, Schärfe CPI, Rodrigues JPGLM et al (2014) Sequence co-evolution gives 3D contacts and structures of protein complexes. eLife 3:1–45. https://doi.org/10.7554/eLife.03430

18. Rodriguez-Rivas J, Marsili S, Juan D, Valencia A (2016) Conservation of coevolving protein interfaces bridges prokaryote-eukaryote homologies in the twilight zone. Proc Natl Acad Sci U S A 113:15018–15023. https://doi.org/10.1073/pnas.1611861114

19. Gueudré T, Baldassi C, Zamparo M et al (2016) Simultaneous identification of

specifically interacting paralogs and interprotein contacts by direct coupling analysis. Proc Natl Acad Sci U S A 113:12186–12191. https://doi.org/10.1073/pnas.1607570113

20. Baker FN, Porollo A (2016) CoeViz: a web-based tool for coevolution analysis of protein residues. BMC Bioinformatics 17:119. https://doi.org/10.1186/s12859-016-0975-z

21. Huntley RP, Sawford T, Mutowo-Meullenet P et al (2015) The GOA database: gene ontology annotation updates for 2015. Nucleic Acids Res 43:D1057–D1063. https://doi.org/10.1093/nar/gku1113

22. Berezin C, Glaser F, Rosenberg J et al (2004) ConSeq: the identification of functionally and structurally important residues in protein sequences. Bioinformatics 20:1322–1324. https://doi.org/10.1093/bioinformatics/bth070

Chapter 5

De Novo Design of Ligands Using Computational Methods

**Venkatesan Suryanarayanan, Umesh Panwar, Ishwar Chandra,
and Sanjeev Kumar Singh**

Abstract

De novo design technique is complementary to high-throughput virtual screening and is believed to contribute in pharmaceutical development of novel drugs with desired properties at a very low cost and time-efficient manner. In this chapter, we outline the basic de novo design concepts based on computational methods with an example.

Key words ADME, De novo ligand design, Drug discovery, Molecular docking, Molecular modeling, Synthetic feasibility, VEGFR2

1 Introduction

The process of drug discovery has evolved manifold from adventitious invention to more rational approaches. From the past three decades computer-aided drug discovery/design (CADD) has played a key role in the development of therapeutically important small molecules [1, 2]. The explosion of the genomics data post-sequencing and the three-dimensional crystallography structures of various proteins (receptors/targets) has expedited the discovery of medicinally significant small molecules. Structure-based drug design and ligand-based drug design with the aid of different computational techniques like virtual screening, molecular docking, molecular dynamics simulation, in silico adsorption, distribution, metabolism, excretion, and toxicity (ADMET) evaluations are the primarily used methods for finding potential drug candidates. De novo drug design is a computational technique wherein novel molecular structures with desired pharmacological properties are generated from the beginning or scratch. De novo in Latin literally means "from new," "afresh," or "a new-fangled." Besides finding new molecules it is also used to produce novel molecular scaffolds and bioisosteric equivalent for already determined or undesired fragments. It not only generates chemical starting points/

Mohini Gore and Umesh B. Jagtap (eds.), *Computational Drug Discovery and Design*, Methods in Molecular Biology, vol. 1762, https://doi.org/10.1007/978-1 4939-7756-7_5, © Springer Science+Business Media, LLC, part of Springer Nature 2018

hypotheses but also enables to secure intellectual property rights and in the identification of new molecules significantly eliciting a response to targets which till now have not been the focus of drug discovery efforts. The classes of computational methods for the de novo design are mentioned below [3–6]:

(a) Fragment positioning methods	Identifies a specific position of atom or fragment in binding sites
(b) Site point connection methods	Identifies a unique site location for placing fragments in the binding sites
(c) Fragment connection methods	Connects the fragments at particular position within binding sites
(d) Library construction methods	Builds a library of fragments with desirable information
(e) Molecule growth methods	Keep atoms or fragments at different places within binding sites of target and growing them by joining with other atoms/fragments with various coordinations
(f) Random connection methods	Connect the fragments in random way

For fruitful candidate design, three paradigms acknowledged by de novo design program are (1) structure construction of the candidate compounds (atom/fragment based), (2) evaluation of the molecule class, i.e., its fitness (based on 3D receptor-ligand docking and scoring or ligand-based similarity measure) and (3) methodically examining the search space or difficulty of optimization (based on depth-first/breadth first search, evolutionary algorithms, exhaustive structure enumeration). These constitute the modern de novo design approach to implement the chemical structure generation process [7, 8].

Complete data linked to ligand receptor interaction forms the *primary target constraints* for the candidate compounds as these input are used in scoring the property evaluation of the generated structures. The designed compound with some target affinity and drug-likeness is proposed. Clusters of the virtual structures are accompanied by simulated organic synthesis steps in order to draw prospective synthesis route for each generated structures. Shape constraints and noncovalent ligand–receptor interactions especially the hydrogen bonding forms the principal interaction site [9]. Atom-based or fragment-based methods are used to assemble the molecules based on the receptor interaction sites. Fragment-based approach narrows the search space effectively. Moreover, if fragment molecules frequently arise in drug molecules then drug-likeness of designed compounds will be high. Fragments

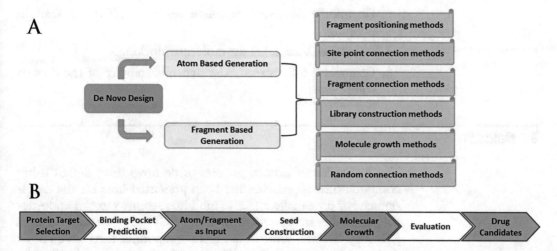

Fig. 1 (a) Schematic representation of de novo drug design methods and (b) de novo design strategy in LigBuilder V2.0

matching the interaction sites are grown and linked based on the connecting rules. Predicted ligands are ranked by estimated binding energy, structural complication and synthetic viability [3, 10, 11]. Successful application of de novo drug design has been studied in thrombin inhibitors, thymidylate synthase inhibitors, carbonic anhydrase II inhibitors, antitrypanosomiasis, estrogen receptor antagonists, and antifungal and some antiviral agents [12–22].

In this chapter, we portray the basic idea of de novo design strategy to design an effective potent drug like candidate against the biological targets. The art of de novo design is epitomized with an example of vascular endothelial growth factor receptor-2 (VEGFR-2) tyrosine kinase inhibitors build using computational methods. An elementary scheme of de novo drug design is represented in schematic diagram, shown in Fig. 1.

2   Materials

1. RCSB protein Data Bank (PDB) to obtain protein structure.
2. Chimera1.9 for refinement of ligand and receptor structure and also for molecular visualization and interaction analysis.
3. Modeller 9.15 for adding missing residues.
4. LigBuilder V2.0 to design new molecules.
5. FAF-Drugs2 to examine absorption, distribution, metabolism, and toxicity of the molecules.

6. Chemically advanced template search (CATS) for scaffold hopping.

7. AutoDock Vina 1.1.2 for molecular docking.

8. Gromacs 4.5.5 to study the dynamic stability of the docked compounds.

3 Methods

The basic idea of general process of de novo drug design using computational approaches has been presented here for the development of potentially effective inhibitor against vascular endothelial growth factor receptor-2 (VEGFR-2) tyrosine kinase [23, 24]. Besides, some of designed compounds through de novo design software are listed in Table 1. In the past couple of years, many of de novo design packages have been created with more futuristic arts in drug discovery and development, represented in Table 2. In addition, some more facts could be utilized for better enhancement of de novo design approaches (*see* **Notes 1** and **2**).

3.1 Generation of VEGFR-2 Tyrosine Kinase Inhibitors Using De Novo Design Strategy

Here, a case study of de novo designed inhibitors for the biological target vascular endothelial growth factor receptor-2 (VEGFR-2) tyrosine kinase using LigBuilder V2.0 is presented, which utilizes fragment-based algorithm for constructing new chemical inhibitors. The X-ray crystallographic coordinates of human VEGFR-2 tyrosine kinase domain with pyrrolopyrimidine inhibitor was retrieved from the Protein Data Bank (PDB code: 3VHE) [23].

3.1.1 Preliminary Requirements

3.1.2 Preprocessing of Targeted Protein

Preprocessing of targeted protein was successfully employed to assign missing hydrogens, for removing unnecessary water molecules and for the separation of protein–ligand along with charge calculation by Gasteiger using Chimera 1.9, and also for adding the missing residues and side chains by Modeller 9.15 [78, 79] (*see* **Note 3**).

3.1.3 Binding Site Prediction and Ligand Generation

The design of the fresh ligand is based on the active site information in the 3D structure of receptor. LigBuilder V2.0 [60], which is a cavity detection method, was utilized to determine the binding sites. Next the LigBuilder V2.0's function "Extract" was carried out to generate the seeds in the form of pyrrolo[3,2-d]pyrimidine, benzene, and urea from the original ligand. Finally, the linking mode strategy of BUILD was applied to create new designs of molecules from prepositioned to positioned seed structure with different pieces. This process was continued until all the fragments in each piece were linked by rational bonds into a single molecule. Later the evaluation of protein–ligand binding affinity using an

Table 1
Examples of various generated compounds through de novo design approaches

S. No.	Structure of compound	Target	Software used	Reference
1		Thrombin inhibitors	Automated combinatorial docking and LUDI	[25]
2		Antifungal	MCSS and Ludi	[8]
3		HIV-1 RT	SYNOPSIS	[8]
4		CDK4 inhibitors	Legend, LUDI, leapfrog	[8]
5		HIV protease	BREED	[26]
6		Human Cannabinoid Receptor 1 inhibitors	TOPAS	[27]

(continued)

Table 1
(continued)

S. No.	Structure of compound	Target	Software used	Reference
7		HDAC inhibitors	PhDD (Pharmacophore-based de novo design method of drug-like molecules)	[28]
8		CDK2 inhibitors	PhDD (Pharmacophore-based de novo design method of drug-like molecules)	[28]
9		Integrase inhibitors	PhDD (Pharmacophore-based de novo design method of drug-like molecules)	[28]
10		PfDHODH inhibitors	SPROUT	[29]
11		FKBP-12 ligands	LUDI	[30]
12		Trypsin inhibitors	DOGS (Design of Genuine Structures)	[31]

(continued)

Table 1
(continued)

S. No.	Structure of compound	Target	Software used	Reference
13		PPARα agonist	SQUIRREL (sophisticated QUantification of InteRaction RELationships)	[32]
14		PPARα agonist	SQUIRREL (sophisticated QUantification of InteRaction RELationships)	[32]
15		Hypothetical inhibitors for COX-2	LigBuilder	[33]
16		Hypothetical inhibitors for COX-2	LigBuilder	[33]
17		5HT$_{1B}$ antagonist	NovoFLAP	[34]

Table 2
List of De novo design software or programs.

S. No.	De novo design software or program	Year of publication	Concept of function	Receptor (R)/Ligand (L) based	Reference
1	HSITE or 2D skeletons	1989	Steric constraints and hydrogen bonds	R	[35]
2	3D skeletons	1990	Steric constraints and hydrogen bonds	R	[36]
3	Diamond lattice	1990	Steric constraints and hydrogen bonds	R	[36]
4	Legend	1991	Force field	R	[37]
5	Builder v1	1992	Combinatorial searching based on empirical scoring	R	[38]
6	LUDI	1992	Combinatorial searching based on empirical scoring	R	[39]
7	NEWLEAD	1993	Steric constraints	R	[40]
8	GroupBuild	1993	Force field	R	[41]
9	SPLICE	1993	Steric constraints	R	[42]
10	GenStar	1993	Steric constraints	R	[43]
11	CONCEPTS	1993	Empirical scoring	R	[44]
12	SPROUT	1993	Solvent accessible surface, electrostatic and hydrophobic interactions, hydrogen bond	R	[45]
13	MCSS & hook	1994	Nonpolar interactions with van der Waals potential	R	[46]
14	GrowMol	1994	Empirical scoring	R	[47]
15	Chemical genesis	1995	Combined score of shape, grid based, and scalar constraints	R and L	[48]
16	PRO_LIGAND	1995	Empirical scoring	R and L	[49]
17	DLD	1995	Potential energy function without electrostatic interactions	R	[50]
18	SMoG	1996	Knowledge based scoring	R	[51]
19	CONCERTS	1996	Force field	R	[52]
20	RASSE	1996	Force field using chemical rules	R	[53]
21	PRO_SELECT	1997	Empirical scoring	R	[54]
22	Skelgen	1997	Geometric and chemical constraints	R	[55]
23	Nachbar	1998	QSAR prediction based on target specific topology descriptor	L	[56]
24	Globus	1999	Molecular similarity function	L	[57]

(continued)

Table 2
(continued)

S. No.	De novo design software or program	Year of publication	Concept of function	Receptor (R)/Ligand (L) based	Reference
25	DycoBlock	1999	Force field and solvent accessible surface	R	[58]
26	LEA	2000	QSAR prediction based on 3D descriptors	L	[59]
27	LigBuilder	2000	Empirical scoring	R	[60]
28	TOPAS	2000	Molecular similarity function	L	[61]
29	F-DycoBlock	2001	Force field and solvent accessible surface	R	[62]
30	ADAPT	2001	Based on weighted sum of dock score, clogP, MM, number of rotatable bonds and hydrogen bonds	R	[63]
31	Pellegrini & field	2003	QSAR prediction based on target specific	R	[64]
32	SYNOPSIS	2003	Electrical dipole moment and empirically derived HIV-RT scoring	R	[65]
33	CoG	2004	Molecular similarity scoring	L	[66]
35	Nikitin	2005	Hydrogen bond, grid based electrostatic interaction	R	[67]
36	LEAD3D	2005	Molecular docking with independent property	R	[68]
37	Flux	2006	Stochastic searching with ligand-based similarity scoring	L	[69, 70]
38	GANDI	2008	Force field	R and L	[71]
39	COLIBREE	2008	Based on chemical advance template search topological pharmacophore similarity	L	[72]
40	SQUIRReLnovo	2008	Shape and pharmacophoric features based generation	L	[32]
41	Hecht & Fogel	2009	GOLD fitness scoring	L	[73]
42	MED-hybridise	2009	MED sumo score	R	[74]
43	MEGA	2009	Multi objective fitness scoring	R	[75]
44	AutoGrow	2009	Molecular docking score	R	[76]
45	NovoFLAP	2010	Ligand-based scoring with structural and pharmacophoric features	L	[34]
46	PhDD	2010	Pharmacophore-based de novo design	L	[28]

(continued)

Table 2
(continued)

S. No.	De novo design software or program	Year of publication	Concept of function	Receptor (R)/Ligand (L) based	Reference
47	DOGS	2010	Ligand-based scoring with structural and pharmacophoric features	L	[31]
48	iScreen	2011	Based on molecular docking	R	[77]

empirical scoring function (SCORE 2.0) [80] and bioavailability by a set of chemical rules with parameters: molecular weight, logP, H-bond donor, H-bond acceptor, 160–500,–0.4–5.6, 2–10, and 2–10 was performed.

3.1.4 *ADMET Prediction, Scaffold Hopping, Molecular Docking, and Simulation Studies*

FAF-Drugs2, an open source web server appliance was used for investigating the ADMET properties of the designed molecules [81] (*see* **Note 4**). All pharmacokinetic properties were set up within the acceptable range of Lipinski's rule of five. Scaffold hopping was executed using "Chemically advanced template search (CATS)" to identify matching compounds [82], where two known VEGFR-2 tyrosine kinase inhibitors Sorafenib and Axitinib were used as template structures. Further, the newly designed molecules along with known candidate Sorafenib were taken into the molecular docking platform with the receptor VEGFR-2 tyrosine kinase and the binding energy was calculated using AutoDock Vina 1.1.2 [83] (*see* **Note 5**). Finally, the top ranked protein–ligand complexes based on the lowest binding energy were simulated for 50 ns to explore the dynamic behavior and its interatomic interactions that facilitate the complex stability using Gromacs 4.5.5 software [84]. Thus, top four chemical entities were provided which were novel compounds toward the target VEGRF-2 tyrosine kinase for anti-cancer drug design (*see* **Note 6–8**).

4   Notes

1. The nature of search algorithm from a variety of de novo design software could provide different kinds of molecules with detailed knowledge of chemical properties. It is possible to get an optimized compound with improved activity and functionality with a different framework than the existing.

2. Several software are available which are free, while others are commercial [85–88]. These could predict the active sites or druggable pockets within the target (protein).

3. Targeted protein's preprocessing and refinement can be perform by other tools like Schrodinger Protein preparation wizard (https://www.schrodinger.com/protein-preparation-wizard) and 3D refine web server (http://sysbio.rnet.missouri.edu/3Drefine/) [89–91].

4. The physical–chemical and pharmaceutical properties [92] can also be predicted for de novo designed ligands using some tools like QikProp (https://www.schrodinger.com/qikprop) [93], TOPKAT (http://accelrys.com/products/collaborative-science/biovia-discovery-studio/qsar-admet-and-predictive-toxicology.html) [94] SwissADME (https://www.swissadme.ch) [95] and admetSAR (http://lmmd.ecust.edu.cn:8000/) [96]. These tools are effective and possess wide range of properties to predict more insights on the ligands.

5. Prior to docking study, the newly designed compounds could be prepared using LigPrep utility of Schrodinger's package [89, 97], which produces all feasible tautomeric, stereochemical, and ionization variants of the participation molecules followed by energy minimization to achieve structures with optimized geometry.

6. The synthetic accessibility of a compound can be predicted with the help of several computational approaches such as myPresto—Medicinally Yielding PRotein Engineering SimulaTOr program suite (http://presto.protein.osaka-u.ac.jp/myPresto4/) and SYLVIA (https://www.mn-am.com/products/sylvia) [98].

7. Prediction of binding free energy of the newly designed against protein target through MM/GBSA [Molecular Mechanics Generalized Born Surface Area continuum solvation] would give higher clarity than docking scores in silico or in vitro processing [99]

8. Characterization of newly designed ligands through Density functional theory calculation on chemical properties such as molecular electrostatic potential (MESP), highest occupied molecular orbitals (HOMOs) and lowest unoccupied molecular orbitals (LUMOs), and aqueous solvation energy would provide key mechanistic insights on ligands which will we very useful in screening the newly designed ligands before further processing [100].

Acknowledgment

SKS thanks Department of Biotechnology (DBT), New Delhi for providing financial support. VS and UP gratefully acknowledge DST (New Delhi) for INSPIRE Senior Research Fellowship

(No. DST/INSPIRE Fellowship/2012/482) and Alagappa University for AURF (No. Ph.D./1122/AURF FELLOWSHIP/ 2015) respectively.

References

1. Song CM, Lim SJ, Tong JC (2009) Recent advances in computer-aided drug design. Brief Bioinform 10:579–591
2. Clark DE, Pickett SD (2000) Computational methods for the prediction of 'drug-likeness'. Drug Discov Today 5:49–58
3. Loving K, Alberts I, Sherman W (2010) Computational approaches for fragment-based and *de novo* design. Curr Top Med Chem 10:14–32
4. Moon JB, Howe WJ (1991) Computer design of bioactive molecules: a method for receptor-based *de novo* ligand design. Proteins 11:314–328
5. Joseph-McCarthy D (1999) Computational approaches to structure-based ligand design. Pharmacol Ther 84:179–191
6. Aparoy P, Reddy KK, Reddanna P (2012) Structure and ligand based drug design strategies in the development of novel 5- LOX inhibitors. Curr Med Chem 19:3763–3778
7. Po-Ssu H, Boyken SE, Baker D (2016) The coming of age of *de novo* protein design. Nature 537:320–327
8. Schneider G, Fechner U (2005) Computer-based *de novo* design of drug-like molecules. Nat Rev Drug Discov 4:649–663
9. Hartenfeller M, Schneider G (2011) Enabling future drug discovery by *de novo* design. Wiley Interdiscip Rev Comput Mol Sci 1:742–759
10. Butina D, Segall MD, Frankcombe K (2002) Predicting ADME properties *in silico*: methods and models. Drug Discov Today 7: S83–S88
11. Takeda S, Kaneko H, Funatsu K (2016) Chemical-space-based *de novo* design method to generate drug-like molecules. J Chem Inf Model 56:1885–1893
12. Jain SK, Agrawal A, Stahl M, Schneider P (2004) De novo drug design: an overview. Indian J Pharm Sci 66:721–728
13. Hilpert K, Ackermann J, Banner DW, Gast A, Gubernator K, Hadváry P, Labler L, Müller K, Schmid G, Tschopp TB, Waterbeemd HVD (1994) Design and synthesis of potent and highly selective thrombin inhibitors. J Med Chem 37:3889–3901
14. Webber SE, Bleckman TM, Attard J, Deal JG, Kathardekar V, Welsh KM, Webber S, Janson CA, Matthews DA, Smith WW, Freer ST, Jordan SR, Bacquet RJ, Howland EF, Booth CLJ, Ward RW, Hermann SM, White J, Morse CA, Hilliard JA, Bartlett CA (1993) Design of thymidylate synthase inhibitors using protein crystal structures: the synthesis and biological evaluation of a novel class of 5-substituted quinazolinones. J Med Chem 36:733–746
15. Greer J, Erickson JW, Baldwin JJ, Varney MD (1994) Application of the three-dimensional structures of protein target molecules in structure-based drug design. J Med Chem 37:1035–1054
16. Baldwin JJ, Ponticello GS, Anderson PS, Christy ME, Murcko MA, Randall WC, Schwam H, Sugrue MF, Springer JP, Gautheron P, Grove J, Mallorga P, Viadert MP, McKeever BM, Navia MA (1989) Thienothiopyran-2-sulfonamides: novel topically active carbonic anhydrase inhibitors for the treatment of glaucoma. J Med Chem 32:2510–2513
17. Verlinde CL, Callens M, Van Calenbergh S, Van Aerschot A, Herdewijn P, Hannaert V, Michels PA, Opperdoes FR, Hol WG (1994) Selective inhibition of trypanosomal glyceraldehyde-3-phosphate dehydrogenase by protein structure-based design: toward new drugs for the treatment of sleeping sickness. J Med Chem 37:3605–3613
18. Von Itzstein M, Wu WY, Kok GB, Pegg MS, Dyason JC, Jin B, Van Phan T, Smythe ML, White HF, Oliver SW, Colman PM, Varghese JN, Ryan DM, Woods JM, Bethell RC, Hotham VJ, Cameron JM, Penn CR (1993) Rational design of potent sialidase-based inhibitors of influenza virus replication. Nature 363:418–423
19. Diana GD, Treasurywala AM, Bailey TR, Oglesby RC, Pevear DC, Dutko FJ (1990) A model for compounds active against human Rhinovirus-14 based on X-ray crystallography data. J Med Chem 33:1306–1311
20. Diana GD, Treasurywala A (1991) Design of compounds active against HRV-14. Drug News Perspect 4:517–523
21. Schmidt JM, Mercure J, Tremblay GB, Pagé M, Kalbakji A, Feher M, Dunn-Dufault R, Peter MG, Redden PR (2003) *De novo*

design, synthesis, and evaluation of novel nonsteroidal phenanthrene ligands for the estrogen receptor. J Med Chem 46:1408–1418

22. Haitao Ji et al (2003) Structure-based *de novo* design, synthesis, and biological evaluation of non-azole inhibitors specific for Lanosterol 14α-Demethylase of fungi. J Med Chem 46:474–485

23. Liu YZ, Wang XL, Wang XY, Yu RL, Liu DQ, Kang CM (2016) *De novo* design of VEGFR-2 tyrosine kinase inhibitors based on a linked-fragment approach. J Mol Model 22:222

24. Kankanala J, Latham AM, Johnson AP, Homer-Vanniasinkam S, Fishwick CW, Ponnambalam S (2012) A combinatorial *in silico* and cellular approach to identify a new class of compounds that target VEGFR2 receptor tyrosine kinase activity and angiogenesis. Br J Pharmacol 166:737–748

25. Böhm HJ, Banner DW, Weber L (1999) Combinatorial docking and combinatorial chemistry: design of potent non-peptide thrombin inhibitors. J Comput Aided Mol Des 13:51–56

26. Pierce AC, Rao G, Bemis GW (2004) BREED: generating novel inhibitors through hybridization of known ligands. Application to CDK2, P38, and HIV protease. J Med Chem 47:2768–2775

27. Rogers-Evans M, Alanine AI, Bleicher KH, Kube D, Schneider G (2004) Identification of novel cannabinoid receptor ligands via evolutionary *de novo* design and rapid parallel synthesis. QSAR Comb Sci 23:426–430

28. Huang Q, Li LL, Sheng-Yong Y (2010) PhDD: a new pharmacophore-based *de novo* design method of drug-like molecules combined with assessment of synthetic accessibility. J Mol Graph Model 28:775–787

29. Heikkilä T, Thirumalairajan S, Davies M, Parsons MR, McConkey AG, Fishwick CWG, Johnson AP (2006) The first *de novo* designed inhibitors of plasmodium falciparum dihydroorotate dehydrogenase. Bioorg Med Chem Lett 16:88–92

30. Babine RE, Bleckman TM, Kissinger CR, Showalter R, Pelletier LA, Lewis C, Tucker K, Moomaw E, Parge HE, Villafranca JE (1995) Design synthesis and X-ray crystallographic studies of novel FKBP-12 ligand. Bioorg Med Chem Lett 5:1719–1724

31. Heartenfeller M, Zettl H, Walter M, Rupp M, Reisen F, Proschak E, Wegen S, Stark H, Schneider G (2012) DOGS: reaction-driven *de novo* design of bioactive compounds. PLoS Comput Biol 8:1–12

32. Proschak E, Sander K, Zettl H, Tanrikulu Y, Rau O, Schneider P, Schubert-Zsilavecz M, Stark H, Schneider G (2009) From molecular shape to potent bioactive agents II: fragment-based *de novo* design. ChemMedChem 4:45–48

33. Dhanjal JK, Sreenidhi AK, Bafna K, Katiyar SP, Goyal S, Grover A, Sundar D (2015) Computational structure-based *de novo* design of hypothetical inhibitors against the anti-inflammatory target COX-2. PLoS One 10:e0134691

34. Damewood JR, Lerman CL, Masek BB (2010) NovoFLAP: a ligand-based *de novo* design approach for the generation of medicinally relevant ideas. J Chem Inf Model 50:1296–1303

35. Danziger DJ, Dean PM (1989) Automated site-directed drug design: a general algorithm for knowledge acquisition about hydrogen bonding regions at protein surfaces. Proc R Soc Lond B Biol Sci 236:101–113

36. Lewis RA (1990) Automated site-directed drug design: approaches to the formation of 3D molecular graphs. J Comput Aided Mol Des 4:205–210

37. Nishibata Y, Itai A (1991) Automatic creation of dug candidate structures based on receptor structure. Starting point for artificial lead generation. Tetrahedron 47:8985–8990

38. Lewis RA, Roe DC, Huang C, Ferrin TE, Langridge R, Kuntz ID (1992) Automated site-directed drug design using molecular lattices. J Mol Graph 10:66–78

39. Böhm HJ (1992) The computer program LUDI: a new simple method for the de-novo design of enzyme inhibitors. J Comput Aided Mol Des 6:61–78

40. Tschinke V, Cohen NC (1993) The NEW-LEAD program: a new method for the design of candidate structures from pharmacophoric hypothesis. J Med Chem 36:3863–3870

41. Rotstein SH, Murcko MA (1993) Group build: a fragment-based method for *de novo* drug design. J Med Chem 36:1700–1710

42. Ho CMW, Marshall GR (1993) SPLICE: a program to assemble partial query solutions from three-dimensional database searches into novel ligands. J Comput Aided Mol Des 7:623–647

43. Rotstein SH, Murcko MA (1993) GenStar: a method for *de novo* drug design. J Comput Aided Mol Des 7:23–43

44. Pearlman DA, Murcko MA (1993) CONCEPTS: new dynamic algorithm for *de novo* design suggestion. J Comput Chem 14:1184–1193

45. Gillett VJ, Myatt G, Zsoldos Z, Johnson AP (1995) SPROUT, HIPPO and CAESA: tools for de novo structure generation and estimation of synthetic accessibility. Perspect Drug Discov Des 3:34–50

46. Eisen MB, Wiley DC, Karplus M, Hubbard RE (1994) HOOK: a program for finding novel molecular architectures that satisfy the chemical and steric requirements of a macromolecule binding site. Proteins 19:199–221

47. Bohacek RS, McMartin C (1994) Multiple highly diverse structures complementary to enzyme binding sites: results of extensive application of a de novo design method incorporating combinatorial growth. J Am Chem Soc 116:5560–5571

48. Glen RC, Payne AWR (1995) A genetic algorithm for the automated generation of molecules within constraints. J Comput Aided Mol Des 9:181–202

49. Clark DE, Frenkel D, Levy SA, Li J, Murray CW, Robson B, Waszkowycz B, Westhead DR (1995) PRO-LIGAND: an approach to de novo molecular design. 1. Application to the design of organic molecules. J Comput Aided Mol Des 9:13–32

50. Miranker A, Karplus M (1995) An automated method for dynamic ligand design. Proteins 23:472–490

51. DeWitte RS, Shakhnovich EI (1996) SMoG de novo design method based on simple, fast, and accurate free energy estimates. 1. Methodology and supporting evidence. J Am Chem Soc 118:11733–11744

52. Pearlman DA, Murcko MA (1996) CONCERTS: dynamic connection of fragments as an approach to de novo ligand design. J Med Chem 39:1651–1663

53. Luo Z, Wang R, Lai L (1996) RASSE: a new method for structure-based drug design. J Chem Inf Comput Sci 36:1187–1194

54. Murray CW, Clark DE, Auton TR, Firth MA, Li J, Sykes RA, Waszkowycz B, Westhead DR, Young SC (1997) PRO_SELECT: combining structure-based drug design and combinatorial chemistry for rapid lead discovery. 1. Technology. J Comput Aided Mol Des 11:193–207

55. Todorov NP, Dean PM (1997) Evaluation of a method for controlling molecular scaffold diversity in de novo ligand design. J Comput Aided Mol Des 11:175–192

56. Nachbar RB (2000) Molecular evolution: automated manipulation of hierarchical chemical topology and its application to average molecular structures. Genet Program Evolvable Mach 1:57–94

57. Globus A, Lawton J, Wipke WT (1999) Automatic molecular design using evolutionary algorithms. Nanotechnology 10:290–299

58. Liu H, Duan Z, Luo Q, Shi Y (1999) Structure based ligand design by dynamically assembling molecular building blocks at binding site. Proteins 36:462–470

59. Douguet D, Thoreau E, Grassy G (2000) A genetic algorithm for the automated generation of small organic molecules: drug design using an evolutionary algorithm. J Comput Aided Mol Des 14:449–466

60. Wang R, Gao Y, Lai L (2000) LigBuilder: a multi-purpose program for structure-based drug design. J Mol Model 6:498–516

61. Schneider G, Lee ML, Stahl M, Schneider P (2000) De novo design of molecular architectures by evolutionary assembly of drug-derived building blocks. J Comput Aided Mol Des 14:487–494

62. Zhu J, Fan H, Liu H, Shi Y (2001) Structure based ligand design for flexible proteins: application of new F-Dyco block. J Comput Aided Mol Des 15:979–996

63. Pegg SCH, Haresco JJ, Kuntz ID (2001) A genetic algorithm for structure-based de novo design. J Comput Aided Mol Des 15:911–933

64. Pellegrini E, Field MJ (2003) Development and testing of a de novo drug-design algorithm. J Comput Aided Mol Des 17:621–641

65. Vinkers HM, de Jonge MR, Daeyaert FF, Heeres J, Koymans LM, van Lenthe JH, Lewi PJ, Timmerman H, Van Aken K, Janssen PA (2003) SYNOPSIS: SYNthesize and OPtimize system in silico. J Med Chem 46:2765–2773

66. Brown N, McKay B, Gilardoni F, Gasteiger J (2004) A graph-based genetic algorithm and its application to the multi objective evolution of median molecules. J Chem Inf Comput Sci 44:1079–1087

67. Nikitin S, Zaitseva N, Demina O, Solovieva V, Mazin E, Mikhalev S, Smolov M, Rubinov A, Vlasov P, Lepikhin D, Khachko D, Fokin V, Queen C, Zosimov V (2005) A very large diversity space of synthetically accessible compounds for use with drug design programs. J Comput Aided Mol Des 19:47–63

68. Douguet D, Munier-Lehmann H, Labesse G, Pochet S (2005) LEA3D: a computer-aided ligand design for structure-based drug design. J Med Chem 48:2457–2468

69. Fechner U, Schneider G (2006) Flux (1): a virtual synthesis scheme for fragment based de novo design. J Chem Inf Model 46:699–707

70. Fechner U, Schneider G (2007) Flux (2): comparison of molecular mutation and cross-over operators for ligand-based *de novo* design. J Chem Inf Model 47:656–667

71. Dey F, Cafl isch A (2008) Fragment-based *de novo* ligand design by multi objective evolutionary optimization. J Chem Inf Model 48:679–690

72. Hartenfeller M, Proschak E, Schüller A, Schneider G (2008) Concept of combinatorial *de novo* design of drug-like molecules by particle swarm optimization. Chem Biol Drug Des 72:16–26

73. Hecht D, Fogel GB (2009) Novel *in silico* approach to drug discovery via computational intelligence. J Chem Inf Model 49:1105–1121

74. Moriaud F, Doppelt-Azeroual O, Martin L, Oguievetskaia K, Koch K, Vorotyntsev A, Adcock SA, Delfaud F (2009) Computational fragment-based approach at PDB scale by protein local similarity. J Chem Inf Model 49:280–294

75. Nicolaou CA, Apostolakis J, Pattichis CS (2009) *De novo* drug design using multiobjective evolutionary graphs. J Chem Inf Model 49:295–307

76. Durrant JD, Amaro RE, McCammon JA (2009) AutoGrow: a novel algorithm for protein inhibitor design. Chem Biol Drug Des 73:168–178

77. TY T, Chang KW, Chen CY (2011) iScreen: world's first cloud-computing web server for virtual screening and *de novo* drug design based on TCM database@Taiwan. J Comput Aided Mol Des 25:525–531

78. Pettersen EF, Goddard TD, Huang CC, Couch GS, Greenblatt DM, Meng EC, Ferrin TE (2004) UCSF chimera—a visualization system for exploratory research and analysis. J Comput Chem 25:1605–1612

79. Eswar N, Webb B, Marti-Renom MA, Madhusudhan MS, Eramian D, Shen MY, Pieper U, Sali A (2007) Comparative protein structure modeling using MODELLER. Curr Protoc Protein Sci 50(2.9):2.9.1–2.9.31

80. Wang R, Liu L, Lai L, Tang Y (1998) SCORE: a new empirical method for estimating the binding affinity of a protein-ligand complex. Mol Model Ann 4:379–394

81. Lagorce D, Sperandio O, Galons H, Miteva MA, Villoutreix BO (2008) FAF-Drugs2: free ADME/tox filtering tool to assist drug discovery and chemical biology projects. BMC Bioinformatics 9:396

82. Reutlinger M, Koch CP, Reker D, Todoroff N, Schneider P, Rodrigues T, Schneider G (2013) Chemically advanced template search (CATS) for scaffold-hopping and prospective target prediction for 'orphan'-molecules. Mol Inform 32:133–138

83. Trott O, Olson AJ (2010) AutoDock Vina: improving the speed and accuracy of docking with a new scoring function, efficient optimization, and multithreading. J Comput Chem 31:455–461

84. Hess B, Kutzner C, Van Der Spoel D, Lindahl E (2008) GROMACS 4: algorithms for highly efficient, load-balanced, and scalable molecular simulation. J Chem Theory Comput 4:435–447

85. Schrödinger Release 2017–1: SiteMap, Schrödinger, LLC, New York, NY, 2017

86. Selvaraj C, Priya RB, Lee JK, Singh SK (2015) Mechanistic insights of SrtA-LPXTG blockers targeting the transpeptidase mechanism in Streptococcus mutans. RSC Adv 5:100498–100510

87. Yang J, Roy A, Zhang Y (2013) Protein-ligand binding site recognition using complementary binding-specific substructure comparison and sequence profile alignment. Bioinformatics 29:2588–2595

88. Singh S, Prabhu SV, Suryanarayanan V, Bhardwaj R, Singh SK, Dubey VK (2016) Molecular docking and structure based virtual screening studies of potential drug target, CAAX prenyl proteases, of Leishmania donovani. J Biomol Struct Dyn 34(11):2367–2386

89. Sastry GM, Adzhigirey M, Day T, Annabhimoju R, Sherman W (2013) Protein and ligand preparation: Parameters, protocols, and influence on virtual screening enrichments. J Comput Aid Mol Des 27:221–234

90. Bhattacharya D, Nowotny J, Cao R, Cheng J (2016) 3Drefine: an interactive web server for efficient protein structure refinement. Nucleic Acids Res 44:W406–W409

91. Reddy KK, Singh SK (2015) Insight into the binding mode between N-methyl Pyrimidones and prototype foamy virus integrase-DNA complex by QM-polarized ligand docking and molecular dynamics simulations. Curr Top Med Chem 15:43–49

92. Aarthy M, Panwar U, Selvaraj C, Singh SK (2017) Advantages of structure-based drug design approaches in neurological disorders. Curr Neuropharmacol 15(8):1136–1155. https://doi.org/10.2174/1570159X15666170102145257

93. Schrödinger Release 2017–1: QikProp, Schrödinger, LLC, New York, NY, 2017

94. Mombelli E (2008) An evaluation of the predictive ability of the QSAR software packages, DEREK, HAZARDEXPERT and TOPKAT, to describe chemically-induced skin irritation. Altern Lab Anim 36:15–24

95. Daina A, Michielin O, Zoete V (2017) SwissADME: a free web tool to evaluate pharmacokinetics, drug-likeness and medicinal chemistry friendliness of small molecules. Sci Rep 7:42717

96. Cheng F, Li W, Zhou Y, Shen J, Wu Z, Liu G, Lee PW, Tang Y (2012) admetSAR: a comprehensive source and free tool for assessment of chemical ADMET properties. J Chem Inf Model 52:3099–3105

97. Suryanarayanan V, Singh SK (2015) Assessment of dual inhibition property of newly discovered inhibitors against PCAF and GCN5 through insilico screening, molecular dynamics simulation and DFT approach. J Recept Signal Transduct Res 35:370–380

98. Fukunishi Y, Kurosawa T, Mikami Y, Hv N (2014) Prediction of synthetic accessibility based on commercially available compound databases. J Chem Inf Model 54:3259–3267

99. Genheden S, Ulf R (2015) The MM/PBSA and MM/GBSA methods to estimate ligand-binding affinities. Expert Opin Drug Discov 10:449–461

100. Bochevarov AD, Harder E, Hughes TF, Greenwood JR, Braden DA, Philipp DM, Rinaldo D, Halls MD, Zhang J, Friesner RA (2013) Jaguar: a high-performance quantum chemistry software program with strengths in life and materials sciences. Int J Quantum Chem 113:2110–2142

Chapter 6

Molecular Dynamics Simulation and Prediction of Druggable Binding Sites

Tianhua Feng and Khaled Barakat

Abstract

Binding site identification and druggability evaluation are two essential steps in structure-based drug design. A druggable binding site tends to have high binding affinity to drug-like molecules. Predicting such sites can have a significant impact on a drug design campaign. This chapter focuses on summarizing the different methods that are used to predict druggable binding sites. The chapter also discusses the importance of including protein flexibility in the search process and the use of molecular dynamics simulations to address this aspect. Case studies from the literature are also summarized and discussed. We hope that this chapter would provide an overview on the different methods employed in binding site identification evaluation.

Key words Conformational ensemble, Cosolvent molecular dynamic simulation, Druggability, Hot spot, Protein flexibility

1 Introduction

Proteins are dynamical entities in nature. They interact with each other or with small molecule compounds to execute their function or to transfer a signal [1]. These interactions usually take place through hot spots on the surface of the proteins [2]. In many cases these hot spots cluster into one region, forming a binding site, which can specifically fit the interacting partner. These binding sites have been always considered as attractive targets to develop target-specific drugs [3–5]. However, not every binding site is suitable to develop a drug. One should think about the druggability of a binding site prior to searching for a compound that can fit within the site [6]. Druggability of binding sites emerged in the recent years [7] and was first defined as the ability of a protein linked to a particular disease to bind a small drug-like molecule with high affinity and specificity [8, 9].

Although using an automated approach to predict the "druggability" of a binding site is still difficult [10], computational

Mohini Gore and Umesh B. Jagtap (eds.), *Computational Drug Discovery and Design*, Methods in Molecular Biology, vol. 1762, https://doi.org/10.1007/978-1-4939-7756-7_6, © Springer Science+Business Media, LLC, part of Springer Nature 2018

methods are becoming more promising in this aspect. These computational methods are usually composed of two subsequent stages, namely, identifying the binding site and, subsequently, characterizing its druggability [10, 11]. The site identification phase aims at analyzing the distribution of all hot spots on the target, and employs both structure-based methods and sequence-based methods. On the other hand, the druggability of a binding site can be characterized different druggability indexes, as described below.

In general, binding sites can be classified into three major types. The first includes catalytic sites or enzymatic binding sites [12]. These binding sites usually possess specific catalytic functions, allowing it to interact with a substrate and execute chemical reactions, transforming the substrate into a new product. The second class comprises allosteric binding sites [13–18], which are not inducing any catalytic activity, however, interacting with these sites can indirectly impact the function, dynamics, or distribution of conformations of the target, which can indirectly modulate its activity [19]. The third and the most complicated class of binding sites are usually termed as cryptic binding sites. They are almost hidden and rarely can appear on the surface of the protein. They usually occupy a small portion of the conformational ensemble of the target and are only partly detectable in the unbound target [20]. Identifying cryptic sites may require a great deal of structural and conformational analysis of the target (Fig. 1).

Binding site recognition methods can hardly identify all potential binding sites, especially, if the search process involves only a single static structure. An experimental crystal structure is an average in time and space of protein dynamics. A binding site can be easily hidden in a crystal structure, and can be only identified when its dynamical properties are taken into account. In this context, the flexibility of the target plays a significant role in binding site formation and identification [21] and studying these conformational dynamics is an essential step in this process. One way to study and reveal these dynamics is to use molecular dynamics (MD)

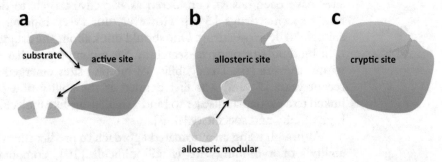

Fig. 1 Different types of binding sites include (**a**) the active site, (**b**) allosteric site, which can change their conformation before (pink) and after (blue) binding with allosteric modular, and (**c**) cryptic binding site, which can occasionally open (blue)

simulations [22]. The snapshots extracted from the MD trajectory represent multiple conformers of the protein structure, involving both backbone and side chain dynamics. These extracted conformations can reveal hidden spots within a crystal structure.

This chapter focuses on binding site identification approaches, with an emphasis on structure-based methods. It also discusses the use of MD simulations in identifying these sites, understanding their dynamicity and evaluating their druggability. Finally a few case studies are summarized, followed by a summary and conclusion of our findings. We hope this chapter would shed light on recent advances in this hot area and will be of great use for interested researchers.

2 Binding Site Identification and Druggability Evaluation Methods

As mentioned above, the prediction of druggable binding sites involves two stages. Firstly, one should identify all potential binding sites within and on the surface of the target structure. This is followed by the ranking of these sites in terms of their druggability.

2.1 Binding Site Identification Methods

The last few years witnessed the development of a few reliable structure-based methods to identify binding sites [23]. These structural methods can be categorized into two main classes, geometric-based methods (e.g., PASS [24], POCKET [25], LigSite [26]), and energy-based methods (e.g., GRID [27], Q-SiteFinder [28]) (*see* **Note 1**). Several reviews comprehensively describe these two approaches [10, 11, 23, 29], though they will be briefly summarized below.

2.1.1 Geometric-Based Methods

Geometric-based methods recognize a binding site based on its geometric parameters. Two example parameters that are commonly used in this aspect are the depth and surface area of the binding site. In this context, Hajduk et al. defined a term, called pocket compactness, as the ratio of the pocket volume to the pocket surface area [3]. The optimal value for this parameter is usually in the range of 0.4. Larger values correspond to more spherical shaped pockets and smaller values represent more elongated shaped pockets. The residual composition of a binding site, which includes polarization, charges, and H-bonds, are also important geometrical parameters to characterize binding sites. By using these various parameters one can identify potential binding sites and provide further druggability assessment (Fig. 2).

For protein–protein interactions (PPIs), the geometric descriptors are usually smaller compared to those of catalytic/active sites, which are usually formed by major, large, and deep binding clefts. An important study in this regard is the work by Bourgeas et al. They extracted the best descriptors, geometrical parameters, and

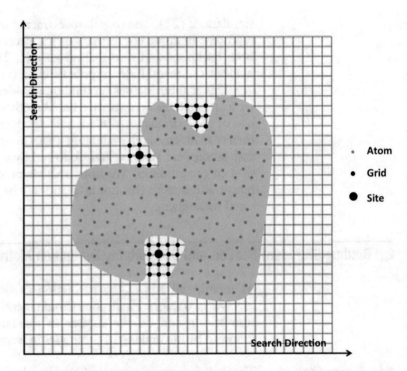

Fig. 2 Geometric-based binding site identification mechanism. The approach scans the grid points outside the protein for protein–solvent–protein and surface–solvent–surface events. When the regions reach the threshold of requirement, they can be labeled as potential binding sites

residue properties for PPIs, and used this information to guide their search for binding sites in heterodimer complexes [30]. The 2P2I database gathers geometry information of interfaces, which comes from known druggable PPIs' interfaces. They summarize several different properties of these interfaces after compared with general PPI interfaces. The druggable PPIs' interfaces are smaller, more hydrophobic, and composed by fewer pockets. Additionally, the druggable PPIs interfaces have less salt bridges and charged residues, but more hydrogen bonds at the interface [30].

2.1.2 Energy-Based Methods

Energy-based methods employ molecular docking as the main tool to identify and characterize the binding sites on proteins. These methods dock multiple probes to potential pockets and calculate their binding free energies. These predicted energies reflect the strength of the interactions of these probes within the target [31]. Fragment-based mapping algorithm (FTMAP) is a popular energy-based method. FTMAP was a developed version of its predecessor, computational solvent mapping (CS-map) [32].

FTMAP uses a diverse library of 16 small organic molecules as probes to search the whole target protein surface for potential binding sites [7, 33]. These small organic probes have different

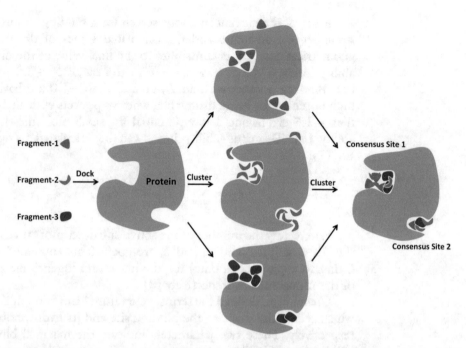

Fig. 3 Probe-based binding site identification mechanism. Different types of drug-like fragments dock randomly on the protein surface. The first clusters are ranked based on their binding free energy. After the second turn of clustering, multiple types of fragments are gathering around the consensus sites (CS)

hydrophobicity and hydrogen bond capacities, allowing them to interact with many parts on the protein surface. A fast Fourier transform correlation approach is implemented to sample millions of receptor–probe complexes. These complexes are clustered within the same probe type, and the generated clusters are ranked based on their binding energies. The method extracts top-ranking clusters from different types of probe and regroups them again. The consensus sites (CSs) represent putative hot spots, where multiple probes congregate. The CSs containing the largest number of probe clusters are considered the main hot spots (Fig. 3) [31]. The FTMAP method has been developed as web server, which is linked to the protein data bank (PDB) and generates a file containing the CSs and their congregated probes for a given target [34].

2.2 Druggability Evaluation Methods

Once a binding site is identified, the next stage focuses on the evaluation of its druggability. In general, this is usually accomplished by analyzing the binding site using various geometrical descriptors and binding free energy analysis. All these calculations are summarized in what is termed as a druggability index. A druggability index, I_D, provides a measure of the potential of a given binding site to accommodate a small-molecule candidate drug.

Most of the current methods search for a binding site using a static protein structure and the calculated values of the various geometrical descriptors contribute to the final value of the druggability index. Typical I_D values are in the range of -3.0 to 0.0 [8]. Binding pockets with an I_D greater than -1.0 are having a high potential for being druggable, whereas pockets with an I_D less than -1.5 are having a low potential for small-molecule druggability [8]. The druggability index can be calculated using the Eq. (1):

$$I_D = \sum_{i=1}^{N} [a_i X_i + b_i \log(X_i)] \tag{1}$$

Where N is the number of the active-site descriptors used, X_i is the ith descriptor, and a_i and b_i are coefficients (obtained from fitting to experimental data) for the linear and logarithmic terms of the ith parameter, respectively [8].

Cheng et al. defined the terms, "curvature" and "lipophilicity," which reflect the shape of the binding site and its hydrophobicity, respectively. These two parameters indicate the maximal binding affinity for drug-like compounds [35–37]. Other binding sites' identification methods use different geometrical descriptors. An example is the Dscore method, which forms a linear function of three pocket properties: size, enclosure (akin to an average degree of buriedness), and hydrophilicity [11, 38]. Another druggability evaluation method, which originated from NMR-Based fragment screening, try to mimic the hit rates concept, This hit rate method relies on the assumption that sites that bind with a higher proportion of fragments are also more likely to deliver high-affinity, non-covalent drug-like leads [3]. The FTMAP is an example of such methods and it can estimate the maximal binding affinity, while evaluating the druggability of a given target toward a particular compound.

2.3 Importance of Protein Flexibility

All the methods described above do not take the protein flexibility into account, making them very limited in identifying and studying complicated and hidden binding sites (see **Note 2**). For example, many studies have shown that the druggability index can vary significantly, when calculating the same index for the same target, but for a different state (i.e., free vs. bound structures) [8]. This is clearly demonstrated in highly dynamical proteins [39]. For example, the unbound Bcl-xL protein cannot accommodate the Bak peptide, which is normally associated with a low druggability index ($I_D = -2.0$). On the contrary, the bound conformation is much wider and deeper, which is reflected by a much higher druggability index ($I_D = -0.5$) (Fig. 4) [8].

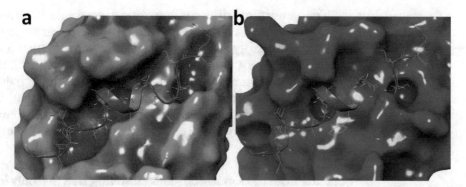

Fig. 4 Structure of Bcl-xL in (**a**) unbound (orange surface, PDB ID: 2LP8) and (**b**) bound (blue surface) conformation. The Bak peptide (green ribbon, side chains show) is detected with the Bcl-xL by using NMR (PDB ID: 2LPC) and superimposed onto the unbound conformation. Based on the geometric feature, the binding site can be recognized as high druggability in bound conformation (**a**). However, the same binding site of unbound Bcl-xL is identified as low druggability in (**b**). Generated by Maestro

A more complicated example is the discovery of a hidden trench in HIV integrase, which is not accessible within the available crystal structure [40]. Other examples include the identification of uncharacterized binding sites on the Cruzain, a therapeutic target for Chagas' disease [41] and the identification of novel transient allosteric binding sites in Ras proteins, a hallmark of diverse cancers [42].

All these examples emphasize the importance of introducing protein flexibility in the search process for a binding site. In this context, MD simulations can be used to explore the dynamicity of the target protein [43, 44]. The method became very popular in studying protein structures and in extracting conformational ensembles of these targets. These simulations can be carried out in the context of the solvent, ions, and various physiological parameters. In this way, one will not only able to identify and understand the flexibility of a given binding site, but will be also able to explore its interaction with water molecules and ions. Moreover, by analyzing the MD trajectory, one can also measure the persistence of the binding site, duration of the hydrogen bonds, and varying depth and width of the binding site.

2.4 Generation of Conformation Ensemble

A conformational ensemble is a group of structures from the same target with different conformations, reflecting the flexibility of the backbone and side chains. In the early 1990s, Pang and Kozikowski made the first attempt to extract multiple conformations of the acetycholinesterase enzyme from MD trajectories. Since this moment, MD simulations become the most common way to generate such structural ensembles [45]. The depth and the shape of a given protein pocket can be assessed during the simulation and transient cavities can be identified and explored [44].

The generation of a conformational ensemble involves two steps. First is to run an MD simulation on the target structure to generate a trajectory. This atomic trajectory can be either a single extensive trajectory, coming from a single simulation, or multiple trajectories combined together to form a single long trajectory [23]. The two approaches can lead to different outcomes, and it seems that using multiple simulations can provide more improved conformational sampling over the use of a single MD trajectory [31].

The next step, involves the clustering of the long trajectory obtained from the simulation. This clustering step not only identifies representative conformations for the target protein, but is also used to reduce the computational time in subsequent binding site evaluation steps [38]. The most common way for clustering protein conformations is using RMSD-based methods. Other methods may also involve principal component analysis (PCA) [46], non-negative matrix factorization (NMF) [47], and independent component analysis (ICA) [46, 48].

2.5 The Sampling Problem

In many cases and depending on the plasticity of the target, a binding site that is not obviously present in a crystal structure may appear after a short simulation time. For example, Eyrisch and Helms identified transient pockets on the protein surface after 10 ns of MD simulation [20]. However, in most cases, conventional MD simulations cannot access these sites, and a significantly long MD simulation may be required to sample the conformational space of the target (*see* **Notes 3** and **4**). This is mainly due to the entrapment of the protein structure in a local minimum within the energy surface and not being able to cross the high-energy barriers separating these minima (Fig. 5) [49].

In this case, one has two options: running a very long MD simulation (in the 100 s of ns scale) or using other MD simulations methods that are designed to solve this sampling problem such as Replica Exchange MD (REMD) [50], accelerated Molecular Dynamic (aMD) [49, 51], Free Energy Perturbation (FEP), Metadynamics-Based Methods, and Steered Molecular Dynamic (SMD) [21]. These methods can provide significant improvement over conventional MD methods, although they require huge computational resources. A good sampling of the protein structure is important to identify binding sites. If the sampling is not sufficiently done to fully explore all possible target conformations, one may miss a very valuable binding site on the target. Many reviews have focused on these different MD methods, and interested readers are directed to these references [21, 22, 52–54].

2.6 Cosolvent Molecular Dynamics Simulations

Flooding a protein structure with different probes during MD simulations emerged as a new way to detect binding sites while taking into account their flexibility. A promising example of such methods is the cosolvent MD simulation approach. In this method,

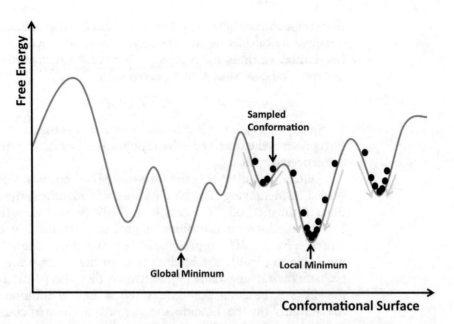

Fig. 5 The free-energy surface of protein. The local and global minimums are separated by free-energy barriers. During the MD simulations, conformations of targeted protein are sampled. The conformations cannot pass some large barriers and have to gather around local minimums. Because protein does not reach global minimum, the MD simulations are insufficient sampling

the protein structure is soaked in different concentrations of different explicit solvents, allowing these solvent molecules to diffuse and interact with hot spots on the protein surface. In this way, cosolvent MD simulations have two major advantages over the traditional binding site recognition methods, described above. First, cosolvent MD simulations do not require a training set to run. Meaning that, the method can be applied to all types of protein structures, without a prior knowledge about similar protein structures or potential binding sites [55]. The second and, perhaps, the most important feature of cosolvent MD simulations is that it fully accommodates protein flexibility, solvent effects and many other parameters during the simulation (*see* **Note 5**).

The used organic solvents can have different chemical properties and shapes, allowing the study of different possible interactions with the protein and also helping in predicating the maximum binding affinity for any identified binding site [1, 7, 9, 10]. During a typical simulation the different solvent molecules are spontaneously distributed and concentrated around possible binding sites. The elapsed time for solvent molecules to occupy the binding site is directly related to its druggability [9]. In this context, the identified binding sites are ranked by the occupation time and the increase in the local density of the interacting organic molecules. The druggability is also assessed by the maximum binding affinity as predicted from these interactions [35]. The maximum binding affinity can be obtained by calculating the associated free energy, ΔG_i. It counts the number of times the different solvents are attracted to a given hot spot and compares with expected value.

$$\Delta G_i = -k_B T \ln(N_i/N_o) \qquad (2)$$

In Eq. (2), k_B is the Boltzmann constant, T is the temperature, N_i represents the observed solvent population, while N_o represents the expected value.

Different studies using the cosolvent MD simulation technique helped in identifying new binding sites and identified the limitations of the method. For example, in 2009, Seco et al. performed MD simulations on five different proteins, dissolved in explicit binary solvents, 20% isopropanol–water (volume/volume). They were able to identify the binding sites on the target proteins and evaluate their druggability [9]. However, they also pointed out to the effect of the simulation time as well as the low diffusion rate of the solvents on the binding site prediction. In particular, they concluded that a low diffusion rate can limit solvent exchange and can also prevent the solvent probes from diffusing into cavities and gaps within the protein structure [9, 56].

2.7 Site Identification by Ligand Competitive Saturation

Guvench et al. developed a more refined MD-based method, namely the site identification by ligand competitive saturation (SILCS). The method uses explicit ternary solvents, comprising benzene, isopropanol, and water. The objective of combining these different solvent molecules was to provide a precise division of affinity properties among hydrophobic groups, aromatic groups, hydrogen bond donors, and hydrogen bond acceptors [57, 58]. They validated the SILCS method using a full flexible simulation for Bcl-6. While including different solvent molecules improved the prediction of interaction energies, it did not overcome the diffusions' limitation [36]. Raman et al. brought up an improvement to the SILCS method in 2013, where more diverse solvent molecules were used [59].

A related approach, with some distinct technical details, is called MixMD and involved an explicitly binary solvent, 50% acetonitrile–water (weight/weight). In enhanced method, Lexa et al. added isopropanol too into the MixMD approach and tested on five proteins. They indicated multiple short MD simulations might be more efficient in sampling binding sites than few but long MD simulations [58]. These two methods have been successfully applied to ligand design and reproducing crystallographic binding sites of small organic molecules [56].

A similar method, named MDmix, employed two binary solvent systems, 20% acetonitrile–water and 20% isopropanol–water (volume/volume). Two proteins were tested, namely, the heat shock protein 90 N-terminal domain (Hsp90) and the HIV-1 protease (HIVpr). MDmix method showed more accurate interaction map and provided affordable water displaceability predictions compared with normal energy-based methods, such as Grid [27, 56].

2.8 WaterMap

WaterMap is another MD-based approach for binding site identification. The method employs explicit water as the only solvent molecules interacting with the protein. WaterMap relies on the tendency for druggable binding sites to have a higher density of thermodynamic unstable hydration sites. Accordingly, the method uses statistical analysis techniques to identify these locations within a given target [60].

3 Cases Studies

Following the description of the different MD-based methods for binding site identification, the next section will provide recent case studies from the literature.

3.1 A Catalytic Site Problem: Viral Neuraminidase

As mentioned above, catalytic active sites are the primary type of druggable targets in drug development and they always have significant geometric features over allosteric sites. Neuraminidase enzymes represent an example of such targets and are usually targeted as the antigenic determinants on the surface of the influenza virus. Neuraminidase has one catalytic site that cleaves sialic acid and promotes new virus particles release [61]. Oseltamivir and zanamivir are both effective orthosteric inhibitors that bind to the active site (Fig. 6).

Neuraminidase exhibits a high degree of selectivity among structurally similar compounds. The N1 subtype specifically binds

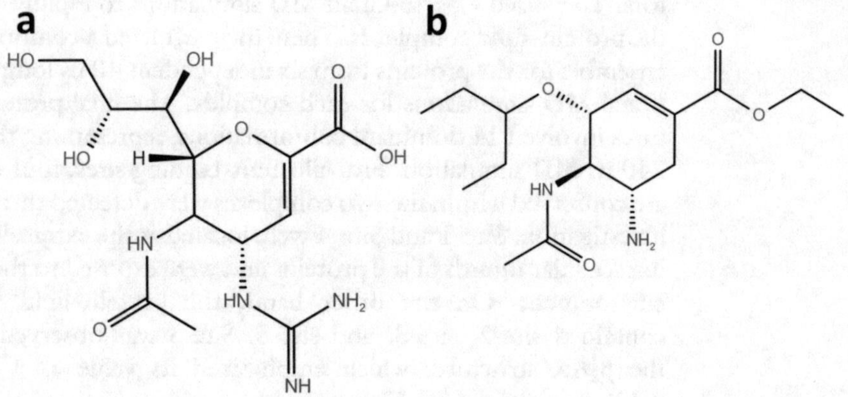

Fig. 6 2D chemical structure of oseltamivir (**a**) and zanamivir (**b**). They are both orthosteric inhibitors bind to the active site of neuraminidase. Generated by Maestro

with Tamiflu and mutations at the binding site can cause resistance against the drug. Therefore, enhancing drug selectivity and searching for novel binding sites are important research areas for influenza treatment. In the search for new binding sites in Neuraminidase for the H5N1 strain, Landon et al. combined extended explicit solvent molecular dynamics (MD) and computational solvent mapping (CS-Map) techniques to identify putative "hot-spots" within flexible binding regions of N1 neuraminidase. They used representative conformations of the N1 binding region as extracted from the clustering of 40 ns MD trajectories. They then employed CS-Map to assess the ability of small solvent-sized molecules to bind close to the sialic acid binding region. Mapping analyses of the dominant MD conformations revealed the presence of additional hot spot around binding region. Hot spot analysis provided further support for the feasibility of developing high-affinity inhibitors that were capable of binding to these regions, which appeared to be unique to the N1 strain [62]. Furthermore, MD simulations also revealed the function of crystal water molecules in the active site. Interestingly, Landon et al. found that more potent ligands did not interact strongly with these cocrystallized water molecules [61, 62]. They were also able to study the effects of mutations on the interactions with these compounds [63].

3.2 An Allosteric Site Problem: G-Protein Coupled Receptor (GPCR)

G-protein coupled receptors (GPCRs) are major targets for drug development [64]. They are associated with approximately 30% of current drugs and are linked to many diseases related to cardiovascular and central nervous systems and cancer [31, 33, 64, 65]. GPCRs are transmembrane proteins with a conservative topology composition, comprising of seven transmembrane alpha-helixes, and highly dynamics structure [33, 66]. Ivetac and McCammon used an ensemble-based approach combined with the FTMAP algorithm to study binding sites in two different GPCRs, namely, the β_1 (β_1AR) and the β_2 (β_2AR) adrenergic receptors. They used Coarse-Grain MD simulations to rapidly assemble the protein–lipid complexes. Then, they extracted a conformational ensemble for the proteins from six independent 40 ns long conventional MD simulations for each complex. The final protein structures involved 14 dominant conformations, representing the whole 240 ns MD simulation. Five allosteric binding sites, four of which are conserved within the two complexes were detected through this investigation. Site-1 and Site-4 were located at the extracellular and intracellular mouth of the proteins and were exposed to the solvent environment. On the other hand, the protein–lipid interface contained site-2, site-3, and site-5. Site-5 was observed only in the β_2AR structure, which emphasized its value as a selective β_2AR-targeted pocket [31].

3.3 A Cryptic Site Problem: Bcl-xL Protein

As discussed above, a cryptic site is defined as a hidden binding site when the protein is in the free/unbound state [20, 21]. Cimermancic et al. used machine learning to predict new cryptic sites based on the features of available cryptic sites [67]. These features included their amino acid sequences, structures, and dynamical attributes. Their major finding was that cryptic sites tend to be as conserved in evaluation as traditional binding pockets but are also less hydrophobic and more flexible [67]. Oleinikovas et al. characterized several additional characteristics for cryptic sites. They concluded that the appearance of a cryptic site does not correspond to a local minimum in the computed conformational free energy landscape. They also found that temperature-based enhanced sampling approaches, such as Parallel Tempering, do not improve the situation, as the entropic term does not help in the opening of these sites. Interestingly, they found that a conventional MD simulation can occasionally lead to the opening of a cryptic site [9, 21].

As the Bcl-2 family of proteins, Bcl-xL is a key regulator of programmed cell death [68]. MD simulations were performed on the apo-Bcl-xL structure in water and in cosolvent to detect binding sites on the protein. In water, the binding site of the apo-Bcl-xL had relatively minor conformational changes. Simulations of three holo-Bcl-xL structures in water, however, showed that the protein exhibited significant dynamic transition of conformations, including burying of several solvent exposed hydrophobic residues in the binding groove. In contrast, the apo-Bcl-xL in cosolvent, the hydrophobic surface tends to exposing itself to the interface, which is similar to the tendency in the crystal complex of Bcl-xL. However, the free energy differences of the Bcl-xL conformations obtained from both solation methods were small, which indicates the perturbation of cosolvent molecules is acceptable to Bcl-xL structure in relatively short MD simulations [58]. Furthermore, the novel binding hot spots that were revealed by cosolvent MD simulation did not find in the cocrystallized complex [39]. Taken together, this study suggested that cosolvent is very capable method in identifying cryptic sites, particularly, for flexible and hydrophobic targets.

4 Conclusion

The surface of a protein target encompasses many hot spots. These spots are essential in mediating the interactions between the target protein and other proteins as well as small molecule drugs. A binding site is formed by the grouping of these hot spots within the surface of the protein. There are many types of such sites. The most complicated ones include cryptic and allosteric sites. Both types do not induce direct effects on the activity of the target protein; however, they indirectly influence the activity by inducing conformational changes within the protein structure.

Identifying these sites and evaluating their druggability is very complicated. Current tools employ both geometrical-based and energy-based approaches to identify a binding site and assess its druggability. While these methods can easily study catalytic sites, they can poorly identify and study more complicated sites. This is mainly due to the fact that they rely on a static structure of the target protein, while an accurate prediction of these sites requires the accommodation of protein flexibility during the binding site search process. It also requires studying the structural dynamics of the different hot spots for a protonated time scale.

In this context, molecular dynamics (MD) simulations became an important tool in structure-based drug design to understand backbone and side chain flexibilities for a given target. MD simulations can be combined with current binding site identification tools to study every single snapshot. This approach led to the successful identification of novel sites in important targets.

This chapter focuses on overviewing the different methods used to identify and evaluate binding sites within a given target. It also highlights the importance of incorporating protein flexibility within the search process and the use of MD simulation in this process.

5 Notes

1. Traditional binding site identification methods can be classified into either geometrical-based or energy-based methods. These methods employ a static structure of the target protein and identify hot spots on its surface.

2. Accounting for the protein flexibility can significantly improve the binding site identification outcomes. Molecular dynamics (MD) simulations is a reliable tool to explore the protein dynamics and help identify cryptic sites that are now obviously shown in a crystal structure.

3. Despite the great benefit of using MD simulations to accommodate for protein flexibility, MD simulations are limited. The main limitation of MD is due to its reliance on a force field to describe the atomic interactions within the simulated system. This is a classical representation of the system, which only allows the study of the atoms movements, without any reference to their electronic dynamics. Although this simplification improves the computational speed for MD simulations and also allows the expansion of its size, this approximation does not allow the simulation of bond breakage and bond formation reactions.

4. Theoretically, multiple short MD simulations are better than one extensive MD simulation. This is mainly because multiple MD simulations can search different directions of the conformational space.

5. Cosolvent MD simulations use small molecules to search for potential binding sites. These molecular probes can help us in revealing buried binding sites.

References

1. Nisius B, Sha F, Gohlke H (2012) Structure-based computational analysis of protein binding sites for function and druggability prediction. J Biotechnol 159(3):123–134

2. Wells JA, McClendon CL (2007) Reaching for high-hanging fruit in drug discovery at protein-protein interfaces. Nature 450 (7172):1001–1009

3. Hajduk PJ, Huth JR, Tse C (2005) Predicting protein druggability. Drug Discov Today 10 (23–24):1675–1682

4. Barakat KH, Mane JY, Tuszynski JA (2011) Virtual screening: an overview on methods and applications, in handbook of research on computational and systems biology. In: Liu L, Wei D, Li Y, Lei H (eds) Handbook of research on computational and systems biology. IGI Global, New York, pp 28–60

5. Ahmed M, Wang F, Levin A et al (2015) Targeting the Achilles heel of the hepatitis B virus: a review of current treatments against covalently closed circular DNA. Drug Discov Today 20(5):548–561

6. Barakat K (2014) Computer-aided drug design. J Pharma Care Health Sys 1(4):1000e113

7. Bakan A, Nevins N, Lakdawala AS, Bahar I (2012) Druggability assessment of allosteric proteins by dynamics simulations in the presence of probe molecules. J Chem Theory Comput 8(7):2435–2447

8. Brown SP, Hajduk PJ (2006) Effects of conformational dynamics on predicted protein druggability. ChemMedChem 1(1):70–72

9. Seco J, Luque FJ, Barril X (2009) Binding site detection and druggability index from first principles. J Med Chem 52(8):2363–2371

10. Henrich S, Salo-Ahen OM, Huang B, Rippmann FF, Cruciani G, Wade RC (2010) Computational approaches to identifying and characterizing protein binding sites for ligand design. J Mol Recognit 23(2):209–219

11. Halgren TA (2009) Identifying and characterizing binding sites and assessing druggability. J Chem Inf Model 49(2):377–389

12. Barakat KH, Law J, Prunotto A et al (2013) Detailed computational study of the active site of the hepatitis C viral RNA polymerase to aid novel drug design. J Chem Inf Model 53 (11):3031–3043

13. Viricel CM, Ahmed M, Barakat K (2015) Human PD-1 binds differently to its human ligands: a comprehensive modeling study. J Mol Graph Model 57C:131–142

14. Ahmed M, Barakat K (2015) Baby steps toward modelling the full human programmed Death-1 (PD-1) pathway. Receptors Clin Investig 2 (3)

15. Barakat KH, Huzil JT, Jordan KE, Evangelinos C, Houghton M, Tuszynski J (2013) A computational model for overcoming drug resistance using selective dual-inhibitors for aurora kinase A and its T217D variant. Mol Pharm 10(12):4572–4589

16. Gajewski MM, Tuszynski J, Barakat K, Huzil JT, Klobukowski M (2013) Interactions of laulimalide, peloruside, and their derivatives with the isoforms of β-tubulin. Can J Chem 91 (7):511–517

17. Gentile F, Tuszynski JA, Barakat KH (2016) New design of nucleotide excision repair (NER) inhibitors for combination cancer therapy. J Mol Graph Model 65:71–82

18. Hu G, Wang K, Groenendyk J (2014) Human structural proteome-wide characterization of cyclosporine a targets. Bioinformatics 30 (24):3561–3566

19. McClendon CL, Friedland G, Mobley DL, Amirkhani H, Jacobson MP (2009) Quantifying correlations between allosteric sites in thermodynamic ensembles. J Chem Theory Comput 5(9):2486–2502

20. Eyrisch S, Helms V (2007) Transient pockets on protein surfaces involved in protein-protein interaction. J Med Chem 50(15):3457–3464

21. Oleinikovas V, Saladino G, Cossins BP, Gervasio FL (2016) Understanding cryptic pocket formation in protein targets by enhanced sampling simulations. J Am Chem Soc 138 (43):14257–14263

22. Ganesan A, Coote ML, Barakat K (2017) Molecular dynamics-driven drug discovery: leaping forward with confidence. Drug Discov Today 22(2):249–269

23. Perot S, Sperandio O, Miteva MA, Camproux AC, Villoutreix BO (2010) Druggable pockets and binding site centric chemical space: a paradigm shift in drug discovery. Drug Discov Today 15(15–16):656–667

24. Brady GP Jr, Stouten PF (2000) Fast prediction and visualization of protein binding pockets with PASS. J Comput Aided Mol Des 14 (4):383–401

25. Levitt DG, Banaszak LJ (1992) POCKET: a computer graphics method for identifying and displaying protein cavities and their surrounding amino acids. J Mol Graph 10(4):229–234

26. Hendlich MF, Rippmann BG (1997) LIG-SITE: automatic and efficient detection of potential small molecule-binding sites in proteins. J Mol Graph Model 15(6):359–363. 389

27. Goodford PJ (1985) A computational procedure for determining energetically favorable binding sites on biologically important macromolecules. J Med Chem 28(7):849–857

28. Laurie AT, Jackson RM (2005) Q-SiteFinder: an energy-based method for the prediction of protein-ligand binding sites. Bioinformatics 21 (9):1908–1916

29. Villoutreix BO, Kuenemann MA, Poyet JL (2004) Drug-like protein-protein interaction modulators: challenges and opportunities for drug discovery and chemical biology. Mol Inform 33(6–7):414–437

30. Bourgeas R, Basse MJ, Morelli X, Roche P (2010) Atomic analysis of protein-protein interfaces with known inhibitors: the 2P2I database. PLoS One 5(3):e9598

31. Ivetac A, McCammon JA (2010) Mapping the druggable allosteric space of G-protein coupled receptors: a fragment-based molecular dynamics approach. Chem Biol Drug Des 76 (3):201–217

32. Landon MR, Lancia DR, Yu J, Thiel SC, Vajda S (2007) Identification of hot spots within druggable binding regions by computational solvent mapping of proteins. J Med Chem 50 (6):1231–1240

33. Miao Y, Nichols SE, McCammon JA (2014) Mapping of allosteric druggable sites in activation-associated conformers of the M2 muscarinic receptor. Chem Biol Drug Des 83 (2):237–246

34. Kozakov D, Grove LE, Hall DR et al (2015) The FTMap family of web servers for determining and characterizing ligand-binding hot spots of proteins. Nat Protoc 10(5):733–755

35. Cheng AC, Coleman RG, Smyth KT et al (2007) Structure-based maximal affinity model predicts small-molecule druggability. Nat Biotechnol 25(1):71–75

36. Makley LN, Gestwicki JE (2013) Expanding the number of 'druggable' targets: non-enzymes and protein-protein interactions. Chem Biol Drug Des 81(1):22–32

37. Fauman EB, Rai BK, Huang ES (2011) Structure-based druggability assessment--identifying suitable targets for small molecule therapeutics. Curr Opin Chem Biol 15 (4):463–468

38. Craig IR, Pfleger C, Gohlke H, Essex JW, Spiegel K (2011) Pocket-space maps to identify novel binding-site conformations in proteins. J Chem Inf Model 51(10):2666–2679

39. Yang CY, Wang S (2011) Hydrophobic binding hot spots of Bcl-xL protein-protein interfaces by Cosolvent molecular dynamics simulation. ACS Med Chem Lett 2 (4):280–284

40. Schames JR, Henchman RH, Siegel JS, Sotrifer CA, Ni H, McCammon A (2004) Discovery of a novel binding trench in HIV integrase. J Med Chem 47(8):1879–1881

41. Durrant JD, Keranen H, Wilson BA, McCammon JA (2010) Computational identification of uncharacterized cruzain binding sites. PLoS Negl Trop Dis 4(5):e676

42. Grant BJ, Lukman S, Hocker HJ et al (2011) Novel allosteric sites on Ras for lead generation. PLoS One 6(10):e25711

43. Schmidtke P, Bidon Chanal A, Luque FJ, Barril X (2011) MDpocket: open-source cavity detection and characterization on molecular dynamics trajectories. Bioinformatics 27 (23):3276–3285

44. Grove LE, Hall DR, Beglov D, Vajda S, Kozakov D (2013) FTFlex: accounting for binding site flexibility to improve fragment-based identification of druggable hot spots. Bioinformatics 29(9):1218–1219

45. De Vivo M, Masetti M, Bottegoni G, Cavalli A (2016) Role of molecular dynamics and related methods in drug discovery. J Med Chem 59 (9):4035–4061

46. Lukman S, Nguyen MN, Sim K, Teo JC (2017) Discovery of Rab1 binding sites using an ensemble of clustering methods. Proteins 85 (5):859–871

47. Lee DD, Seung HS (1999) Learning the parts of objects by non-negative matrix factorization. Nature 401(6755):788–791

48. Hyvarinen A, Oja E (2000) Independent component analysis: algorithms and applications. Neural Netw 13(4–5):411–430

49. Ortiz-Sanchez JM, Nichols SE, Sayyah J, Brown JH, McCammon JA, Grant BJ (2012) Identification of potential small molecule binding pockets on rho family GTPases. PLoS One 7(7):e40809

50. Sugita Y, Okamoto Y (2000) Replica-exchange multicanonical algorithm and multicanonical replica-exchange method for simulating systems with rough energy landscape. Chem Phys Lett 329(3–4):261–270

51. Voter AF (1997) Hyperdynamics: accelerated molecular dynamics of infrequent events. Phys Rev Lett 78(20):3908–3911

52. Kerrigan JE (2013) Molecular dynamics simulations in drug design. Methods Mol Biol 993:95–113

53. Mortier J, Rakers C, Bermudez M, Murgueitio MS, Riniker S, Wolber G (2015) The impact of molecular dynamics on drug design: applications for the characterization of ligand-macromolecule complexes. Drug Discov Today 20(6):686–702

54. Zhao H, Caflisch A (2015) Molecular dynamics in drug design. Eur J Med Chem 91:4–14

55. Li H, Kasam V, Tautermann CS, Seeliger D, Vaidehi N (2014) Computational method to identify druggable binding sites that target protein-protein interactions. J Chem Inf Model 54(5):1391–1400

56. Alvarez-Garcia D, Barril X (2014) Molecular simulations with solvent competition quantify water displaceability and provide accurate interaction maps of protein binding sites. J Med Chem 57(20):8530–8539

57. Guvench O, MacKerell AD Jr (2009) Computational fragment-based binding site identification by ligand competitive saturation. PLoS Comput Biol 5(7):e1000435

58. Lexa KW, Carlson HA (2011) Full protein flexibility is essential for proper hot-spot mapping. J Am Chem Soc 133(2):200–202

59. Raman EP, Yu W, Lakkaraju SK, MacKerell AD Jr (2013) Inclusion of multiple fragment types in the site identification by ligand competitive saturation (SILCS) approach. J Chem Inf Model 53(12):3384–3398

60. Beuming T, Che Y, Abel R, Kim B, Shanmugasundaram V, Sherman W (2012) Thermodynamic analysis of water molecules at the surface of proteins and applications to binding site prediction and characterization. Proteins 80(3):871–883

61. Masukawa KM, Kollman PA, Kuntz ID (2003) Investigation of neuraminidase-substrate recognition using molecular dynamics and free energy calculations. J Med Chem 46(26):5628–5637

62. Landon MR, Amaro RE, Baron R et al (2008) Novel druggable hot spots in avian influenza neuraminidase H5N1 revealed by computational solvent mapping of a reduced and representative receptor ensemble. Chem Biol Drug Des 71(2):106–116

63. Shu M, Lin Z, Zhang Y, Wu Y, Mei H, Jiang Y (2011) Molecular dynamics simulation of oseltamivir resistance in neuraminidase of avian influenza H5N1 virus. J Mol Model 17(3):587–592

64. Dror RO, Pan AC, Arlow DH et al (2011) Pathway and mechanism of drug binding to G-protein-coupled receptors. Proc Natl Acad Sci U S A 108(32):13118–13123

65. Overington JP, Al-Lazikani B, Hopkins AL (2006) Opinion - how many drug targets are there? Nat Rev Drug Discov 5(12):993–996

66. Kappel K, Miao Y, McCammon JA (2015) Accelerated molecular dynamics simulations of ligand binding to a muscarinic G-protein-coupled receptor. Q Rev Biophys 48(4):479–487

67. Cimermancic P, Weinkam P, Rettenmaier TJ (2016) CryptoSite: expanding the druggable proteome by characterization and prediction of cryptic binding sites. J Mol Biol 428(4):709–719

68. Petros AM, Olejniczak ET, Fesik SW (2004) Structural biology of the Bcl-2 family of proteins. Biochim Biophys Acta 1644(2–3):83–94

Chapter 7

Virtual Ligand Screening Using PL-PatchSurfer2, a Molecular Surface-Based Protein–Ligand Docking Method

Woong-Hee Shin and Daisuke Kihara

Abstract

Virtual screening is a computational technique for predicting a potent binding compound for a receptor protein from a ligand library. It has been a widely used in the drug discovery field to reduce the efforts of medicinal chemists to find hit compounds by experiments.

  Here, we introduce our novel structure-based virtual screening program, PL-PatchSurfer, which uses molecular surface representation with the three-dimensional Zernike descriptors, which is an effective mathematical representation for identifying physicochemical complementarities between local surfaces of a target protein and a ligand. The advantage of the surface-patch description is its tolerance on a receptor and compound structure variation. PL-PatchSurfer2 achieves higher accuracy on apo form and computationally modeled receptor structures than conventional structure-based virtual screening programs. Thus, PL-PatchSurfer2 opens up an opportunity for targets that do not have their crystal structures. The program is provided as a stand-alone program at http://kiharalab.org/plps2. We also provide files for two ligand libraries, ChEMBL and ZINC Drug-like.

  Key words Drug discovery, Molecular surface, Protein–ligand interaction, Three-dimensional Zernike descriptor, Virtual screening, 3DZD

1 Introduction

Virtual screening is a computational technique that searches active compounds for a target protein from a large virtual compound library [1]. It has been widely used to help the efforts of medicinal chemists to experimentally test and synthesize a large number of compounds by reducing the chemical space to explore. The technique is classified into two categories: ligand-based virtual screening (LBVS) and structure-based virtual screening (SBVS). LBVS compares the compounds in library with known drugs that have been previously discovered. Therefore, to use LBVS, prior knowledge of the known drugs is required. LBVS methods compare ligands in their 1D [2, 3], 2D [4, 5], or 3D structure representations [6, 7]. On the other hand, SBVS methods use the 3D

Mohini Gore and Umesh B. Jagtap (eds.), *Computational Drug Discovery and Design*, Methods in Molecular Biology, vol. 1762, https://doi.org/10.1007/978-1-4939-7756-7_7, © Springer Science+Business Media, LLC, part of Springer Nature 2018

structure of a target receptor protein and compute complementarities between the ligand binding pocket of the receptor and ligands in a library. The fit of a ligand to the binding pocket of the receptor is measured by estimating the binding energy in protein–ligand docking [8–10] or by evaluating geometrical matching of pharmacophores [11, 12]. One of the most widely used classes of SBVS methods is protein–ligand docking. In protein–ligand docking, interaction between a receptor and a ligand is evaluated by sampling binding poses of the ligand in the pocket and calculating the binding affinity of the poses. Generally the binding affinity is computed with a pairwise atom-based energy function.

Here, we explain how to use our novel SBVS method, PL-PatchSurfer2 [13]. Instead of employing an atomic-based interaction description, this program adopts molecular surface description. Four physicochemical features of molecules, both a receptor and ligands, are calculated and assigned on the surface: geometric shape, the electrostatic potential, hydrogen bonding ability (donors or acceptors), and the hydrophobicity. The complementarity between a pocket and a ligand is calculated by comparing chemical characters of local surface patches. A schematic illustration of PL-PatchSurfer2 is shown in Fig. 1.

The chemical features on each surface patch of a receptor and ligands are converted to three-dimensional Zernike descriptors (3DZD). 3DZD is a rotationally invariant representation of a 3D function in the Euclidean space (i.e., physicochemical properties mapped on the 3D molecular surface), which is essentially a vector

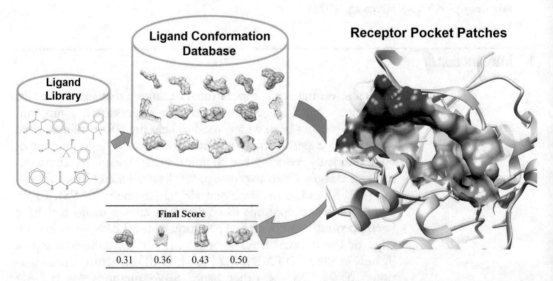

Fig. 1 Illustration of PL-PatchSurfer2. Multiple three-dimensional conformations of ligands are generated by OMEGA. The surfaces of each ligand in a conformation and a receptor pocket are divided into patches. Local surface patches between the binding pocket of the protein and ligands are matched and the ligands are ranked in an ascending order of their scores

of coefficients from a series expansion of the 3D function into 3D Zernike basis function [14]. Our group has applied 3DZD to solve various structural biology problems, such as ligand similarity calculation [15], pocket–pocket comparison [16], electron microscopy density map comparison [17], and protein–protein docking [18]. An asset of PL-PatchSurfer2 is that it is tolerant to conformational changes of a receptor protein. Thus, the program showed better performance than conventional protein–ligand docking programs including AutoDock Vina [13], when the receptor structure is computationally modeled or in an apo-form, which can be substantially different from the ligand-bound form of the protein.

2 Materials

PL-PatchSurfer2 is available for academic users at our lab website, http://kiharalab.org/plps2/ (Fig. 2). The program and associated files are compressed in a file named *PLPS.tar.gz* and can be downloaded from a link shown as label 1 in Fig. 2. To decompress the file, in a GUI interface, right-click and select an option for decompress or double click to decompress the file. In Linux command line, type *tar –zxf PLPS.tar.gz*. All binary files are for the Linux OS.

Decompressing the file creates a directory named *PL-PatchSurfer2*. In the directory, there are four directories and *README* file. *apbs_tool* gives utilities to run APBS [19], which will be described later, *bin* and *scripts* contain executable files and python scripts to

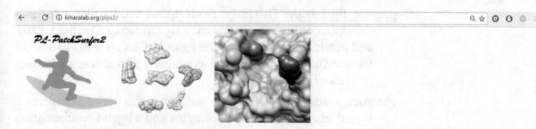

PL-PatchSurfer2: A virtual screening program based on local surface matching

PL-PatchSurfer2 is a protein ligand virtual screening program that uses local surface matching between ligand and receptor pocket. It uses three-dimensional Zernike descriptor to calculate complementarity of the patches. Detailed description of the program is given in the reference below:

• W.-H. Shin, C. W. Christoffer, J. Wang, and D. Kihara*, PL-PatchSurfer2: Improved Local Surface Matching-Based Virtual Screening Method that is Tolerant to Target and Ligand Structure Variation. J. Chem. Info. Model. 56(9): 1676-91 (2016).

Binary executable files, running python scripts, and example can be freely downloadable at the following link.

PL-PatchSurfer2 **1**

Pre-generated ligand library from ZINC Druglike subset and ChEMBL19.

ZINC Druglike (123472 molecules, 18GB)
ChEMBL19 (80159 molecules, 17GB) **2**

Contact Information

If you have any questions or suggestions, please feel free to contact us (dkihara@purdue.edu).

Fig. 2 The PL-PatchSurfer2 webpage

run PL-PatchSurfer2, and *example* provides a step-by-step example of a virtual screening process. The details of the required program and input file will be described in next section.

On the PL-PatchSurfer2 webpage, pregenerated ligand library files are also made available (Label 2 of Fig. 2). *druglike.tar.gz* and *chembl.tar.gz* contain preprocessed files for ~120,000 and ~80,000 compounds, respectively. The libraries can be used for a virtual screening after decompressing file by typing *tar –zxf druglike.tar. gz* or *chembl.tar.gz*. Descriptions of how to use them will be given in Methods.

2.1 Input Files and Python Scripts of PL-PatchSurfer2

PL-PatchSurfer2 requires a receptor structure file and ligands files to be screened against. The input receptor structure file should be in the PDB format without any hetero atoms in the HETATM fields. To define a binding pocket of the protein, a cognate ligand that is cocrystallized ligand should also be given in PDB format. Ligand files need to be in the MOL2 format, which contains the atom information, coordinates, and charge information. The final output of the program is a text file that has a ranking of the compounds.

To execute a virtual screening experiment, the following Python scripts will be used, which locate in the *scripts* directory:

prepare_receptor.py: This script takes a protein PDB file and a cognate ligand PDB file as inputs and generates an SSIC file that contains patch information of the protein binding pocket. The format of SSIC file is shown in Subheading 3.

prepare_ligands.py: This script reads ligand MOL2 files, generates multiple conformations for each ligand using OMEGA [20], and produces SSIC files of the ligands. SSIC is a PL-PatchSurfer specific file format and contains information of surface patches of a molecule.

compare_seeds.py: As its name indicates, this script compares a ligand-binding pocket of a receptor and a ligand conformation by the Auction algorithm [21]. It takes SSIC files of the pocket and the ligand as input.

rank_ligands.py: PL-PatchSurfer2 offers two scoring options that evaluate the fit between a binding pocket and a ligand: The Lowest Conformation Score (LCS) and The Boltzmann-weighted Score (BS). LCS ranks ligands using the best scoring conformation of a ligand, whereas BS sorts ligands by a Boltzmann-weighted scoring scheme [13].

2.2 Required Programs to Run PL-PatchSurfer2

In order to run PL-PatchSurfer2, five external programs are required: PDB2PQR, APBS, OPEN BABEL, XLOGP3, and OMEGA. A brief explanation of each program is given below. These programs can be replaced alternative ones with the same function.

APBS and PDB2PQR: APBS [19] calculates molecular surface and the electrostatic potential on molecular surface by solving the Poisson-Boltzmann equation. PDB2PQR convert a PDB file to a PQR-format file, an input file of APBS by adding atom charge and radius information to the PDB file. The programs can be obtained from http://www.poissonboltzmann.org/.

XLOGP3: The aim of this program to estimate log*P* value of a molecule [22] and assigns a log*P* value to each atom. PL-PatchSurfer2 calculates a hydrophobic field [23] from atomic log*P* values and assigns the field on a molecular surface. XLOGP3 is downloadable at http://www.sioc-ccbg.ac.cn/skins/ccbgwebsite/software/xlogp3/.

OMEGA: To consider ligand flexibility, we use OMEGA [20] to generate multiple conformations of a ligand molecule from a single MOL2 file. For academic users, a 1-year license is offered, and the program can be obtained from http://eyesopen.com.

OPEN BABEL [24]: This program is for converts file formats of ligand files and used internally in the python scripts. It can be downloaded from http://openbabel.org/

3   Methods

PL-PatchSurfer2 first computes SSIC files of a ligand binding pocket of a receptor and ligands, which contain surface patch information. The input receptor structure and ligand structures need to be prepared in the PDB and in the MOL2 format, respectively. Once the SSIC files are computed, the patches are compared between the binding pocket and ligands and the ligands are ranked by the score that evaluates compatibility between the pocket and ligands. The overview of PL-PatchSurfer2 is illustrated in Fig. 3.

3.1   Receptor Binding Pocket File Preparation

To run PL-PatchSurfer2, an SSIC file of a ligand binding pocket of a receptor protein needs to be prepared, which contains information about the position, the distribution, and physicochemical properties of surface patches represented in 3DZD. To prepare the SSIC file, three files are required: a receptor structure PDB file, a cognate ligand to define a binding pocket also in the PDB format, and an input file, which lists file locations etc. A receptor PDB file and a cognate ligand file can be obtained by any structure viewer such as UCSF Chimera [25]. Otherwise, it can be obtained using *split_lig.py* in the *script* directory in command window as follows:

```
python split_lig.py [PDB file] [Chain ID] [Ligand ID]
```

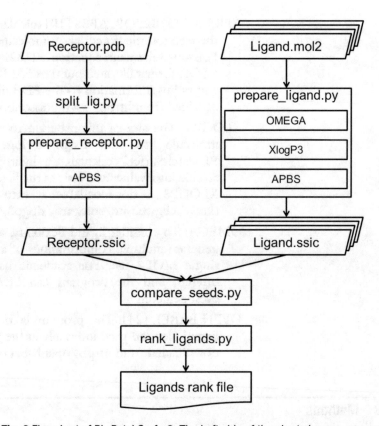

Fig. 3 Flowchart of PL-PatchSurfer2. The Left side of the chart shows a process for generating an SSIC file for a receptor, while the right side shows the ligand library preparation steps. "split_lig.py" extracts a cocrystallized ligand from a receptor PDB file. "prepare_receptor.py" detects a binding pocket from the extracted ligand, runs APBS to calculate pocket surface and electrostatic potential, and generates a receptor SSIC file. On the ligand side, multiple conformations of a ligand are generated by OMEGA, atomic log$P$ values are assigned by XlogP3, and molecular surface and the electrostatic potential are calculated by APBS. All these steps for ligand are executed in "prepare_ligand.py". A complementarity between the receptor and the ligands are calculated by "compare_seeds.py." "rank_ligands.py" gives the final result, a rank of the ligands in the library

[PDB file] is a name of PDB file that has a receptor and a ligand structure. [Chain ID] should be matched to a chain name in PDB file, and [Ligand ID] should also be matched to a three-letter code of a ligand in the PDB file. The script identifies ligand coordinates in the PDB file and writes them in a file named *xtal-lig.pdb*. The coordinates of the receptor structure without the ligand is written in *rec.pdb*.

The current version of PL-PatchSurfer2 requires a cocrystallized ligand structure with the receptor protein to define a receptor binding pocket. If the receptor structure does not have a bound ligand, such as a computationally modeled structure or an apo structure, the user can provide a potential bound ligand from a homologous protein structure found in the PDB database (*see* **Note 1**) or provide a center position of the putative binding pocket identified by a ligand binding site prediction program, such as VisGrid [26] (*see* **Note 1**).

After splitting the receptor and the ligand into separate PDB files, the SSIC file of the receptor is generated by running *prepare_receptor.py* in the *scripts* directory:

```
python prepare_receptor.py [Input file]
```

An example of the input file is shown below (*rec_prep.in* in the *example* directory):

```
PLPS_path ~/project/PL-PatchSurfer2/
PDB2PQR_path ~/apps/pdb2pqr
APBS_path /apps/apbs/apbs-1.4/bin
BABEL_path /usr/bin
receptor_file rec.pdb
ligand_file xtal-lig.pdb
```

The top line, *PLPS_path*, shows the path of PL-PatchSurfer2 is installed. Similarly, following three lines designate the locations of programs. They can be changed to match the user's environment. The last two lines, *receptor_file* and *ligand_file* are file names of the receptor and its cognate ligand.

The output of this script is an SSIC format file named after the input structure file. For example, if the PDB file's name is *rec.pdb*, then the output is named as *rec.ssic*. This file contains information of patches: the coordinates of the patch center, 3DZDs of chemical features (shape, electrostatic potential, hydrogen bonding, and hydrophobicity), and the distribution of geodesic distance of patches. An example of SSIC file is given below:

```
68 72 144 144 144
5.632 10.269 10.834
 0 72 0.16617 0.00000 0.26899 0.27014 0.01290 0.01691 0.20478 0.21539 0.21553
0.04274 ...
 3 144 0.04947 0.00000 0.07677 0.07714 0.00725 0.00944 0.05392 0.05716 0.05732
0.02009 ...
 5 144 0.00000 0.00000 0.00000 0.00000 0.00000 0.00000 0.00000 0.00000 0.00000
0.00000 ...
 6 144 0.00337 0.00000 0.00726 0.00726 0.00004 0.00006 0.01014 0.01017 0.01017
0.00022 ...
68 0 12 10 8 13 5 5 13 8 14 17 17 21 20 15 22 21 25 23 24 20 24 24 28 26 21 30 28
27 28 32 30 27 30 37 31 35 29 28 31 27 26 32 24 21 20 22 22 17 24 27 23 22 19 25 18
17 24 27 16 13 16 12 11 13 17 18 21
```

The first line indicates that the pocket is composed of 68 patches and chemical features, shape, electrostatic potential, hydrogen bonding, and hydrophobicity, are converted to 72-, 144-, 144-, and 144-dimensional 3DZD vectors, respectively. The second line is a (x, y, z) coordinate of the center of the patch. The following four lines starting with *0 72*, *3 144*, *5 144*, and *6 144* show 3DZD vectors of the geometric shape, the electrostatic potential, the hydrogen bonding, and the hydrophobicity. The last line, *11 13 17 18 21*, is a histogram of geodesic distance between the patch the patch center to the other patch centers of the pocket with a bin size of 1.0 Å. *convert_ssic_to_pdb.py* helps visualizing location of patches by generating PDB files that contains the coordinates of patch centers (*see* **Note 2**).

3.2 Ligand File Preparation

Similar to the receptor, input files for ligands should be prepared in the SSIC format from their MOL2 format files. A MOL2 file can be converted from a SMILES string, a one-dimensional representation of a molecule, using OpenBabel [24]. Alternatively, it can be also obtained from a public accessible library such as ZINC [27], ChEMBL [28], and PubChem [29].

Ligands files are prepared using *prepare_ligands.py* in the *scripts* directory, in the similar way as the receptor preparation:

```
python prepare_ligands.py [Input file]
```

The input file should have contents shown below (*lig_prep.in* in *example* directory):

```
PLPS_path ~/project/PL-PatchSurfer2/
PDB2PQR_path ~/apps/pdb2pqr
APBS_path /apps/apbs/apbs-1.4/bin
BABEL_path /usr/bin
XLOGP3_path ~/apps/XLOGP3/bin/
OMEGA_path ~/apps/openeye/arch/Ubuntu-12.04-x64/omega
n_conf 50
ligand_file ZINC03833861.mol2
ligand_file ZINC03815630.mol2
```

Up to the fourth line from the top of the file are the locations of the programs: PL-PatchSurfer2, PDB2PQR, APBS, and OPEN BABEL. The fifth and the sixth lines show the locations of programs, XLOGP3 and OMEGA. *n_conf* is a parameter for OMEGA. The program generates multiple conformations of a ligand to reflect its flexibility and *n_conf* determines the maximum number of conformations to be produced. Ligand MOL2 files are listed after that, with *ligand_file* as a header of a line. There is no limit for the number of ligands to process.

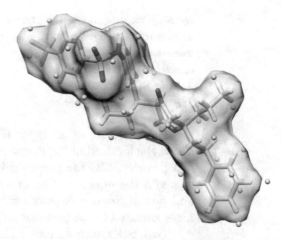

Fig. 4 Seed points of local surface patches distributed on the surface of a compound, ZINC03815630. There are 35 patches and blue dots show the centers of the patches (seed points)

Running the scripts will generate a directory, for each ligand in the ligand list in the *lig_prep.in* file, each of which contains conformation files in the PDB format and patch information files in the SSIC format. Thus, the number of directories generated equals the number of ligands in the library. Patches of a ligand conformation are generated and distributed along the molecular surface as Fig. 4. An example of a ligand SSIC file is given below. This is the same format as a receptor SSIC file:

```
35 72 144 144 144
8.908 0.088 1.140
0  72 0.14882 0.00000 0.25880 0.25937 0.00286 0.00380 0.22792 0.23418 0.23420
0.01081...
3 144 0.03049 0.00000 0.05685 0.05688 0.00016 0.00043 0.05894 0.05928 0.05928
0.00070...
5 144 0.00000 0.00000 0.00000 0.00000 0.00000 0.00000 0.00000 0.00000 0.00000
0.00000...
6 144 0.05316 0.00000 0.09245 0.09265 0.00102 0.00136 0.08142 0.08365 0.08366
0.00386...
35 0 4 4 20 7 5 20 28 25 23 23 29 8 20 24 28 28 16 13 12 18 12 14 19 8 12 18 14
28 31 27 16 29 5 17
```

3.3 Comparing Patches

After generating SSIC files of a receptor and ligands, complementarities between are measured to find active ligands. In PL-Patch-Surfer, the auction algorithm [21] is employed to match surface patches between the protein and each ligand. To compare and identify compatible surface patches between a receptor and ligands, *compare_seeds.py* in *scripts* is executed as follows.

```
python compare_seeds.py [Input file]
PLPS_path ~/project/PL-PatchSurfer2/
receptor_file rec.ssic
n_conf 50
ligand_dir ZINC03833861
ligand_dir ZINC03815630
```

The structure of an input file is shown above. The first line shows the location of PL-PatchSurfer2 is installed, and *receptor_file* is a protein SSIC file prepared in the receptor preparation step. *n_conf* is the number of maximum conformations for each ligand and *ligand_dir* is a directory for ligand conformations and SSIC files generated in the previous step.

Two types output files will be generated by executing the python script. The first set of output files are named as a combination of a receptor name, ligand name, and the conformation number. For example, for a case that a receptor's name is ERa and a ligand's name is estrogen, output file names will be ERa_estrogen_-conf_01.dat for the first conformation of the ligand. If the user runs this script with the same parameter as the provided example, the output file name will be rec_ZINC03815630_conf_01.dat and so on. They are saved in the directory of ligand conformations. An example of the output file is illustrated below.

```
54 19 0.373 0.277 0.227 0.287 0.197 0.127 0.297 0.000 14.097
59 16 0.328 0.349 0.160 0.249 0.294 0.095 0.169 0.000 12.716
60 26 0.412 0.240 0.223 0.273 0.108 0.102 0.190 0.360 14.616
61 7 0.324 0.223 0.178 0.227 0.153 0.111 0.249 0.000 17.601
62 8 0.398 0.235 0.286 0.328 0.189 0.074 0.156 0.000 12.513
65 22 0.382 0.307 0.186 0.259 0.194 0.232 0.199 0.000 8.476
SUM: 8.807 AVG: 0.275 avgRP: 2.915 navgRP: 1.872 AVGSd 0.226 0.142 0.186 0.214
```

The first two columns except for the last line are patch indices of the receptor protein and the ligand in a certain conformation that are paired by the auction algorithm. The next four columns show a total score of matched pairs, and three individual terms of the score (weighted sum of 3DZD difference, geodesic distance distribution difference, and geodesic distance difference between matched pairs). Values in the next four columns show the 3DZD differences (dissimilarity) of the two patches in terms of shape, the electrostatic potential, hydrophobicity, and hydrogen bond term, from left to right, respectively. The last column is the Euclidean distance of the patch centers. The last line summarizes the score of the two patches by averaging three scoring terms used in PL-PatchSurfer2: 3DZD difference, geodesic distance difference, and approximate position difference calculated by the geodesic distance histogram [13].

Another output is a summary file provided for each ligand screened. It is named as a combination of the receptor file name and the ligand name, for example, *rec_ZINC03815630.dat*. The file lists the conformation of the ligand and the four scoring terms.

```
 1  0.37611  0.18108  0.13645  0.45588
 2  0.35956  0.18906  0.12975  0.50000
 3  0.38208  0.18667  0.15510  0.47059
 4  0.39500  0.19485  0.16095  0.42647
 5  0.39779  0.19794  0.13975  0.50000
 6  0.40681  0.19178  0.15785  0.47059
 7  0.40150  0.19709  0.14375  0.50000
 8  0.38156  0.19872  0.13715  0.47059
 9  0.41342  0.18456  0.12550  0.47059
10  0.39468  0.19456  0.13200  0.50000
```

The first column is the conformation index. Following columns are 3DZD difference, APPD (approximate position difference), GRPD (geodesic distance difference), and size difference between the pocket and a ligand in that conformation, respectively. The overall score of a conformation is calculated as a weighted sum of these four values.

3.4 Ranking Ligands

The last step of PL-PatchSurfer2 is ranking ligands for the target binding pocket in the receptor. The top ranked ligands are predicted to bind to the target binding pocket. The program provides two options for scoring ligands: the lowest conformer score, which ranks ligands based on the lowest scored conformer among conformations examined, and the Boltzmann weighted scoring, which averages the scores given to different conformations of each ligand by putting exponential weight to each conformation.

$$\text{Boltzmann-Weighted Score } (P, L)$$

$$= \frac{\sum_{C}^{N_{\text{conf}}} \text{CS}(P, C) \times \exp[-\beta \times \text{CS}(P, C)]}{\sum_{C}^{N_{\text{conf}}} \exp[-\beta \times \text{CS}(P, C)]}$$

where P, L, and C stand for pocket, ligand, and ligand in a certain conformation, respectively. $\text{CS}(P,C)$ is a *Conformer Score*, the score between the pocket P and the ligand in the conformation C. N_{conf} is the number of ligand conformations. β determines a weight to be given to each conformer, which is set to 1.

To execute ranking of ligands, run *rank_ligands.py* in the *scripts* directory as follows:

```
python rank_ligands.py [input file]
```

An example of an input file is illustrated below (*lcs.in* provided in the *example* directory):

```
receptor_file rec.ssic
scoring_type lcs
ligand_dir ZINC03833861
ligand_dir ZINC03815630
output_file lcs.rank
```

receptor_file, *ligand_dir*, and *output_file* are the names of the receptor SSIC file, the ligand conformation directories, and the output file that has a ranked list of screened ligands. *scoring_type* designates the type of the scoring function, either *lcs* or *bs*, for the lowest conformer score or the Boltzmann-weighted score, selected by the user.

The output file of *bs* scoring type has two columns. The first column shows the name of the ligands, while the second column shows the score of ligands. The ligands are sorted by the score in the ascending order.

```
ZINC03815630 0.69811
ZINC03833861 0.70995
```

The output of *lcs* scoring function has three columns. Between the columns of ligand names and the score is situated an additional column which shows the index of the conformations of the ligand that gave the lowest score.

```
ZINC03815630 1 0.66714
ZINC03833861  31 0.67820
```

3.5 Virtual Screening Using Pregenerated Ligand Sets

On the web site of PL-PatchSurfer2 (http://kiharalab.org/plps2/), we provide two pregenerated ligand sets: Drug-like (*druglike.tar.gz*) and ChEMBL19 (*chembl.tar.gz*). Both sets are preselected sets provided in the ZINC library (http://zinc.docking.org). The Drug-like set is composed of ligands that satisfy "Lipinski's Rule of Five" [30], which are four chemical properties of compounds that are suitable for drugs. The ChEMBL19 dataset was selected from ChEMBL [28], which is an open compound library with bioactivity information collected from medicinal chemistry literature. The pre-selection of the two datasets was performed using the SUBSET 1.0 algorithm [31]. The Drug-like dataset were filtered with 90% Tanimoto similarity cutoff and the ChEMBL19 dataset were filtered with 80% Tanimoto similarity cutoff. The Drug-like and ChEMBL19 set have 123472 and 80159 compounds, respectively.

To use the database, decompress by a command *tar –zxf [tar.gz file]*. In the directory, *gen_input.py* makes input files for comparing patches and ranking ligands. Four parameters should be given to run the python script.

```
python gen_input.py [Receptor SSIC] [PL-PatchSurfer2 path]
[Scoring function] [Rank file]
```

Receptor SSIC is the name of the pocket SSIC file. *PL-Patch-Surfer2 path* is a location of the program. The user may choose type of scoring function by typing *lcs* for lowest conformer or *bs* for Boltzmann-weighted in [*Scoring function*]. [*Rank file*] is an output file name that will contain the ranking of the ligands in the library. It can be any file name the user wishes to have. The outputs of this python script are *compare_seeds.in* and *rank_ligands.in*, which are input files to run *compare_seeds.py* and *rank_ligands.py*, respectively.

3.6 Case Study

In this section, we will show an example of virtual screening using PL-PatchSurfer2. The target protein is a SRC kinase (PDB ID: 2SRC). SRC kinase phosphorylates tyrosine of other proteins [32]. The activation of the SRC pathway is related to colon, liver, lung, breast, and pancreatic cancer [33]. The three-dimensional structure bound with phosphoaminophosphonic acid-adenylate ester, an inhibitor of ATP-dependent phosphorylation, is shown in Fig. 5. The active 60 compounds of this target were mixed with 1740 nonactive compounds in the library. The ratio between actives and decoys are 1:29. Nonactive compounds were randomly chosen from the DUD dataset [34]. In this example, the ligands were scored and ranked by the lowest conformer scoring scheme.

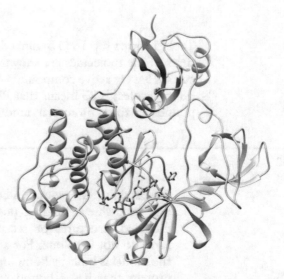

Fig. 5 The crystal structure of human SRC kinase bound with phosphoaminophosphonic acid-adenylate ester, an analog of ATP (PDB ID: 2SRC)

Table 1
Top 18 ligands ranked by the lowest conformer score

Rank	Class	ZINC ID	Score
1	Active	ZINC03815379	0.49045
2	Active	ZINC03815551	0.51416
3	Active	ZINC03815482	0.51647
4	Active	ZINC03815493	0.53378
5	Active	ZINC03815508	0.53546
6	Active	ZINC03815483	0.53770
7	Active	ZINC03815489	0.54398
8	Active	ZINC03815307	0.54499
9	Active	ZINC03815505	0.56146
10	Active	ZINC03815507	0.56395
11	Active	ZINC03815525	0.56614
12	Active	ZINC03815490	0.56656
13	Decoy	ZINC02196955	0.56680
14	Active	ZINC03815503	0.56779
15	Active	ZINC03832351	0.57083
16	Decoy	ZINC03631303	0.57389
17	Decoy	ZINC00766404	0.57602
18	Active	ZINC03815545	0.57719

Table 1 shows top 18 (1%) ranked ligands. Two-dimensional structures of the molecules are shown in Fig. 6. Among top 18 molecules, 15 were active compounds. The enrichment factor at 1% (top 18 molecules) is 25 means that PL-PatchSurfer2 finds active compounds 25 times more than random selection at top 1%.

4   Notes

1. PL-PatchSurfer2 requires a bound ligand in the receptor protein to define a binding pocket. However, computationally modeled structures or receptors in their apo (ligand-free) form do not have one. For a computational protein model, if the model is built by homology modeling based on a template protein that has a bound cognate ligand, superimpose the modeled structure on to the template structure and use the

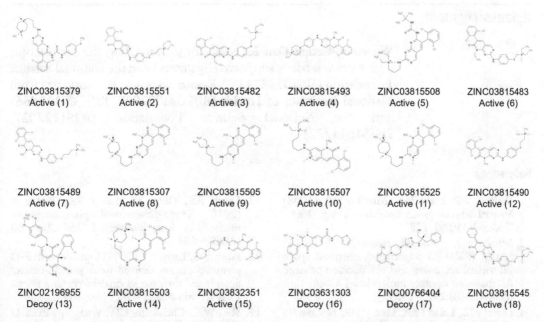

| ZINC03815379 | ZINC03815551 | ZINC03815482 | ZINC03815493 | ZINC03815508 | ZINC03815483 |
| Active (1) | Active (2) | Active (3) | Active (4) | Active (5) | Active (6) |

| ZINC03815489 | ZINC03815307 | ZINC03815505 | ZINC03815507 | ZINC03815525 | ZINC03815490 |
| Active (7) | Active (8) | Active (9) | Active (10) | Active (11) | Active (12) |

| ZINC02196955 | ZINC03815503 | ZINC03832351 | ZINC03631303 | ZINC00766404 | ZINC03815545 |
| Decoy (13) | Active (14) | Active (15) | Decoy (16) | Decoy (17) | Active (18) |

Fig. 6 Two-dimensional structures of top 1% ligands identified by PL-PatchSurfer2 for SRC kinase. The number indicates the rank of the ligand assigned by PL-PatchSurfer2. ZINC ID is shown for each ligand. The numbers in parentheses are the rank of ligands

cognate ligand of the template structure as the input parameter used in Subheading 3.1.

If there are no homologous structures that have bound ligand, or if apo-form of a binding pocket is used, provide the binding pocket center position in *pkt_cntr.pdb* in the *scripts* directory. Then, replace the line *ligand_file* in *rec_prep.in* from *xtal-lig.pdb* to *pkt_cntr.pdb*.

2. To visualize the patch location on a binding pocket or on a ligand molecule, PL-PatchSurfer2 provides *convert_ssic_-to_pdb.py* in the *scripts* directory, a python script that extracts seed point (center of patch) coordinates from the SSIC file. Executing the script gives a PDB format file of seed point coordinates:

```
python convert_ssic_to_pdb.py [SSIC file] [Output PDB
file]
```

Output PDB file can be any file name the user wish to use for an output file. Use any molecular structure viewer, such as PyMol, and load the output file and a three-dimensional structure file of a molecule (a protein or a ligand), from which SSIC file was generated, to visualize the seed position of patches distributed on the molecular surface.

Acknowledgment

We acknowledge Dan K. Ntala for proofreading the manuscript. This work was partly supported by grants from the National Science Foundation (IIS1319551). D.K. also acknowledges supports from National Institutes of Health (R01GM097528, R01GM123055) and the National Science Foundation (IOS1127027, DMS1614777).

References

1. Walters WP, Stahl MT, Murcko MA (1998) Virtual screening—an overview. Drug Discov Today 3(4):160–178

2. Schwartz J, Awale M, Reymond JL (2013) SMIfp (SMILES fingerprint) chemical space for virtual screening and visualization of large databases of organic molecules. J Chem Info Model 53(8):1979–1989

3. Durant JL, Leland BA, Henry DR, Nourse JG (2002) Reoptimization of MDL keys for use in drug discovery. J Chem Inf Comput Sci 42(6):1273–1280

4. Raymond JW, Gardiner EJ, Willett P (2002) RASCAL: calculation of graph similarity using maximum common edge subgraphs. Comput J 45(6):631–644

5. Bender A, Mussa HY, Glen RC (2004) Similarity searching of chemical databases using atom environment descriptors (MOLPRINT 2D): evaluation of performance. J Chem Inf Comput Sci 44(5):1708–1718

6. Ballester PJ, Richards WG (2007) Ultrafast shape recognition to search compound databases for similar molecular shapes. J Comput Chem 28(10):1711–1723

7. Hawkins PCD, Skillman AG, Nicholls A (2007) Comparison of shape-matching and docking as virtual screening tools. J Med Chem 50(1):74–82

8. Jain AN (2007) Surflex-dock 2.1: robust performance from ligand energetic modeling, ring flexibility, and knowledge-based search. J Comput-Aided Mol Des 21(5):281–306

9. Trott O, Olson AJ (2010) AutoDock Vina: improving the speed and accuracy of docking with a new scoring function, efficient optimization, and multithreading. J Comput Chem 31(2):455–461

10. Allen WJ, Balius TE, Mukherjee S, Brozell SR, Moustakas DT, Lang PT, Case DA, Kuntz ID, Rizzo RC (2015) DOCK 6: impact of new features and current docking performance. J Comput Chem 36(15):1132–1156

11. Leach AR, Gillet VJ, Lewis RA, Taylor R (2010) Three-dimensional pharmacophore methods in drug discovery. J Med Chem 53(2):539–558

12. Wolber G, Langer T (2005) LigandScout: 3-D pharmacophores derived from protein-bound ligands and their use as virtual screening filters. J Chem Info Model 45(1):160–169

13. Shin WH, Christoffer CW, Wang J, Kihara D (2016) PL-PatchSurfer2: improved local surface matching-based virtual screening method that is tolerant to target and ligand structure variation. J Chem Info Model 56(9):1676–1691

14. Novotni M, Klein R (2003) 3D Zernike descriptors for content based shape retrieval. In: Proceedings of eighth ACM symposium on solid modeling and applications, Washington, pp 216–225

15. Shin WH, Zhu X, Bures MG, Kihara D (2015) Three-dimensional compound comparison methods and their application in drug discovery. Molecules 20(7):12841–12962

16. Zhu X, Xiong Y, Kihara D (2015) Large-scale binding ligand prediction by improved patch-based method Patch-Surfer2.0. Bioinformatics 31(5):707–713

17. Esquivel-Rodriguez J, Xiong Y, Han X, Gang S, Christoffer CW, Kihara D (2015) Navigating 3D electron microscopy maps with EM-SURFER. BMC Bioinf 16:181

18. Venkatraman V, Yang YD, Sael L, Kihara D (2009) Protein-protein docking using region-based 3D Zernike descriptors. BMC Bioinf 10:407

19. Baker NA, Sept D, Joseph S, Holst MJ, McCammon JA (2001) Electrostatics of nanosystems: application to microtubules and the ribosome. Proc Natl Acad Sci U S A 98(18):10037–10041

20. Hawkins PCD, Skillman AG, Warren GL, Ellingson BA, Stahl MT (2010) Conformer generation with OMEGA: algorithm and validation using high quality structures from the

protein databank and Cambridge Structural Database. J Chem Info Model 50(4):572–584

21. Sael L, Kihara D (2012) Detecting local ligand-binding site similarity in nonhomologous proteins by surface patch comparison. Proteins 80 (4):1177–1185

22. Cheng T, Zhao Y, Li X, Lin F, Xu Y, Zhang X, Li Y, Wang R (2007) Computation of octanol–water partition coefficients by guiding an additive model with knowledge. J Chem Info Model 47(6):2140–2148

23. Heiden W, Moeckel G, Brickmann J (1993) A new approach to analysis and display of local lipophilicity/hydrophilicity mapped on molecular surfaces. J Comput-Aided Mol Des 7 (5):503–514

24. O'Boyle NM, Banck M, James CA, Morley C, Vandermeersh T, Hutchison GR (2011) Open Babel: an open chemical toolbox. J Cheminf 3:33

25. Pettersen EF, Goddard TD, Huang CC, Couch GS, Greenblatt DM, Meng EC, Ferrin TE (2004) UCSF chimera—a visualization system for exploratory research and analysis. J Comput Chem 25(13):1605–1612

26. Li B, Turuvekere S, Agrawal M, La D, Ramani K, Kihara D (2008) Characterization of local geometry of protein surfaces with the visibility criterion. Proteins 71(2):670–683

27. Irwin JJ, Sterling T, Mysinger MM, Bolstad ES, Coleman E (2012) ZINC: a free tool to discover chemistry for biology. J Chem Inf Model 52(7):1757–1768

28. Bento AP, Gaulton A, Hersey A, Bellis LJ, Chambers J, Davies M, Krüger FA, Light Y, Mak L, McGlinchey S, Nowotka M, Papadatos G, Santos R, Overington JP (2014) The ChEMBL bioactivity database: an update. Nucleic Acids Res 42(D1):D1083–D1090

29. Kim S, Thiessen PA, Bolton EE, Chen J, Fu G, Gindulyte A, Han L, He J, He S, Shoemaker BA, Wang J, Yu B, Zhang J, Bryant SH (2016) PubChem substance and compound databases. Nucleic Acids Res 44(D1):D1202–D1213

30. Lipinski CA (2000) Drug-like properties and the causes of poor solubility and poor permeability. J Pharmacol Toxicol Methods 44 (1):235–249

31. Volgt JH, Blenfalt B, Wang S, Nicklaus MC (2001) Comparison of the NCI open database with seven large chemical structural databases. J Chem Inf Comput Sci 41(3):702–712

32. Wheeler DL, Iida M, Dunn EF (2009) The role of Src in solid tumors. Oncologist 14 (7):667–678

33. Dehm SM, Bonham K (2004) SRC gene expression in human cancer: the role of transcriptional activation. Biochem Cell Biol 82 (2):263–274

34. Huang N, Shoichet BK, Irwin JJ (2006) Benchmarking sets for molecular docking. J Med Chem 49(23):6789–6801

Chapter 8

Fragment-Based Ligand Designing

Shashank P. Katiyar, Vidhi Malik, Anjani Kumari, Kamya Singh, and Durai Sundar

Abstract

Fragment-based drug design strategies have been used in drug discovery since it was first demonstrated using experimental structural biology techniques such as nuclear magnetic resonance (NMR) and X-ray crystallography. The underlying idea is that existing or new chemical entities with known desirable properties may serve both as tool compounds and as starting points for hit-to-lead expansion. Despite the recent advancements, there remain challenges to overcome, such as assembly of the synthetically feasible structures, development of scoring functions to correlate structure and their activities, and fine tuning of the promising molecules. This chapter first covers the theoretical background needed to understand the concepts and the challenges related to the field of study, followed by the description of important protocols and related software. Case studies are presented to demonstrate practical applications.

Key words 3D QSAR, De novo, Fragment growing, Fragment linking, High-throughput screening, Ligand-based drug design, Structure-based drug design

1 Introduction

Fragment-based drug discovery has shown its potential with the success stories of development of some early inhibitors like urokinase inhibitors, p38 MAP kinase inhibitors, cyclic nucleotide phosphodiesterases inhibitors, and HSP90 inhibitors [1–4]. Number of compounds developed by fragment based approach have successfully faced the Phase-I clinical trials. Contributing to the list are (1) a factor Xa inhibitor from Lilly (LY-517717), (2) a Bcl-xL inhibitor from Abbott (ABT263), (3) kinase inhibitor from Astex (AT9283), (4) an HSP90 inhibitor from a collaboration between Novartis and Vernalis (NVP-AUY-922), and (5) a PPAR agonist from Plexxikon (PLX-204). De novo designing, on the other hand, despite sharing the common characteristics with fragment-based drug discovery has not shown same level of success. Many of the concepts and objectives of de novo are similar to those of fragment-based. First, both the approaches depend on the small chemical

Mohini Gore and Umesh B. Jagtap (eds.), *Computational Drug Discovery and Design*, Methods in Molecular Biology, vol. 1762, https://doi.org/10.1007/978-1-4939-7756-7_8, © Springer Science+Business Media, LLC, part of Springer Nature 2018

building material to start with and develop novel blocks with drug-like properties. Next, developed blocks are screened for the initial desired properties such as biological activity, pharmacokinetic properties at an initial stage of the project. Further, screened molecular blocks with desirable properties are prolonged by either growing or linking. A set of ligands with desirable properties can be obtained by the iteration of the above steps. Hence frequently, the term de novo or fragment-based drug designing are used interchangeably. To avoid confusion, this chapter only uses the term de novo, instead of using two separate names of similar approaches.

Computer aided de novo drug discovery process has complemented the experimental combinatorial chemistry by providing cost-effective and time saving approach to explore vast chemical space. Cox-2, factor Xa, CDK4, carbonic anhydrase II, and HIV protease are among few scientifically proven examples [5–9]. A de novo molecule design software is challenged by virtually infinite chemical search space to start with. The estimated number of chemically feasible molecules is in order of 10^{60} to 10^{1000} for the selection of promising candidates [10–12]. Despite boost in computational power and advent of high-throughput screening (HTS), exhaustive searching is not feasible for such a large chemical space. Hence, the search in de novo design process focuses on principle of local optimization rather than concentrating on global optimization and does not systematically construct, evaluate, and compare each and every individual compound. In such case, the covered space is called "practical" optimum. Therefore, most of the software work in nondeterministic way and rely on stochastic structure optimization. As chemists from different background will most likely consider different molecules as "lead molecule," similarly repeated runs from same software that rely on stochastic optimization will generate different lead molecules. Hence, it becomes important to include as much chemical structure search space as possible. There are two important aspects of a de novo software; search algorithm and the scoring function. In a way, search algorithms mimic a medicinal chemist and a scoring function analogically performs as an assay to evaluate the activity. Ideally, computational approaches or in silico experiments provide routes that facilitate identification of high quality molecular structures with easiest possible synthetic process. The chances of identifying "promising candidate" without getting lost into the vast chemical space depend on two design strategies: positive design and the negative design strategy. Positive design strategy limits the search space within small region of molecules with high probable drug-like molecules. Negative design defines the "unwanted" region by identifying adverse properties and unwanted structures [13, 14].

Once a library of potential molecules is generated, the molecules can further be engineered to avoid issues that prevent a chemical series from delivering low quality molecules. Such engineering techniques need to keep all the good properties of the molecules to further identify and remove the unwanted properties. Because a property of a molecule is often associated directly with its associated functional groups and chains, parts of the molecules responsible for the unwanted properties are either removed or replaced with favorable parts. The process is called "rescaffolding" or "scaffold hopping" when the central part of the molecule is replaced with the other chemical motif [15–18]. Scaffold hopping might be an anticipated outcome of a de novo process in order to obtain a library of lead molecules with potentially improved properties.

Identification of new lead molecule using the de novo experiments can be advanced by two approaches: structure-based de novo computational drug design (SBDND) and ligand-based de novo drug design (LBDND). SBDND makes use of available tertiary structure of the target protein, which can be solved experimentally or computationally. SBDND can be achieved by either a ligand growing or linking approach. In ligand growing method, a fragment is docked into the binding site of target protein and extended by adding favorable functional groups to it. The linking method is similar but instead of docking one, multiple small fragments are docked within and adjacent to the binding pocket of the target molecule and linked with each other to form one complex molecule. Availability of the target protein structure helps in screening fragments at both the search and scoring steps. In the absence of protein tertiary structure, the structure–activity relationship (SAR) information about the existing active and inactive compounds can be exploited using an approach called LBDND. Quantitative structure–activity relationships based on three-dimensional structures of molecules (3D QSAR) is an important and widely used method in LBDND. New Molecules are built using the fragment library constructed using known molecules with high biological activity.

This chapter focuses on both concepts of computer based molecular de novo design methods and general protocols to perform the study based on SBDND. By discussing the case studies involved in successful developments of lead and hit molecules, the potential of this approach will be highlighted.

2 Concepts and Challenges

The basic concept behind identifying a new lead molecule is generating a new molecule using the fragment of existing active fragments. Therefore, final product depends extensively, first on the initial material and second on their rearrangement to create something new with different activity. Any de novo software or algorithm must address three basic questions: assembly or clustering of candidate fragments, evaluation of their features and activity, and sampling of the search space optimally. The performance of any software depends on how well it performs these three basic operations. The biggest challenge lies in exploring the vast space generated as a result of combinatorial explosion by the number of element types and their arrangement possibilities in 2D space, i.e., topology. Furthermore, the problem gets more complex when a single topology has variety of conformations in 3D space. Hence, it makes it impossible for any software to perform an exhaustive search. The ability of a software to reduce the chemical space without sacrificing on possible leads including other algorithmic decisions ultimately decides its quality of outcome results. A de novo drug design program face following constraints while developing underlying algorithms.

2.1 Design Constraint: Primary Target

The first design constraint to be encountered comes from the target of interest. The type of input, specific for the biological target has to be decided first [19]. This constraint is directly connected to the quality assessment of the candidate fragments because the constraints extracted from fragments are used for the scoring of generated structures [20]. All the ligand–receptor-related information contributes to the formation of primary target constraint. The ligand–receptor-related information can be inferred by the exploration of the receptor binding site to reveal possible ligand-binding points or regions and extraction of complementarity information between receptor and ligands. In doing so, the design process is made biased toward specific region of primary target such as binding site based on the ligand–receptor interactions and key receptor–ligand interactions. Analysis of electrostatic regions, hydrogen bond (H-bond) donor and acceptor regions, hydrophilic and hydrophobic regions, π–cation and π–anion interactions as well as noncanonical interactions is critical to identify key ligand interactions. Receptor regions having H-bonding potential are of special interest due to the directional nature of H-bond acceptor and donor, which often form key interaction sites. Aromatic stack pairing at the catalytic site of proteins has been shown to play critical role for the selectivity and specificity of a protein target toward a particular type of molecules [21]. Aromatic residues play important role in enhancing the affinity by both π–π or π–ionic interactions and shape complementarity. These interactions allow the allocation of ligand atoms with a defined orientation and with a complementarity within a small region of space. The accuracy of constraints comes from the accuracy of the primary target structure. Therefore, it is important to consider the most accurate target protein structure. In the absence of experimental structures, computationally predicted structures of primary target can be used. However, there remains greater scope for errors in computationally predicted structures; previous studies have reported its successful applications in structure-based programs [22–24].

In the absence of target structure, LBDND approach can be used by gathering constraints from the known active and inactive ligands of primary target [25]. Furthermore, ligands contain the hidden information about the target binding pocket that can be revealed by the superimposition of 3D ligand structures over each other and generating a pseudoreceptor binding pocket image [26]. Finally, 3D QSAR model based on selective and common pharmacophores can be generated to quickly facilitate the search of ligands [27].

There are many methods reported to explore the receptor binding site for SBDND such as "rule based approach," "grid-based methodology," and flooding of protein binding sites with fragments [28–33].

2.2 Design Constraint: Secondary Target

A drug should not only be an active molecule but should also be biologically active. Possession of suitable drug-like properties such as absorption, distribution, metabolism, excretion, and toxicity (ADMET properties) makes an active molecule to be biologically active. Constrains other than those that define binding affinity are considered secondary constraints. The overall de novo scoring is adjusted accordingly based on the weightage of secondary constraints. The prediction models can be as simple as *Lipinski's rule of five* or as complex as deriving the bioavailability based on cell line studies [34, 35].

2.3 Scoring Function

Scoring functions are used (1) to control and direct the ligand design process and (2) to estimate the binding affinity and rank the generated novel molecules. The scoring function must be accurate enough to avoid false positive and false negative selections from the chemical space and fast enough to quickly explore the vast chemical space at the same time. In SBDND, scoring functions take advantage of available 3D coordinate information about the target molecule and are very similar to those used for molecular docking process. All the quality assessment scoring functions are approximations and their algorithms can be classified into three categories (1) explicit force-field methods, (2) empirical scoring functions, and (3) knowledge based scoring functions. Explicit force-field methods are computationally more demanding but are expected to produce more accurate results. Empirical scoring functions are based on the weightage sum of the receptor–ligand interaction types, where few interactions are favored over other and unfavorable interactions leads to penalty. The interaction types include the H-bonds, electrostatic interactions, hydrophobic interactions, and also inclusion of aromatic interactions in recent years. Empirical methods provide the computational speed without sacrificing much on the accuracy, and are specifically effective in ranking the molecules. Knowledge based scoring functions are based on the statistical analysis between ligand–receptor complex structures.

The existing receptor–ligand information is explored and exploited to generate frequency database of each possible atom pairs and models are trained using advanced statistical methods such as support vector machine and deep learning.

In the case of LBDND, the information is derived from the structure–activity relationship data of known biologically active molecules. The 3D-pharmacophore models are used to extract the features of active molecules, responsible for the biological activity. Using such pharmacophore, a pseudoreceptor model is feasible to exploit to come up with a scoring function as an alternative to the SBDND [36, 37].

2.4 Structural Sampling

To start the process of de novo ligand design, either a single atom or a fragment or the library of fragments can work as building block. Atom-based approach generates more diverse chemical space as compared to the fragment based approach but also increases the possible solutions and makes harder to choose the right compounds. Therefore, increasing the chemical space can be advantageous in the absence of diverse fragment library, otherwise, increasing the chemical search space may require higher computation power. Fragment based design strategies, on the other hand, limit the chemical search space and provide easier opportunity to select the potential candidates. Such a reduction is called "meaningful reduction," if fragment library is diverse enough to cover most of the fragments that occur in drug molecules. However, an atom is a subset of fragment and there is no limit defined for the size of a fragment. The general relationship is that smaller the fragment size, bigger the combinatorial space problem. The structural sampling deals with the expansion of building blocks. There are several approaches for the growth and expansion of the initial seed fragment, such as linking, growing, random structure mutations, lattice-based sampling, and graph-based sampling [38–40]. Linking, growing, and random structure mutations are used for the SBDND while in the absence of interactions site for LBDND, graph-based sampling particular are of high significance [41]. The most of LBDND depends on topological molecular graph and evolutionary algorithms [42].

2.5 Combinatorial Search Strategies

As discussed above, the smaller the fragment size, the bigger the combinatorial explosion issue. Though larger fragment libraries limit the search space, they also have their own limitation, as a fragment library must be diverse enough. Under such contradictory advantages, de novo design experiments have to tackle combinatorial explosion related problems. There is no optimal solution available with right blend to fulfill both the demands. Combinatorial search algorithms are designed to offer practical solution by giving up at least one of the advantages. There are three types of algorithms used based on the input design: 'Breath-first and depth-first search', 'Monte Carlo and Metropolis criterion' and 'Evolutionary algorithms' [36, 39, 43, 44].

After the briefings on the concepts of de novo drug designing, protocols and software related to de novo drug design are defined further in this chapter.

3   Methodology

In silico drug designing methods are not restricted by the constraints that govern experimental approaches. The combination of both these methods has led to the discovery of many lead molecules. The strategy of drug discovery involves execution of multistep computational approaches (Fig. 1). Although many software based on different algorithms are available, here we discuss only selected widely popular software (MacroModel, LigBuilder, QikProp, etc.) used in representative steps of structure-based in silico drug designing process.

3.1   Construction of the Fragment Libraries

Thorough sampling of the chemical space is highly dependent on the fragments present in the library. Hence, successful lead generation requires construction of quality fragment libraries. Designing a good fragment library depends on a number of factors like diversity, complexity, selectivity, reactivity, solubility, and efficiency of the fragments. Computational steps involved in generation of fragment library are discussed below:

1. *Selection of the two-dimensional atomic structure of the fragment*
   While selecting the 2D structure of the virtual fragments, various points must be taken into account. There should be no significant change in the properties of the fragment when it is made a part of the molecule. Commercial availability of synthetic intermediates or synthetic feasibility of the fragment must be ensured. Sometimes, known ligands are deconstructed as components for creating fragments.

2. *Generation of the three-dimensional conformers*
   Use of rigid fragments during simulation studies of the same gives rise to the need of generating multiple 3D structures as the atomic structures are usually flexible [45]. Selection of 2D structure should be in a way that it has minimum number of rotatable bonds eliminating the requirement of many simulations due to large number of conformers. MacroModel has a system conformational search module used for this purpose [46]. After identification of conformers, energy minimization of structure coordinates is performed.

3. *Assignment of force field atom types to fragment atoms*
   The simulations of fragment–protein complex make use of molecular mechanics force field. Hence, designating force field

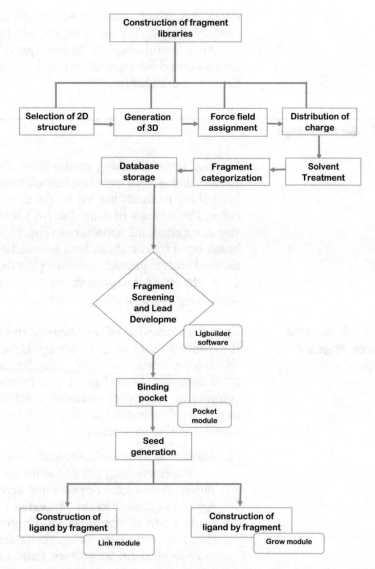

Fig. 1 Graphical depiction of the methodology for structure-based de novo drug designing

atom types helps in determining the parameters to be used for each atom. If the protein is considered to be static and fragments are treated rigid, only nonbonded parameters are needed. Generally, for such a procedure, AMBER force field is used [47]. Performance of AMBER for studying protein–fragments interactions has already being reported [48–51].

4. *Distribution of charge*

This step involves the calculation of point charges of atoms for all the 3D conformers generated. Gaussian is used to perform single point calculation as the geometry of the fragment is already known [52]. The combination of 6-31G(d) set [53] and B3LYP method [54] is also used for hybrid function.

5. *Execution of symmetry operation*

In order to maintain the symmetry for the fragment plane and to account for errors, the operation is done on the atomic coordinates with their point charges.

6. *Solvent treatment for simulation studies*

Either continuum dielectric, cosimulated explicit water molecules or solvent correction factor that is based on the solvation energies can be used for treatment of the solvent. This specific solvent correction procedure is aimed to simulate the fragments in vacuo.

7. *Creation of category field for the fragment*

Extraction of the fragments from the library is facilitated by adding various labels to categorize the fragments.

8. *Storage of fragment in the database*

Depending on the compatibility of the software used for simulation studies of the fragment–protein complex, the fragments are stored in the database in specific formats.

3.2 Screening of Fragment Libraries and Developing Leads Through Fragment Growing or Linking

After preparation of fragment libraries, the next step in the SBDND is to analyze the binding pocket of target protein in order to build a pharmacophore model and develop seed structures for construction of potential lead molecules. Experimentally determined high-resolution structure of target molecule is a prerequisite to carry out binding pocket analysis. If cocrystallized structure of protein–ligand complex exists, then it is an ideal structure to start with for fragment library screening. In the absence of experimentally solved structure, computational techniques can be employed to model the structure of protein based on homology with crystal structures deposited in PDB (Protein Data Bank) [55]. Though various software are available for carrying out binding site analysis and generation of seed structure, we describe the different modules of LigBuilder that can be used for the same [56]:

1. *Binding pocket analysis of the target protein*

Binding pocket analysis should not only aim at defining the shape of the protein but also its hypothetical key interaction sites. It should specify hydrogen bond acceptor, hydrogen bond donor and hydrophobic interaction sites that can be used to develop pharmacophore model. Derived pharmacophore model can be used as a query structure for fragment screening. *POCKET* is one of the modules of LigBuilder that is designed to analyze the binding pocket of protein and generate pharmacophore model of protein binding site. It uses a command line prompt and requires a parameter file as input that includes all the information required to run *POCKET.* Simple command line for running *POCKET* is:

```
#Pocket parameter_file.index
```

Parameter file contains information about the input files, i.e., LIGAND_FILE (Mol2 file of ligand of target protein), RECEPTOR_FILE (PDB file of target protein) and PARA-METER_DIRECTORY (path to directory "parameter" that includes all force field parameters used by LigBuilder). It also includes information about the program's output such as POCKET_ATOM_FILE (includes information about atoms of the binding pocket), POCKET_GRID_FILE (contain information about grids inside the binding pocket) and KEY_SI-TE_FILE (describes the key interaction sites of binding pocket).

2. *Generation of seed from reference molecules*

Successful drug discovery initially requires identification of seed molecules for generation of lead compounds. Preparation of seed is generally done by identification of the substructures present in the active compounds. These desirable molecules are not present in fragment libraries. The seed molecules are arranged in a hierarchical manner to traverse the chemical space completely. For this purpose a reference structure that already has its biological activity established is used as an input. The seeds are generated by the fragmentation of the reference structure. This generation of seed molecules gives rise to an initial set comprising of individual structures.

3. *Construction of ligand molecule through fragment growing*

GROW, a LigBuilder module, uses the seed structures and binding pocket site information for the generation of ligand molecule by growing seed structure through addition of fragments from fragment library. It employs genetic algorithm for evolution of fragments into lead-like molecules. Addition of fragments to seed molecules yields initial structures that are manipulated by fragment mutation or crossover for several generations, to yield lead molecule similar to reference molecule but with different scaffold and better interactions with target molecule [56, 57]. Command line for running *GROW* is:

```
#grow Parameter_file_for_grow.index
```

Parameter file for *GROW* includes information about all the input files, output files, and setting up manipulations related to growing, linking and mutation. It also includes parameters required for running genetic algorithms like number of generation, size of population, number of parent molecules, similarity cutoff, and percentage of elitism (*see* **Note 1**).

4. *Construction of ligand molecule through fragment linking*

    Fragment linking is useful in case of larger binding site and involves the covalent linking of two or more fragments, placed at distinct location within same binding pocket, via linkers [58]. It is a powerful strategy for optimizing low affinity fragment molecules into high affinity lead molecules. However, it is difficult to obtain same binding mode of both fragments in the final optimized product because of limitations of linker molecule [59]. Similar to *GROW* module, *LINK* module of Lig-Builder also uses seed structure to construct lead molecule but unlike *GROW*, seed structure for *LINK* consist of more than one small fragment. These fragments are linked by *LINK* into single heavy molecule having higher affinity with target protein. *LINK* also uses genetic algorithm for evolution of fragments into drug-like molecule by linking them with different linker molecules. Simple command line to run *LINK* is:

    ```
    #link link_parameter-file.index
    ```

    Parameter file for *LINK* includes same constraints as the one described for *GROW* (*see* **Note 2**). Ligand molecules generated by *LINK* and *GROW* are reported in LIG file of LigBuilder (*see* **Note 3**).

3.3 Evaluation of Physicochemical and Pharmacokinetic Properties of Lead Molecules

The structural and biological properties of the lead molecules must be evaluated to identify the potential of the lead molecules. The efforts directed toward creating synthetic molecules have greatly been aided by the molecular descriptors calculated using various tools. QikProp is one such prediction program that was developed by Professor William L. Jorgensen. QikProp predicts descriptors of physical significance and properties that are pharmaceutically relevant [60]. It also provides with an option to compare the properties of a molecule with those of already known drugs. Generated structure of de novo molecule is fed as an input to the QikProp tool. Running QikProp module generates file containing property data, structural information, and reference values. Analysis of the descriptors is done on the basis of the recommended values to perform screening of the lead compounds.

3.4 De novo Ligand Design Software

Since the advent of de novo drug discovery, many computer programs have been used to aid the complex process. The main objective of all the software remains the same; however, their scoring functions and sampling algorithms vary and keep evolving with time to come up with an optimal solution between accuracy and speed. Table 1 lists some of the widely used SBDND and LBDND based de novo software.

Table 1
List of de novo structure-based and ligand-based lead designing software

Structure-based approach			Ligand-based approach		
	Building block	**Scoring function**		**Building block**	**Scoring function**
LigMerge	Fragment	–	NEWLEAD	–	–
LigBuilder	Fragment	Empirical scoring function	PhDD	Fragments	Pharmacophore model
LEGEND	Atom	Force field	TOPAS	–	
LUDI	Fragment	Empirical scoring function	CoG	–	–
SPROUT	Fragment	SASA, electrostatic	Flux	–	–
BREED	Fragment	–	LEA3D	Fragment	Composite fitness function
AlleGrow	Fragment	Empirical and force field	Globus	Fragment	All-atom-pairs-shortest-path descriptor
SYNOPSIS	Fragment	Empirical	Nachbar	Fragment	Target specific QSAR
iScreen	Fragment	LEA3D's scoring function	PRO_LIGAND	–	–
DycoBlock	Fragment	Force field and SASA	SkelGen	–	–
GANDI	Fragment	Force field			

Various software have been developed based on different objectives, and hence, their starting building material and the scoring functions have also been mentioned

4   Case Studies

Various fragment based drug designing approaches have shifted the focus of pharmaceutical industries and academia from high throughput screening to structural biology based designing of drug molecules. Several successful attempts of de novo designing of ligand molecules have already been published in the last few years. Some of them are discussed here to give a brief overview of how one proceeds with drug designing studies.

4.1 Structure-Based De Novo Design Against COX-2

Cyclooxygenase-2 (COX-2) is an enzyme that catalyzes the formation of prostaglandins in a two-step process and has different active sites to perform its cyclooxygenase and peroxidase activity. Two isoforms of COX enzyme, COX-1 and COX-2, share high structural homology but engage in different roles. To be precise, COX-1 is involved in keeping housekeeping functions, whereas COX-2 induces inflammatory responses. Various anti-inflammatory drugs like Bextra, Vioxx, Celebrex, and many more were designed to inhibit COX-2 activity, but most of them additionally interact with COX-1 and induces gastrointestinal and cardiovascular side effects. Therefore, need for development of novel anti-inflammatory drug molecules with high selectivity toward COX-2 emerges. To accomplish this, computational SBDND approach was used by Dhanjal *et al.* [24].

SBDND approach requires structure of the target molecule and small compound library. Structures of human COX enzymes were not available in PDB. MODELLER v9.11 was used to model COX-1 and COX-2 structure based on homology with template molecule prostaglandin H2 synthase-1 of *Ovis aries* (PDBID: 1CQE) and Cox-2 of *Mus musculus* (PDBID: 1PXX). Modeled protein structures were stabilized by 15 ns long molecular dynamics simulations (MDS) in aqueous environment using Desmond software of Schrodinger suite [61]. An average representative structure was obtained from stable trajectories of simulation. The next requirement was to generate small compound library, which were accomplished using LigBuilder. 3D structures of eleven COX-2 inhibitors were obtained from NCBI-PubChem database to prepare seed structures using *extract* program of LigBuilder. Thirty-seven seed structures generated by *extract* were then linked and grown by *build* program into 1135 and 1522 potential lead molecules respectively, drug-like properties of which was simultaneously evaluated by software. Similarities between various derivatives were found by calculating Tanimoto coefficients, which gives a set of 2657 unique drug-like molecules, out of which 35 top scoring molecules were selected to check their binding affinity with COX-2 protein.

Ligand molecules were prepared using LigPrep and protein structure was prepared using protein preparation wizard of Schrodinger suite [62]. Glide XP docking protocol was used to dock ligand molecules at COX-2 active site and compounds showing binding efficiency greater than 8 kcal/mol were selected and docked against COX-1 active site [63]. Two compounds showing least binding affinity with COX-1 were selected for further analysis, namely, C_773 (IUPAC name:5,5-dihydrogenio-3-[(1Z)-1-[4-({3-hydroxy-4-[hydroxy(λ3-oxidanidylidene)methyl]phenyl} carbamoyl)phenyl]prop-1-en-1-yl]-1*H*-1,2,4-triazol-2-ium) and C_997 (IUPAC name: (3R)-3-carbamoyl-5-[(1Z)-1-{4-[(4-carboxy-3-hydroxyphenyl)carbamoyl]phenyl}prop-1-en-1-yl]-3*H*-1,2,4-triazol-1-ium). Molecular dynamic simulations of both docked complexes were carried out to get more realistic insight into the protein–ligand interactions. Both ligands were interacting with conserved residues that play a key role in reaction mechanism of COX-2 enzyme, thereby suggesting their potential to specifically block the function of COX-2 isoform of COX enzyme (Table 2).

Table 2
Docking scores of predicted compounds docked against COX-1 and COX-2 and three already available drug molecules docked against COX-2

Ligand	Docking score for COX-2	Docking score for COX-1	Hydrogen bonds interactions formed with COX-2 residues after MDS	Hydrophobic interactions formed with COX-2 residues after MDS
C_773	−10.298	−3.806	Asn 361and Phe 515	Phe 195, Gly 213, Val 214, Val 330, Val 335, Ile 363, Phe 367, Leu 370, Trp 373, Met 508, Val 509, Gly 512, Ser 516, Gly 519, Leu 520, Asn 523
C_997	−8.688	−3.435	Asn 361 and Met 508	Phe 195, His 212, Gly 213, Ile 363, Phe 367, Leu 370, Tyr 371, Phe 504, Gly 512, Ala 513, Ser 516, Gly 519, Leu 520, Asn 523
Valdecoxib	−9.458	–	–	–
Celecoxib	−9.878	–	–	–
Rofecoxib	−9.767	–	–	–

Interactions formed by predicted molecules with COX-2 protein residues after molecular dynamic simulations are also listed

Binding free energy calculation of both ligand–protein complexes were carried out using MM-GBSA, which gives binding free energy estimation of −80.063 kcal/mol for C_773 and −73.791 kcal/mol for C_997. Binding efficiency of predicted drug molecules were also compared with already available anti-inflammatory drug molecule (Bextra, Celebrex, and Vioxx) using same protocol (Table 2). It was found that both predicted molecules show similar binding affinity as those of already available drug molecules with high specificity toward COX-2 enzyme.

Docking and simulation studies showed that the predicted compounds were showing good affinity and selectivity toward COX-2. This does not imply that predicted compounds are potential lead molecules until they satisfy all physicochemical and pharmacokinetic properties of drug-like molecule. ADMET properties of C_773 and C_997 were predicted using Qikprop tool of Schrodinger suite and webserver admetSAR. Both molecules passed all five criteria of Lipinski's rule and their solvent accessible surface area (SASA) was within reference range suggested by QikProp. Blood–brain barrier (BBB) permeability was also predicted negative ensuring its administration safe for brain. Knowing that both predicted molecules satisfy all drug-likeliness properties, synthetic accessibility of these compounds was also checked in order to rule out the risk of failure at the time of chemical synthesis. "Synthetic Accessibility" program of myPresto (Medicinally Yielding PRotein

Engineering SimulaTOr) suite was used to calculate SA (synthetic accessibility) score. SA score of 4.680 and 5.036 was obtained for C_773 and C_997 respectively, indicating feasibility of their chemical synthesis. This in silico study reported two de novo designed potential anti-inflammatory drug molecules, which can be further explored to check whether they have potential to overcome limitations posed by clinically available drug molecules.

4.2 Computational Fragment Based Designing of p38 Inhibitor

With the discovery of p38 MAPK as the key factor in the production of various pro-inflammatory molecules, numerous efforts were focused toward designing p38 inhibitors. It became the focal point for drug discovery as blocking of p38 exhibited the potential to downregulate the pro-inflammatory mediators TNF-alpha, IL-beta, and COX-2. *Locus Pharmaceuticals* tried to explore the opportunity of regulating signal transduction process by targeting p38 by fragment-based drug discovery method. The approach was mainly aimed at creating a small molecule which was orally available and nontoxic, and did not bind at the ATP site of p38.

The initial study results from two groups; Bayer and Boehringer Ingelheim (BI) intensely led to conflicting views at *Locus* on whether to target the ATP site or not. The molecules discovered at Bayer exemplified allosteric inhibitors that instead of binding at the ATP site, were binding at the conserved DFG (Asp-Phe-Gly) motif. Yet the compounds had poor in vivo profile due to planar hydrophobic nature. Subsequently the BI group reported increase in solubility of DFG-binding molecules with the addition of morpholino-ATP binding moiety to these compounds. In addition to this BIRB-796 was shown to have low affinity for 11 other kinases [64]. Thus, to work this out, *Locus* decided to test BIRB-796 after synthesizing it. They ran point assays against panel of kinases and the four isoforms of p38. Inhibition of all p38 isoforms was observed and the other significant finding was that a key hydrogen bond was formed between BIRB-796 and ATP-site. This led to the proposal of a hypothesis that the lack of selectivity might be resulting from this specific interaction. The idea was to make a superior derivative of BIRB-796 with high affinity for ATP site, but did not participate in the specific hydrogen bond formation.

The technology that was used to discover fragments, which did not make hydrogen bond with methionine in the ATP site but still had high affinity for it, was called simulated annealing of chemical potential (SACP). The technology was run on BI crystal structure (PDB ID: 1KV2). SACP method involves Monte Carlo procedure which ranks the binding affinity of different fragments in relative order for a specific site in the protein. It is possible to generalize the procedure as an automated protocol to identify hotspots in protein that can make nonbonded interactions of high affinity. For the algorithm, the only input is the structure of the protein and the fragments that are to be simulated. An illustrative protocol for the same is given below [65]

1. Generating a random number (RanX) with values ranging from 0 to 1.

2. If RanX < 0.5, the fragment is inserted into the protein simulation and if Ran X > 0.5, the fragment is deleted. Both these cases are trial moves with a probability assigned to each attempted insertion and attempted deletion.

    The calculation of the probability involves energy of the system (depends on insertion or deletion of the fragment), chemical potential of the simulation cell (the only parameter which can be adjusted), gas constant, and the temperature. Adjustment of high value of the chemical potential dramatically enhances the chances of inserting a fragment, whereas low value tends to evacuate the fragments from the simulation cell. For each value of the chemical potential approximately five million simulation steps are performed.

3. Independent running of SACP on a panel of fragments is done which gives distinct binding pattern for each fragment on the protein.

4. The individual simulations are combined together to predict fragment binding with high affinity, clustering of the fragments and exclusion of water.

The simulation results of SACP predicted that diphenylether and its derivatives will bind in the hinge region without forming a hydrogen bond at the ATP site. On the basis of SACP results, Locus performed experiments and found that p38 is blocked by two closely related diphenylether molecules having different modes of binding in ATP site although their affinity was comparable. This made Locus sure of not targeting the ATP site, as none of the compounds had isoform specificity.

The fragment-based protocols finally shifted their focus to develop compounds that binds purely to DFG motif. Hence, the goal was to create a low molecular weight (<450 Da), soluble, nonplanar, DFG binding compound. The compound must also have the potential to inhibit p38 in cell assays with submicromolar efficacy. To achieve the same, they tried replacing one of the functional groups to reduce the molecular weight of the Bayer compound. The phenyl moiety in Bayer was found to mimic the phenylalanine of the conserved DFG triplet which binds in the p38 allosteric site. Predictions of the SACP simulations showed that free binding of energy for some aliphatic heterocyclic compounds were comparable to that of phenyl groups. They confirmed the predictions of substituting the phenyl group by dioxothiomorpholine and diazepanone using inhibition assays and cocrystallography.

Yet the p38 project was a failure as it was shown that isoform selective p38 inhibitor was less effective in treating rheumatoid arthritis than methotrexate [66]. Finally, Locus felt that not more than one order of magnitude in potency must be lost when going from a protein inhibition assay to cell assay and addition of blood to the cell assay must lead to only an additional loss of one order of magnitude in potency.

4.3 Computational Study for Structure-Based Designing of Novel Hepatitis C Virus Helicase Inhibitor

Hepatitis C virus (HCV) causes hepatitis C infection that could lead to hepatic disorders such as cirrhosis subsequently progressing to hepatocellular carcinoma. Current therapy includes direct antiviral agents, which is associated with several side effects and are expensive.

The case study is a pragmatic methodology for de novo based ligand drug discovery to design potential inhibitors for HCV NS3 helicase [67]. The crystal structure PDB 1A1V that was cocrystallized with DNA strand attached to the helicase domain was chosen for the study.

The first step involved finding the binding site for ligand. Therefore, the amino acids involved in the enzyme activity were explored and Arg393 was found conserved. Arg393 plays a significant role in enzymatic activity as mutation of this particular amino acid caused unfavorable impact on the enzyme activity. The nucleic acid was detached from the structure, due to which the neighboring residues came in direct contact to the solvent. Furthermore it was found that at a distance of nearly 10 Å the sulfur atom of Cys431 is in synergy with mercaptoethanol molecule of crystallized H_2O. This made it clear that Cys431 can covalently bond with a suitable small molecule. By these observations it was proposed that a molecule can be a potential inhibitor of helicase if it is interacting with Arg393 in addition to making covalent bond with Cys431.

The Ligbuilder software was used to design the ligand. The first step is to look for the binding site in the protein structure. Design of ligand involves identification of seed molecule for generation of lead compound. After which it constructs number of molecules by linking the most suitable fragments to the growing structures. The resultant series of structures were complex and difficult to obtain synthetically. To solve this problem, screening of fragment library was performed to select residues with least possibility to generate chiral centers after the combining process. For lead molecule to interact with the desired residue an atomic wall with no physical properties was formed. This reduced the complexity of the resultant structure, and it was able to interact with Arg393. Additionally there was an interaction with A481 with no functional group attached and in close proximity with Cys431. This represented a suitable basic scaffold for further functionalization.

The in silico design process was optimized by employing a different approach. A series of virtual libraries was created using

Molecular Operating Environment (MOE). This was achieved by altering the linking group between the two aromatic rings and at the same time substituting one of the carboxylic groups with Michael's acceptor. The next step is to dock these molecules into the binding site which was done using the software FLEXX. The scoring was done on the potential of the molecule to interact with the two arginine residues and to situate the vinyl ketone in such a position that it is in close proximity to Cys431. The best structures were presented with:

1. Michael's acceptor located 5 Å away from the sulfur atom of Cys431.
2. Addition of side chain with more interaction sites.

Further, to assess the stability of the protein–ligand complex MDS was performed. The 1 ns simulation presented with a relatively stable interaction. On the other hand it was observed that there was steric hindrance due to the presence of aromatic ring which led the compound to drift away from Cys431 almost 6–7 Å. Hence a smaller heterocycle ring was needed to be found that could replace benzene. Moreover in MDS it was observed that the linker side chain was not beneficial, hence was detached in later molecules. Finally, a pyrrole derivative was chosen as a potential inhibitor. The structure presented following key interactions:

1. Formation of H bond between ester moiety and R393.
2. Formation of H bond between Arg481 and the carbonyl group of the vinyl ketone.
3. In MDS distance between the sulfur of Cys431 and the Michael's acceptor of <4 Å was found to be stable.
4. Formation of H bond between NH of pyrrole and carbonyl group of Val432 acted as a stabilizing factor.

The compound was synthesized to evaluate its activity in helicase assay.

5 Summary

Fragment based or de novo drug designing has proven to be an indispensable tool in tedious and complex process of drug discovery. In the past decade, computational de novo methods have evolved to aid the process for time and cost saving. Computational fragment screening provides an effective investigation of the chemical space, and identification of more valuable hits as compared to the traditional screening approach. Computational methods overcome the limitations of the experimental approach by avoiding the need of material, solubility concerns, and higher time and cost, but at the cost of accuracy. Here, we have discussed the challenges in de novo drug discovery that leaves abundant space for innovation and discovery in the future.

6   Notes

1. Growing of fragments using *GROW* module is a time-consuming step, it employs genetic algorithm to evolve molecules. Increasing the number of generation will increase the computational time required; but at the same time, will generate molecules with high potency. Usually 10–20 generations of genetic algorithm are enough for this step.

2. *LINK* module also utilizes genetic algorithm for linking molecules and time consumed is proportional to the number of generations assigned for genetic algorithm. Unlike *GROW*, large number of generations ranging from 25,000 to 30,000 will be required which makes it more time-consuming step.

3. Ligand molecules generated by modules *GROW* and *LINK* are in LIG format. *PROCESS* script provided in LigBuilder can be used to analyze and filter generated ligands or can be used to convert them to Mol2 format to analyze them using other software like QikProp.

References

1. Nienaber VL, Richardson PL, Klighofer V, Bouska JJ, Giranda VL, Greer J (2000) Discovering novel ligands for macromolecules using X-ray crystallographic screening. Nat Biotechnol 18(10):1105–1108

2. Card GL, Blasdel L, England BP, Zhang C, Suzuki Y, Gillette S, Fong D, Ibrahim PN, Artis DR, Bollag G, Milburn MV, Kim S-H, Schlessinger J, Zhang KYJ (2005) A family of phosphodiesterase inhibitors discovered by cocrystallography and scaffold-based drug design. Nat Biotechnol 23(2):201–207

3. Hartshorn MJ, Murray CW, Cleasby A, Frederickson M, Tickle IJ, Jhoti H (2005) Fragment-based lead discovery using X-ray crystallography. J Med Chem 48(2):403–413. https://doi.org/10.1021/jm0495778

4. Jensen MR, Schoepfer J, Radimerski T, Massey A, Guy CT, Brueggen J, Quadt C, Buckler A, Cozens R, Drysdale MJ, Garcia-Echeverria C, Chène P (2008) NVP-AUY922: a small molecule HSP90 inhibitor with potent antitumor activity in preclinical breast cancer models. Breast Cancer Res 10

(2):R33–R33. https://doi.org/10.1186/bcr1996

5. Gehlhaar DK, Moerder KE, Zichi D, Sherman CJ, Ogden RC, Freer ST (1995) De novo design of enzyme inhibitors by Monte Carlo ligand generation. J Med Chem 38(3):466–472

6. Stewart KD, Loren S, Frey L, Otis E, Klinghofer V, Hulkower KI (1998) Discovery of a new cyclooxygenase-2 lead compound through 3-D database searching and combinatorial chemistry. Bioorg Med Chem Lett 8(5):529–534

7. Han Q, Dominguez C, Stouten PF, Park JM, Duffy DE, Galemmo RA Jr, Rossi KA, Alexander RS, Smallwood AM, Wong PC, Wright MM, Luettgen JM, Knabb RM, Wexler RR (2000) Design, synthesis, and biological evaluation of potent and selective amidino bicyclic factor Xa inhibitors. J Med Chem 43(23):4398–4415

8. Honma T, Hayashi K, Aoyama T, Hashimoto N, Machida T, Fukasawa K, Iwama T, Ikeura C, Ikuta M, Suzuki-

Takahashi I, Iwasawa Y, Hayama T, Nishimura S, Morishima H (2001) Structure-based generation of a new class of potent Cdk4 inhibitors: new de novo design strategy and library design. J Med Chem 44 (26):4615–4627

9. Grzybowski BA, Ishchenko AV, Kim CY, Topalov G, Chapman R, Christianson DW, Whitesides GM, Shakhnovich EI (2002) Combinatorial computational method gives new picomolar ligands for a known enzyme. Proc Natl Acad Sci U S A 99(3):1270–1273. https://doi.org/10.1073/pnas.032673399

10. Schneider G (2002) Trends in virtual combinatorial library design. Curr Med Chem 9:2095–2101

11. Dobson CM (2004) Chemical space and biology. Nature 432:824–828

12. Lipinski C, Hopkins A (2004) Navigating chemical space for biology and medicine. Nature 432:855–861

13. Richardson JS, Richardson DC (1989) The de novo design of protein structures. Trends Biochem Sci 14:304–309

14. Richardson JS (1992) Looking at proteins: representations, folding, packing, and design. Biophys J 63:1185–1209

15. Bohm HJ, Flohr A, Stahl M (2004) Scaffold hopping. Drug Discov Today Technol 1 (3):217–224. https://doi.org/10.1016/j.ddtec.2004.10.009

16. Renner S, Schneider G (2006) Scaffold-hopping potential of ligand-based similarity concepts. ChemMedChem 1(2):181–185. https://doi.org/10.1002/cmdc.200500005

17. Mauser H, Guba W (2008) Recent developments in de novo design and scaffold hopping. Curr Opin Drug Discov Devel 11(3):365–374

18. Langdon SR, Ertl P, Brown N (2010) Bioisosteric replacement and scaffold hopping in lead generation and optimization. Mol Inform 29 (5):366–385. https://doi.org/10.1002/minf.201000019

19. Loving K, Alberts I, Sherman W (2010) Computational approaches for fragment-based and de novo design. Curr Top Med Chem 10(1):14–32

20. Schneider G, Fechner U (2005) Computer-based de novo design of drug-like molecules. Nat Rev Drug Discov 4(8):649–663

21. Katiyar SP, Bakkiyaraj D, Karutha Pandian S (2011) Role of aromatic stack pairing at the catalytic site of gelonin protein. Biochem Biophys Res Commun 410(1):75–80. https://doi.org/10.1016/j.bbrc.2011.05.107

22. Shacham S, Marantz Y, Bar-Haim S, Kalid O, Warshaviak D, Avisar N, Inbal B, Heifetz A, Fichman M, Topf M, Naor Z, Noiman S, Becker OM (2004) PREDICT modeling and in-silico screening for G-protein coupled receptors. Proteins 57(1):51–86. https://doi.org/10.1002/prot.20195

23. Hillisch A, Pineda LF, Hilgenfeld R (2004) Utility of homology models in the drug discovery process. Drug Discov Today 9 (15):659–669. https://doi.org/10.1016/S1359-6446(04)03196-4

24. Dhanjal JK, Sreenidhi AK, Bafna K, Katiyar SP, Goyal S, Grover A, Sundar D (2015) Computational structure-based de novo design of hypothetical inhibitors against the anti-inflammatory target COX-2. PLoS One 10 (8):e0134691. https://doi.org/10.1371/journal.pone.0134691

25. Fechner U, Schneider G (2006) Flux (1): a virtual synthesis scheme for fragment-based de novo design. J Chem Inf Model 46 (2):699–707. https://doi.org/10.1021/ci0503560

26. Lloyd DG, Buenemann CL, Todorov NP, Manallack DT, Dean PM (2004) Scaffold hopping in de novo design. Ligand generation in the absence of receptor information. J Med Chem 47(3):493–496. https://doi.org/10.1021/jm034222u

27. Pasha FA, Muddassar M, Beg Y, Cho SJ (2008) DFT-based de novo QSAR of phenoloxidase inhibitors. Chem Biol Drug Des 71 (5):483–493. https://doi.org/10.1111/j.1747-0285.2008.00651.x

28. Goodford PJ (1985) A computational procedure for determining energetically favorable binding sites on biologically important macromolecules. J Med Chem 28(7):849–857

29. Miranker A, Karplus M (1991) Functionality maps of binding sites: a multiple copy simultaneous search method. Proteins 11(1):29–34. https://doi.org/10.1002/prot.340110104

30. Bohm HJ (1992) LUDI: rule-based automatic design of new substituents for enzyme inhibitor leads. J Comput Aided Mol Des 6 (6):593–606

31. Mills JE, Dean PM (1996) Three-dimensional hydrogen-bond geometry and probability information from a crystal survey. J Comput Aided Mol Des 10(6):607–622

32. Pearlman DA (1999) Free energy grids: a practical qualitative application of free energy perturbation to ligand design using the OWFEG method. J Med Chem 42(21):4313–4324

33. Halgren TA (2009) Identifying and characterizing binding sites and assessing druggability. J Chem Inf Model 49(2):377–389. https://doi.org/10.1021/ci800324m

34. Lipinski CA, Lombardo F, Dominy BW, Feeney PJ (2001) Experimental and computational approaches to estimate solubility and permeability in drug discovery and development settings. Adv Drug Deliv Rev 46 (1–3):3–26

35. Kumar R, Sharma A, Varadwaj PK (2011) A prediction model for oral bioavailability of drugs using physicochemical properties by support vector machine. J Nat Sci Biol Med 2 (2):168–173. https://doi.org/10.4103/0976-9668.92325

36. Clark DE, Frenkel D, Levy SA, Li J, Murray CW, Robson B, Waszkowycz B, Westhead DR (1995) PRO-LIGAND: an approach to de novo molecular design. 1. Application to the design of organic molecules. J Comput Aided Mol Des 9(1):13–32

37. Pellegrini E, Field MJ (2003) Development and testing of a de novo drug-design algorithm. J Comput Aided Mol Des 17 (10):621–641

38. Lewis RA (1990) Automated site-directed drug design: approaches to the formation of 3D molecular graphs. J Comput Aided Mol Des 4(2):205–210

39. Nishibata Y, Itai A (1991) Automatic creation of drug candidate structures based on receptor structure. Starting point for artificial lead generation. Tetrahedron 47(43):8985–8990. https://doi.org/10.1016/S0040-4020(01)86503-0

40. Yuan Y, Pei J, Lai L (2011) LigBuilder 2: a practical de novo drug design approach. J Chem Inf Model 51(5):1083–1091. https://doi.org/10.1021/ci100350u

41. Schneider G, Lee ML, Stahl M, Schneider P (2000) De novo design of molecular architectures by evolutionary assembly of drug-derived building blocks. J Comput Aided Mol Des 14 (5):487–494

42. Globus A, Lawton J, Wipke T (1999) Automatic molecular design using evolutionary techniques. Nanotechnology 10(3):290–299

43. Luo Z, Wang R, Lai L (1996) RASSE: a new method for structure-based drug design. J Chem Inf Comput Sci 36(6):1187–1194

44. Nachbar RB (2000) Molecular evolution: automated manipulation of hierarchical chemical topology and its application to average molecular structures. Genet Program Evol Mach 1(1–2):57–94. https://doi.org/10.1023/a:1010072431120

45. Moore W Jr (2005) Maximizing discovery efficiency with a computationally driven fragment approach. Curr Opin Drug Discov Devel 8 (3):355–364

46. Mohamadi F, Richards NG, Guida WC, Liskamp R, Lipton M, Caufield C, Chang G, Hendrickson T, Still WC (1990) MacroModel—an integrated software system for modeling organic and bioorganic molecules using molecular mechanics. J Comput Chem 11 (4):440–467

47. Weiner SJ, Kollman PA, Case DA, Singh UC, Ghio C, Alagona G, Profeta S, Weiner P (1984) A new force field for molecular mechanical simulation of nucleic acids and proteins. J Am Chem Soc 106(3):765–784

48. Ludington J, Fujimoto T, Hollinger F (2004) Determining partial atomic charges for fragments used in de novo drug design. Paper presented at the American Chemical Society, Washington, DC

49. Clark M, Guarnieri F, Shkurko I, Wiseman J (2006) Grand canonical Monte Carlo simulation of ligand–protein binding. J Chem Inf Model 46(1):231–242

50. Clark M, Meshkat S, Talbot GT, Carnevali P, Wiseman JS (2009) Fragment-based computation of binding free energies by systematic sampling. J Chem Inf Model 49(8):1901–1913

51. Moffett K, Konteatis Z, Nguyen D, Shetty R, Ludington J, Fujimoto T, Lee K-J, Chai X, Namboodiri H, Karpusas M (2011) Discovery of a novel class of non-ATP site DFG-out state p38 inhibitors utilizing computationally assisted virtual fragment-based drug design (vFBDD). Bioorg Med Chem Lett 21 (23):7155–7165

52. Frisch MJ, Trucks GW, Schlegel HB, Gill PMW, Johnson BG, Robb MA, Cheeseman MJR, Keith TA, Petersson GA, Montgomery JA, Raghavachari K, Al-Laham MA, Zakrzewski VG, Ortiz JV, Foresman JB, Cioslowski J, Stefanof BB, Nanayakkara A, Challacombe M, Peng CY, Ayala PY, Chen W, Wong MW, Andres JL, Replogle ES, Gomperts R, Martin RL, Fox DJ, Binkley JS, Defrees DJ, Baker J, Stewart JP, Head-Gordon M, Gonzalez C, Pople JA (1998) Gaussian 98, revision a. 7. Gaussian. Inc, Pittsburgh, PA

53. Hariharan PC, Pople JA (1973) The influence of polarization functions on molecular orbital hydrogenation energies. Theoretica Chimica Acta 28(3):213–222

54. Becke AD (1988) Density-functional exchange-energy approximation with correct asymptotic behavior. Phys Rev A 38 (6):3098–3100

55. Bernstein FC, Koetzle TF, Williams GJ, Meyer EF, Brice MD, Rodgers JR, Kennard O, Shimanouchi T, Tasumi M (1977) The protein data bank. Eur J Biochem 80(2):319–324

56. Wang R, Gao Y, Lai L (2000) LigBuilder: a multi-purpose program for structure-based drug design. Mol Model Annu 6 (7–8):498–516

57. de Kloe GE, Bailey D, Leurs R, de Esch IJ (2009) Transforming fragments into candidates: small becomes big in medicinal chemistry. Drug Discov Today 14(13):630–646

58. Rees DC, Congreve M, Murray CW, Carr R (2004) Fragment-based lead discovery. Nat Rev Drug Discov 3(8):660–672

59. Kumar A, Voet A, Zhang K (2012) Fragment based drug design: from experimental to computational approaches. Curr Med Chem 19(30):5128–5147

60. Schrödinger L (2013) Small-molecule drug discovery suite 2013–3: QikProp, version 3.8. Schrödinger, LLC, New York

61. Schrödinger Release (2014) 1: Desmond molecular dynamics system, version 3.7. DE Shaw Research, New York, NY, Maestro-Desmond Interoperability Tools, version 3

62. Schrödinger Release (2013) 1: Schrödinger Suite 2013 Protein Preparation Wizard. Epik version 2:2013

63. Schrödinger L (2013) Small-molecule drug discovery suite 2013–3: Glide, version 6.1. Schrödinger, LLC, New York

64. Pargellis C, Tong L, Churchill L, Cirillo PF, Gilmore T, Graham AG, Grob PM, Hickey ER, Moss N, Pav S (2002) Inhibition of p38 MAP kinase by utilizing a novel allosteric binding site. Nat Struct Mol Biol 9(4):268–272

65. Guarnieri F (2015) Designing a small molecule erythropoietin mimetic. Methods Mol Biol 1289:185–210

66. Cohen SB, Cheng TT, Chindalore V, Damjanov N, Burgos-Vargas R, DeLora P, Zimany K, Travers H, Caulfield JP (2009) Evaluation of the efficacy and safety of pamapimod, a p38 MAP kinase inhibitor, in a double-blind, methotrexate-controlled study of patients with active rheumatoid arthritis. Arthritis Rheumatol 60(2):335–344

67. Kandil S, Biondaro S, Vlachakis D, Cummins A-C, Coluccia A, Berry C, Leyssen P, Neyts J, Brancale A (2009) Discovery of a novel HCV helicase inhibitor by a de novo drug design approach. Bioorg Med Chem Lett 19 (11):2935–2937

Chapter 9

Molecular Dynamics as a Tool for Virtual Ligand Screening

Grégory Menchon, Laurent Maveyraud, and Georges Czaplicki

Abstract

Rational drug design is essential for new drugs to emerge, especially when the structure of a target protein or catalytic enzyme is known experimentally. To that purpose, high-throughput virtual ligand screening campaigns aim at discovering computationally new binding molecules or fragments to inhibit a particular protein interaction or biological activity. The virtual ligand screening process often relies on docking methods which allow predicting the binding of a molecule into a biological target structure with a correct conformation and the best possible affinity. The docking method itself is not sufficient as it suffers from several and crucial limitations (lack of protein flexibility information, no solvation effects, poor scoring functions, and unreliable molecular affinity estimation).

At the interface of computer techniques and drug discovery, molecular dynamics (MD) allows introducing protein flexibility before or after a docking protocol, refining the structure of protein–drug complexes in the presence of water, ions and even in membrane-like environments, and ranking complexes with more accurate binding energy calculations. In this chapter we describe the up-to-date MD protocols that are mandatory supporting tools in the virtual ligand screening (VS) process. Using docking in combination with MD is one of the best computer-aided drug design protocols nowadays. It has proved its efficiency through many examples, described below.

Key words Affinity, Clustering, Docking, Drug design, Interaction energy, Molecular dynamics, Protein–ligand complex, Virtual screening

---

1 Introduction

Virtual ligand screening has become an important tool in the world of rational drug design and early development process in the last decades, but remains a very challenging task. The complexity of such a research requires more and more accurate and sophisticated computational techniques and material to achieve a successful active and biologically relevant compound discovery program.

In contrast with an experimental high-throughput assay, knowledge of the experimental 3D structure of a target protein or enzyme (or at least a high quality model based on homologous proteins) is a prerequisite to a rational approach in drug discovery. This information is brought through the well-known NMR, X-ray

Mohini Gore and Umesh B. Jagtap (eds.), *Computational Drug Discovery and Design*, Methods in Molecular Biology, vol. 1762, https://doi.org/10.1007/978-1-4939-7756-7_9, © Springer Science+Business Media, LLC, part of Springer Nature 2018

crystallography, and molecular modeling approaches [1–16], and more recently through the cryo-electron microscopy [17]. There is no unique protocol or solution for dealing with a drug discovery problem but the general workflow of a virtual ligand screening campaign can be compared to a "funnel strategy" and usually starts with a high-throughput docking experiment, with filtered and enriched ligand libraries and a set of representative 3D protein structures determined with the previously mentioned techniques. See Fig. 1 for a general schematic overview of this procedure. Computational docking allows finding the best position, orientation and theoretical affinity of a ligand in the binding pocket of a target receptor [18–21]. However, docking methods also face major issues, especially considering that the mechanisms of protein–ligand recognition and binding are dynamic processes. Although flexible docking protocols easily predict different ligand conformations, the docking protocols and output results cannot account for full protein flexibility, induced-fit, and solvent effects, nor for protein–ligand complex stability and accurate binding free energy estimation. In that situation, flexible docking technique can

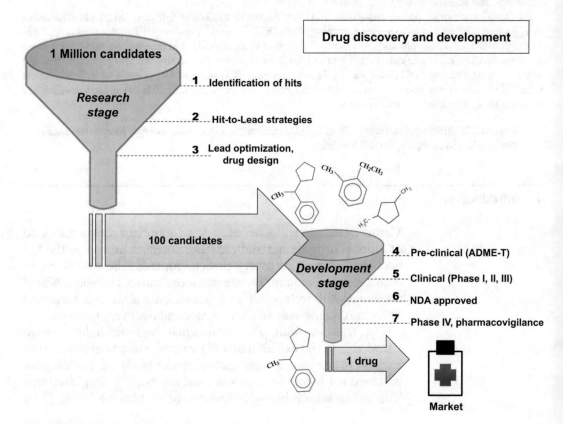

Fig. 1 A general schematic illustration of the funnel-like approach to drug discovery. This chapter deals with virtual screening, representing the first step of this method

be used to afford protein flexibility during the ligand binding event but it is only limited to a small number of residues usually in the proximity of the binding pocket. Thus, it cannot take into account important conformational changes occurring during drug binding (induced-fit effect) [22–25]. Furthermore, docking scoring functions, which allow discriminating and ranking the compounds according to their predicted binding affinity, are limited in accuracy and can be often misleading [26–30]. MD is a powerful tool which helps to overcome these critical limitations, and is generally implemented before and after docking.

MD is a computational simulation of a complex biological system which describes motions, interactions, and dynamics at the atomic level by choosing a "force field" describing all the interatomic interactions and by integrating the Newtonian equations which give position and speed of atoms over time [31–34]. As protein and protein–ligand motions would involve highly complex and computationally expensive quantum mechanics (QM) calculations, MD aims at approximating these QM terms and movements governed by probability functions through Newtonian physics and by implementing force-fields that are parameterized to fit physicochemical knowledge obtained from experimental data. Before docking, MD allows a conformational sampling and clustering of a protein or enzyme to account for protein dynamics and the conformational selection by a ligand [35, 36]. This allows facing the limitations of a "static" experimental structure by docking molecules to a representative set of protein's conformations. In some other cases where it is not obvious to find a proper binding site, it allows the detection of cryptic or allosteric cavities that were not present in the initial experimentally determined structure [37]. MD is also used as a second-step filtering process to further validate a protein–ligand complex obtained from docking by determining the stability of the complex from a trajectory, identifying persistent interatomic interactions and by estimating the binding free energy (Fig. 2). This more accurate protein-complex evaluation and validation allows better ranking of the hit molecules and further reduces the time and cost during experimental testing as well as the number of false positives and negatives [38]. Finally, by including the induced-fit and solvent effects, we can work with a more realistic model, which may apply even to a membrane-like environment in the case of membrane proteins [39]. These MD procedures will be described in detail in Subheading 3.

Docking and MD approaches are highly complementary computational methods for drug screening. But in a way similar to docking, MD also faces its own limitations. The current issues concern the high computational cost and approximations in the force-fields used, even if considerable improvements have been made in computer power and algorithmic efficiency [40–44]. Subheading 3 will present protocols to prepare a protein and MD files,

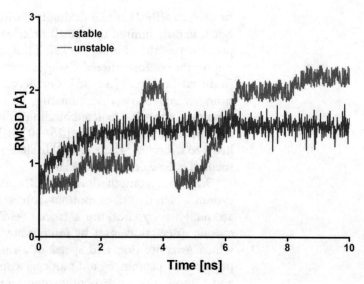

Fig. 2 Example of stability analysis (RMSD vs time) for a stable molecule (blue) and an unstable one (red) within a target protein, along a 10 ns MD trajectory

to launch an MD simulation, to analyze the MD trajectories, to extract representative receptor structures and use them in docking of a library of filtered molecules and finally to validate the putative complexes by calculating their stability, detecting interatomic interactions and by computing ligand affinity parameters.

In this chapter we describe the general virtual ligand screening workflow by implementing docking coupled with MD simulations. Each step, from the preparation of the receptor and ligand input files to the validation of the complexes is described in detail and gives the reader an overview of a complete and general strategy which is broadly used by computational biologists to find new binding molecules with pharmacological interest. We especially emphasize the need to use the information on molecular flexibility during a virtual screening procedure, which is mandatory to fully explain and predict a binding event between a receptor and a putative binding molecule.

2   Materials

The existing MD and VS software runs on a variety of platforms, but in this chapter we will focus on the programs we have used in our laboratory. Some of the other existing options will be given in references, but this is not meant to be an exhaustive review. The calculations have been performed on Desktop Workstations operating under the Linux OS (Centos 6.6), equipped with NVidia Titan Black GPU cards (http://www.nvidia.com/gtx-700-

graphics-cards/gtx-titan-black). The MD procedures outlined below have been developed with the Amber 14 and AmberTools 13 suite of programs [45] but may work with other versions of the software. Some of the data conversion was done with the Open-Babel program (http://openbabel.org/wiki/Main_Page). The docking has been performed with the AutoDock Vina program [46] using the AutoDock Tools [47] as well as with the OpenEye software suite (OpenEye Scientific Software, Santa Fe, NM, http://www.eyesopen.com). Chemical structures were drawn with MarvinSketch from ChemAxon (Marvin 6.1.5, 2013, http://www.chemaxon.com). Visualization has been done with Pymol v.1.8 (https://www.pymol.org) and Vida v.4.3 (OpenEye).

3   Methods

The objective of this chapter is to describe in detail how to perform virtual screening preserving the flexibility of both the receptor and the ligand. The receptor's flexibility is mimicked by docking to a representative set of receptor's structures, which can be obtained from the clustering analysis of an MD trajectory. The ligand's flexibility depends on the number of the rotatable bonds. This problem is routinely handled by the recent software. The MD runs are executed on GPU cards rather than on CPUs in order to profit from the acceleration of the calculation offered by hugely increased numbers of processing units present in GPUs. Details of the procedures which refer specifically to GPU computing will be mentioned explicitly in the text below.

3.1 Preparation of the Receptor's Input Files

1. Obtain the PDB file of the protein you are interested in. Typically, it will come from the PDB database (http://www.rcsb.org, http://www.pdb.org/) if the structure was experimentally determined using X-ray, NMR, or cryo-EM studies, or it can be obtained by homology modeling [48–50]. The NMR files include protons, the others usually only heavy atoms (*see* **Note 1**).

2. Add missing residues. Unstructured loops and other flexible regions of the receptor may not appear in crystallographic PDB files. The MD software, however, needs a complete molecule. We use mainly MODELLER v. 9 [48] to fill in the structural gaps. The python script "loop.py", supplied with examples of MODELLER's use, can be used for this purpose. Alter the line:

```
self.residue_range('X:A', 'Y:A')
```

to define your own region to model, substituting X, Y, and A by the relevant residue range and chain symbol, respectively.

The input PDB file must contain the residues to be modeled, but their atomic coordinates may be arbitrary. The easiest way to achieve this is to create a linear chain with the missing residues in the extended conformation as a separate molecule, then paste it in the original PDB file. Finally, launch the following script (here called "Run_Modeller_Loop") to generate N models, numbered from MOD_FROM to MOD_TO (this allows adding new models to the set of the existing ones):

```
#!/bin/sh
#
# Usage: Run_Modeller_Loop input_file MOD_FROM MOD_TO
#
fname=$1
from=$2
to=$3

cp $fname input.pdb
i=$from
while [ $i -le $to ]
do
echo "Model #"$i
  python loop.py $i > $i.log
  ((i++))
done
```

At the end the best model can be extracted according to the optimized energy score, e.g., with the command:

```
grep -H OBJECTIVE loop* | sort -n -k6
```

This produces sorted entries with the best models at the top of the list. This approach uses only command lines, but there is a graphic user interface (GUI) alternative: the Super-Looper web site (http://bioinf-applied.charite.de/super looper). The relatively easy Java-based interface allows the selection of the gap region and the residue sequence to be added. It then searches its database for a sequence match. The score is attributed according to the similarity of the database sequence to the one given in the input, and according to the satisfaction of the spatial constraints of the loop within the sequence (*see* **Note 2**).

3. Clean the PDB file. Remove the CONECT records and all protons if they exist (as is the case with NMR structures). Add TER records after the last residue of each molecular entity (polypeptide chain, cofactor, ligand) you wish to include in the MD. Look for structure-embedded disordered water

molecules. Remove all but one population of them. Similarly, look for residues which exist in alternate conformations (ALYS, BLYS, etc.). Select one of them for further processing, removing the rest. Also, correct partially built residues, such as surface side-chains with atoms missing as a result of local disorder.

4. Decide on the protonation state of residues such as HIS and CYS (in some cases ASP and GLU side chains may also be protonated). HIS becomes HID, HIE or HIP, if protonated in position delta, epsilon or both, respectively. Deprotonated cysteines and those bound to metal atoms become CYM, while those involved in disulphide bridges become CYX (*see* **Note 3**).

5. To create a disulphide bridge, use a tleap command such as "bond mol.X.SG mol.Y.SG", where mol is the object holding the protein structure, while X and Y stand for the residue numbers of cysteines involved. The residue numbers typically start from the first number in the PDB file and continue sequentially through chains and all extras, such as ions and ligands. Type "desc mol" in tleap to see all residue numberings. We use tleap rather than xleap to be independent of the graphical platform used, and to be able to include this command in batch scripts. We launch tleap on a predefined set of scripts (e.g., "tleap –f script.txt"). An example of a tleap script follows:

```
source leaprc.ff03              #(make sure that this is in the path of the program)
set default PBradii mbondi2     #(for affinity calculations; see Subheading 3.7)
mol=loadpdb prot.pdb            #(loads the cleaned and completed PDB file)
list                            #(checks the contents)
check mol                       #(there should be no missing parameters)
bond mol.10.SG mol.20.SG        #(example of a bridge between Cys10 and Cys20)
saveamberparm mol rec.prmtop rec.inpcrd   #(create topology files)
savepdb mol rec.pdb             #(optionally save the new PDB file)
quit
```

In the above the saveamberparm command allows keeping the topology of the receptor, which will be needed at the analysis stage. The script checks if the structure and topology are correct (*see* **Note 4**). Should this not be the case, error messages will appear, helping to identify the source of the problem, which should be corrected before continuing.

6. If there are ions present in the structure (Mg^{2+}, Zn^{2+}, ...), treat each as a separate residue (i.e., insert TER before and after each line on which an ion is placed). Change the atom and residue names to those recognized by the force field used, such as ff03 in the example above (e.g., for chlorine: use "Cl–" in the fields of both atom and residue names).

3.2 Preparation of MD Input Files

1. Prepare the whole system for the MD simulations in tleap by creating a solvated periodic box and adding charge neutralizing ions. The script may look like this:

```
source leaprc.ff03
set default PBradii mbondi2
mol=loadpdb prot.pdb
check mol
charge mol                    #(determine the net charge of the system)
bond mol.10.SG mol.20.SG      #(example of a bridge between Cys10 and Cys20)
solvatebox mol TIP3PBOX 10    #(create a cubic periodic box with 10Å between the
                                protein and the box edge)
addions mol Na+ 0             #(neutralize charges; use either Na+ or Cl-)
saveamberparm mol sys.prmtop sys.inpcrd   #(create topology files)
savepdb mol sys.pdb           #(optionally save the new PDB file)
quit
```

2. The MD protocol we follow executes first of all a rapid minimization of the solvent by the steepest descent algorithm. The solute is restrained by a harmonic potential with the force constant equal to 100 kcal/mol/Å^2. The typical values of different parameters are given in the script below:

```
Initial energy minimization—step 1 (solvent only)
 &cntrl
    imin=1, ncyc=500, maxcyc=500,
    ntb=1, cut=12, ntr=1
/
Hold the solute fixed
100.0
RES 1 291
END
END
```

In the above, 291 is the number of residues of the receptor including any cofactor or ligand residues, and should be adjusted as needed. As for the choice of the cutoff, the general rule is that the box size should be at least twice the cutoff plus a margin of 1–2 Å. Since the distance between a protein and the box edge is 10 Å on each side, the box size is twice this value plus the diameter of the protein, in total ca. 40 Å in this example. Since the cutoff was defined as 12 Å, the above rule is satisfied. For the description of other parameters, see the relevant manuals on the Web page http://ambermd.org/doc12.

The second stage is a more thorough minimization, where the initial 500 iterations of the steepest descent are followed by 1500 iterations (maxcyc-ncyc) of the conjugate gradient algorithm. This time the minimization includes solute under weak restraints (force constant equal to 10 kcal/mol/Å^2):

```
Initial  energy  minimization-step  2  (solvent  and  restrained
solute)
 &cntrl
   imin=1, ncyc=500, maxcyc=2000,
   ntb=1, cut=12, ntr=1
/
Weak restraints
10.0
RES 1 291
END
END
```

In the third stage we perform a short MD run of the *NVT* ensemble (ntb = 1), i.e., keeping the number of molecules (*N*), volume (*V*), and temperature (*T*) constant. The integration step is equal to 1 fs, and during the run we increase the temperature from 0 K to 300 K:

```
MD 20 ps with weak restraints and step of 1 fs
 &cntrl
   imin=0, irest=0, ntx=1,
   ntb=1, cut=12, ntr=1,
   ntc=2, ntf=2,
   tempi=0.0, temp0=300.0,
   ntt=3, gamma_ln=1.0,
   nstlim=20000, dt=0.001,
   ioutfm=1, ntxo=2,
   ntpr=1000, ntwx=1000, ntwr=1000
/
Weak restraints
10.0
RES 1 291
END
END
```

The ioutfm = 1 keyword indicates the binary output trajectory in the NetCDF format. Similarly, ntxo = 2 creates the restart file in the NetCDF format. The keywords ntpr, ntwx and ntwr define the frequency of writing to the output file, to the trajectory file and to the restart file, respectively. In this case we see new output every 1000 steps of 1 fs each, i.e., with the interval of 1 ps. In the next stage of the protocol we perform a somewhat longer MD run on the NPT ensemble (ntb = 2), i.e., keeping the number of molecules (*N*), pressure (*P*), and temperature (*T*) constant. We use the integration step of 2 fs. It is during this simulation that the system starts shrinking if the initial density was not optimal:

```
MD 100 ps NPT at 300 K; no restraints; step 2 fs
 &cntrl
   imin=0, irest=1, ntx=7,
   ntb=2, pres0=1.0, ntp=1,
   taup=2.0,
   cut=12, ntr=0,
   ntc=2, ntf=2,
   tempi=300.0, temp0=300.0,
   ntt=3, ig=-1, gamma_ln=1.0,
   nstlim=50000, dt=0.002,
   ioutfm=1, ntxo=2,
   ntpr=1000, ntwx=1000, ntwr=1000
 /
&ewald skinnb=4.0d0 /
```

In the above we have added the &ewald section with one keyword (skinnb) whose value we wish to modify. Its default value is 2 Å and it corresponds to an extension of the cutoff in which the nonbond neighbor list is created. When the system is being equilibrated, it may shrink more than the size of this parameter. This causes no problems if calculations are done on CPUs, but the GPU code is not the same and may cause an execution error. To avoid it, we altered the skinnb parameter. This value is not necessarily optimal, so its fine-tuning for each specific case is encouraged. Finally, in the final stage of the protocol we initiate a production run of 100 ns:

```
Production run: MD 100 ns NPT at 300 K; output once every 10 ps
 &cntrl
   imin=0, irest=1, ntx=7,
   ntb=2, pres0=1.0, ntp=1,
   taup=2.0,
   cut=12, ntr=0,
   ntc=2, ntf=2,
   tempi=300.0, temp0=300.0,
   ntt=3, ig=-1, gamma_ln=1.0,
   nstlim=50000000, dt=0.002,
   ioutfm=1, ntxo=2,
   ntpr=5000, ntwx=5000, ntwr=5000
 /
&ewald skinnb=4.0d0 /
```

In this case the output will be written to files every 5000 steps of 2 fs each, i.e., once every 10 ps. This gives 100 frames of the whole system per nanosecond. If the system is large, it will produce huge output trajectory files. It is for this reason that we use the NetCDF format, which roughly halves the original volume of the ASCII files (*see* **Note 5**).

3.3 Running the MD Simulation

1. Create a script that will launch all MD stages automatically. Here is an example of such a script, named "Run_pmemd_cuda":

```sh
#!/bin/sh
#
# Setup of AMBER CUDA jobs.
# Each job needs:
# - mdinX (X is the current job number)
# - $BASE.prmtop (topology file)
# - ${BASE}Y.rst (Y=X-1, coordinate file)
# NOTE: the 1st coordinate file may be the original inpcrd
file.
#
# Each job creates:
# - ${BASE}X.out (output file)
# - ${BASE}X.rst (last coordinates)
# - ${BASE}X.mdcrd (trajectory)
#
# The CUDA version launches the tasks on a GPU. To select a
given
# device, use deviceQuery, then set CUDA_VISIBLE_DEVICES.
#
echo -n "Total number of jobs: "
read Njobs
echo -n "ID of the 1st job [1]: "
read MDfirst
echo -n "Basename for I/O files: "
read BASE
echo "List of available GPUs:"
deviceQuery -noprompt | egrep '^Device' |
while read dev; do
  echo " "$dev
done
echo -n "Enter device #: "
read GPU
export CUDA_VISIBLE_DEVICES=$GPU
#
echo "Launching jobs on GPU #"$GPU"..."
if [ 0$MDfirst -eq "0" ]
then
  MDfirst=1
fi
```

```
                    MDlast=$Njobs
                    MDcurr=$MDfirst
                    MDinp=0

                    while [ $MDcurr -le $MDlast ]
                    do
                      echo -n "Job $MDcurr started on "
                      date
                      let "MDinp = ${MDcurr} - 1"

                      $AMBERHOME/bin/pmemd.cuda -O -i mdin$MDcurr \
                                        -o $BASE$MDcurr.out \
                                        -p $BASE.prmtop \
                                        -c $BASE$MDinp.rst \
                                            -ref $BASE$MDinp.rst \
                                        -r $BASE$MDcurr.rst \
                                            -inf mdinfo$MDcurr \
                                        -x $BASE$MDcurr.mdcrd

                      let "MDcurr = ${MDcurr} + 1"
                    done

                    echo -n "Jobs finished on "
                    date
```

The deviceQuery command comes with the CUDA Toolkit (https://developer.nvidia.com/cuda-toolkit), which has to be installed before using any GPU-related software. The CUDA version should correspond to the one with which the software was developed. If multiple GPU cards are to be used in parallel, the list of selected devices (variable "GPU" in the script above) contains comma-separated identifiers (e.g., "0,1"), and the first line of the launch command should be:

```
mpirun -n NGPUS $AMBERHOME/bin/pmemd.cuda.MPI -O -i mdin
$MDcurr \
```

where NGPUS is the number of GPU cards supposed to work in parallel on a given task. In order to adjust the input MD files to the above script, rename the file sys.inpcrd (*see* Subheading 3.2, **step 1**) to sys0.rst before the start of the simulations (*see* **Note 6**).

2. Log files from each stage of the simulation should be inspected for possible problems. If the first MD stage fails, it may be due to the failure of the first two minimization steps to remove the hot spots in the initial structure. Consequently, the input structure has to be examined and corrected. Ideally, the simulation would terminate without problems. However, large

systems require long computation times, often weeks to months long. If a power failure occurs, the MD run is terminated prematurely. In order to restart the calculation, we can use the rst files saved with predefined frequencies. Suppose the production run is interrupted. First, check the length of the trajectory already calculated, by consulting the simulation time at the end of the sys5.out file. Then, copy mdin5 file to a new file called mdin6 and adjust the parameter nstlim so as to obtain the initially desired length of the simulation after completing this new stage. Then simply launch the script Run_pmemd_-cuda again, specifying the total number of stages to be 6 and beginning simulations from stage #6. The program will use the existing sys5.rst as input and continue the calculation of the trajectory. If desired, the two trajectories, sys5.mdcrd and sys6.mdcrd, can be combined by the ptraj or cpptraj utility program.

3.4 Analysis of the MD Trajectory

1. Monitor the time dependence of such variables as potential energy, density, and volume. The analysis will be performed on the equilibrated part of the trajectory, where these parameters are stable. To do it, use a Perl script from the Amber website, available at the address http://archive.ambermd.org/200507/att-0228/process_mdout.perl. It produces text files whose contents can be visualized by any plotting software. By looking at the graphs one can see from which frame the trajectory can be considered stable. This and all subsequent frames to the end of the trajectory will be used in clustering to find representative and distinct structures of the receptor.

2. The clustering procedure involves several steps. We will use the kclust routine from the MMTSB software package, available from http://blue11.bch.msu.edu/mmtsb/Main_Page. In the first step we extract individual frames from the trajectory and put them as PDB files in a subdirectory. Run the following command: "ptraj sys.prmtop ptraj_PDB.in", where the last argument is the file name containing the following lines:

```
trajin sys5.mdcrd 3001 10000 1
# remove solvent and ions
strip :291-999999
# remove trans & rot
center :1-290 mass origin
image origin center familiar
# best fit to the first frame
rms first mass :1-290@CA,C,N
# put all the pdb frames in a subdirectory
trajout PDB/frame.pdb pdb
```

To obtain the same result with the newer command cpptraj (Amber 14) add the keyword multi at the end of the last line. The example above assumes that the production run sys5.mdcrd is in the current directory and that the equilibrated trajectory spans frame numbers from 3001 to 10,000. The increment is equal to 1, hence all 7000 frames will be extracted. Also, the receptor in the example above has 290 residues. You should adjust these numbers to your specific case.

The second step adjusts the file numbering format to the input requirements of the kclust program. The numbers should have leading zeros and be written with five characters. This is done by the script below:

```
#! /bin/csh
set DIR='PDB'
set ff = `ls -1 ${DIR}/*.pdb.* | head -1`
set fnam = $ff:r
set numfil = `ls -1 ${DIR}/*.pdb.???? | wc -1`
if( $numfil != 0)then
foreach fnam (${DIR}/*.pdb.????)
set fr=$fnam:r
set fnum=$fnam:e
mv $fnam $fr.0$fnum
echo $fnam $fr.0$fnum
end
endif
set numfil = `ls -1 ${DIR}/*.pdb.??? | wc -1`
if( $numfil != 0)then
 foreach fnam (${DIR}/*.pdb.???)
   set fr=$fnam:r
   set fnum=$fnam:e
   mv $fnam $fr.00$fnum
   echo $fnam $fr.00$fnum
 end
endif
set numfil = `ls -1 ${DIR}/*.pdb.?? | wc -1`
if( $numfil != 0)then
 foreach fnam (${DIR}/*.pdb.??)
   set fr=$fnam:r
   set fnum=$fnam:e
   mv $fnam $fr.000$fnum
   echo $fnam $fr.000$fnum
 end
endif
set numfil = `ls -1 ${DIR}/*.pdb.? | wc -1`
```

```
if( $numfil != 0)then
 foreach fnam (${DIR}/*.pdb.?)
   set fr=$fnam:r
   set fnum=$fnam:e
   mv $fnam $fr.0000$fnum
   echo $fnam $fr.0000$fnum
 end
endif
ls -1 ${DIR}/*.pdb* > framelist
```

The second line of the script defines the PDB subdirectory and should point at the one used in the previous step. The file created at the end of the script ("framelist") contains the list of all frames to be used in subsequent clustering.

In the third step we launch kclust and create an output file ("kclust.out") with the results:

```
#!/bin/sh
rad=2.0
list='framelist'
kclust -mode rmsd -centroid -cdist -heavy -lsqfit -radius $rad \
      -maxerr 1 -iterate ${list} > kclust.out
ncl='grep Cluster kclust.out | wc -l'
echo Found $ncl clusters
```

In the above, the name of the file with the list of frames ("framelist") should match the one used in the previous step. The rad parameter is the radius in Å, defining the size of a cluster. If a structure has RMSD distance from the centroid that is larger than rad Å, it will not be included in the current cluster. By controlling this parameter, we control the number of generated clusters.

In the fourth step we extract the centroids from the list of clusters:

```
#!/bin/sh
awk -f extract_centroids.awk kclust.out | tee centroids.stat
```

Here we use an awk script ("extract_centroids.awk", available from http://ambermd.org/tutorials/basic/tutorial3/files/extract_centroids.awk):

```
BEGIN{b0=2;}
{centind=index($1,"#Centroid");
 c=$2;
 getline;centind=index($0,"#Centroid");
 FIL0 = sprintf("centroid%2.2d.member.dat",c);
 while(centind != 1){
   print $1,$3 > FIL0 ;
```

```
        getline;centind=index($0,"#Centroid");
    }
    numcent=0; print $2,$1,NR-b0;
    c=$2;
    getline; endrec = index("End",$0);
    while( endrec != 1 ){
      FIL = sprintf("centroid%2.2d.pdb",c);
      print > FIL;
      getline; endrec = index($0,"#End");
    }
    b0=NR+2;
}
```

However, since the centroid structures have no physical meaning, we shall search for best cluster members, i.e., those of the clustered structures that are the closest to the centroids in the RMSD sense. Here is the fifth step of the procedure:

```
#!/bin/csh
set list='framelist'

rm -f best_members.out
foreach file ('ls *.member.dat')
    set i=$file:r
    set j=$i:r
    set num='sort -nk2 $file | head -1 | cut -f1 -d' ''
    set rms='sort -nk2 $file | head -1 | cut -f2 -d' ''
    set i=1
    foreach name ('cat $list')
    if ($i == $num) then
      set m=$name:e
      echo 'Best member in' $j':' ID = $m '(rmsd = '$rms')'
      echo 'Best member in' $j':\
            ' ID = $m '(rmsd = '$rms')' >> best_members.out
      cp $name ${j}_best_member.pdb
    endif
    set i='expr $i + 1'
    end
end
```

Please note that at the beginning of the script we specify explicitly the name of the file with the frame list, defined at the clustering step. The output is saved in the text file best_members. out. It lists the identifiers of the best structures in each cluster along with their corresponding RMSD values (*see* **Note** 7).

As a result, we now have a relatively short list, containing representative structures of the receptor (one per each cluster found), which will be used in subsequent docking.

3.5   Virtual Screening of Ligands and Multiple Receptor Structures

In this chapter, we will deal with two possible virtual screening strategies. The first uses Fred [51] and the associated OpenEye software (*see* Subheading 2) and considers both the ligand and the receptor to be rigid. This significantly increases the speed of the calculation, at the cost of precision. It is therefore usual to use several starting conformations for each ligand to be evaluated. The second strategy considers flexible ligand but rigid receptor, and relies on AutoDockVina [46], in which case a single conformation of each ligand is included in the library. It should be noted that Vina can, in principle, define some receptor's side-chains as being flexible, but this significantly increases the computation time and is not appropriate to fully mimic the conformational adaptation of the receptor to the ligand binding.

1. Preparation of files for docking.

   Download the chemical compounds library you are interested in or use in-house preassembled libraries. Most of the online chemical structures libraries are freely accessible for downloading (e.g., ZINC database, [52] and most of the compounds should be commercially available. These files have often an .sdf or .mol2 extension. First of all, generate 3D coordinates for the molecules. If you are planning to use Auto-Dock Vina, split them into .pdbqt files via OpenBabel with added hydrogens, removed salts and charges corresponding to the protonation state at physiological pH. The following commands can be used:

   ```
   obabel –isdf drugs.sdf –omol2 –O drugs.mol2 –r –h –p7.2 --gen3d
   obabel –imol2 drugs.mol2 –opdbqt –O drugs.pdbqt –m
   ```

   Filter your molecules according to selected physicochemical properties (e.g., Lipinski's rule of five). The Screening Assistant v.2 (http://sa2.sourceforge.net) can be used to remove known reactive compounds (covalent binders), warheads (noncovalent binders) and to eliminate PAINS (Pan-Assay Interference) compounds [53]. Alternatively, you can use the programs from the OpenEye software suite to enumerate tautomeric states for each molecule, to filter them, calculate partial atomic charges and to generate low-energy conformers:

   ```
   tautomers -in drugs.sdf -out taut_drugs.sdf
   filter -i taut_drugs.sdf -o filt_drugs.sdf -typecheck
   fixpka -i filt_drugs.sdf -o fixpka_drugs.sdf
   molcharge -method am1bccsym fixpka_drugs.sdf drugs.mol2
   omega2 drugs.mol2 drugs.oeb.gz
   ```

2. The "cleaned" chemical library is then submitted to rigid-receptor docking on a set of receptor's representative structures (extracted as previously described from MD trajectories). When defining the receptor molecular entity, it should be kept in mind that water molecules might be important for ligand recognition and binding, although this is difficult or even impossible to predict. It might therefore be useful to run virtual screening several times both with and without selected water molecules in the putative ligand binding site. The volume within which the search for the optimal ligand position will be performed has to be defined by creating a box, characterized by the coordinates of its center and the sizes in each dimension. This can easily be done with the "make_receptor" GUI of the OpenEye software. Walking through the "Molecules," "Box," "Shape," and, optionally, the "Constraints" menus will create all information necessary for the docking. Save the result in an .oeb file (.oeb.gz if compressed). If using Vina, generate a grid for each receptor structure with the AutoDock Tools. By doing this, you will place the center of the grid at the pocket's center of mass and use a spacing of 1 Å. Save the grid size and coordinates for the use in docking configuration input files.

Docking with OpenEye can be accomplished with the following example of a command line:

```
fred -rec rec.oeb.gz -dbase drugs.oeb.gz -dock_resolution
High \
      -hitlist_size 100 -numposes 20
```

Note that the product of hitlist_size and numposes should not exceed 10000. The command above uses a set of options, whose default values are listed below:

```
-docked docked.oeb.gz
-undocked undocked.oeb.gz
-score score.txt
-report report.txt
-settings settings.param
-status status.txt
-annotate false (for VIDA display; per atom score breakdown)
-prefix fred     (prefix of all output files)
```

It is also possible to launch the docking in parallel, on multiple CPUs. For example, to launch docking on N processors, replace the "fred" command with "oempirun -np N fred".

Docking with Vina can be performed on multiple CPU cores, but the program has been parallelized under OpenMP (http://openmp.org) and it works on shared memory architectures. In order to use it with chemical libraries containing large numbers of ligands, we prefer to launch Vina on a computer cluster in a typical distributed memory environment, running single-core copies of Vina, each working on a different ligand. This is accomplished by launching an array job, available in many queuing systems, such as SGE (https://arc.liv.ac.uk/trac/SGE) or PBS Professional (http://www.pbsworks.com). Ask your system manager for a generic script for your machine. Here is an example of a script that submits an array job to a cluster with the SGE queue system:

```
#!/bin/sh
# Submit an AutoDock array job, with each Vina running on 1 CPU
# and working on a different ligand, taken from a list of
files.

echo -n "Enter name of directory with input file(s): "
read indir
echo -n "Enter name of directory for output file(s): "
read outdir
echo -n "Number of concurrent jobs to run [no limit]: "
read nconc
echo -n "Job's queue identifier: "
read jid


Nmax=9999
# check nconc
if [ 0$nconc -eq "0" ]
then
  nconc=`echo $Nmax`
fi


# create a list of ligands
ls -1 ${indir}/*.pdbqt > filelist
nlig=`cat filelist | wc -l`


# create input file for qsub, in the current directory
cat << END > $jid
#!/bin/sh
#$ -o out -j y
#$ -cwd


LIGAND=\`awk "NR==\$SGE_TASK_ID" filelist\`
lnam=\`echo \$LIGAND | rev | cut -f1 -d"/" | cut -f2- -d"." |
rev\`
```

```
vina --config vina.conf --cpu 1 --ligand \$LIGAND \
     --out ${outdir}/\${lnam}_out.pdbqt \
     --log ${outdir}/\${lnam}_log.dat

END
# launch the job
qsub -R y -V -t 1-$nlig -tc $nconc $jid
```

In the above, SGE_TASK_ID is a unique identifier attributed to each processor and initialized by the system at the beginning of the program's execution. The number of simultaneously running jobs is limited to nconc (option –tc for the qsub command) in order to keep the cluster available for other users. An example of the input file vina.conf is given below:

```
# specify cpu, ligand, out & log on the command line

receptor = receptor.pdbqt
center_x = 4.531
center_y = -23.703
center_z = 66.949

size_x = 42.0
size_y = 42.0
size_z = 45.0

num_modes = 20
exhaustiveness = 100
energy_range = 5
```

Adapt the names of files and the grid size/center coordinates to your case.

3. At the end of the docking process, rank your molecules for each structure according to their Vina scores (in kcal/mol) in the output log files and a selected threshold value (*see* **Note 8**). You can also create a script to extract and rank only the first conformer for each molecule (presumed to be the most stable conformer), as in the example below:

```
#!/bin/sh
outdir = "results"    (adapt this line to your case)
nlig=`ls -1 $outdir/*log.dat | wc -l`
i=1
rm -f x_tmp
ls -1 $outdir/*log.dat |
while read fnam; do
  nrj=`grep '^ 1' $fnam | cut -c10-20`;
```

```
echo $nrj $fnam >> x_tmp;
i=`expr $i + 1`;
done
sort -n -k1 x_tmp > sorted_NRG
rm x_tmp
```

The output file sorted_NRG contains the sorted list of the ligands, best on top. Inspect the intermolecular contacts and select a number of candidates for the following steps. Then, run MD simulation to validate the selected protein–ligand complexes.

Visualization of the OpenEye docking results can be done with Vida, e.g., with the command "vida docked.oeb.gz". One can also save the structures in the mol2 format (as one single file) to view them with Pymol (as individual models).

3.6 Validation of Complexes by MD Simulations

1. Putative complex structures resulting from docking studies should be validated from the point of view of their stability. The MD simulation performed even for a relatively short stretch of time (10–20 ns) can give a wealth of information about the behavior of the ligand within the binding site, as well as about the nature of the intermolecular contacts.

   The preparation of input data for MD simulation of complex structures is similar to the procedure described above for the receptor. The difference is that a new molecule (ligand) has to be added to the system and we need its topology. In general, it will require the use of a different force field. In what follows we assume that ligands are small organic molecules which can be treated by the general Amber force field (GAFF) [54].

   We start with a PDB file of a ligand molecule. Make sure that the ligand is protonated. Use the antechamber utility to generate the first of the tleap input files:

```
antechamber -nc 0 -rn LIG -I lig.mol2 -fi mol2 -o lig.prep \
            -fo prepc -c bcc -s 2
```

   The meaning of the options is as follows: ns = net charge, rn = residue name, i = input file, fi = format of the input file, o = output file, fo = format of the output file (prepc or prepi), c = charge model, s = output verbosity. When the lig.prep file is ready, we check if all force field parameters are available:

```
parmchk -i lig.prep -f prepc -o lig.frcmod
```

   The contents of the output frcmod file should be examined, and if problems occur, they should be fixed before continuing (*see* **Note 9**).

166   Grégory Menchon et al.

In the next step, use tleap to create topology and coordinate files for the ligand. The following script shows an example of tleap's input:

```
source leaprc.ff03        (for basic definitions)
source leaprc.gaff         (for the ligand)
set default PBradii mbondi2
loadamberprep lig.prep      (antechamber-generated file)
loadamberparams lig.frcmod     (parmchk-generated file)
check LIG                  (there should be no error messages)
saveamberparm LIG lig.prmtop lig.inpcrd   (save the ligand topology)
savepdb LIG lignew.pdb        (use this file to add ligand to the receptor)
quit
```

Note that we are using the same residue name (LIG) as the one we defined for antechamber (*see* **Note 10**).

2. Prepare a receptor–ligand complex by combining protein and ligand in a single PDB file (e.g., "complex.pdb"). Copy the ligand's PDB file at the end of the receptor's PDB file. Attribute a unique chain identifier to the ligand's residues. Insert TER records after each molecule. Then, run tleap on the following script:

```
source leaprc.ff03
source leaprc.gaff
set default PBradii mbondi2
loadamberprep lig.prep
loadamberparams lig.frcmod
mol=loadpdb complex.pdb
# add modifications, such as disulfide bonds, if any
check mol
# the unit should be OK, except warnings about close
contacts.
# They will be removed by subsequent energy minimizations.
saveamberparm mol cpl.prmtop cpl.inpcrd (save topology)
savepdb mol cpl.pdb
# saves newly assigned residue numbers, protons included
quit
```

If the script terminates without errors, the complex structure is correct. See the contents of the output cpl.pdb file for newly assigned residue numbers (containing protons). Solvate the system and add charge neutralizing ions if necessary, by completing the above script with the solvatebox and addions commands, as discussed in Subheading 3.2 (*see* **Note 11**). This will produce topology files for the whole system, with names such as sys.prmtop, sys.inpcrd and sys.pdb.

3. Launch MD simulation following the recipes in Subheadings 3.2 and 3.3. The procedures for the complex are identical as for the receptor alone. In the two initial energy minimization steps of the procedure, the ligand should be considered as part of the protein, i.e., it should be restrained. Given that ligands are very small compared with the receptor, there will be no noticeable differences in MD execution times. The above steps should be repeated for all ligands obtained from the docking procedure.

4. The final validation of structures comes from the analysis of MD trajectories of the studied complexes. A stable complex should be characterized by a low root mean square deviation (RMSD) value for the ligand throughout the entire trajectory. However, the RMSD criterion is not sufficient to conclude about the stability of the complex. In spite of thermal fluctuations, the ligand should remain in the same position within the binding site, showing persistent intermolecular contacts. The information about the amplitude of atomic thermal motions can be obtained from the root mean square fluctuations (RMSF). The intermolecular contacts can be determined from the analysis of atomic proximities, which also permit to observe the formation of intermolecular hydrogen bonds. The analysis makes use of the ptraj (or cpptraj) utility, which can be run with the command "ptraj complex.prmtop ptraj.in", where the contents of the input script ptraj.in depend on the profile of the analysis. To obtain the values of RMSD and RMSF, the following example can be used:

```
trajin complex5.mdcrd 1 999999
strip :292-999999
center :1-290 mass origin
image origin center familiar
rms first mass out RMSD-rec.txt time 10 :1-290@C,N,CA
rms first mass out RMSD-lig.txt time 10 :291 nofit
atomicfluct out RMSF-lig.txt :291
```

In this example we read all frames from the input trajectory, then discard all components except the complex (in this example the receptor has 290 residues and the ligand has only one residue, #291). We superpose each frame on the first one using the mass-weighted receptor's backbone and calculate RMSD for the receptor. Then, using the previous superposition, we compute the ligand's RMSD from the dispersion of all of its atoms. The time step (10 ps) is meant to set the units on the X-axis of the generated plot. This graph will tell us if the gravity center of the ligand remains in the same position, but not whether the pose is stable. If ligand moves within the binding site, its atoms will show high values of RMSF. The last line of the above script produces a file containing RMSF of atomic fluctuations. Finally, there remains the question of intermolecular contacts. These can be obtained from the following script:

```
trajin complex5.mdcrd 3001 10000 10
#-- Donors from standard amino acids
donor mask :GLN@OE1
donor mask :GLN@NE2
donor mask :ASN@OD1
donor mask :ASN@ND2
donor mask :TYR@OH
donor mask :ASP@OD1
donor mask :ASP@OD2
donor mask :GLU@OE1
donor mask :GLU@OE2
donor mask :SER@OG
donor mask :THR@OG1
donor mask :HIS@ND1
donor mask :HIE@ND1
donor mask :HID@NE2

#-- Acceptors from standard amino acids
acceptor mask :ASN@ND2 :ASN@HD21
acceptor mask :ASN@ND2 :ASN@HD22
acceptor mask :TYR@OH :TYR@HH
acceptor mask :GLN@NE2 :GLN@HE21
acceptor mask :GLN@NE2 :GLN@HE22
acceptor mask :TRP@NE1 :TRP@HE1
acceptor mask :LYS@NZ :LYS@HZ1
acceptor mask :LYS@NZ :LYS@HZ2
acceptor mask :LYS@NZ :LYS@HZ3
acceptor mask :SER@OG :SER@HG
acceptor mask :THR@OG1 :THR@HG1
acceptor mask :ARG@NH2 :ARG@HH21
acceptor mask :ARG@NH2 :ARG@HH22
acceptor mask :ARG@NH1 :ARG@HH11
acceptor mask :ARG@NH1 :ARG@HH12
acceptor mask :ARG@NE :ARG@HE
acceptor mask :HIS@NE2 :HIS@HE2
acceptor mask :HIE@NE2 :HIE@HE2
acceptor mask :HID@ND1 :HID@HD1

acceptor mask :HIP@ND1,NE2 :HIP@HE2,HD1
#-- Backbone donors and acceptors for this particular molecule
# N-H for prolines do not exist so are not in the mask
# in this example res181 is supposed to be PRO and excluded
donor mask @O
acceptor mask :2-180,182-290@N :2-290@H
```

```
# Terminal residues have different atom names
donor mask @OXT
acceptor mask :1@N :1@H1
acceptor mask :1@N :1@H2
acceptor mask :1@N :1@H3
#
hbond print .05 series hbt time 10 distance 3.5 angle 120.0 \
    out hbond.dat solventdonor WAT O solventacceptor WAT O H1 \
        solventacceptor WAT O H2
```

The generic version of the example above is downloadable from the address http://ambermd.org/tutorials/basic/tutorial3/files/analyse_hbond.ptraj. Adjust it according to your needs. The output file ("hbond.dat") contains information about the formation and breaking of hydrogen bonds throughout the trajectory. The total combined information should be used to assess the stability of the studied complex.

3.7 Estimation of Ligand Affinity

One of the most attractive features offered by the analysis of an MD trajectory is the estimation of the protein–ligand interaction energy. This in turn should be linked to ligand affinity. Unfortunately, this is a very complex issue and not yet sufficiently resolved in practice. Theoretically, the intermolecular interaction energy can be calculated from the difference between the energy of the complex and the sum of energies of its individual components. The Gibbs free energy of the system is the sum of the enthalpic and the entropic terms. The force field-based energy is an approximation to the enthalpic term of the free energy expression [55–57]. The entropic term is often as important as the enthalpic one, but there are enormous difficulties in computing it, and so in practice it is usually neglected. This simplification nevertheless allows comparison of similar ligands, for which the entropic terms may not vary too much. In spite of these difficulties, several methods are frequently used. The most popular approach in evaluating intermolecular interaction energy is the molecular mechanics (MM) combined with the Poisson-Boltzmann (PB) or generalized Born (GB) and surface area (SA) continuum solvation methods (MM-PBSA and MM-GBSA) [58]. Other, more sophisticated methods have also been developed, such as interactive Linear Interaction Energy (iLIE) approach [59–61], but they require calibration on a known set of ligands with experimentally determined affinities, which constitutes a major limitation. Moreover, they require more time to run, which is prohibitive in virtual screening, where affinities for many ligands have to be determined in a relatively short time. In what follows we focus on the most widely used MM-PBSA and MM-GBSA methods, as available in the Amber software suite. These methods are based on the implicit solvent approach and need as input the separate trajectories of unsolvated complex, of the protein and of the ligand. In practice, this information is extracted from the MD trajectory of the solvated protein–ligand complex. Consequently, the program requires the corresponding topologies, which have already been generated with tleap in intermediate steps of the procedure (files named sys.prmtop, cpl. prmtop, rec.prmtop, and lig.prmtop, corresponding to the solvated system, the unsolvated complex, the receptor, and the ligand, respectively).

1. Use the MMPBSA.py.MPI [62] program to profit from multi-core systems. The script below demonstrates its use in calculating the protein–ligand intermolecular energy with both the MM-PBSA and the MM-GBSA methods:

```sh
#!/bin/sh

echo -n "Input script name: [mmpbsa_py.in] "
read INSCRIPT
if [ -z $INSCRIPT ]
then
  INSCRIPT="mmpbsa_py.in"
fi

echo -n "Solvated prmtop file: [sys.prmtop] "
read SYSFILE
if [ -z $SYSFILE ]
then
  SYSFILE="sys.prmtop"
fi

echo -n "Complex prmtop file: [cpl.prmtop] "
read CPLFILE
if [ -z $CPLFILE ]
then
  CPLFILE="cpl.prmtop"
fi

echo -n "Receptor prmtop file: [rec.prmtop] "
read RECFILE
if [ -z $RECFILE ]
then
  RECFILE="rec.prmtop"
fi

echo -n "Ligand prmtop file: [lig.prmtop] "
read LIGFILE
if [ -z $LIGFILE ]
```

```
then
  LIGFILE="lig.prmtop"
fi

echo -n "Trajectory file (name with ext.): "
read MDCRD
if [ -z "$MDCRD" ]
then
  echo "*** Error: Trajectory files must be specified expli-
citly."
  exit
fi

echo -n "Number of CPUs to use: [4] "
read NPROC
if [ -z $NPROC ]
then
  NPROC=4
fi

echo "Launching MMPBSA.py.MPI on $NPROC CPUs."
echo -n "JOB STARTED on "
date

mpiexec -np $NPROC $AMBERHOME/bin/MMPBSA.py.MPI -O -i $IN-
SCRIPT \
                        -o out_binding.dat \
                        -do out_decomp.dat \
                        -sp $SYSFILE \
                        -cp $CPLFILE \
                        -rp $RECFILE \
                        -lp $LIGFILE \
                        -y $MDCRD > out.log

echo -n "JOB FINISHED on "
date
exit 0
```

Note that there are two output files with predefined names: out_binding.dat and out_decomp.dat. The first one contains information on binding energies and the second one lists energy decomposition details. An example of the input script for per-residue energy decomposition (mmpbsa_py.in) is given below:

```
MMPBSA input file for running per-residue decomposition
&general
  startframe=3001, endframe=5000, interval=2,
```

```
/
&gb
# for igb=5, use "set default PBradii mbondi2"
# in scripts producing prmtop files
# for igb=7, use "set default PBradii bondi" (not for nucleic
acids)
  igb=5, saltcon=0.010
/
&pb
  istrng=0.010,
  indi=4,
/
&decomp
  idecomp=1, print_res='1-303', csv_format=0,
  dec_verbose=2,
/
```

The &pb and &gb sections refer to the MM-PBSA and the MM-GBSA methods, respectively (*see* **Note 12**). As usual, adjust the relevant variables as needed.

2. In order to perform pairwise energy decomposition, use the above script with the following minor modifications: set idecomp to 3, and dec_verbose to 0 (otherwise the output will be too voluminous). In both cases the output can be sorted to focus on residues important for the intermolecular interactions.

3.8 Concluding Remarks

In conclusion, docking and MD are fully complementary. Docking is fast and inexpensive, and MD allows taking into account a full system flexibility giving more reliable and "realistic" interaction and affinity information. MD is not an easy task and its protocols are constantly improving with better algorithms and force fields, and in parallel with better computer performance, allowing today to simulate a protein in the microsecond timescale and in complex membrane-like environments. Docking with simultaneous MD calculation would be an appropriate solution with all steps included in one pass, but would currently take too long to simulate and would face difficulties in the interpretation if the system got trapped in local minima. Implementing MD protocols within a virtual ligand screening process is necessary to increase the hit compounds discovery success rate and enter a well-known "hit-to-lead" strategy to obtain molecules with higher affinity and specificity against medically relevant biological targets.

The choice of methods presented in this chapter has been dictated by our own experience, but there are numerous alternative approaches, which the readers are encouraged to explore [63–70, 72].

The archive containing the scripts presented in this chapter is available for download from the following URL: http://cribligand.ipbs.fr/cheminfo-scripts.html.

4   Notes

1. PDB files from NMR studies usually contain 20 superposed structures. Pick the first one, as it should have the least constraint violations. The choice is not critical because the MD will relax the molecule and drive it to equilibrium.

2. The loop modeling as described above works up to the loop length of 30 residues. For longer loops a different strategy has to be adopted. One can model loops incrementally, a fragment at a time. Another possibility is to run an MD simulation with the loop as a separate chain, with distance constraints on loop termini to obtain spatial proximity to the receptor, then running the MD again to equilibrate the loop incorporated in the structure.

3. If you want to simulate deprotonated HIS, *see* ref. 71.

4. tleap renumbers residues beginning from 1. Subsequent residue referencing (e.g., for the "bond" command) must take this into account.

5. If multiple GPU cards are supposed to execute the MD protocol, the first two stages (i.e., the two consecutive minimizations) have to be performed on a single card. At the time of the writing this part of the code is not yet parallelized for GPUs. Multiple GPU cards can work on the MD protocol beginning with the third stage, i.e., from the short MD run with sample heating.

6. In order to use GPUs for MD, install the appropriate version of NVidia's CUDA library on your system, then compile the CUDA version of the software (e.g., Amber's pmemd.cuda). This will create a binary compatible with your hardware. There is a problem in NVidia's software with the detection of GPU cards and the assignment of unique identifiers. The order in which GPU cards are detected is different depending on whether we launch a command from a terminal (nvidia-smi), from a GUI interface (nvidia-settings) or via the CUDA library (deviceQuery). In each case the identifiers of GPU cards may be different, which is confusing. However, in practice only the output from deviceQuery is valid for the launch of the GPU software.

7. The kclust program handles up to 50000 files. In practice, this is not a significant limitation. However, its output contains an error: the PDB files written by kclust show residue numbers in

columns 24–27, instead of columns 23–26. Pymol displays them correctly, but VMD does not. This can be corrected by shifting the residue numbers by one column to the left.

8. Currently there are over 30 scoring functions, which represent diverse approaches to the calculation of ligand affinity [30]. It is a good idea to rescore your results with several different functions and accept ligands as hits only if there is a consensus, i.e., when ligands score well with most of the methods.

9. When preparing ligands with the antechamber utility, the program sometimes fails on PDB files. In this case try the mol2 format. However, it is likely that the reasons of these problems come from erroneous or ambiguous definition of the ligand's structure. If the initial structure is not optimized, the missing CONECT records may be the reason of the failure.

10. When preparing a complex PDB file with several ligands, make sure that each ligand has a different chain identifier and also that you use different residue numbers for different ligands. Otherwise Amber complains about split residues.

11. Adding charge neutralizing ions to the system can be done using the addions command. Another version exists: addions2. It is longer in execution, but it uses a more sophisticated algorithm for placement of ions within the periodic box.

12. When comparing intermolecular energy values calculated with different versions of the Amber software and different scripts supplied with it, we obtain results which are not necessarily in agreement, sometimes not even qualitatively. The most coherent results we have obtained in our calculations come from Amber 14 (as compared to versions 9 and 12). We compared the results of energy calculations with the Generalized Born (GB) and Poisson–Boltzmann (PB) methods by the two most commonly used scripts supplied with the Amber software: mm_pbsa.pl written in Perl (PL), and MMPBSA.py, written in Python (PY). The tests were performed on eight different receptor-ligand systems (data not published). The results of the GB method as calculated by the PL and PY scripts are comparable (within ±10%) for half of the studied systems. In two of the remaining cases, the PL script gave a result 20–30% higher than the PY script, in the other two the PL script clearly broke down, giving unrealistic values. Therefore, we prefer to trust the results of GB calculations with the PY script.

The calculations using the PB method with the PL script are consistent with the rest of the results and provide reasonable values for the cases for which the GB method has not worked. By way of contrast, the PB method used with the PY script always gives results which are scaled by a factor of ½ with respect to all the other values. If we multiply each PB

(PY) result by the empirical factor of 2, we get consistent and coherent results for the full set of the studied systems. Since these corrected values are overall closer to those calculated by the GB method of the same PY script (as compared to the GB/PB values from the PL script), we have a preference for using the PY script, under the condition of doubling the PB values. This particular requirement may not be necessary in newer versions of AmberTools, but we have been unable to test it for lack of access.

Acknowledgment

We acknowledge financial support from PICT—GenoToul platform of Toulouse, CNRS, Université de Toulouse-UPS, European structural funds, the Midi-Pyrénées region, CNRS. G.M. was supported by Ph.D. fellowships from Ministère de l'enseignement supérieur et de la Recherche (3 years) and from Ligue Nationale Contre le Cancer (1 year). We thank Alain Milon and Pascal Demange for their critical reading of the manuscript, which improved its final quality.

References

1. Tarcsay A, Paragi G, Vass M, Jojart B, Bogar F, Keseru GM (2013) The impact of molecular dynamics sampling on the performance of virtual screening against GPCRs. J Chem Inf Model 53:2990–2999

2. Barakat KH, Jordheim LP, Perez-Pineiro R, Wishart D, Dumontet C, Tuszynski JA (2012) Virtual screening and biological evaluation of inhibitors targeting the XPA-ERCC1 interaction. PLoS One 7:e51329

3. De Vivo M, Masetti M, Bottegoni G, Cavalli A (2016) Role of molecular dynamics and related methods in drug discovery. J Med Chem 59:4035–4061

4. Durrant JD, McCammon JA (2011) Molecular dynamics simulations and drug discovery. BMC Biol 9:71–79

5. Galeazzi R (2009) Molecular dynamics as a tool in rational drug design: current status and some major applications. Curr Comput Aided Drug Des 5:225–240

6. Hospital A, Goni JR, Orozco M, Gelpi JL (2015) Molecular dynamics simulations: advances and applications. Adv Appl Bioinform Chem 8:37–47

7. Jiang L, Zhang X, Chen X, He Y, Qiao L, Zhang Y, Li G, Xiang Y (2015) Virtual screening and molecular dynamics study of potential negative allosteric modulators of mGluR1 from Chinese herbs. Molecules 20:12769–12786

8. Kundu A, Dutta A, Biswas P, Das AK, Ghosh AK (2015) Functional insights from molecular modeling, docking, and dynamics study of a cypoviral RNA dependent RNA polymerase. J Mol Graph Model 61:160–174

9. Mirza SB, Salmas RE, Fatmi MQ, Durdagi S (2016) Virtual screening of eighteen million compounds against dengue virus: combined molecular docking and molecular dynamics simulations study. J Mol Graph Model 66:99–107

10. Moroy G, Sperandio O, Rielland S, Khemka S, Druart K, Goyal D, Perahia D, Miteva MA (2015) Sampling of conformational ensemble for virtual screening using molecular dynamics simulations and normal mode analysis. Future Med Chem 7:2317–2331

11. Naresh KN, Sreekumar A, Rajan SS (2015) Structural insights into the interaction between molluscan hemocyanins and phenolic substrates: an in silico study using docking and molecular dynamics. J Mol Graph Model 61:272–280

12. Nichols SE, Baron R, Ivetac A, McCammon JA (2011) Predictive power of molecular

dynamics receptor structures in virtual screening. J Chem Inf Model 51:1439–1446

13. Nichols SE, Riccardo B, McCammon JA (2012) On the use of molecular dynamics receptor conformations for virtual screening. Methods Mol Biol 819:93–103

14. Okimoto N, Futatsugi N, Fuji H, Suenaga A, Morimoto G, Yanai R, Ohno Y, Narumi T, Taiji M (2009) High-performance drug discovery: computational screening by combining docking and molecular dynamics simulations. PLoS Comput Biol 5:e1000528

15. Rodriguez-Bussey IG, Doshi U, Hamelberg D (2016) Enhanced molecular dynamics sampling of drug target conformations. Biopolymers 105:35–42

16. Sliwoski G, Kothiwale S, Meiler J, Lowe EW Jr (2014) Computational methods in drug discovery. Pharmacol Rev 66:334–395

17. Bartesaghi A, Merk A, Banerjee S, Matthies D, Wu X, Milne JLS, Subramaniam S (2015) 2.2 Å resolution cryo-EM structure of β-galactosidase in complex with a cell-permeant inhibitor. Science 348:1147–1151

18. Hughes JP, Rees S, Kalindjian SB, Philpott KL (2011) Principles of early drug discovery. Br J Pharmacol 162:1239–1249

19. Kuenemann MA, Sperandio O, Labbe CM, Lagorce D, Miteva MA, Villoutreix BO (2015) In silico design of low molecular weight protein-protein interaction inhibitors: overall concept and recent advances. Prog Biophys Mol Biol 119:20–32

20. Ramirez D (2016) Computational methods applied to rational drug design. Open Med Chem J 10:7–20

21. Rognan D (2015) Rational design of protein-protein interaction inhibitors. Med Chem Commun 6:51–60

22. B-Rao C, Subramanian J, Sharma SD (2009) Managing protein flexibility in docking and its applications. Drug Discov Today 14:394–400

23. Cavasotto CN, Abagyan RA (2004) Protein flexibility in ligand docking and virtual screening to protein kinases. J Mol Biol 337:209–225

24. Durrant JD, McCammon JA (2010) Computer-aided drug-discovery techniques that account for receptor flexibility. Curr Opin Pharmacol 10:770–774

25. Totrov M, Abagyan R (2008) Flexible ligand docking to multiple receptor conformations: a practical alternative. Curr Opin Struct Biol 18:178–184

26. Feher M (2006) Consensus scoring for protein–ligand interactions. Drug Discov Today 11:421–428

27. Politi R, Convertino M, Popov K, Dokholyan NV, Tropsha A (2016) Docking and scoring with target-specific pose classifier succeeds in native-like pose identification but not binding affinity prediction in the CSAR 2014 benchmark exercise. J Chem Inf Model 56:1032–1041

28. Quiroga R, Villarreal MA (2016) Vinardo: a scoring function based on autodock vina improves scoring, docking, and virtual screening. PLoS One 11:e0155183

29. Wang Z, Sun H, Yao X, Li D, Xu L, Li Y, Tian S, Hou T (2016) Comprehensive evaluation of ten docking programs on a diverse set of protein–ligand complexes: the prediction accuracy of sampling power and scoring power. Phys Chem Chem Phys 18:12964–12975

30. Seifert MHJ (2009) Targeted scoring functions for virtual screening. Drug Discov Today 14:562–569

31. Leach AR (2001) Molecular modelling: principles and applications, 2nd edn. Pearson, Dorchester

32. Ryckaert J-P, Ciccotti G, Berendsen HJC (1977) Numerical integration of the cartesian equations of motion of a system with constraints: molecular dynamics of n-alkanes. J Comput Phys 23:327–341

33. Schlick T (2002) Molecular modeling and simulation: an interdisciplinary guide. Springer, New York

34. Stanley N, De Fabritiis G (2015) High throughput molecular dynamics for drug discovery. Silico Pharmacol 3:3–6

35. Lin JH, Perryman AL, Schames JR, McCammon JA (2003) The relaxed complex method: accommodating receptor flexibility for drug design with an improved scoring scheme. Biopolymers 68:47–62

36. Sinko W, Lindert S, McCammon JA (2013) Accounting for receptor flexibility and enhanced sampling methods in computer-aided drug design. Chem Biol Drug Des 81:41–49

37. Cala O, Remy M-H, Guillet V, Merdes A, Mourey L, Milon A, Czaplicki G (2013) Virtual and biophysical screening targeting the gamma-tubulin complex – a new target for the inhibition of microtubule nucleation. PLoS One 8:e63908

38. Alonso H, Bliznyuk AA, Gready JE (2006) Combining docking and molecular dynamic simulations in drug design. Med Res Rev 26:531–568

39. Mori T, Miyashita N, Im W, Feig M, Sugita Y (2016) Molecular dynamics simulations of biological membranes and membrane proteins

using enhanced conformational sampling algorithms. Biochim Biophys Acta 1858:1635–1651

40. Arthur EJ, Brooks CL III (2016) Efficient Implementation of constant pH molecular dynamics on modern graphics processors. J Comput Chem 37:2171–2180

41. Ge H, Wang Y, Li C et al (2013) Molecular dynamics-based virtual screening: accelerating the drug discovery process by high-performance computing. J Chem Inf Model 53:2757–2764

42. Iakovou G, Hayward S, Laycock SD (2015) Adaptive GPU-accelerated force calculation for interactive rigid molecular docking using haptics. J Mol Graph Model 61:1–12

43. Kazachenko S, Giovinazzo M, Hall KW, Cann NM (2015) Algorithms for GPU-based molecular dynamics simulations of complex fluids: applications to water, mixtures, and liquid crystals. J Comput Chem 36:1787–1804

44. Kutzner C, Pall S, Fechner M, Esztermann A, de Groot BL, Grubmüller H (2015) Best bang for your buck: GPU nodes for GROMACS biomolecular simulations. J Comput Chem 36:1990–2008

45. Salomon-Ferrer R, Case DA, Walker RC (2013) An overview of the Amber biomolecular simulation package. WIREs Comput Mol Sci 3:198–210

46. Trott O, Olson AJ (2010) AutoDock Vina: improving the speed and accuracy of docking with a new scoring function, efficient optimization, and multithreading. J Comput Chem 31:455–461

47. Morris GM, Huey R, Lindstrom W, Sanner MF, Belew RK, Goodsell DS, Olson AJ (2009) AutoDock4 and AutoDockTools4: automated docking with selective receptor flexibility. J Comput Chem 30:2785–2791

48. Eswar N, Eramian D, Webb B, Shen M-Y, Sali A (2008) Protein structure modeling with MODELLER. In: Kobe B, Guss M, Huber T (eds) Structural proteomics. High-throughput methods. Methods in molecular biology, vol 426. Humana, Totowa, NJ, pp 145–159

49. Song Y, DiMaio F, Wang RY-R, Kim D, Miles C, Brunette T, Thompson J, Baker D (2013) High resolution comparative modeling with RosettaCM. Structure 21:1735–1742

50. Kelley LA, Mezulis S, Yates CM, Wass MN, Sternberg MJ (2015) The Phyre2 web portal for protein modeling, prediction and analysis. Nat Protoc 10:845–858

51. McGann M (2011) FRED pose prediction and virtual screening accuracy. J Chem Inf Model 51:578–596

52. Irwin JJ, Shoichet BK (2005) ZINC-a free database of commercially available compounds for virtual screening. J Chem Inf Model 45:177–182

53. Baell J, Walters MA (2014) Chemical con artists foil drug discovery. Nature 513:481–483

54. Wang J, Wolf RM, Caldwell JW, Kollman PA, Case DA (2004) Development and testing of a general amber force field. J Comput Chem 25:1157–1174

55. Chong S-H, Ham S (2015) Structural versus energetic approaches for protein conformational entropy. Chem Phys Lett 627:90–95

56. Kassem S, Marawan A, El-Sheikh S, Barakat KH (2015) Entropy in bimolecular simulations: a comprehensive review of atomic fluctuations-based methods. J Mol Graph Model 62:105–117

57. Procacci P (2016) Reformulating the entropic contribution in molecular docking scoring functions. J Comput Chem 37:1819–1827

58. Genheden S, Ryde U (2015) The MM/PBSA and MM/GBSA methods to estimate ligand-binding affinities. Expert Opin Drug Discovery 10:449–461

59. Vosmeer CR, Pool R, van Stee MF, Peric-Hassler L, Vermeulen NPE, Geerke DP (2014) Towards automated binding affinity prediction using an iterative linear interaction energy approach. Int J Mol Sci 15:798–816

60. Rosendahl Kjellgren E, Skytte Glue OE, Reinholdt P, Egeskov Meyer J, Kongsted J, Poongavanam V (2015) A comparative study of binding affinities for 6,7-dimethoxy-4-pyrrolidylquinazolines as phosphodiesterase 10 A inhibitors using the linear interaction energy method. J Mol Graph Model 61:44–52

61. Stjernschantz E, Oostenbrink C (2010) Improved ligand-protein binding affinity predictions using multiple binding modes. Biophys J 98:2682–2691

62. Miller BR III, McGee TD, Swails JM, Homeyer N, Gohlke H, Roitberg AE (2012) MMPBSA.py: an efficient program for end-state free energy calculations. J Chem Theory Comput 8:3314–3321

63. Borhani DW, Shaw DE (2012) The future of molecular dynamics simulations in drug discovery. J Comput Aided Mol Des 26:15–26

64. Decherchi S, Masetti M, Vyalov I, Rocchia W (2015) Implicit solvent methods for free energy estimation. Eur J Med Chem 91:27–42

65. Le L (2012) Incorporating molecular dynamics simulations into rational drug design: a case study on influenza a neuraminidases. In: Pérez-Sánchez H (ed) Bioinformatics. InTech, Rijeka

66. Mortier J, Rakers C, Bermudez M, Murgueitio MS, Riniker S, Wolber G (2015) The impact of molecular dynamics on drug design: applications for the characterization of ligand–macromolecule complexes. Drug Discov Today 20:686–702

67. Tautermann CS, Seeliger D, Kriegl JM (2015) What can we learn from molecular dynamics simulations for GPCR drug design? Comput Struct Biotechnol J 13:111–121

68. Zhao H, Caflisch A (2015) Molecular dynamics in drug design. Eur J Med Chem 91:4–14

69. Okimoto N, Suenaga A, Taiji M (2016) Evaluation of protein–ligand affinity prediction using steered molecular dynamics simulations. J Biomol Struct Dyn 7:1–11

70. Li MS, Mai BK (2012) Steered molecular dynamics—a promising tool for drug design. Curr Bioinformatics 7:342–351

71. Pang Y-P, Xu K, El Yazal J, Prendergast FG (2000) Successful molecular dynamics simulation of the zinc-bound farnesyltransferase using the cationic dummy atom approach. Protein Sci 9:1857–1865

72. Menchon G, Bombarde O, Trivedi M et al (2016) Structure-based virtual ligand screening on the XRCC4/DNA ligase IV interface. Sci Rep 6:22878–22890

Chapter 10

Building Molecular Interaction Networks from Microarray Data for Drug Target Screening

Sze Chung Yuen, Hongmei Zhu, and Siu-wai Leung

Abstract

Potential drug targets for the disease treatment can be identified from microarray studies on differential gene expression of patients and healthy participants. Here, we describe a method to use the information of differentially expressed (DE) genes obtained from microarray studies to build molecular interaction networks for identification of pivotal molecules as potential drug targets. The quality control and normalization of the microarray data are conducted with R packages *simpleaffy* and *affy*, respectively. The DE genes with adjusted P values less than 0.05 and log fold changes larger than 1 or less than -1 are identified by *limma* package to construct a molecular interaction network with InnateDB. The genes with significant connectivity are identified by the Cytoscape app *jActiveModules*. The interactions among the genes within a module are tested by *psych* package to determine their associations. The gene pairs with significant association and known protein structures according to the Protein Data Bank are selected as potential drug targets. As an example for drug target screening, we demonstrate how to identify potential drug targets from a molecular interaction network constructed with the DE genes of significant connectivity, using a microarray dataset of type 2 diabetes mellitus.

Key words Differentially expressed genes, Drug targets, Microarray, R, Type 2 diabetes mellitus

1 Introduction

Microarrays are a high-throughput technology to determine differential gene expression [1, 2]. For example, the Affymetrix platform can detect the expression of 20,000–40,000 genes simultaneously [3]. Its capability is adequate to cover major genes in human genome [4, 5]. Affymetrix applies a probe set to interrogate a single gene. The expression ratios estimated from significantly different signal intensities within a probe set should be consistent [6].

Microarray technology allows researchers to detect dysregulation in gene expression that would help diagnose and understand

Mohini Gore and Umesh B. Jagtap (eds.), *Computational Drug Discovery and Design*, Methods in Molecular Biology, vol. 1762, https://doi.org/10.1007/978-1-4939-7756-7_10, © Springer Science+Business Media, LLC, part of Springer Nature 2018

the molecular mechanism of diseases [7, 8]. Identification of dys-regulated genes, i.e., differentially expressed (DE) genes, could also help identify potential drug targets. Determination of DE genes would require special statistical analysis to avoid or correct biases due to violation of statistical assumptions (e.g., sample sizes and multiple testing). For example, moderated t-statistic [9] can avoid bias due to small sample sizes in determining the variance from many selected genes.

Building a molecular interaction network from a list of DE genes would be a daunting task due to the sheer volume of data. A molecular interaction network is usually characterized by its community structure [10]. The molecules (represented as nodes in a network), e.g., genes or proteins, found in a module could be enriched for their possible biological functions [11]. The molecules involved in the mechanism of a disease are likely interacting with one another in modules [12]. In such a module, the molecular interactions are significantly correlated in suggesting strong associations of the DE genes with the disease.

To illustrate how this method works, we take type 2 diabetes mellitus (T2DM) for example. There are more than 380 million people diagnosed with T2DM worldwide [13]. The prevalence is increasing, and expected to affect more than 550 million people by 2030. More than 4 million T2DM patients died in 2011 [13]. T2DM patients suffer from insulin resistance and β-cell dysfunction, resulting in hyperglycemia [14, 15]. T2DM causes severe vascular complications, including atherosclerosis and diabetic nephropathy [16]. It costs 5–10% of total expenditure in health care in many countries [17]. Insulin is synthesized by pancreatic β-cells and released in response to elevation of blood glucose level [18]. There is a strong genetic predisposition associated with T2DM, i.e., are expected to have T2DM and the risk would surge to 40% or 70% depending on whether one parent or both parents have diabetes [19]. Genetic studies [20–22] found many genes related to β-cell function, including TCF7L2 for increasing insulin secretion, PPARG for insulin sensitivity. However, the genetics of T2DM has not been fully elucidated. DE genes are thus crucial to understanding the pathogenic mechanism and identifying potential drug targets of T2DM. The following sections describe a method to identify potential drug targets by building molecular interaction networks from microarray data.

2 Materials

A microarray dataset, which comprises gene expression information obtained from patients and healthy participants, is selected to identify potential drug targets. Microarray dataset GSE25724 is downloaded from Gene Expression Omnibus (GEO), contributed by

```
#Install affy package
source("https://bioconductor.org/biocLite.R")
biocLite("affy")


#Install RColorBrewer package
install.packages("RColorBrewer")


#Install simpleaffy package
source("https://bioconductor.org/biocLite.R")
biocLite("simpleaffy")


#Install limma package
source("https://bioconductor.org/biocLite.R")
biocLite("limma")


#Install hgu133a.db package
source("https://bioconductor.org/biocLite.R")
biocLite("hgu133a.db")


#Install psych package
install.packages("psych")
```

Fig. 1 Installation of R packages

Bugliani M, including a total of 13 samples, 7 samples from non-T2DM and 6 samples from T2DM [23]. Also, this microarray dataset is compliant with the Minimum Information About a Microarray Experiment (MIAME) guideline [24]. Its microarray platform is Affymetrix Human Genome U133A Array.

R is downloaded from https://cran.r-project.org/bin/windows/base. RStudio is downloaded from https://www.rstudio.com/products/rstudio/download. Cytoscape [25] is downloaded from http://www.cytoscape.org.

The R packages, *affy* [26], *RColorBrewer* [27], *simpleaffy* [28], *limma* [29], *hgu133a.db* [30], and *psych* [31], should be installed (Fig. 1).

3 Methods

3.1 Quality Control

All downloaded .CEL files are saved in a single file (e.g., the file can be named by the GEO number GSE25724). The raw data of .CEL files are read by *affy* package of R software (Fig. 2).

The intensities of all arrays provide some information about the quality of the arrays. The package *RColorBrewer* is used to provide color-coded quality control plots. The arrays in the same color indicates that they are from the same group, i.e., healthy or T2DM. The label are put on the x-axis at the size of 50% smaller, by setting las=3, cex.axis=0.5, respectively. The box plots show the relative medians among all arrays (Fig. 3).

The quality control of these files is conducted with *simpleaffy* package of R software. The parameter "usemid=T" suggests that 3′ to mid ratios for β-actin and GAPDH are used, instead of 3′–5′ ratios for β-actin and GAPDH (*see* **Note 1**).

The median of GSM631755.CEL is higher, compared with the others. The quality control plot provides the information of several quality control metrics, including average background, number of genes called present, scale factor, 3′ to mid ratios for β-actin and GAPDH (Fig. 4). The direction of scaling factor for GSM631755.CEL is significantly different from the others, and it is close to the boundary. The average background for GSM631755.CEL is also higher than the others, suggesting that a greater signal is detected from the array. The GSM631755.CEL is then removed from the data set.

The arrays are saved into a new file (i.e., the file can be named cleanerrawdata). Again, we need to set the working directory, read the arrays, assess the intensities, and conduct the quality control (Fig. 5a).

The medians of intensities are similar across all 12 arrays (Fig. 5b). The average background, number of genes called present, and scale factor are similar across 12 arrays (Fig. 5c). The hybridization control gene is called present in each array, indicating good quality of hybridization. The high ratios of 3′ to mid for β-actin and GAPDH from diabetic samples indicate unsatisfactory

a
```
#Read the .CEL files by affy

library(affy)

rawfiles<-list.celfiles()

rawdata<-ReadAffy(filenames=rawfiles)
```

b
```
> rawfiles
 [1] "GSM631755.CEL.gz" "GSM631756.CEL.gz" "GSM631757.CEL.gz" "GSM631758.CEL.gz" "GSM631759.CEL.gz" "GSM631760.CEL.gz"
 [7] "GSM631761.CEL.gz" "GSM631762.CEL.gz" "GSM631763.CEL.gz" "GSM631764.CEL.gz" "GSM631765.CEL.gz" "GSM631766.CEL.gz"
[13] "GSM631767.CEL.gz"
```

Fig. 2 Access to .CEL files. (**a**) R code for reading .CEL files. (**b**) A list of .CEL files available in the folder

a

```
#Intensity of .CEL files
library("RColorBrewer")
usr.col=brewer.pal(9, "Set1")
mycols=rep(usr.col, each=7,6)
boxplot(rawdata, col=mycols, las=3, cex.axis=0.5,
names=sampleNames(rawdata), main="Rawdata")
```

b

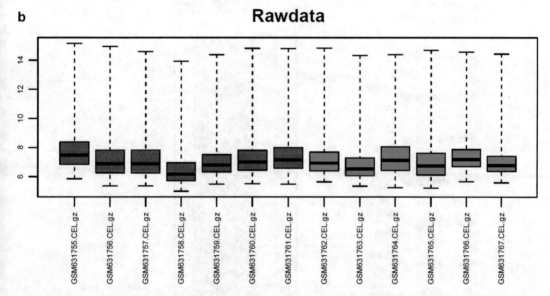

Fig. 3 Intensities of arrays. (**a**) R code for showing the intensity of all arrays. (**b**) The intensities of all arrays are shown in box plots

RNA quality, while the RNA quality from nondiabetic samples is acceptable. It is possible that there is contamination during sample collection for diabetic samples. Although these arrays are not perfect in quality, they can be used for the subsequent analysis.

3.2 Normalization

The noisy signals from the experiments should be removed by data normalization. The intensities from arrays are processed through background correction, normalization, and probe-specific correction. The probe set-level data are on log scale. There are several methods of background correction, normalization, probe-specific correction, and summarization provided by *affy* package [32]. The background data can be corrected by *rma* method (Fig. 6) but should be conjugated with *pmonly* method for probe-specific correction. The data summarized by *medianpolish* method should not be used after *subtractmm* method for probe-specific

a

```
#Quality plot of .CEL files
library("simpleaffy")
rawdata.qc<-qc(rawdata)
plot(rawdata.qc, usemid=T)
```

b

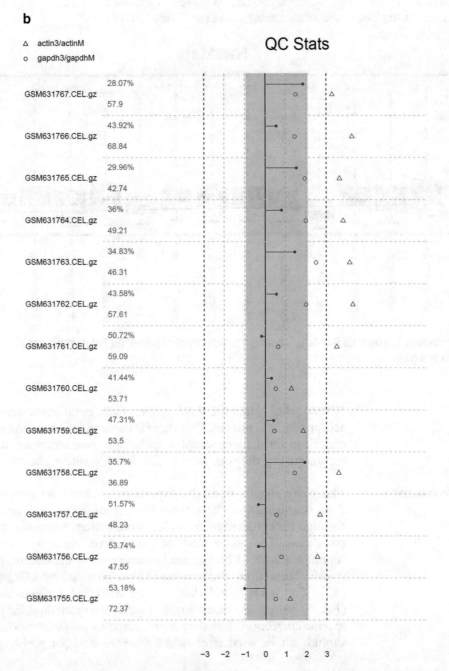

Fig. 4 Quality control of arrays. (**a**) R code for quality control of all arrays. (**b**) A summary of quality control metrics for all arrays

correction [26]. Compared with other processes, the results of different normalization methods are significantly different, and should be compared before making decision.

Figure 6 shows the box plots of the arrays after background correction by *rma* method and normalization by three different methods. Compared with the other two normalization methods, the *quantile* normalization method gives better results.

a

```
CELfiles<-list.celfiles()

cleanerdata<-ReadAffy(filenames=CELfiles)

cleanerdat.qc<-qc(cleanerdata)

mycols=rep(usr.col, each=6,6)

boxplot(cleanerdata, col=mycols, las=3, cex.axis=0.5,
names=sampleNames(cleanerdata), main="Cleanerdata")

plot(cleanerdat.qc,usemid=T)
```

b

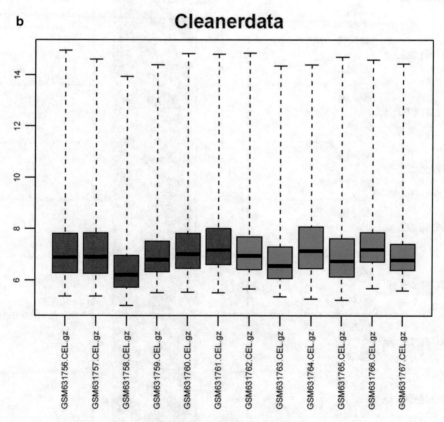

Fig. 5 Intensities and qualities of cleaner data. (**a**) R code for showing the intensity and quality control of cleaner data. (**b**) The intensities of 12 arrays are shown in box plots. (**c**) A summary of quality control metrics for 12 arrays

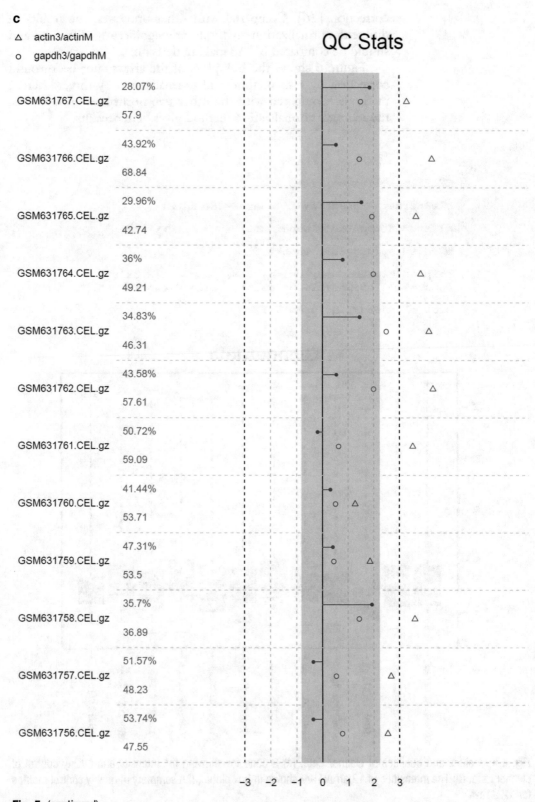

Fig. 5 (continued)

```
#Normalization

cleanerdata.rma<-bg.correct(cleanerdata, method="rma")

cleanerdata.qtl<-normalize(cleanerdata.rma, method="quantiles")

cleanerdata.con<-normalize(cleanerdata.rma, method="constant")

cleanerdata.inv<-normalize(cleanerdata.rma,
method="invariantset")

usr.col<-rep(c("red", "blue"), each=6)

usr.line<-rep(1:6, 2)

boxplot(cleanerdata.rma, col=usr.col, las=3, cex.axis=0.5,
main="Background corrected")

boxplot(cleanerdata.qtl, col=usr.col, las=3, cex.axis=0.5,
main="Quantiles")

boxplot(cleanerdata.con, col=usr.col, las=3, cex.axis=0.5,
main="Constant")

boxplot(cleanerdata.inv, col=usr.col, las=3, cex.axis=0.5,
main="Invariantset")
```

b

Background corrected

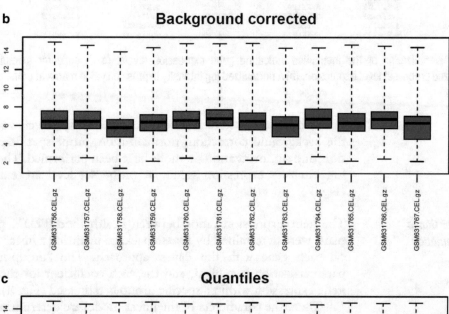

c

Quantiles

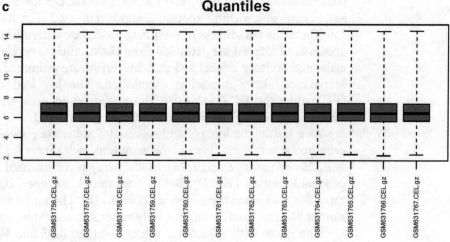

Fig. 6 Background correction and normalization. (**a**) R code for background correction and different normalization methods of cleaner data. (**b**) The boxplots of probe intensities of the background corrected data. (**c**) The boxplots of probe intensities of the background corrected data after normalization by *quantile*, *constant*, and *invariantset* methods

a

```
#Extracting the normalized probe set level expression

cleanerdata.exp<-expresso(cleanerdata, bgcorrect.method="rma",
normalize.method="quantiles", pmcorrect.method="pmonly",
summary.method="medianpolish")

eDat<-exprs(cleanerdata.exp)

write.csv(eDat, "eDat.csv", row.name=T)
```

b

```
> head(eDat)
           GSM631756.CEL.gz GSM631757.CEL.gz GSM631758.CEL.gz GSM631759.CEL.gz GSM631760.CEL.gz GSM631761.CEL.gz
1007_s_at          9.467514         9.500710         8.972834         9.435623         8.836636        10.013943
1053_at            4.789688         4.555502         4.490585         4.574391         4.947794         4.572832
117_at             4.822821         4.965472         5.631986         7.138396         5.372570         5.186308
121_at             7.299549         7.192399         8.157408         7.855879         8.233287         7.795211
1255_g_at          3.047725         3.209085         3.358505         3.178422         3.478595         3.432940
1294_at            6.015173         5.510424         7.190681         5.966142         6.321872         6.017257
           GSM631762.CEL.gz GSM631763.CEL.gz GSM631764.CEL.gz GSM631765.CEL.gz GSM631766.CEL.gz GSM631767.CEL.gz
1007_s_at          8.944723         9.073658         9.633117         9.069653        10.432395         8.844459
1053_at            4.416152         4.420022         4.304997         4.200602         4.485369         4.678686
117_at             5.229100         5.561861         6.320910         5.579605         5.325763         5.925421
121_at             7.561463         8.206571         8.734240         9.076341         8.348982         8.211676
1255_g_at          3.339058         3.561640         3.616025         3.667329         3.677484         3.763625
1294_at            6.282208         6.589050         7.426195         6.935302         7.295641         6.588507
```

Fig. 7 Normalization of the intensities indicating gene expression levels. (**a**) R code for extracting the normalized probe-set level expression. (**b**) A normalized log intensity expression value matrix at probe set level

The preprocessed data should be stored in an object as soon as the background correction, normalization, probe-specific correction, and summarization methods have been performed. Then, the log intensity expression values at probe set level are extracted (Fig. 7).

3.3 DE Genes Determination

The gene expression ratios between healthy and T2DM participants were determined by *limma* package by fitting a linear model on each gene with the Bayes' approach. The "group-means" parametrization is applied, and the each coefficient for the mean gene expression within a specific group is estimated (Fig. 8).

Then, the parameters of the linear model are determined. The contrasts of interest are extracted from the coefficient vectors. The estimated contrast effects and standard errors are estimated, and a hierarchical Bayes' model is established. The log fold change (FC) and adjusted P value for the probe set in each array are obtained by setting the parameter lfc=0, p.value=1.

As a result, the log FC and adjusted P value are provided for each probe set in csv format. We annotate each probe set by the *hgu133a.db* package according to the array platform used in the original literature (Fig. 9). Before annotation, we open the geneExp file, and name the probe set column ID. The probe sets that cannot be annotated or duplicatively annotated should be omitted.

The genes with adjusted P values less than 0.05 and log FCs larger than 1 or less than -1 were considered DE genes. There are 701 DE genes identified according to these criteria. We copy the

a

```
#"group-means" parametrization

library(limma)

TS <- gl(2,6, labels=c("control", "disease"))

design <- model.matrix(~0+TS)

colnames(design) <- levels(TS)

design


#DE genes determination

fit <- lmFit(eDat, design)

cont.matrix <- makeContrasts(contrast=disease-
control,levels=design)

cont.matrix

fit <- contrasts.fit(fit, cont.matrix)

fit <- eBayes(fit)

geneExp<-topTable(fit, coef="contrast", number=nrow(eDat),
adjust.method="fdr",lfc=0, p.value=1, confint=TRUE)

write.csv(geneExp, "geneExp.csv", row.name=T)
```

b

```
> design
    control disease
1         1       0
2         1       0
3         1       0
4         1       0
5         1       0
6         1       0
7         0       1
8         0       1
9         0       1
10        0       1
11        0       1
12        0       1
attr(,"assign")
[1] 1 1
attr(,"contrasts")
attr(,"contrasts")$TS
[1] "contr.treatment"
```

c

```
> head(geneExp)
                logFC       CI.L        CI.R   AveExpr           t     P.Value   adj.P.Val          B
218692_at   -1.864939 -2.3181081 -1.4117703  7.214989  -8.907891  7.800707e-07  0.01693743  5.833888
215416_s_at -1.099884 -1.4019703 -0.7977977  6.726232  -7.881089  2.972381e-06  0.01693743  4.721687
207098_s_at -1.970107 -2.5122282 -1.4279861  5.510403  -7.866181  3.033352e-06  0.01693743  4.704449
208631_s_at -1.309779 -1.6805747 -0.9389841  7.015531  -7.646000  4.106838e-06  0.01693743  4.446055
211465_x_at  1.041787  0.7416131  1.3419602  7.969387   7.512366  4.950111e-06  0.01693743  4.285705
210027_s_at -1.258768 -1.6257043 -0.8918320  8.612511  -7.425498  5.595661e-06  0.01693743  4.180020
```

Fig. 8 Group-means parameterization of DE genes. (**a**) R code for group-means parametrization. (**b**) R code for group-means parameterization of DE genes. (**c**) The estimated statistics of the probe sets

190   Sze Chung Yuen et al.

a

```
#Gene annotation
library(hgu133a.db)
hgu133a <- hgu133aENTREZID
annot<-read.csv("geneExp.csv")
annot$ENTREZ<-unlist(as.list(hgu133a[annot$ID]))
annot<-annot[!is.na(annot$ENTREZ),]
annot<-annot[!duplicated(annot$ENTREZ),]
head(annot)
write.csv(annot, "annot.csv", row.name=T)
```

b

```
> head(annot)
          ID     logFC      CI.L       CI.R  AveExpr         t  P.Value adj.P.Val        B ENTREZ
1   218692_at -1.864939 -2.3181081 -1.4117703 7.214989 -8.907891 7.80e-07 0.01693743 5.833888  55638
2 215416_s_at -1.099884 -1.4019703 -0.7977977 6.726232 -7.881089 2.97e-06 0.01693743 4.721687  30968
3 207098_s_at -1.970107 -2.5122282 -1.4279861 5.510403 -7.866181 3.03e-06 0.01693743 4.704449  55669
4   208631_s_at -1.309779 -1.6805747 -0.9389841 7.015531 -7.646000 4.11e-06 0.01693743 4.446055   3030
5 211465_x_at  1.041787  0.7416131  1.3419602 7.969387  7.512366 4.95e-06 0.01693743 4.285705   2528
6 210027_s_at -1.258768 -1.6257043 -0.8918320 8.612511 -7.425498 5.60e-06 0.01693743 4.180020    328
```

Fig. 9 Gene annotation. (**a**) R code for gene annotation. (**b**) Results of gene annotation

data of Entrez IDs, log FCs, and adjusted *P* values to a .txt file named DEgenes.

3.4 Network Analysis

Over 300,000 experimentally validated molecular interactions are included in InnateDB [33, 34]. They are curated according to MIMIx standards [35]. We conduct a network analysis by uploading the DEgenes file to InnateDB (Fig. 10).

To determine the relationship among the genes, we conduct correlation analysis to determine the interactions among uploaded genes. If we are strict in controlling the data quality, we can return the curated interactions only. If we would like to find more interactions among uploaded genes, we should include the interactions predicted by orthology.

3.5 Module Identification

The network generated by InnateDB is downloaded in XGMML format and visualized by Cytoscape (Fig. 11). The node and edge attributes include GO terms and number of supporting publications.

Through *jActiveModules* (*see* **Note 2**) [36], the connected region with significant changes in gene expression is identified as a module (Fig. 12).

As the size of the first module is larger than the others, we only select the first module for subsequent analysis.

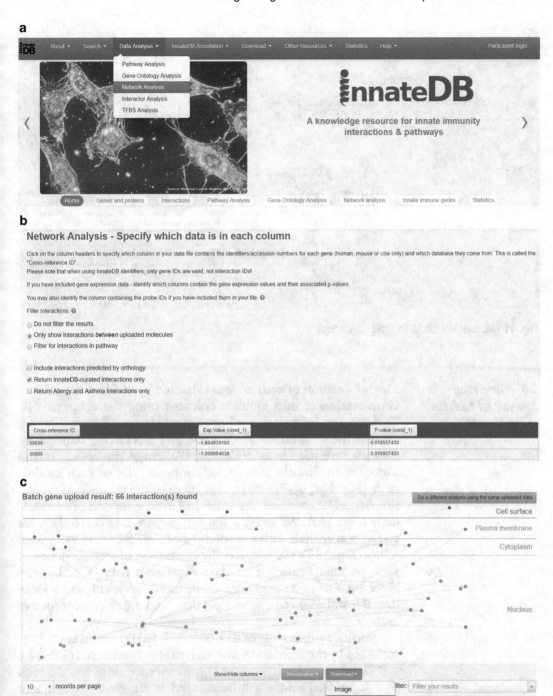

Fig. 10 Network analysis using InnateDB. (**a**) Overview of InnateDB. (**b**) Uploading the genes for constructing network and setting the criteria for the interaction to be shown. (**c**) Downloading the network analysis result

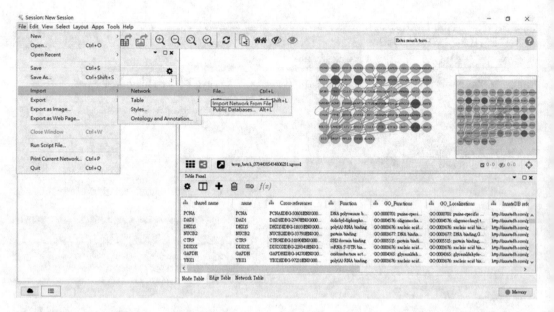

Fig. 11 Network visualization using Cytoscape

3.6 Correlation Analysis for Each Node in the Module

The information of each node is extracted by dividing the column Cross-references into multiple columns using the character "|". To keep the information of gene symbols and Entrez IDs, we rename the column to NodeName and ENTREZ, respectively. And we save the file as nodes.csv. We merge the nodes.csv and annot.csv to find the corresponding probe IDs of each module node (Fig. 13a, b). We also merge them to the normalized expression data eDat.csv to call the individual expression data of a module node (Fig. 13c). We save the file and prepare it as corNod.csv for correlation analysis with the columns of ENTREZ and expression values (Fig. 13d). We calculate the correlation of module nodes by *psych* package according to their expression data (Fig. 14) (*see* **Note 3**). The node pairs with correlation coefficient values more than 0.9 and adjusted *P* values less than 0.01 are chosen for further analysis.

Finally, a submodule of six nodes with EDD protein as the center tested by the correlation analysis is manually extracted (Table 1).

The six proteins represented by the submodule of 6 nodes with significant correlations will be selected as targets for subsequent drug design. Their 3D protein structures (if available) can be collected from the Protein Data Bank.

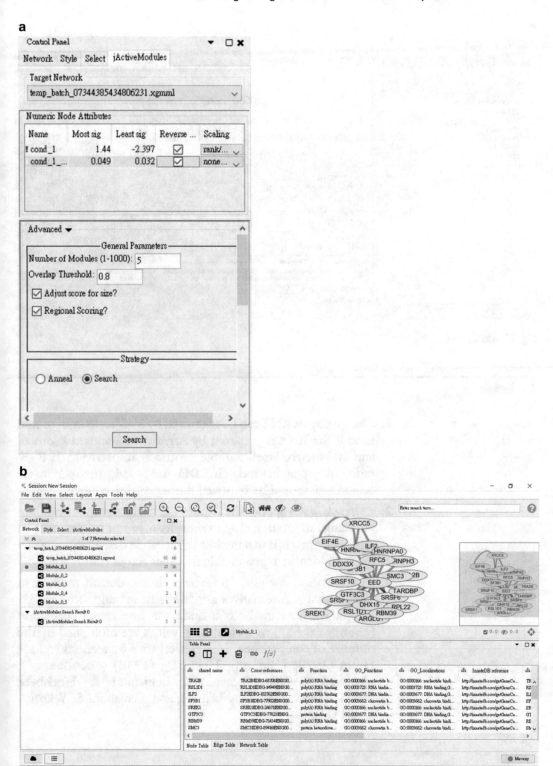

Fig. 12 Modules identification using *jActiveModules*. (**a**) Settings of *jActiveModules*. (**b**) Results. (**c**) Extraction of a node list from a module

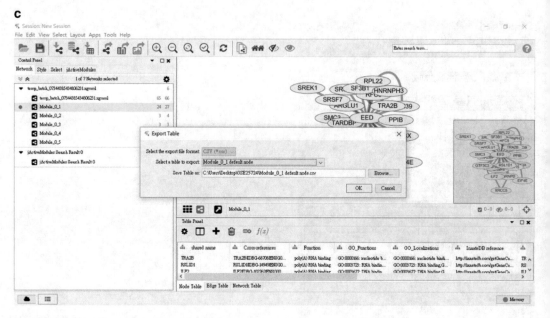

Fig. 12 (continued)

4 Notes

1. The quality of RNA can be measured by 3′–5′ ratio or 3′ to mid ratio if the RNA is prepared by Affymetrix Standard Protocol and Affymetrix Small Sample protocol, respectively. If 3′–5′ ratios for β-actin and GAPDH are used, the parameter usemid=T should be removed during quality control.

2. *jActiveModules* applies the Monte Carlo algorithm for random sampling, suggesting that the results may not be the same in different runs. It is worthwhile to repeat *jActiveModules* several times to identify reproducible modules across runs.

3. In correlation analysis, "pearson" is the default method in *psych* package. Alternatives are "spearman" and "kendall". The adjustment methods include the Bonferroni correction ("bonferroni") in which the p-values are multiplied by the number of comparisons. Less conservative corrections include Holm (1979) ("holm"), Hochberg (1988) ("hochberg"), Hommel (1988) ("hommel"), Benjamini & Hochberg (1995) ("BH" or its alias "fdr"), and Benjamini & Yekutieli (2001) ("BY").

a

```
#Merge nodes.csv and annot.csv
dat1=read.csv("annot.csv", header=TRUE)
dat2=read.csv("nodes.csv", header=TRUE)
dat3=merge(dat2,dat1,all=FALSE)
head(dat3)
#Merge to eDat.csv
dat0=read.csv("eDat.csv",header=TRUE)
dat4=merge(dat3,dat0,all=FALSE)
head(dat4)
write.table(dat4, "corNod.txt",sep="\t")
```

b

```
> head(dat3)
  ENTREZ NodeName        ID      logFC        CI.L        CI.R  AveExpr         t
1   1654    DDX3X 212515_s_at -1.852172 -2.899426 -0.8049185 5.184590 -3.828245
2   1665    DHX15 201386_s_at -1.895391 -2.779423 -1.0113589 6.849807 -4.640888
3   1977    EIF4E 201435_s_at -1.478243 -2.185667 -0.7708193 5.878045 -4.523103
4   3184   HNRNPD   213359_at -1.278655 -1.941032 -0.6162788 5.446006 -4.178485
5   3189  HNRNPH3 208990_s_at -1.023753 -1.563276 -0.4842299 7.422457 -4.107291
6   3608     ILF2 200052_s_at -2.110900 -3.031823 -1.1899766 6.794812 -4.961518
     P.Value  adj.P.Val           B
1 0.002161098 0.04322778 -1.24540793
2 0.000485328 0.03319827  0.15015816
3 0.000599868 0.03444220 -0.04724306
4 0.001125581 0.03760509 -0.63498697
5 0.001283951 0.03760509 -0.75811860
6 0.000275061 0.03317504  0.67753471
```

c

```
> head(dat4)
           ID ENTREZ NodeName     logFC      CI.L       CI.R  AveExpr         t     P.Value
1 200052_s_at   3608     ILF2 -2.110900 -3.031823 -1.1899766 6.794812 -4.961518 0.000275061
2 200892_s_at   6434    TRA2B -1.958388 -2.985437 -0.9313385 6.709252 -4.127411 0.001236995
3   201054_at  10949  HNRNPA0 -1.816894 -2.611058 -1.0227299 6.271544 -4.952103 0.000279633
4 201071_x_at  23451    SF3B1 -1.568726 -2.308947 -0.8285045 9.293485 -4.587286 0.000534343
5 201386_s_at   1665    DHX15 -1.895391 -2.779423 -1.0113589 6.849807 -4.640888 0.000485328
6 201435_s_at   1977    EIF4E -1.478243 -2.185667 -0.7708193 5.878045 -4.523103 0.000599868
   adj.P.Val           B GSM631756.CEL.gz GSM631757.CEL.gz GSM631758.CEL.gz GSM631759.CEL.gz
1 0.03317504  0.67753471         7.671156         7.693495         6.157461         9.157913
2 0.03760509 -0.72326556         7.570453         7.835555         5.879375         8.722206
3 0.03317504  0.66226541         6.918733         7.346952         6.362259         7.431084
4 0.03335230  0.06055692        10.067922        10.331854         9.566085        10.290492
5 0.03319827  0.15015816         7.297146         7.916906         6.179498         8.764839
6 0.03444220 -0.04724306         6.232459         7.161909         5.419905         6.861800
  GSM631760.CEL.gz GSM631761.CEL.gz GSM631762.CEL.gz GSM631763.CEL.gz GSM631764.CEL.gz
1         8.707541         7.714004         5.953533         5.238972         5.448127
2         9.083341         7.039745         6.329260         5.136560         5.705173
3         7.690004         7.330916         5.417941         4.210278         5.359792
4        10.481912         9.728824         9.238712         7.996113         7.788087
5         9.066692         7.559933         5.863444         5.584520         5.471066
6         7.841860         6.185069         5.320540         5.385624         4.901127
  GSM631765.CEL.gz GSM631766.CEL.gz GSM631767.CEL.gz
1         5.216224         6.166645         6.412669
2         4.992325         6.307029         5.910002
3         5.456785         6.852136         4.881651
4         7.892486         9.858226         8.281108
5         5.900113         6.450409         6.143116
6         5.108118         4.904167         5.213968
```

d

	A	B	C	D	E	F	G	H	I
1	ENTREZ	GSM631756	GSM631757	GSM631758	GSM631759	GSM631760	GSM631761	GSM631762	GSM631763
2	3608	7.671156	7.693495	6.157461	9.157913	8.707541	7.714004	5.953533	5.238972
3	6434	7.570453	7.835555	5.879375	8.722206	9.083341	7.039745	6.32926	5.13656
4	10949	6.918733	7.346952	6.362259	7.431084	7.690004	7.330916	5.417941	4.210278
5	23451	10.06792	10.33185	9.566085	10.29049	10.48191	9.728824	9.238712	7.996113
6	1665	7.297146	7.916906	6.179498	8.764839	9.066692	7.559933	5.863444	5.58452
7	1977	6.232459	7.161909	5.419905	6.8618	7.84186	6.185069	5.32054	5.385624
8	5985	5.563448	6.00655	5.347524	5.283309	5.715193	5.005635	5.119601	4.021878

Fig. 13 Correlation of module nodes. (**a**) R code for file preparation. (**b**) The results of merge nodes.csv and annot.csv. (**c**) Results of merging to eDat.csv. (**d**) Use of corNod.csv for correlation calculation

```
#Correlation calculation

dat5=read.csv("corNod.csv",header=TRUE,row.name=1)

dat5=t(dat5)

library(psych)

corrT<-corr.test(dat5,adjust="BH")
```

Fig. 14 R code for correlation analysis

Table 1
Gene pairs in a module with significant correlation

ID2	Label2	Label1	ID1	Correlation coefficient	Adjusted P value
6432	SRSF7	EED	8726	0.902914	0.003226
6434	TRA2B	EED	8726	0.914704	0.004676
10,772	SRSF10	EED	8726	0.930143	0.000129
23,451	SF3B1	EED	8726	0.917909	0.00014
26,156	RSL1D1	EED	8726	0.936396	4.24E-06

References

1. Schena M, Shalon D, Davis R, Brown P (1995) Quantitative monitoring of gene expression patterns with a complementary DNA microarray. Science 270:467–470

2. Bumgarner R (2013) DNA microarrays: types, applications and their future. Curr Protoc Mol Biol 6137:1–17

3. Affymetrix (2007) Data sheet: genechip human genome U133 arrays. Proc Natl Acad Sci U S A 2007:1–8

4. Lander ES, Linton LM, Birren B et al (2001) Initial sequencing and analysis of the human genome. Nature 409:860–921. https://doi.org/10.1038/35057062

5. Venter JC, Adams MD, Myers EW et al (2001) The sequence of the human genome. Science 291:1304–1351. https://doi.org/10.1126/science.1058040

6. Wang Y, Miao ZH, Pommier Y et al (2007) Characterization of mismatch and high-signal intensity probes associated with Affymetrix genechips. Bioinformatics 23:2088–2095. https://doi.org/10.1093/bioinformatics/btm306

7. Palacios G, Quan P, Jabado OJ et al (2007) Panmicrobial oligonucleotide array for diagnosis of infectious diseases. Emerg Infect Dis 13:73–81. https://doi.org/10.3201/eid1301.060837

8. Cowell JK, Hawthorn L (2007) The application of microarray technology to the analysis of the cancer genome. Curr Mol Med 7:103–120. https://doi.org/10.2174/156652407779940387

9. Smyth G (2004) Linear models and empirical Bayes methods for assessing differential expression in microarray experiments linear models and empirical bayes methods for assessing differential expression in microarray experiments. Stat Appl Genet Mol Biol 3:1–26. https://doi.org/10.2202/1544-6115.1027

10. Watts DJ, Strogatz SH (1998) Collective dynamics of 'small-world' networks. Nature 393:440–442. https://doi.org/10.1038/30918

11. Hartwell LH, Hopfield JJ, Leibler S et al (1999) From molecular to modular cell biology. Nature 402:C47–C52. https://doi.org/10.1038/35011540

12. Barabási A-L, Gulbahce N, Loscalzo J (2011) Network medicine: a network-based approach to human disease. Nat Rev Genet 12:56–68. https://doi.org/10.1038/nrg2918.Network

13. IDF diabetes atlas–Home. http://www.diabetesatlas.org/

14. Beckman JA, Paneni F, Cosentino F et al (2013) Diabetes and vascular disease: pathophysiology, clinical consequences, and medical therapy: part II. Eur Heart J 34:2444–2456. https://doi.org/10.1093/eurheartj/eht142

15. Creager MA, Lüscher TF, Cosentino F et al (2003) Diabetes and vascular disease. Pathophysiology, clinical consequences, and medical therapy: part I. Circulation 108:1527–1532. https://doi.org/10.1161/01.CIR.0000091257.27563.32

16. Jung CH, Baek AR, Kim KJ et al (2013) Association between cardiac autonomic neuropathy, diabetic retinopathy and carotid atherosclerosis in patients with type 2 diabetes. Endocrinol Metab (Seoul) 28:309–319. https://doi.org/10.3803/EnM.2013.28.4.309

17. Lin Y, Sun Z (2010) Current views on type 2 diabetes. J Endocrinol 204:1–11. https://doi.org/10.1677/JOE-09-0260

18. Fu Z, Gilbert ER, Liu D (2013) Regulation of insulin synthesis and secretion and pancreatic Beta-cell dysfunction in diabetes. Curr Diabetes Rev 9:25–53. https://doi.org/10.2174/157339913804143225

19. Majithia AR, Florez JC (2009) Clinical translation of genetic predictors for type 2 diabetes. Curr Opin Endocrinol Diabetes Obes 16:100–106. https://doi.org/10.1097/MED.0b013e3283292354

20. Prokopenko I, McCarthy MI, Lindgren CM (2008) Type 2 diabetes: new genes, new understanding. Trends Genet 24:613–621. https://doi.org/10.1016/j.tig.2008.09.004

21. Ridderstråle M, Groop L (2009) Genetic dissection of type 2 diabetes. Mol Cell Endocrinol 297:10–17. https://doi.org/10.1016/j.mce.2008.10.002

22. Stančáková A, Laakso M (2016) Genetics of type 2 diabetes. Endocr Dev 31:203–220. https://doi.org/10.1159/000439418

23. Dominguez V, Raimondi C, Somanath S et al (2011) Class II phosphoinositide 3-kinase regulates exocytosis of insulin granules in pancreatic?? Cells. J Biol Chem 286:4216–4225. https://doi.org/10.1074/jbc.M110.200295

24. Brazma A, Hingamp P, Quackenbush J et al (2001) Minimum information about a microarray experiment (MIAME)-toward standards for microarray data. Nat Genet 29:365–371. https://doi.org/10.1038/ng1201-365

25. Yeung N, Cline MS, Kuchinsky A et al (2008) Exploring biological networks with Cytoscape software. Curr Protoc Bioinformatics. https://doi.org/10.1002/0471250953.bi0813s23

26. Gautier L, Cope L, Bolstad BM et al (2004) Affy – analysis of Affymetrix GeneChip data at the probe level. Bioinformatics 20:307–315. https://doi.org/10.1093/bioinformatics/btg405

27. Neuwirth E. (2014) RColorBrewer: ColorBrewer palettes. *R Packag version 11–2*: https://cran.R--project.org/package=RColorBrewer. https://cran.r-project.org/web/packages/RColorBrewer/index.html

28. Wilson CL, Miller CJ (2005) Simpleaffy: a bioconductor package for Affymetrix quality control and data analysis. Bioinformatics 21:3683–3685. https://doi.org/10.1093/bioinformatics/bti605

29. Ritchie ME, Phipson B, Wu D et al (2015) Limma powers differential expression analyses for RNA-sequencing and microarray studies. Nucleic Acids Res 43:e47. https://doi.org/10.1093/nar/gkv007

30. Carlson M (2016) hgu133a.db: Affymetrix Human Genome U133 Set annotation data (chip hgu133a)

31. Revelle W (2017) Psych: procedures for personality and psychological research. Northwestern University, Evanston, Illinois, USA. https://CRAN.R-project.org/package=psych Version = 1.7.5

32. Gautier L, Irizarry R, Cope L (2009) Description of affy. Changes 2009:1–29

33. Breuer K, Foroushani AK, Laird MR (2013) InnateDB: systems biology of innate immunity and beyond–recent updates and continuing curation. Nucleic Acids Res 41:1228–1233. https://doi.org/10.1093/nar/gks1147

34. Lynn DJ, Winsor GL, Chan C (2008) InnateDB: facilitating systems-level analyses of the mammalian innate immune response. Mol Syst Biol 4:218. https://doi.org/10.1038/msb.2008.55

35. Orchard S, Salwinski L, Kerrien S (2007) The minimum information required for reporting a molecular interaction experiment (MIMIx). Nat Biotechnol 25:894–898. https://doi.org/10.1038/nbt1324

36. Cline MS, Smoot M, Cerami E (2007) Integration of biological networks and gene expression data using Cytoscape. Nat Protoc 2:2366–2382. https://doi.org/10.1038/nprot.2007.324

Chapter 11

Absolute Alchemical Free Energy Calculations for Ligand Binding: A Beginner's Guide

Matteo Aldeghi, Joseph P. Bluck, and Philip C. Biggin

Abstract

Many thermodynamic quantities can be extracted from computer simulations that generate an ensemble of microstates according to the principles of statistical mechanics. Among these quantities is the free energy of binding of a small molecule to a macromolecule, such as a protein. Here, we present an introductory overview of a protocol that allows for the estimation of ligand binding free energies via molecular dynamics simulations. While we focus on the binding of organic molecules to proteins, the approach is in principle transferable to any pair of molecules.

Key words Free energy, Computer simulations, Molecular dynamics, Alchemical transitions, Protein–ligand binding, Binding free energy, Binding affinity, Drug design, Molecular modeling

1 Introduction

The accurate prediction of the affinity of a drug for its target protein has long been a central objective of structure-based drug design. As such, many computational approaches that try to calculate or approximate binding free energy have been developed [1, 2]. These range from fast scoring functions [3], to implicit-solvent approaches based on the postprocessing of simulation snapshots [4], to the more rigorous yet computationally expensive free energy methods [2]. In particular, alchemical free energy calculations based on all-atom molecular dynamic (MD) simulations in explicit solvent are one of the approaches that operate at the highest level of theoretical rigor, calculating free energy differences from well-founded statistical mechanics principles and naturally including entropic and solvent effects. These calculations are based on a thermodynamic cycle that include a series of nonphysical intermediate states (hence the name *alchemical*), from which the free energy difference between two physical end states can be recovered

Mohinl Gore and Umesh B. Jagtap (eds.), *Computational Drug Discovery and Design*, Methods in Molecular Biology, vol. 1762, https://doi.org/10.1007/978-1-4939-7756-7_11, © Springer Science+Business Media, LLC, part of Springer Nature 2018

as the sum of the free energy differences between all pairs of alchemical intermediate states [5]. Here, we will focus in particular on absolute binding free energy (ABFE) calculations that make use of such an alchemical cycle, in which the ligand is nonphysically "removed" from the solution environment and "inserted" into the protein's binding site. Note that the term *absolute* refers to the fact that a binding free energy ΔG_b, rather than a binding free energy difference ($\Delta\Delta G_b$), is being calculated.

The advantage of the alchemical approach as compared to computationally cheaper ones is that it is expected to be more accurate due to its ability to return the exact binding free energy for the physical model used [1, 2, 6]. As will become evident in this chapter, however, this comes at a high computational cost. The method is also in principle general, meaning it can be applied to any protein–ligand pair, as long as the sampling challenges can be addressed. Potential applications of the approach are the ranking of ligands with different scaffolds binding to a specific protein, the accurate rescoring of docking poses, and the prediction of ligand selectivity [7, 8].

Here, we present a guide on how to carry out alchemical ABFE calculations based on a standard protocol that uses equilibrium MD simulations. In particular, we focus on the more practical aspects of setting up the calculations alongside a brief overview of the theory and technical details. Throughout the text, we direct the reader who would like to further explore certain technical topics toward more specialized reviews and chapters. Despite this being a guide that aims to explain how to set up and run the calculations in simple terms, at this point in time these calculations should still be considered an advanced approach. Consequently, we recommend that the reader first familiarize themselves with ligand parametrization and simulations of protein–ligand complexes. Some experience with solvation free energy calculations may also be beneficial, as these represent part of the thermodynamic cycle used for the binding free energy calculations.

The chapter is organized as follows. First, we provide an overview of the theoretical aspects of binding free energy, including its definition, how it can be extracted from computer simulations, and the alchemical thermodynamic cycle we will use to calculate it. Then, we touch upon the software and hardware requirements for the calculations. Finally, we discuss the protocol step by step, pointing out potential pitfalls and issues. In Subheading 5, we show how certain steps can be carried out using the Gromacs 2016 simulations package. This chapter is accompanied by a tutorial (Absolute Binding Free Energy—Gromacs 2016) available on www.alchemistry.org, where the reader can find the input files needed to practice with an example calculation.

2 Theory

Here we review some theoretical and methodological concepts that underlie the use of computer simulations for the calculation of binding free energies. We provide only a brief overview of some key concepts and, due to the practical nature of the chapter, this section is not meant to be exhaustive. The reader can find a more extensive appraisal of theoretical aspects in one of the many excellent reviews and textbooks written on the subject and here referenced [9–13]. The book by Chipot and Pohorille [9] is particularly comprehensive.

2.1 Definition of Binding Free Energy

The reversible binding of a ligand (L) to a protein (P) to form a complex (PL) can be described by the following chemical reaction:

$$P + L \rightleftharpoons PL$$

At equilibrium, the binding constant K°_b defines the ratio of the product and reactants concentrations in solution:

$$K^\circ_b = c^\circ \frac{[PL]}{[L][P]} \tag{1}$$

where square brackets indicate a concentration, and c° is the standard state concentration, which is typically defined as 1 mol/L. Since this definition of standard state does not change the numerical value of K°_b (as it is multiplied by one) it is customary to omit c° when discussing equilibrium constants. However, it is important to remember that the binding constant is a dimensionless quantity (without c° it would have units of inverse concentration), and it is dependent on the chosen standard state. For a single ligand binding event, K°_b is associated to the binding free energy by the following well-known equation.

$$\Delta G^\circ_b = -k_B T \ln K^\circ_b \tag{2}$$

where k_B is the Boltzmann constant, and T is the temperature. For a mole of ligand, the gas constant ($R = N_A k_B$, where N_A is the Avogadro constant) is used instead of k_B. From the above discussion of the standard state, it follows that the binding free energy is also thus defined with respect to the chosen standard state.

The equilibrium constant can also be expressed as the ratio of probabilities ($\mathcal{P}$) for the system being in either the bound or unbound state, so that $K^\circ_b = \mathcal{P}_1/\mathcal{P}_0$, where "1" denotes the bound (PL) state, and "0" the unbound ($P + L$) state. The probability of finding the system in the bound versus unbound state is determined by the ratio of their partition functions Q_1 and Q_0, where the partition function of a system in the isothermal-isobaric (NPT) ensemble is defined as follows.

$$Q_{\text{NPT}} = \frac{1}{N! h^{3N}} \iiint e^{-\beta[H(x,p)+pV]} dV dx dp \qquad (3)$$

with N being the number of particles, $\beta = 1/(k_B T)$, x and p the coordinates and momenta, H the Hamiltonian, p the pressure, V the volume, and h the Planck's constant. The Hamiltonian of a system consists of a potential energy term $U(x)$ that depends on the particles' coordinates, and a kinetic term $K(p)$ that depends on their momenta. However, since we are considering the free energy difference of a process in which neither the temperature or particles' masses change, the kinetic contribution to the Hamiltonian is constant. Therefore, only the configurational part of the partition function needs to be considered in this case, and the Gibbs binding free energy can be expressed as follows.

$$\Delta G_b^\circ = -k_B T \ln \frac{\int_{V_1} \int_{\Gamma_1} e^{-\beta[U_1(x)+pV_1]} dV dx}{\int_{V_0} \int_{\Gamma_0} e^{-\beta[U_0(x)+pV_0]} dV dx} \qquad (4)$$

where V_1 and V_0 are the container volumes, while Γ_1 and Γ_2 are the *phase space volumes* of the bound and unbound states, respectively. However, due to the limited compressibility of water, at 1 atm the effect of changes in average volume on the binding free energy is negligible [11, 14]. This means that the pV component of the free energy can be ignored without major effects on the results, and that the Helmholtz free energy closely approximates the Gibbs free energy.

$$\Delta G_b^\circ \cong \Delta A_b^\circ = -k_B T \ln \frac{\int_{\Gamma_1} e^{-\beta U(x)} dx}{\int_{\Gamma_0} e^{-\beta U(x)} dx} \qquad (5)$$

This definition assumes the existence of separate and well-defined "bound" and "unbound" states, which is valid for tight and specific binders, but might not be justified in the case of very weak and nonspecific binders [11]. The partition function for a complex system has no analytical solution and thus simulations need to be used to sample the accessible phase space. The whole phase space is computationally difficult to sample but, when calculating free energy *differences*, inaccessible high-energy regions will quite often not be sampled for either state of interest, resulting in a cancellation of errors that allow ΔG to be calculated.

When comparing binding free energies, it is important to keep in mind that, as mentioned previously, the binding constant depends upon a reference concentration. This dependence is due to the connection between available volume and entropy [15]. It is therefore necessary to refer to the same standard state when comparing binding free energies. A standard concentration $c^\circ = 1$ mol/L corresponds to a standard volume $V^\circ = 1660$ Å^3 (the volume occupied by one molecule at the concentration of

1 mol/L). As the 1 M standard state is the most widely adopted, it follows that it is simplest to calculate the binding free energy with respect to this standard state. However, during a free energy calculation the protein–ligand system is not simulated at c°, and thus a correction is needed to recover the standard binding free energy. If ΔG_b is the binding free energy calculated using a simulated box of volume V, the standard binding free energy $\Delta G^\circ{}_b$ can be recovered as follows [15]:

$$\Delta G_b^\circ = \Delta G_b - k_B T \ln \frac{V}{V^\circ} \tag{6}$$

where V° is the standard volume of 1660 Å^3, which corresponds to a standard concentration $c^\circ = 1$ mol/L.

2.2 Estimating Free Energy Differences from Equilibrium Simulations

Given the relationship $K_b^\circ = \mathcal{P}_1/\mathcal{P}_0$, one could think of straightforwardly calculating the difference in free energy between two states of a system by counting the number of configurations in both states. That is, for binding free energies, by counting the number of bound versus unbound configurations during a simulation. This approach is however only feasible when sufficient statistics can be collected, i.e., when the system can transition between the two states of interest many times within the timeframe of the simulation. Despite great improvements in simulation performance in the last few decades, this is still not computationally feasible with unbiased simulations due to the timescales involved in the binding/unbinding process. Several other approaches have thus been developed to estimate free energy differences using data that can be collected via molecular dynamics simulations. Here, we focus only on the main approaches used to estimate free energy differences from equilibrium simulations and that are relevant for alchemical pathways. Approaches that estimate free energy from nonequilibrium transitions between end states are also available, and reviews of such methods can be found elsewhere [9, 16].

2.2.1 Perturbation Approaches

One of the most well-known methods to estimate free energy differences is based on perturbation theory, and relies on the following formula introduced by Zwanzig [17].

$$\Delta G_{0,1} = -k_B T \ln \left\langle e^{-\beta(U_1(x) - U_0(x))} \right\rangle_0 \tag{7}$$

The equation shows that the free energy difference can be calculated as the logarithm of the ensemble average of the exponential of the Boltzmann weighted potential energy difference between the two states. From the subscript of the ensemble average it is possible to note how the potential energy difference is evaluated for the same reference ensemble; i.e., equilibrium sampling is carried out for one state, here labeled "0," and the energies are computed for both thermodynamic states "0" and "1" over the same configurations. The above formula applies to the *forward* transformation $0 \rightarrow 1$; it is also possible to calculate the free energy difference for the *backward* transformation $1 \rightarrow 0$. While the two expressions are equivalent, in practice their convergence properties may not be the same [9, 18], and the difference in the two resulting ΔG values is referred to as *hysteresis*. As mentioned previously, the kinetic part of the Hamiltonian does not contribute toward the free energy as temperature and masses are unvaried, and the pressure-volume contribution is only marginal, so that here we consider only the potential energy contribution to the Hamiltonian for simplicity.

The approach based on Eq. 7 can be referred to as *exponential averaging* (EXP), however, the term *free energy perturbation* (FEP) is often used too. Note that FEP is also at times used to refer to alchemical free energy methods in general, where *perturbation* in this case refers to the perturbation in the chemical identity and interactions of the atoms themselves. Despite the above equation being exact, it has been shown that EXP converges only slowly with the amount of data collected, and an average that appears to have converged may only indicate poor overlap between the two states studied [19, 20].

The free energy obtained via EXP for either the forward or reverse direction converges to the same result in the limit of infinite sampling. A simple way to improve EXP is thus to simply perform the calculation in both directions and average the results. However, because of a direct relationship between the distributions of potential energy differences in the forward and reverse directions, Bennet could derive a more robust and statistically optimal way to use information from both directions [21]. The *Bennett's Acceptance Ratio* (BAR) provides a maximum likelihood estimate of the free energy given the samples from the two states [22, 23]. Studies have shown the superiority of the BAR over EXP in molecular simulations: significantly less phase space overlap between states is required in order to converge results as compared to EXP [19, 20]. Note, however, that BAR requires sampling and energy evaluation of the system configurations from both states to estimate the free energy difference.

As phase space overlap affects the reliability of the estimate, free energy differences are most often calculated by simulating several intermediate states in addition to the two end states, in order to increase the overlap between each pair of states. A multistate extension of BAR, called the *multistate Bennett's Acceptance Ratio* (MBAR), has been proposed by Shirts et al. [24]. In this approach, a series of weighting functions are derived to minimize the uncertainties in free energy differences between all states considered simultaneously. MBAR reduces to BAR when only two states are considered, and it can also be interpreted as a zero-width weighted histogram analysis method (WHAM) [11, 24]. MBAR has the lowest variance among the methods discussed here, and is likely the most reliable estimator for the type of free energy calculations described in this chapter [24, 25].

EXP and BAR are available in popular simulation packages such as Gromacs [26], Amber [27], and NAMD [28]. A python implementation of the MBAR estimator is instead provided by the authors of the original publication at https://github.com/choderalab/pymbar.

2.2.2 Thermodynamic Integration

In the thermodynamic integration (TI) approach, rather than potential energy differences, the data needed to estimate the free energy difference is the derivative of the potential energy with respect to the coupling parameter λ, a continuous variable that describes the series of intermediates states between the two end states $\lambda = 0$ and $\lambda = 1$. From this observable, it is possible to recover the free energy difference with the following formula.

$$\Delta G_{0,1} = \int_{\lambda=0}^{\lambda=1} \frac{\partial U(\lambda, \boldsymbol{x})}{\partial \lambda}\bigg|_{\lambda} \tag{8}$$

The ensemble average $\langle \partial U/\partial \lambda \rangle$ is obtained from an equilibrium simulation performed at a certain value of λ. Numerical integration is then needed to recover the free energy difference between $\lambda = 0$ and $\lambda = 1$. The trapezoidal rule is often used for simplicity, but any numerical integration method can be employed. While λ is a continuous variable, only discrete values of it are sampled, so that there will be a bias in the estimate that depends on how well the chosen values of λ allow for an accurate quadrature. Therefore, while the accuracy of perturbation approaches depends on the overlap of energy distributions, the accuracy of TI depends on the smoothness of the integrand [29, 30].

TI is a popular method for the estimation of free energy differences, as it is robust and accurate while also easy to implement if the simulation code provides $\partial U/\partial \lambda$ values. The *alchemical analysis* tool [30] available at https://github.com/MobleyLab/alchemical-analysis already implements the automated analysis of simulation data collected with Gromacs [26], Amber [31], or Sire (http://siremol.org/), and the estimation of free energy differences using TI, EXP, BAR, and MBAR.

2.3 The Thermodynamic Cycle

For both perturbation and thermodynamic integration methods, several intermediate states are needed in order to obtain a reliable estimate of their free energy difference. In fact, when the two end states are the protein-bound and protein-unbound ligand, it is not possible to obtain a reliable binding free energy estimate by simulating only these two, and a pathway of intermediate states is needed. The computation of a free energy difference thus involves

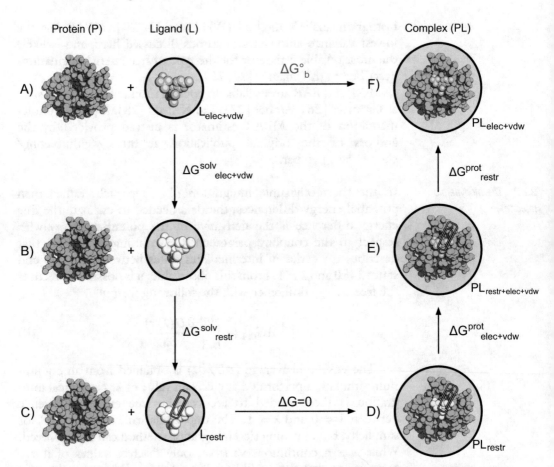

Fig. 1 Thermodynamic cycle used in absolute binding free energy calculations. The fully interacting ligand (orange) in solution at the top left (A) is transformed into a noninteracting solute (B, white) during a series of equilibrium simulations where its electrostatic and van der Waals interactions are scaled to zero, providing the term $\Delta G_{elec+vdW}^{solv}$. The ligand is then restrained while still noninteracting with the environment (C), calculating ΔG_{restr}^{solv}. This state is equivalent to having the noninteracting ligand restrained within the protein cavity (D). The restrained and noninteracting ligand in complex with the protein has its electrostatic and vdW interactions turned back on again (E), giving $\Delta G_{elec+vdW}^{prot}$. The restraints between ligand and protein are then removed (ΔG_{restr}^{prot}), closing the cycle, and the final state is the unrestrained and fully interacting ligand in complex with the protein (F). Reproduced from Aldeghi et al. [7] with permission from The Royal Society of Chemistry

the definition of the path that connects the two end states of interest. Since the free energy is a state function, the nature of the path is unimportant, and we can choose to use a thermodynamic cycle that connects the bound and unbound states through several nonphysical intermediate ones, as shown in Fig. 1. The nonphysical nature of the cycle used is the reason why this type of calculations is typically referred to as *alchemical*. The cycle depicted in Fig. 1 can be discretized in N states, which are independently simulated. These independent simulations are also often referred to as *windows*. Then, the free energy difference between each state i and its successor $i + 1$ can be calculated, and the binding free energy can be recovered as the sum of all these $\Delta G_{i,i+1}$.

$$\Delta G_b = \sum_{i=0}^{i=N-2} \Delta G_{i,i+1} \qquad (9)$$

There are six states along the absolute binding free energy cycle that are conceptually helpful to think of: the two physically meaningful end states (i.e., the bound and unbound states), and four alchemical intermediate states where the ligand is *decoupled* from the environment, i.e., it does not interact with any other molecular species in the simulation. In general, we use the term *decoupled* to indicate a state in which the intermolecular interactions of the ligand have been removed, while the intramolecular interactions are still present; i.e., the atoms in the ligand feel the forces resulting from electrostatic and van der Waals (vdW) interactions with the other atoms in the same molecule. On the other hand, we use the term *annihilated* when also the intramolecular interactions have been removed. Figure 1 shows these intermediate states visually, to help understand their nature and how they connect the two end states together. In the unbound end state (state A), we are considering a ligand that is free in solution. Simulating a box containing only the ligand is computationally efficient and ensures there are no interactions with the protein. This fully interacting ligand in solution (Fig. 1. State A; in orange) is then transformed into a noninteracting solute (Fig. 1. State B; in white) by scaling its electrostatic and vdW interactions to zero through several nonphysical states that can be simulated independently. The ligand is then restrained to limit its accessible sampling volume while still not interacting with the environment (Fig. 1, State C; in white with a paper clip). Restraining the ligand substantially aids the convergence of the calculations. In fact, if the ligand was left unrestrained when decoupled, it could leave the binding pocket and float around the whole simulation box. Then, once its interactions with the environment were turned back on, it would have to go through a physical binding process in order to find its position in the protein again. State C is equivalent to having the noninteracting and restrained ligand within the protein cavity (Fig. 1, State D), since no work is needed to change the relative positions of the completely noninteracting protein and ligand. The decoupled and restrained ligand in complex with the protein has then its electrostatic and vdW interactions turned back on again (Fig. 1, State E). The restraints between ligand and protein are then finally removed, closing the cycle, and reaching the other physical end state, that is, the bound protein–ligand state (Fig. 1, State F).

If the cycle just described is discretized into N intermediate states, it is then possible to recover the binding free energy ΔG_b. Following from the discussion above, the cycle can be split into four main steps, each of them corresponding to the free energy difference of transitioning between the intermediate states high-lighted in Fig. 1. $\Delta G_{\text{elec+vdW}}^{\text{solv}}$ is the free energy of decoupling the ligand from the solution (state A → B), effectively bringing it to gas phase. $\Delta G_{\text{restr}}^{\text{solv}}$ is the free energy of restraining the ligand to a certain portion of phase space while still not interacting with the environment (state B → C). The free energy of placing the noninteracting and restrained ligand into the protein binding pocket (state C → D) is zero, so that it needs not be calculated. $\Delta G_{\text{elec+vdW}}^{\text{prot}}$ is then the free energy of coupling the restrained ligand to the environment again (state D → E), basically bringing the ligand back into the solution while being kept into the protein's binding pocket. Then, finally, $\Delta G_{\text{restr}}^{\text{prot}}$ is the free energy of removing the restraints that kept the ligand in place when not interacting with the environment. Thus, the binding free energy can be recovered as the sum of these four major steps, with the addition of a correction for the 1 M standard state:

$$\Delta G_{\text{b}}^{\circ} = \Delta G_{\text{elec+vdW}}^{\text{solv}} + \Delta G_{\text{restr}}^{\text{solv}} + \Delta G_{\text{elec+vdW}}^{\text{prot}} + \Delta G_{\text{restr}}^{\text{prot}} - k_{\text{B}} T \ln \frac{V}{V^0}$$

(10)

2.3.1 Restraints

The use of restraints is important in the protocol here described as it prevents the ligand from leaving the protein binding pocket while it is not interacting with the environment. This is necessary to make sure that the conformations sampled during the simulations corre-spond to a well-defined bound state. If the ligand were to leave the binding pocket in the windows where it is partially or completely decoupled, and started sampling the whole volume of the box, it would have a large configurational phase space available, leading to convergence issues. The use of restraints aids good phase space overlap between windows and faster convergence [32, 33].

In theory, any type of restraint that keeps the ligand in its bound pose can be used if its free energy contribution is properly accounted for. Also note that the use of restraints somewhat com-plicates the standard state correction, since the volume V does not correspond anymore to the volume of the whole box [15]. In practice, we find the set of restraints proposed by Boresch et al. [32] to be particularly convenient. In summary, this set of restraints not only allows to keep the ligand in a specific orientation relative to the binding pocket [33], but also provides an analytical solution for $\Delta G_{\text{restr}}^{\text{solv}}$, thus reducing the number of simulations to be run. Fur-thermore, the analytical solution also already includes the standard state correction. This set of restraints needs to be harmonic and is comprised by one distance, two angles, and three dihedrals, to be applied between three atoms of the ligand and three of the protein, as shown in Fig. 2. The authors also showed how the exact value of the force constant used for the harmonic restraints should not

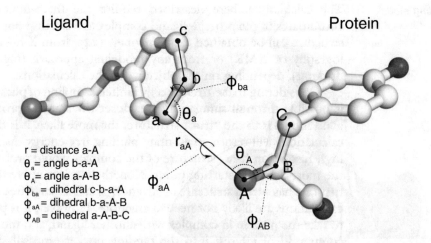

Fig. 2 Set of restraints proposed by Boresch et al. [32] for use in free energy calculations. The atoms and terms involved in this set of restraints are shown. Atoms "a," "b," and "c" belong to the ligand (on the left), while atoms "A," "B," and "C" belong to the protein (on the right)

affect the result, as the effects of different restraint strengths cancels out between $\Delta G_{\text{restr}}^{\text{solv}}$ and $\Delta G_{\text{restr}}^{\text{prot}} + \Delta G_{\text{elec+vdW}}^{\text{prot}}$.

$\Delta G_{\text{restr}}^{\text{prot}}$ needs to be estimated via simulations, running multiple intermediate states where the force constants of the six harmonic restraints are interpolated between their chosen value and zero. On the other hand, $\Delta G_{\text{restr}}^{\text{solv}}$ can be calculated analytically using the following formula (Eq. 32 in Boresch et al. [32]), which also includes the standard state correction:

$$\Delta G_{\text{restr}}^{\text{solv}} - k_B T \ln \frac{V}{V^\circ}$$

$$= k_B T \ln \left[\frac{8\pi^2 V^\circ}{r_{\text{aA}}^2 \cdot \sin \theta_{\text{a}} \cdot \sin \theta_{\text{A}}} \frac{(k_{r_{\text{aA}}} k_{\theta_{\text{a}}} k_{\theta_{\text{A}}} k_{\phi_{\text{ba}}} k_{\phi_{\text{aA}}} k_{\phi_{\text{AB}}})^{1/2}}{(2\pi k_B T)^2} \right] \quad (11)$$

where V° is the standard volume of 1660 Å^3, r_{aA} is the reference value chosen for the distance restraint, θ_{a} and θ_{A} are the reference values of the two angle restraints, and k are the force constants of the harmonic restraints for the one distance (r_{aA}), two angle (θ_{a} and θ_{A}), and three dihedral (ϕ_{ba}, ϕ_{aA}, and ϕ_{AB}) restraints. Later in the text, we will refer to Eq. 11 simply as $\Delta G_{\text{restr}}^{\text{solv}}$, while implicitly assuming it also contains a correction for the standard state.

3   Materials

In this section, we summarize the information and tools that are needed before one can obtain binding free energy predictions as described in this chapter.

3.1 Starting Model Structure

The calculations here described require the three-dimensional coordinates of the protein–ligand complex as a starting point. The structure can be obtained experimentally (e.g., from X-ray crystallography or NMR) or from any modeling approach (e.g., from docking), depending on the objective of the calculations.

Considering that currently only limited sampling of phase space is possible through simulation, the closer the starting protein–ligand model is to the "true" structure, the more likely it is that the calculations will return an accurate binding free energy. As such, a high-resolution X-ray structure of the complex would probably be the most desirable starting point. Nonetheless, it is rarely the case that one has such a structure in advance, as at this stage free energy calculations are likely not needed anymore. However, it is possible to take the protein in complex with another ligand, and model the compound of interest into the binding pocket especially if conserved binding patterns are present and known. Alternatively, it is possible to use docking to generate hypotheses about the binding pose of the ligand of interest, and then use free energy calculations in order to accurately rescore them and identify the most stable pose [7, 34].

In some cases, the structure of the protein might not be experimentally resolved. In this situation, it is still possible to resort to homology modeling. However, the chances of starting from a structure far from equilibrium and possibly trapped in some metastable state are higher, resulting in calculations more likely to return inaccurate results. Good performance in relative binding free energy (RBFE) calculations using homology models has been recently reported [35]. However, ABFE calculations do not benefit from the same error cancellations present in RBFE methods and this usually manifests itself in ways that are indicative of a more pronounced sampling problem [36–38]. In any case, it is evident that the performance of the calculations would be highly dependent on the quality of the model, in particular in the proximity of the binding pocket. Thus, we would suggest extreme care in the interpretation of the results when the confidence on the quality of the starting protein–ligand structure is low—whether this comes from experiments or modeling.

3.2 Software Requirements

As mentioned in Subheading 2, simulations that sample a correct statistical ensemble of system configurations need to be performed. Moreover, depending on the free energy estimator we plan to use, we need to be able to extract the data that will be used for the free energy estimate. There are a number of simulation packages that satisfy these two requirements and are freely available, among which are Gromacs [26], Amber [31], NAMD [39], Sire (http://sire.org) and ProtoMS (http://www.essexgroup.soton.ac.uk/ProtoMS/index.html). Here, we often refer specifically to the setup in Gromacs, as it the code the authors are most familiar with.

3.3 Hardware Requirements	Considering that many intermediate states (windows) need to be simulated, obtaining well-converged ABFE calculations is computationally demanding, despite the calculations being highly parallelizable. The hardware requirements will depend on the details of the system simulated, the specifications of the hardware used, the simulation code, and on how long one is willing to wait for an answer. Here, we assume that a reasonable timeframe for a single calculation is not more than one or 2 days. At the time of writing of this protocol (early 2017), such deadline cannot be met if running the calculations on a modern desktop machine for most protein–ligand systems. Thus, typically, ABFE calculations need to be run on CPU or GPU clusters where at least a few hundred CPUs, or a few tens GPUs, or a mix of those, are available. Nevertheless, algorithmic and hardware improvements might mean that such recommended requirements might soon not apply anymore.

---

4   Methods

4.1 System Preparation	The steps for the preparation of the system to be simulated are not different from the ones needed for any simulation of a protein–ligand complex. First, the protein model typically needs to be refined. X-ray structures may contain missing residues and atoms, which need to be modeled; these include hydrogen atoms, which need to be added at the pH of interest. Similar considerations apply to the ligand, for which pK_a calculations might reveal the protonation state that is dominant in solution. Care should be taken also in checking for the presence of multiple tautomeric states.
4.2 Force Field Choice and Ligand Parameterization	Once the simulation box (including water molecules and ions) is prepared, a potential energy function (force field) needs to be chosen. Among the most commonly used force fields for protein–ligand simulations are the ones from the Amber [40–42] and CHARMM [43–45] families. Although this is not necessarily the case, generally the more recent the force field the more likely it will be accurate given the additional experience collected through its use by the community and consequent refinement by the developers. The standard Amber and CHARMM biomolecular force fields do not contain parameters for organic molecules. Thus, in order to obtain the parameters for these small molecules, the complementary General Amber Force Field (GAFF) [46] and CHARMM General Force Field (CGenFF) [47] need to be used. For both these force fields there are tools that allow automated atom typing, assignment of parameters, and charge derivation [48–50]. It goes without saying that the quality of the ligand parameters is very important for the accurate estimation of their binding free energies. The user can therefore also use more

advanced protocols in order to refine the model of the organic molecule if the available parameters are suspected to be inadequate [51, 52].

4.3 Defining the Intermediate States

The core step in the setup of the calculations is possibly the definition of the alchemical pathway. As depicted in Fig. 1, several intermediate states need to be used to link the bound and unbound states and recover a precise estimate of the binding free energy. Since we will be sampling discrete alchemical states along the path, we need to choose how many intermediate states to have, how they should be distributed along the alchemical path, and for how long to simulate them. From Fig. 1 it is also possible to gather how there will be two sets of simulations during the calculations: one set in which the ligand in solution is simulated (left leg of the cycle in Fig. 1), and one in which the protein–ligand complex is simulated (right leg of the cycle in Fig. 1).

The coupling parameter λ defines the thermodynamic state of the system along the alchemical pathway. This parameter can take any value between zero and one and is used to scale coulombic charges, Lennard–Jones parameters and restraint force constants. Since these are the three sets of parameters that need to be scaled, it is convenient to have distinct coupling parameters: $\lambda_{coul}, \lambda_{vdw}, \lambda_{restr}$. In fact, it is often easier to carry out these three transformation separately, i.e., using a set of windows where only the charges are changed, then a set where only the LJ are changed, and then a third set where only the restraints are modified, as exemplified in Fig. 3. However, as mentioned in Subheading 2.3.1, ΔG_{restr}^{solv} can be calculated analytically so that λ_{restr} apply only to the protein–ligand complex simulations on the right-hand side of the cycle in Fig. 1. For convenience, and to avoid confusion, in Fig. 3 and throughout the text $\lambda = 0$ always indicates the state where the ligand is unrestrained and fully coupled (both in solution and the complex), and $\lambda = 1$ always indicate the state where the ligand is restrained and fully decoupled. We can see in Fig. 1 that for the protein–ligand complex simulations we need to calculate the free energy of coupling the ligand to the environment, i.e., going from the decoupled and restrained state to the coupled and unrestrained state. Nonetheless, it does not matter what is defined as $\lambda = 0$ and $\lambda = 1$, since the equilibrium free energy of coupling (state D → F in Fig. 1) the ligand is simply the opposite of the free energy of decoupling it (state F → D in Fig. 1); we just need to make sure the correct signs are used. When using the EXP estimator, there are also considerations about the forward and reverse calculations, as mentioned in Subheading 2.2.1. However, this is not a concern when using the more robust BAR and MBAR estimators that consider information from multiple states at once.

As mentioned, there are two main sets of simulations to be run: the ligand and complex simulations. Figure 3 shows a simple

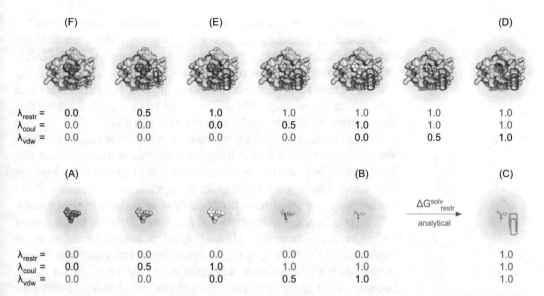

(F) (E) (D)

λ_{restr} =	0.0	0.5	1.0	1.0	1.0	1.0	1.0
λ_{coul} =	0.0	0.0	0.0	0.5	1.0	1.0	1.0
λ_{vdw} =	0.0	0.0	0.0	0.0	0.0	0.5	1.0

(A) (B) (C)

ΔG^{solv}_{restr}
analytical

λ_{restr} =	0.0	0.0	0.0	0.0	0.0	1.0
λ_{coul} =	0.0	0.5	1.0	1.0	1.0	1.0
λ_{vdw} =	0.0	0.0	0.0	0.5	1.0	1.0

Fig. 3 Simplified example of alchemical path and states controlled by the λ parameters. The top row represents the decoupling and restraining of the ligand from the solvated protein–ligand complex; the bottom row represents the decoupling of the ligand from solution. The thermodynamic states (A)–(F) match the states shown in the thermodynamic cycle in Fig. 1. An orange color for the ligand indicates the presence of coulombic interactions with the environment, while a white color their absence; when the vdW surface of the ligand is shown, it indicates the presence of vdW interactions with the environment, while a stick representation of the ligand indicates the absence of vdW intermolecular interactions; a paper clip represents the presence of restraints, with its size proportional to the force constant used. The values of λ_{restr}, λ_{coul}, and λ_{vdw} define the thermodynamic state of the simulation

example of alchemical path that can be used for the calculations. It considers only a very small number of windows just for illustration purposes; in reality many more intermediate states should be used. At the top of this figure, the ligand is decoupled/annihilated from the protein environment, while at the bottom it is decoupled/ annihilated from the solution environment. The columns of λ values for the restraints, coulombic, and Lennard–Jones interactions define each thermodynamic state, that is, each simulation that is carried out. For instance, in state F (corresponding to state F in Fig. 1 too) nothing has changed yet, since all λ values are zero and the simulation is a standard unbiased protein–ligand simulation. Then, in the second complex simulation, the restraints have been turned on partially, while the coulombic and LJ interactions are still fully on; in the third simulation, the restraints have been turned on completely ($\lambda_{restr} = 1$). Then, the coulombic interactions of the ligand start being modified, and between the fourth and fifth simulation of the complex, the ligand charges have been completely decoupled/annihilated. Finally, in the sixth and seventh simulation, the Lennard–Jones interactions of the ligand have also now been decoupled/annihilated, reaching state D where the ligand is fully decoupled and restrained. *See* **Note 1** for how to set up such an alchemical path in Gromacs. The same procedure is carried out for the ligand in solution. In this case, however, the restraints are turned on after the decoupling of the ligand intermolecular interactions. However, as discussed in Subheading 2.3.1, when using the set of restraints proposed by Boresch et al. [32] and described here, these restraining steps do not need to be simulated since this free energy difference can be calculated analytically.

In general, it is difficult to know a priori how many windows should be run and for how long for a specific system that has not been tested before. Test runs are then useful in order to have an idea about phase space overlap, convergence, and precision of the calculations; we will discuss how one can assess these in Subheading 4.6. In practice, the computational resources available play a role as well: the more sampling (i.e., simulation length or number of repeat runs) the better, but if computational efficiency is required (either due to large scale calculations, or limited resources) it becomes even more important to test the calculations in order to find the setup that maximizes precision for the resources available. To provide an idea of what the calculations might involve, for systems containing drug-like ligands binding to small (~110 residues) and fairly rigid proteins, we typically employed 42 windows for the complex and 31 for the ligand simulations, each lasting 10–15 ns.

Ideally, the λ values for the intermediate states should be spaced in such a way that the statistical uncertainty in the free energy difference between neighboring states is equal, as this results in the lowest variance path [53]. In practice, this might be hard to achieve; yet, if the uncertainty of the ΔG between two states is particularly large, it is evident that more windows or tighter spacing is needed. Whether tighter lambda spacing is necessary can also be visually evaluated by looking at the plot of $\langle \partial U / \partial \lambda \rangle$ versus λ used for TI: where the slope of the curve changes more rapidly more windows are needed (an example is shown Fig. 4). The windows used for decoupling the ligand charges can generally be spaced linearly, e.g., $\lambda_{\text{coul}} = [0.0, 0.2, 0.4, 0.6, 0.8, 1.0]$. Using a LJ soft-core potential, λ_{vdw} can also be spaced linearly to start with, and adjusted as needed. However, more windows are typically needed for the LJ than for the charge decoupling. For the restraints, tighter lambda spacing is typically needed when inserting the harmonic potentials [33]. For instance, with $\lambda_{\text{restr}} = 0$ being the state without restraints and $\lambda_{\text{restr}} = 1$ the state with fully coupled restraints, a possible spacing is $\lambda_{\text{restr}} = [0.0, 0.01, 0.025, 0.05, 0.075, 0.1, 0.15, 0.2, 0.35, 0.5, 0.75, 1.0]$.

While the number, spacing, and length of the windows will need to be adapted to the specific system of interest and the desired precision, there are a few rules that should always be followed. Some of these have already been mentioned or alluded to in the

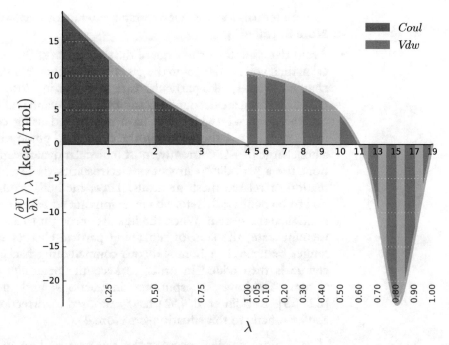

Fig. 4 Thermodynamic integration plot for the decoupling of a ligand from solution. More specifically, it shows the $\langle \partial U / \partial \lambda \rangle$ profile for the decoupling of n-phenylglycinonitrile [54], the ligand used as an example in the tutorial that accompanies this chapter and available on the alchemistry.org website. It is possible to notice the separate decoupling of coulombic and vdW interactions, as well as the fact that the coulombic transformation is smoother than the vdW one

previous paragraphs; here we report them more explicitly and with a brief explanation:

- Use a soft-core potential for decoupling/annihilating the LJ interactions (*see* **Note 2**) [55–58]. Simple scaling schemes for the LJ parameters result in unequal phase space overlap between lambda windows, as well as large forces and numerical instabilities due to a singularity at $r_{ij} = 0$, where i and j are two particles and r the distance between them. Soft-core potentials resolve the instabilities observed during the decoupling of the van der Waals parameters by modifying the LJ equation so that the interaction energy is finite for any configuration.

- Decouple charges and LJ separately (as shown in **Note 1**). Imagine two atoms with opposite partial charges and little repulsion. Even if the charges are small, in the limit of $r_{ij} = 0$, the potential energy of the interaction goes to infinity. This results in large forces and simulation crashes [59, 60]. Thus, a simple way to resolve this issue is to make sure the LJ parameters are decoupled after the charges, or coupled before them, so that when charges are present the repulsive part of the LJ interactions is present too. Another way around this problem is to use a soft-core potential for the electrostatic interactions as well (*see* **Note 3**) [60, 61].

- Avoid changing the net charge of the system across the alchemical path; if you need to, as in the case of decoupling/annihilating charged ligands, take particular care in correcting for artifacts [11, 62]. If you are decoupling/annihilating a ligand that bears a net charge of +1 (which you have neutralized using counter ions), at $\lambda_{\text{coul}} = 1$ the system in the condensed phase will have a net charge of -1. Currently, most molecular dynamics simulations use a periodic treatment of electrostatics via Ewald summation or related mesh methods. These methods require the box to be neutral; therefore counter ions are added in order to neutralize the system. When the ligand is brought to a separate vacuum state, the sum of remaining particle charges will no longer be neutral. A homogeneous compensating background charge is then added in order to keep the neutrality of the system, resulting in spurious interactions and artifacts [62, 63]. Rocklin et al. [62] have proposed a correction that applies exactly to this situation (*see* **Note 4**).

For a more detailed overview of the current best practices related to constructing the alchemical path, we highly recommend the chapter by Shirts [11] and the relevant pages on the Alchemistry website (www.alchemistry.org).

4.4 Defining the Restraints

When using the set of restraints proposed by Boresch et al. [32], one distance, two angle, and three dihedral harmonic restraints between the ligand and the protein need to be defined. Thus, one needs to choose three protein and three ligand atoms to be involved in the restraints, the reference values of the harmonic potentials and their force constants. Since the objective is to keep the position and orientation of the decoupled ligand roughly similar to its known or hypothetical binding pose, we suggest choosing atoms from rigid parts of the ligand and the protein: e.g., three atoms from the protein backbone and three atoms from an aromatic ring in the core of the small molecule (*see* **Note 5**).

The equilibrium values of the distance and angles restraints can be obtained from a small preliminary MD simulation, or also simply set equal to the distance and angles observed in the X-ray or docked ligand structure. In fact, these equilibrium values do not need to represent exactly the minimum energy orientation of the ligand; if the ligand is restrained to a slightly unfavorable orientation, $\Delta G_{\text{restr}}^{\text{prot}}$ will be larger as more work is necessary to fix the ligand in that position, but it will be compensated by $\Delta G_{\text{elec}}^{\text{prot}}$, $\Delta G_{\text{vdw}}^{\text{prot}}$, and $\Delta G_{\text{restr}}^{\text{solv}}$. However, it is important that the target-restrained orientation is not a high-energy state and it is easily accessible from the starting orientation of the ligand. If the target orientation is chosen in such a way that the ligand clashes into the protein, or if the starting orientation is kinetically trapped in a different conformation as compared to the target one, large and unconverged free energy values of $\Delta G_{\text{restr}}^{\text{prot}}$ will be obtained [33, 54]. In our experience we find that, using force constants of $10 \text{ kcal/mol/Å}^2 \text{ [rad}^2\text{]}$, restraining free energies are typically below 2 kcal/mol; in some case they can be larger, but we would suggest that if they exceed 3–4 kcal/mol the simulations should be carefully checked, as this may be symptomatic of either a trapped ligand conformation or an error in the definition of the target orientation.

In their example, Boresch et al. [32] used restraint force constants ranging from 5 to $50 \text{ kcal/mol/Å}^2 \text{ [rad}^2\text{]}$, showing how the correctness of the approach is independent of the stiffness of the restraints. The precision of the restraining free energy may however be affected by restraints that are too loose of too stiff [32]. Thus, in practice, intermediate force constants of about 10 kcal/mol/Å^2 $\text{[rad}^2\text{]}$ have typically been used [7, 8, 54, 64]. **Note 6** shows how protein–ligand restraints can be applied in Gromacs.

4.5 Running the Simulations

At this point the simulations can be started. The rest of the setup is equivalent to a standard unbiased MD simulation, and it is necessary to make sure the correct ensemble is sampled [65]. Remember that anything that can affect the potential energy of the system and the resulting thermodynamic ensemble can also affect the free energy calculations. For instance, the correct Boltzmann distributions of kinetic energies should be generated for both the coupled and decoupled states. Thus, stochastic thermostats that ensure ergodicity and the generation of the correct ensemble, such as the Andersen or Langevin thermostats [66–68], are typically used [69–73]. Similar considerations apply to pressure coupling, so that the Berendsen barostat [74] is avoided in favor of Parrinello–Rahman [75] for the production runs from which data is collected.

In order to be able to analyze the data and estimate the free energy differences at the end of the simulations, it is important that the code stores this information for postprocessing. What data is needed depends upon the free energy estimator of choice (e.g., $\partial U/\partial \lambda$ for TI or ΔU_{ij} for perturbation approaches). If the software allows it, one can also save the data used by all estimators and then compare the results from different approaches (*see* **Note 7**).

Each state, as defined by its λ value, needs then to be minimized and equilibrated independently. This means that if there is a total of N windows, we will need to run N separate minimization, equilibration, and production simulations. This is important because the ligand is present in some simulations, but effectively absent from others, so that the protein and solvent need to adapt to the different environments. All production runs can be run independently, making it easy to parallelize the calculations, or with Hamiltonian replica exchange (HREX) in order to enhance the mixing between states [76, 77] (*see* **Note 8**). The HREX approach has low computational overhead and can result in enhanced sampling, improved phase space overlap and faster convergence, while in the worst case scenario is no different from running the calculations independently [76, 78–80].

4.6 Analyzing the Data

The data collected from all simulations is finally analyzed in order to obtain an estimate of the binding free energy as the sum of the smaller free energy differences along the path. In particular, we need to estimate the two free energy differences for the decoupling of the ligand from solution ($\Delta G^{solv}_{coul+vdw}$) and from the protein–ligand complex ($\Delta G^{prot}_{elec+vdw} + \Delta G^{prot}_{restr}$); these contributions can then be added along with the ΔG^{solv}_{restr} that was obtained analytically to recover the final binding free energy (*see* **Note 9**). Each separate free energy estimate will have its associated uncertainty, which will need to be propagated into the final $\Delta G°_b$. Simulation packages that support alchemical free energy calculations also provide tools for their analysis, using one or more of the estimators previously discussed. Alternatively, the *alchemical-analysis* tool (https://github.com/MobleyLab/alchemical-analysis) is a Python program that implements the automated analysis of free energy calculations performed with Gromacs [26], Amber [31], Sire (http://sire.org), and Desmond [81], and allows easy access to a number of estimators, including MBAR, and the best practices mentioned below (*see* **Note 10**) [24, 30]. An example plot for TI obtained with this tool is shown in Fig. 4.

When analyzing the data obtained from the simulations, it is first important to make sure the samples are not correlated. In practice, $\partial U/\partial \lambda$ and ΔU_{ij} values are typically printed to file frequently, and their values are likely correlated. One could set a particularly low output frequency when setting up the calculations, but this is likely to result in the loss of potentially useful information from the simulations. What is often done is then to calculate the autocorrelation time τ of the time series, and then subsample the data by picking a sample every $1 + 2\tau$ [82]. Once uncorrelated $\partial U/\partial \lambda$ or ΔU_{ij} values have been obtained, they can be fed into different estimators, such as TI and MBAR. Since TI and perturbation approaches use different information for the free energy estimation and have different limitations, comparing the results obtained with the two can be a simple way to check for potential analysis or sampling issues with the calculations.

It is common to exclude from the analysis an initial portion of the simulations, as it is expected to contain nonequilibrated samples. The exact determination of the nonequilibrated region of the simulations is however not trivial. In fact, if extensive equilibration is performed prior the production runs, some system may reach equilibrium before the data needed for the analysis even starts being collected. Nonetheless, it is important to try to exclude nonequilibrated regions of the simulations from the analysis and two main approaches have been proposed for this task. One approach is to plot the convergence of the free energy results in both the "forward" and "reverse" directions, that is, plotting the free energy estimate as a function of the simulated time by including more data while going both from t_0 to t_f, and from t_f to t_0, where t_f is the time of the final snapshot in the simulations [30]. When all data is included, the forward and reverse estimates are the same. If the data have been collected at equilibrium and from the same distributions, and if the calculations have converged, the forward and reverse plots should agree within error. If, when considering the data from the two ends of the simulations, the "forward" and "reverse" free energy estimates converge to two separate and well-defines values, this indicate that nonequilibrated samples have likely been included in the analysis [30]. A different approach, which detects the equilibrated region automatically, has instead recently been proposed by Chodera [83]. In this automated approach, the autocorrelation time is calculated while removing larger portions of the simulation data, and the equilibration time is chosen as the time that maximizes the number of effective uncorrelated samples [83].

Phase space overlap is another property that should be checked when analyzing the results. Poor overlap in specific regions can be resolved by using more, or differently spaced, λ windows. Little overlap does not necessarily lead to wrong free energy estimates, but does result in increased uncertainty; the user should decide what level of uncertainty is acceptable. However, when using perturbation approaches, very poor overlap can result in an underestimate of the variance and an inaccurate free energy estimate [30]. If the MBAR estimator is used, it is possible to obtain an overlap matrix that provides a quantitative estimate of the phase space overlap between simulations [24]. This matrix shows the probability of a sample from state i having been generated in state j, thus providing an indication of the degree of phase space overlap. An example of such an overlap matrix is shown in Fig. 5. The overlap matrix should be tridiagonal, which means that all elements of the main diagonal, as well as the diagonal below and above it, should be nonzero. A value of 0.03 for the tridiagonal elements has been suggested as a threshold to highlight potential phase space overlap issues between two windows [30]. If phase space overlap issues are identified during testing of the free energy protocol for a specific system, it might be possible to adjust the spacing of the λ windows so to increase overlap and reduce the uncertainty of the free energy estimate. If phase space overlap issues are identified instead after running extensive simulations, it is still possible to run additional λ windows in the problematic area of the path, which will be more cost-effective than rerunning the whole calculation with a different

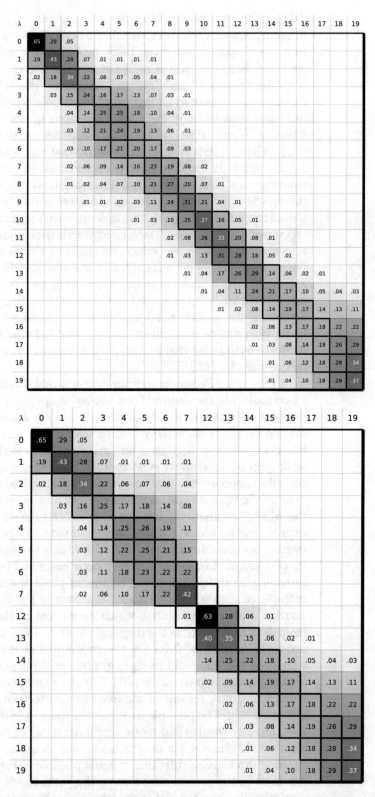

Fig. 5 Overlap matrices for the decoupling of a ligand from solution. The overlap matrix at the top was obtained for the decoupling of n-phenylglycinonitrile from solution using a total of 20 windows, and shows good overlap

spacing. In general, a good phase space overlap is attainable for the decoupling of the ligand from solution, but can be more challenging for the decoupling of the ligand from the complex.

Finally, in some cases it might be necessary to correct for simulation artifacts. We have already mentioned how charged ligands can be problematic, as the net charge of the system changes across windows during the charge annihilation process. This introduces a series of artifacts when using Ewald summation methods for the treatment of electrostatics in periodic systems [62]. In this case, the approach proposed by Rocklin et al. [62], which consists of a few analytical corrections and an implicit-solvent calculation, can be used. Sometimes, a correction for the long-range Lennard–Jones interactions is included too. Some simulation packages, like Gromacs, already include an analytical correction for the long-range LJ interactions, which are generally excluded during the simulations by the use of LJ cutoffs. However, these analytical corrections assume an isotropic system outside the cutoff, which is not valid when simulating protein–ligand complexes (as the cutoff is generally smaller than the largest dimension of the complex). Shirts et al. [84] have proposed a numerical correction to the free energy estimate for such cases. The correction is based on the postprocessing of some of the simulations using a larger LJ cutoff, effectively building an additional thermodynamic cycle on top of the one already used in order to calculate the $\Delta\Delta G$ of going from a system with a short LJ cutoff (where the isotropic assumption fails) to a system with a long LJ cutoff (where the isotropic assumption holds). Note that since the long-range part of the LJ interactions is always attractive, the correction results in the prediction of slightly stronger affinity values; in our experience, for drug-like ligands and using a LJ cutoff of 1.0 nm, this typically amounts to an additional 0.3–0.8 kcal/mol to the binding free energy. Taking these additional interactions into account does not necessarily result in more accurate binding affinity predictions, but it does increase reproducibility by removing the dependence on the cutoff value used. An alternative option to the correction by Shirts et al. [84] is to run the simulation using lattice summation methods also for the LJ interactions, such as the recently proposed LJ-PME approach [85]. In this way, there is no need for a post hoc correction, and the forces arising from these long-range interactions are considered already during the simulation. However, this comes at additional computational cost [85].

Fig. 5 (continued) between each pair of states. The matrix at the bottom was obtained by disregarding the data from four windows (8, 9, 10, and 11), and shows poor overlap between states 7 and 12. In the latter case, it becomes evident that additional simulations or a different λ spacing is needed. The overlap plots have been obtained with the *alchemical analysis* python tool [30]

In this section, we provided a brief overview of how to analyze alchemical free energy results while also mentioning some recommended procedures to check for possible issues affecting the reliability of the estimate. For a more detailed explanation of the best practices and tools available for the analysis of equilibrium free energy calculations, we highly recommend reading the article by Klimovich et al. [30].

4.7 Sampling and Modeling Challenges

As in all MD simulations, issues may arise as a consequence of limited sampling and model inaccuracies. Inadequate sampling might manifest itself as poorly converged free energy estimates, which can be identified through convergence plots and the size of the uncertainty in estimates. Repeating the calculations, possibly using different starting structures, is a simple yet appropriate way to assess the precision of the calculations and highlight possible convergence problems, confirming that the results are reproducible. It is important to assess whether converged results can be obtained within the timescale of the planned calculations for the specific system of interest. Alchemical free energy calculations are expected to be more accurate than implicit solvent end-point methods and scoring functions, [6, 8, 9]. However, they are also sensitive to sampling issues [86] such that they can become unreliable if the phase space explored by the simulations is inadequate for capturing the conformational ensembles that largely determine the binding free energy. Moreover, severe sampling issues due to very slow degrees of freedom that cannot be sampled during the timescale of the simulations can result in apparently converged calculations despite affecting the predicted affinities. This can be the case when the ligand induces conformational changes in the protein. If these changes are known, the problem may be tackled by separately calculating the potential of mean force (PMF) for the conformational change with methods such as umbrella sampling. Mobley et al. [87] used such an approach to take into account the free energy contribution of a valine side chain rearrangement that was not sampled during the alchemical calculations. Lin et al. [88] have used umbrella sampling to calculate the free energy change involved in the large loop rearrangement that is associated with the binding of type-II kinase inhibitors. In many instances, however, similar slow degrees of freedom might be unknown, and left unsampled. The position of structural water molecules can be important as well. If these water molecules are not present in the starting structure for the calculations, but are important for binding, and if diffusion to their most stable location is kinetically hindered, this too can result in convergence issues and biased results. Sampling schemes that try to tackle these issues have been developed or are subject of active research [89–92], but are outside the scope of this discussion.

Considerations about the quality of the starting structure and the modeling of the system's chemistry are important too. For instance, the ligand might have multiple protonation and tautomer states in solution, without a single one being necessarily largely dominant. In addition, the solvent and the protein represent two very different environments, so that pK_a shifts are possible and the protonation states of the ligand or protein residues may change between the unbound and bound states. Currently, this is not inherently captured by typical simulations. These complications might thus require multiple calculations or more advanced protocols that correctly take into account the contributions arising from the presence of multiple molecular species in equilibrium. Furthermore, the suitability of the force field for the molecules studied can clearly have important effects on the accuracy of the calculated affinities. Given the vast chemical space of small drug-like molecules, the transferability of certain parameters, such as those for the torsions, can be problematic and may result in inaccurate energies and relative conformational populations. This, in turn, may affect the binding free energy results in ways that are hard to foresee. Small molecule parameters can be refined, for instance, by targeting quantum mechanical energies [8, 51] but it is up to the user to decide how much human and computational effort to invest in order to validate the quality of the parameters.

5 Notes

In these Notes we describe how specific steps can be carried out in Gromacs 2016. It is however recommended to also refer to the Gromacs manual for additional details, in particular considering possible changes/developments in future versions of the software.

1. In Gromacs, the fictitious alchemical path depicted in Fig. 3 and pertaining to the simulations of the protein–ligand complex could be implemented via options in the mdp file as follows.

```
free-energy     = yes
couple-moltype  = ligand
couple-lambda0  = vdw-q
couple-lambda1  = none
bonded-lambdas  = 0.0  0.5  1.0  1.0  1.0  1.0  1.0
coul-lambdas    = 0.0  0.0  0.0  0.5  1.0  1.0  1.0
vdw-lambdas     = 0.0  0.0  0.0  0.0  0.0  0.5  1.0
```

The `free-energy` flag tells the code we are performing free energy calculations; `couple-moltype` defines the molecule type, as defined in the topology, that is to be (de)coupled.

`couple-lambda0` and `couple-lambda1` define the state of the intermolecular interactions at λ values of zero and one, respectively; in this case we are defining that at lambda zero both coulombic and vdW interactions are on, while they are off at lambda one (i.e., the ligand is decoupled while going from lambda zero to one). `bonded-lambdas` defines the vector of λ_{restr} values, since the restraints can be applied as additional bonded terms between different molecules, as shown in **Note 6**. This vector can be omitted when decoupling the ligand from solution, since for that leg of the cycle the contribution of the restraints can be obtained analytically. `coul-lambdas` and `vdw-lambdas` define instead the lambda vectors for the decoupling of the coulombic and Lennard–Jones interactions. In this example, there are seven states to be simulated, each defined by a column of the vectors above. `init-lambda-state` is then used in the mdp file in order to choose which column is being simulated; for instance, `init-lambda-state = 0` means that the index 0 of the lambda arrays is simulated ($\lambda_{restr} = 0.0$, $\lambda_{coul} = 0.0$, $\lambda_{vdw} = 0.0$), while `init-lambda-state = 3` means that index 3 of the arrays is simulated ($\lambda_{restr} = 1.0$, $\lambda_{coul} = 0.5$, $\lambda_{vdw} = 0.0$). Additionally, the `couple-intramol` flag can be used to decide whether the ligand should be decoupled or annihilated.

2. In Gromacs, the Lennard–Jones soft-core potential by Beutler et al. [55] is implemented and can be used by specifying the following in the mdp file.

```
sc-alpha = 0.5
sc-power = 1
sc-sigma = 0.3
```

These three parameters define the soft-cored Lennard–Jones function [55]. In particular, the alpha parameter needs to be larger than zero for the LJ interactions to be soft-cored. An `sc-alpha` of 0.5, `sc-power` of 1, and `sc-sigma` of 0.3 are typically used values [33, 54, 56, 69, 93].

3. A soft-core potential for the coulombic interactions can be activated in Gromacs with the mdp option `sc-coul`. However, for equilibrium ABFE calculations, it is not clear whether performing the coulombic and vdW transformations simultaneously would result in much better efficiency as compared to performing the transformation separately. In fact, since the charge decoupling process typically shows good overlap between windows and smooth $\langle \partial U / \partial \lambda \rangle$, few windows are usually necessary [61, 93, 94].

4. One might think that in order to keep the neutrality of the box it could also be possible to (de)couple an ion from solution

together with the ligand, so that the change in net charge would be compensated. This is however likely to introduce spurious free energy contributions, due to the fact that the free energy of decoupling an ion from the water box is not the same as the free energy of decoupling it from the box that contains also the protein. Since the environments in the two legs of the ABFE cycle are very different, the two ion decoupling free energies are unlikely to cancel out. Alternatively, the two legs of the cycle could be performed in a single simulation box. However, for the ligand in solution to avoid strong interactions with the protein–ligand complex a very large simulation box is needed. When considering the scaling of MD simulations with the number of particles, it can be seen how the calculations would become computationally much more expensive. In addition, there could still be residual finite size effects that remain unaccounted for [95, 96].

5. In our experience, we have found that including hydrogen atoms (which bonds are typically constrained with the LINCS algorithm) as part of the set of restrained atoms can cause stability issues during the simulation. Therefore, we would suggest choosing a set of heavy atoms only for the protein–ligand restraints.

6. Protein–ligand restraints can now be applied in Gromacs through the use of the [intermolecular_interactions] section at the very end of the topology file. In this section, it is possible to define bonded terms between any atom in the system using global indices (i.e., the indices found in the coordinates file). To generate harmonic restraints, bonds of type 6, angles of type 1, and dihedrals of type 2, can be used (*see* Table 5.5 in the Gromacs manual) as shown in the example below. Furthermore, it is necessary to define the force constants for the restraints in states A and B (i.e., states $\lambda_{restr} = 0$ and $\lambda_{restr} = 1$). One of the two force constants needs to be zero, which corresponds to the state where the restraints are effectively absent. The equilibrium distance/angles can be set to the same value for both states instead. The other force constant should be set to the value chosen, as discussed in Subheading 4.4, for example 10 kcal/mol/Å^2 [rad^2]. Remember that Gromacs uses kJ/mol and nm as units for energy and length. In the example below, *ai, aj, ak,* and *al* are global atom indices (atoms 1, 2, 3 can be ligand atoms, and atoms 4, 5, 6 protein atoms, or vice-versa); type defines the function type used; b_A, th_A, and phi_A are the equilibrium values of distance and angles for the harmonic restraints in state A ($\lambda_{restr} = 0$), and b_B, th_B, and phi_B the ones in state B ($\lambda_{restr} = 1$); k_A is the force constant used in state A ($\lambda_{restr} = 0$), and k_B the one used in state B ($\lambda_{restr} = 1$). The bonded-lambdas vector discussed in **Note 1** will

interpolate between the force constant (and equilibrium positions) in state A and B.

```
[ intermolecular_interactions]
[ bonds ]
; ai  aj  type  bA    kA    bB    kB
   3   4   6    0.5   0.0   0.5   4184.0

[ angles ]
; ai aj ak type  thA    kA    thB    kB
   2  3  4  1    80.0   0.0   80.0   41.84
   3  4  5  1    30.0   0.0   30.0   41.84

[ dihedrals ]
; ai aj ak al type  phiA     kA    phiB     kB
   1  2  3  4  2   -100.0    0.0  -100.0   41.84
   2  3  4  5  2    120.0    0.0   120.0   41.84
   3  4  5  6  2     15.0    0.0    15.0   41.84
```

7. In the Gromacs mdp file, `calc-lambda-neighbors` controls the number of lambda values for which ΔU_{ij} will be calculated. If one wants to use BAR rather than FEP, then the value of `calc-lambda-neighbors` should be set to 1; in order to also use MBAR, a value of -1, which effectively means "all," should be used instead. With the option `dhdl-derivatives` set to "yes" by default when using the free energy code, also the $\partial U/\partial \lambda$ values (needed for TI) will be calculated and stored with the frequency specified by `nstdhdl`. By setting `separate-dhdl-file`=yes, the $\partial U/\partial \lambda$ and ΔU_{ij} values will be printed to a file with default name "dhdl.xvg", which can later be processed with the Gromacs tool `gmx bar` or with the `alchemical_analysis` Python tool [30].

8. Replica exchange can be activated when using `mdrun` in Gromacs with the `--replex` flag, which specifies the frequency of exchange attempts. It has been suggested to set the frequency of the exchanges as high as possible, as long as this does not result in substantial simulation slowdown [76]. With only the `--replex` flag, swaps only between neighboring windows are attempted. Using also the `--nex` command, multiple exchange are performed between any pair of lambda windows, resulting in further mixing between states. A number of swaps between N^3 and N^5, where N is the number of replicas, has empirically been found to provide sufficient mixing [76]. Thus, as an example, for a calculation involving 30 windows, one could use `mdrun --replex 1000 --nex 500000`.

9. In addition to the free energy terms discussed, in certain cases a contribution due to the symmetry should in principle be taken

into account [33]. A symmetry correction applies when: (a) the ligand is symmetric or contains a symmetric moiety; (b) the equivalent (symmetric) orientations or the ligand are not sampled during the simulations, typically due to large energy barriers between the orientations; and (c) the restraints used break the symmetry, such that the normally equivalent orientations of the molecule have different energies due to the biasing potential employed [33]. For a ligand with a number σ_L of symmetric and thus equivalent orientations, this correction amounts to $\Delta G_{sym} = -kT\ln(\sigma_L)$. Thus, at 300 K, for a benzene molecule $\Delta G_{sym} = -kT\ln(12) = -1.48$ kcal/mol; while for a ligand containing a phenyl group $\Delta G_{sym} = -kT\ln(2) = -0.41$ kcal/mol.

10. The *alchemical_analysis.py* script may be run as follows:

```
alchemical_analysis.py -d dhdl_files/ -s 1000 -t 298 -w -g
```

Where the $--$d flag specifies the directory containing the files with the $\partial U/\partial \lambda$ and ΔU_{ij} information from all the windows; the $--$s flag specifies the amount of simulation time (in ps) to discard as equilibration period; $-$t specifies the temperature in Kelvin; $-$w asks for the overlap matrix to be plotted; and $--$g asks for the ΔG between each adjacent state to be plotted. The code defaults to the analysis of Gromacs files, so that in the *dhdl_files* folder it expects to find files that start with "dhdl" and have ".xvg" extension (e.g., *dhdl_1.xvg*, *dhdl_2.xvg*, *dhdl_3.xvg*, etc.); this can however be changed with the $--$p and $--$q flags. Moreover, free energy calculations run with Amber [31], Sire (http://sire.org), or Desmond [81], can still be analyzed by choosing the software with the $--$a flag. The $--$f flag allows instead to plot the free energy estimate as a function of time in both directions. These are just some of the options available, and the reader can find an explanation for all of them by displaying the help message of the script.

Acknowledgments

The EPSRC and Evotec via the Systems Approaches to Biomedical Sciences Doctoral Training Centre (EP/G037280/1) support M.A. J.B. is supported by the EPSRC/MRC via the Systems Approaches to Biomedical Sciences Doctoral Training Centre (EP/G037280/1) with additional support from GSK. We thank David Mobley (University of California, Irvine), John Chodera (MSKCC), and Michael Shirts (University of Colorado, Boulder) for sharing their extensive experience on alchemical free energy calculations through publicly available platforms and personal communications. Work in PCB's laboratory is currently supported by the MRC, BBSRC, and the John Fell Fund. We thank the Advanced Research Computing (ARC) facility, the EPSRC UK National Service for Computational Chemistry Software (NSCCS) at Imperial College London (grant no. EP/J003921/1), and the ARCHER UK National Supercomputing Services for computer time granted via the UK High-End Computing Consortium for Biomolecular Simulation, HECBioSim (http://www.hecbiosim.ac.uk), supported by EPSRC (grant no. EP/L000253/1).

References

1. Mobley DL, Dill KA (2009) Binding of small-molecule ligands to proteins: "what you see" is not always "what you get". Structure 17:489–498

2. Chipot C (2014) Frontiers in free-energy calculations of biological systems. Wiley Interdiscip Rev Comput Mol Sci 4(1):71–89

3. Kitchen DB, Decornez H, Furr JR, Bajorath J (2004) Docking and scoring in virtual screening for drug discovery: methods and applications. Nat Rev Drug Discov 3:935–949

4. Genheden S, Ryde U (2015) The MM/PBSA and MM/GBSA methods to estimate ligand-binding affinities. Expert Opin Drug Discov 10(5):449–461

5. Shirts MR, Mobley DL, Chodera JD (2007) Free energy calculations: ready for prime time? Annu Rep Comput Chem 3:41–59

6. Aldeghi M, Bodkin MJ, Knapp S, Biggin PC (2017) A statistical analysis on the performance of MMPBSA versus absolute binding free energy calculations: bromodomains as a case study. J Chem Inf Model 57:2203–2221

7. Aldeghi M, Heifetz A, Bodkin MJ, Knapp S, Biggin PC (2016) Accurate calculation of the absolute free energy of binding for drug molecules. Chem Sci 7:207–218

8. Aldeghi M, Heifetz A, Bodkin MJ, Knapp S, Biggin PC (2017) Predictions of ligand selectivity from absolute binding free energy calculations. J Am Chem Soc 139:946–957

9. Chipot C, Pohorille A (2007) Free energy calculations: theory and applications in chemistry and biology, vol 86. Springer series in chemical physics. Springer, New York

10. Pohorille A, Jarzynski C, Chipot C (2010) Good practices in free-energy calculations. J Phys Chem B 114(32):10235–10253

11. Shirts MR (2012) Best practices in free energy calculations for drug design. Methods Mol Biol 819:425–467

12. Shirts MR, Mobley DL (2013) An introduction to best practices in free energy calculations. In: Monticelli L, Salonen E (eds) Biomolecular simulations: methods and protocols. Humana Press, Totowa, NJ, pp 271–311

13. Zhou H-X, Gilson MK (2009) Theory of free energy and entropy in noncovalent binding. Chem Rev 109(9):4092–4107

14. Gilson MK, Given JA, Bush BL, McCammon JA (1997) The statistical-thermodynamic basis for computation of binding affinities: a critical review. Biophys J 72(3):1047–1069

15. General IJ (2010) A note on the standard state's binding free energy. J Chem Theory Comput 6(8):2520–2524

16. Gapsys V, Michielssens S, Peters JH, de Groot BL, Leonov H (2015) Calculation of binding free energies. In: Kukol A (ed) Molecular modeling of proteins. Springer New York, New York, NY, pp 173–209

17. Zwanzig RW (1954) High-temperature equation of state by a perturbation method. I. Nonpolar gases. J Chem Phys 22(8):1420–1426

18. Widom B (1963) Some topics in the theory of fluids. J Chem Phys 39(11):2808–2812

19. Lu N, Singh JK, Kofke DA (2003) Appropriate methods to combine forward and reverse free-energy perturbation averages. J Chem Phys 118(7):2977–2984

20. Shirts MR, Pande VS (2005) Comparison of efficiency and bias of free energies computed by exponential averaging, the Bennett acceptance ratio, and thermodynamic integration. J Chem Phys 122(14):144107

21. Bennett CH (1976) Efficient estimation of free energy differences from Monte Carlo data. J Comput Phys 22(2):245–268

22. Shirts MR, Mobley DL, Brown SP (2010) Free-energy calculations in structure-based drug design. In: Merz KM, Ringe D, Reynolds CH (eds) Drug design. Cambridge University Press, Cambridge, pp 61–86

23. Shirts MR, Bair E, Hooker G, Pande VS (2003) Equilibrium free energies from

nonequilibrium measurements using maximum-likelihood methods. Phys Rev Lett 91(14):140601

24. Shirts MR, Chodera JD (2008) Statistically optimal analysis of samples from multiple equilibrium states. J Chem Phys 129:124105

25. Paliwal H, Shirts MR (2011) A benchmark test set for alchemical free energy transformations and its use to quantify error in common free energy methods. J Chem Theory Comput 7 (12):4115–4134

26. Abraham MJ, Murtola T, Schulz R, Páll S, Smith JC, Hess B, Lindahl E (2015) GROMACS: high performance molecular simulations through multi-level parallelism from laptops to supercomputers. SoftwareX 1–2:19–25

27. Homeyer N, Gohlke H (2013) FEW: a workflow tool for free energy calculations of ligand binding. J Comput Chem 34(11):965–973

28. Liu P, Dehez F, Cai W, Chipot C (2012) A toolkit for the analysis of free-energy perturbation calculations. J Chem Theory Comput 8 (8):2606–2616

29. Pham TT, Shirts MR (2011) Identifying low variance pathways for free energy calculations of molecular transformations in solution phase. J Chem Phys 135(3):034114

30. Klimovich P, Shirts M, Mobley D (2015) Guidelines for the analysis of free energy calculations. J Comput Aided Mol Des 29 (5):397–411

31. Case DA, Betz RM, Cerutti DS, Cheatham TE III, Darden TA, Duke RE, Giese TJ, Gohlke H, Goetz AW, Homeyer N, Izadi S, Janowski P, Kaus J, Kovalenko A, Lee TS, LeGrand S, Li P, Lin C, Luchko T, Luo R, Madej BD, Mermelstein D, Merz KM, Monard G, Nguyen H, Nguyen HT, Omelyan I, Onufriev A, Roe DR, Roitberg A, Sagui C, Simmerling CL, Botello-Smith WM, Swails J, Walker RC, Wang J, Wolf RM, Wu X, Xiao L, Kollman PA (2016) AMBER 2016. University of California, San Francisco

32. Boresch S, Tettinger F, Leitgeb M, Karplus M (2003) Absolute binding free energies: a quantitative approach for their calculation. J Phys Chem B 107(35):9535–9551

33. Mobley DL, Chodera JD, Dill KA (2006) On the use of orientational restraints and symmetry corrections in alchemical free energy calculations. J Chem Phys 125(8):084902

34. Evoli S, Mobley DL, Guzzi R, Rizzuti B (2016) Multiple binding modes of ibuprofen in human serum albumin identified by absolute binding free energy calculations. Phys Chem Chem Phys 18(47):32358–32368

35. Cappel D, Hall ML, Lenselink EB, Beuming T, Qi J, Bradner J, Sherman W (2016) Relative binding free energy calculations applied to protein homology models. J Chem Inf Model 56 (12):2388–2400

36. Mobley DL, Graves AP, Chodera JD, McReynolds AC, Shoichet BK, Dill KA (2007) Predicting absolute ligand binding free energies to a simple model site. J Mol Biol 371 (4):1118–1134

37. Mobley DL (2012) Let's get honest about sampling. J Comput Aided Mol Des 26 (1):93–95

38. Mobley DL, Klimovich PV (2012) Perspective: alchemical free energy calculations for drug discovery. J Chem Phys 137(23):230901

39. Phillips JC, Braun R, Wang W, Gumbart J, Tajkhorshid E, Villa E, Chipot C, Skeel RD, Kale L, Schulten K (2005) Scalable molecular dynamics with NAMD. J Comput Chem 26:1781–1802

40. Hornak V, Abel R, Okur A, Strockbine B, Roitberg A, Simmerling C (2006) Comparison of multiple Amber force fields and development of improved protein backbone parameters. Proteins 65(3):712–725

41. Lindorff-Larsen K, Piana S, Palmo K, Maragakis P, Klepeis J, Dror R, Shaw D (2010) Improved side-chain torsion potentials for the Amber ff99SB protein force field. Proteins 78:1950–1958

42. Maier JA, Martinez C, Kasavajhala K, Wickstrom L, Hauser KE, Simmerling C (2015) ff14SB: improving the accuracy of protein side chain and backbone parameters from ff99SB. J Chem Theory Comput 11 (8):3696–3713

43. MacKerell AD, Bashford D, Bellott M, Dunbrack RL, Evanseck JD, Field MJ, Fischer S, Gao J, Guo H, Ha S, Joseph-McCarthy D, Kuchnir L, Kuczera K, Lau FTK, Mattos C, Michnick S, Ngo T, Nguyen DT, Prodhom B, Reiher WE, Roux B, Schlenkrich M, Smith JC, Stote R, Straub J, Watanabe M, Wiórkiewicz-Kuczera J, Yin D, Karplus M (1998) All-atom empirical potential for molecular modeling and dynamics studies of proteins. J Phys Chem B 102(18):3586–3616

44. Mackerell AD (2004) Empirical force fields for biological macromolecules: overview and issues. J Comput Chem 25(13):1584–1604

45. Best RB, Zhu X, Shim J, Lopes PEM, Mittal J, Feig M, MacKerell AD (2012) Optimization of the additive CHARMM all-atom protein force field targeting improved sampling of the backbone φ, ψ and side-chain $\chi(1)$ and

χ(2) dihedral angles. J Chem Theory Comput 8(9):3257–3273

46. Wang J, Wolf RM, Caldwell JW, Kollman PA, Case DA (2004) Development and testing of a general amber force field. J Comput Chem 25 (9):1157–1174

47. Vanommeslaeghe K, Hatcher E, Acharya C, Kundu S, Zhong S, Shim J, Darian E, Guvench O, Lopes P, Vorobyov I, Mackerell Jr AD (2010) CHARMM general force field: a force field for drug-like molecules compatible with the CHARMM all-atom additive biological force fields. J Comput Chem 31 (4):671–690

48. Wang J, Wang W, Kollman PA, Case DA (2006) Automatic atom type and bond type perception in molecular mechanical calculations. J Mol Graph Model 25(2):247–260

49. Vanommeslaeghe K, MacKerell AD (2012) Automation of the charmm general force field (CGenFF) I: bond perception and atom typing. J Chem Inf Model 52(12):3144–3154

50. Vanommeslaeghe K, Raman EP, MacKerell AD (2012) Automation of the CHARMM general force field (CGenFF) II: assignment of bonded parameters and partial atomic charges. J Chem Inf Model 52(12):3155–3168

51. Huang L, Roux B (2013) Automated force field parameterization for nonpolarizable and polarizable atomic models based on ab initio target data. J Chem Theory Comput 9 (8):3543–3556

52. Betz RM, Walker RC (2015) Paramfit: automated optimization of force field parameters for molecular dynamics simulations. J Comput Chem 36(2):79–87

53. Shenfeld DK, Xu H, Eastwood MP, Dror RO, Shaw DE (2009) Minimizing thermodynamic length to select intermediate states for free-energy calculations and replica-exchange simulations. Phys Rev E Stat Nonlin Soft Matter Phys 80(4):046705

54. Boyce SE, Mobley DL, Rocklin GJ, Graves AP, Dill KA, Shoichet BK (2009) Predicting ligand binding affinity with alchemical free energy methods in a polar model binding site. J Mol Biol 394(4):747–763

55. Beutler TC, Mark AE, van Schaik RC, Gerber PR, van Gunsteren WF (1994) Avoiding singularities and numerical instabilities in free energy calculations based on molecular simulations. Chem Phys Lett 222:529–539

56. Steinbrecher T, Mobley DL, Case DA (2007) Nonlinear scaling schemes for Lennard-Jones interactions in free energy calculations. J Chem Phys 127(21):214108

57. Zacharias M, Straatsma TP, McCammon JA (1994) Separation-shifted scaling, a new scaling method for Lennard-Jones interactions in thermodynamic integration. J Chem Phys 100 (12):9025–9031

58. Gapsys V, Seeliger D, de Groot BL (2012) New soft-core potential function for molecular dynamics based alchemical free energy calculations. J Chem Theory Comput 8 (7):2373–2382

59. Pitera JW, van Gunsteren WF (2002) A comparison of non-bonded scaling approaches for free energy calculations. Mol Simul 28 (1–2):45–65

60. Anwar J, Heyes DM (2005) Robust and accurate method for free-energy calculation of charged molecular systems. J Chem Phys 122 (22):224117

61. Steinbrecher T, Joung I, Case DA (2011) Soft-core potentials in thermodynamic integration: comparing one- and two-step transformations. J Comput Chem 32(15):3253–3263

62. Rocklin GJ, Mobley DL, Dill KA, Hünenberger PH (2013) Calculating the binding free energies of charged species based on explicit-solvent simulations employing lattice-sum methods: an accurate correction scheme for electrostatic finite-size effects. J Chem Phys 139:184103

63. Hub JS, de Groot BL, Grubmüller H, Groenhof G (2014) Quantifying artifacts in ewald simulations of inhomogeneous systems with a net charge. J Chem Theory Comput 10 (1):381–390

64. Rocklin GJ, Boyce SE, Fischer M, Fish I, Mobley DL, Shoichet BK, Dill KA (2013) Blind prediction of charged ligand binding affinities in a model binding site. J Mol Biol 425 (22):4569–4583

65. Shirts MR (2013) Simple quantitative tests to validate sampling from thermodynamic ensembles. J Chem Theory Comput 9(2):909–926

66. Goga N, Rzepiela AJ, de Vries AH, Marrink SJ, Berendsen HJC (2012) Efficient algorithms for langevin and DPD dynamics. J Chem Theory Comput 8:3637–3649

67. Andersen HC (1980) Molecular dynamics simulations at constant pressure and/or temperature. J Chem Phys 72(4):2384–2393

68. Schneider T, Stoll E (1978) Molecular-dynamics study of a three-dimensional one-component model for distortive phase transitions. Phys Rev B 17(3):1302–1322

69. Shirts MR, Pitera JW, Swope WC, Pande VS (2003) Extremely precise free energy calculations of amino acid side chain analogs: comparison of common molecular mechanics force

fields for proteins. J Chem Phys 119 (11):5740–5761

70. Kelly E, Seth M, Ziegler T (2004) Calculation of free energy profiles for elementary bimolecular reactions by ab initio molecular dynamics: sampling methods and thermostat considerations. J Phys Chem A 108(12):2167–2180

71. Hess B, van der Vegt NFA (2006) Hydration thermodynamic properties of amino acid analogues: a systematic comparison of biomolecular force fields and water models. J Phys Chem B 110(35):17616–17626

72. Wang J, Deng Y, Roux B (2006) Absolute binding free energy calculations using molecular dynamics simulations with restraining potentials. Biophys J 91(8):2798–2814

73. Bussi G, Parrinello M (2008) Stochastic thermostats: comparison of local and global schemes. Comput Phys Commun 179 (1–3):26–29

74. Berendsen HJC, Postma JPM, van Gunsteren WF, DiNola A, Haak JR (1984) Molecular dynamics with coupling to an external bath. J Chem Phys 81:3684–3690

75. Parinello M, Rahman A (1981) Polymorphic transitions in single crystals – a new molecular dynamics method. J Appl Phys 52:7182–7190

76. Chodera JD, Shirts MR (2011) Replica exchange and expanded ensemble simulations as Gibbs sampling: simple improvements for enhanced mixing. J Chem Phys 2011 (135):194110

77. Bussi G (2014) Hamiltonian replica exchange in GROMACS: a flexible implementation. Mol Phys 112(3–4):379–384

78. Faraldo-Gómez JD, Roux B (2007) Characterization of conformational equilibria through Hamiltonian and temperature replica-exchange simulations: assessing entropic and environmental effects. J Comput Chem 28 (10):1634–1647

79. Wang K, Chodera JD, Yang Y, Shirts MR (2013) Identifying ligand binding sites and poses using GPU-accelerated Hamiltonian replica exchange molecular dynamics. J Comput Aided Mol Des 27:989–1007

80. Woods CJ, Essex JW, King MA (2003) Enhanced configurational sampling in binding free-energy calculations. J Phys Chem B 107 (49):13711–13718

81. Bowers KJ, Chow E, Xu H, Dror RO, Eastwood MP, Gregersen BA, Klepeis JL, Kolossvary I, Moraes MA, Sacerdoti FD, Salmon JK, Shan Y, Shaw DE (2006) Scalable algorithms for molecular dynamics simulations on commodity clusters. In: Proceedings of the 2006 ACMI/IEEE conference on supercomputing. ACM Press, New York

82. Chodera JD, Swope WC, Pitera JW, Seok C, Dill KA (2007) Use of the weighted histogram analysis method for the analysis of simulated and parallel tempering simulations. J Chem Theory Comput 3:26–41

83. Chodera JD (2016) A simple method for automated equilibration detection in molecular simulations. J Chem Theory Comput 12 (4):1799–1805

84. Shirts MR, Mobley DL, Chodera JD, Pande VS (2007) Accurate and efficient corrections for missing dispersion interactions in molecular simulations. J Phys Chem B 111 (45):13052–13063

85. Wennberg CL, Murtola T, Páll S, Abraham MJ, Hess B, Lindahl E (2015) Direct-space corrections enable fast and accurate lorentz–berthelot combination rule Lennard-Jones lattice summation. J Chem Theory Comput 11 (12):5737–5746

86. Lim NM, Wang L, Abel R, Mobley DL (2016) Sensitivity in binding free energies due to protein reorganization. J Chem Theory Comput 12(9):4620–4631

87. Mobley DL, Chodera JD, Dill KA (2007) Confine-and-release method: obtaining correct binding free energies in the presence of protein conformational change. J Chem Theory Comput 3:1231–1235

88. Lin Y-L, Meng Y, Jiang W, Roux B (2013) Explaining why Gleevec is a specific and potent inhibitor of Abl kinase. Proc Natl Acad Sci U S A 110(5):1664–1669

89. Li H, Fajer M, Yang W (2007) Simulated scaling method for localized enhanced sampling and simultaneous "alchemical" free energy simulations: a general method for molecular mechanical, quantum mechanical, and quantum mechanical/molecular mechanical simulations. J Chem Phys 126(2):024106

90. Wang L, Berne BJ, Friesner RA (2012) On achieving high accuracy and reliability in the calculation of relative protein–ligand binding affinities. Proc Natl Acad Sci U S A 109 (6):1937–1942

91. Wang L, Deng Y, Knight JL, Wu Y, Kim B, Sherman W, Shelley JC, Lin T, Abel R (2013) Modeling local structural rearrangements using FEP/REST: application to relative binding affinity predictions of CDK2 inhibitors. J Chem Theory Comput 9(2):1282–1293

92. Ross GA, Bodnarchuk MS, Essex JW (2015) Water sites, networks, and free energies with Grand Canonical Monte Carlo. J Am Chem Soc 137(47):14930–14943

93. Shirts MR, Pande VS (2005) Solvation free energies of amino acid side chain analogs for common molecular mechanics water models. J Chem Phys 122(13):134508

94. Mobley DL, Dumont ML, Chodera JD, Dill KA (2007) Comparison of charge models for fixed-charged force-fields: small molecule hydration free energies in explicit solvent. J Phys Chem B 111:2242–2254

95. Hünenberger PH, McCammon JA (1999) Effect of artificial periodicity in simulations of biomolecules under Ewald boundary conditions: a continuum electrostatics study. Biophys Chem 78:69–88

96. Lin Y-L, Aleksandrov A, Simonson T, Roux B (2014) An overview of electrostatic free energy computations for solutions and proteins. J Chem Theory Comput 10(7):2690–2709

Chapter 12

Evaluation of Protein–Ligand Docking by Cyscore

Yang Cao, Wentao Dai, and Zhichao Miao

Abstract

Protein–ligand docking is a powerful method in drug discovery. The reliability of docking can be quantified by RMSD between a docking structure and an experimentally determined one. However, most experimentally determined structures are not available in practice. Evaluation by scoring functions is an alternative for assessing protein–ligand docking results. This chapter first provides a brief introduction to scoring methods used in docking. Then details are provided on how to use Cyscore programs. Finally it describes a case study for evaluation of protein–ligand docking.

   Key words Binding pocket, Cyscore, CurvatureSurface, Protein–ligand docking, Scoring function

1   Introduction

Protein–ligand docking is prediction of the complex structure formed by a ligand and a target protein with known 3D structures respectively. It has been widely applied to drug discovery and biological studies [1–3]. Modern docking methods, established on the historical "lock-and-key" and "induced-fit" theories, are generally constituted of a search algorithm and a scoring function. The search algorithm explores possible binding positions and orientations, and may account for the flexibility of ligand or protein during the searching, while the scoring function evaluates the binding free energy of conformations generated by the search algorithm. Because the searching and scoring processes are repeated thousands of times in order to find the most energy-favorable binding conformation, docking is computationally expensive. In the last few decades, tens of algorithms have been proposed to overcome docking problem [2, 4–9]. Nowerdays the state-of-the-art docking programs could achieve high accuracy [2, 10, 11], however, failures still appear in practice. One of the main reasons is due to the trade-off between computational speed and prediction accuracy: reducing the number of freedom and

Mohini Gore and Umesh B. Jagtap (eds.), *Computational Drug Discovery and Design*, Methods in Molecular Biology, vol. 1762, https://doi.org/10.1007/978-1-4939-7756-7_12, © Springer Science+Business Media, LLC, part of Springer Nature 2018

using simplified scoring functions may accelerate calculation at the expense of lower accuracy.

The accuracy of docking is often quantified by Root Mean Square Deviation (RMSD) between a docking predicted structure and an experimentally determined one. However, most experimentally determined structures are not available in practice. Alternatively, molecular 3D visualization system, such as Pymol, VMD [12], and Chimera [13], offers intuitive inspections of docking results. To confirm the prediction, interface shape complementarity, hydrophobicity, hydrogen bonding, and other relevant interactions are checked by visualization. Besides, using independent scoring functions is a shortcut for docking evaluation [9, 14]. In contrast to the scoring functions in docking programs, these independent functions are more accurate but time-consuming. They are comprised of more energy terms or employ sophisticated models to fit the experimentally determined binding affinities. A number of independent scoring functions have been proposed in recent years [15–20]. Benchmark assessments showed their power in binding affinity prediction and virtual screening [21].

Cyscore is an independent protein–ligand scoring function developed in our group [15]. It mainly focus on improving the prediction of hydrophobic free energy, which is dominant in most protein–ligand binding [22–25]. Conventionally, hydrophobic free energy is treated as surface tension, which is proportional to interfacial surface area for simplicity and efficiency. However, this model ignores the role of molecular shape and hinders the accurate prediction. Inspired by the thermodynamic research of Tolman [26] and the pioneer work of Nicholls et al. [27, 28], Cyscore takes curvature as the descriptor of shape and quantifies the hydrophobic free energy by a curvature dependent surface area model. Figure 1 illustrates the evaluation of docking by Cyscore on a 106 protein–ligand set, which was generated by a well-known docking software, DOCK6. The differences between predicted and experimentally determined binding structures are quantified by RMSD. The Cyscore of docking results versus RMSD illustrates the relationship between docking accuracy and Cyscore. The figure shows that the RMSD is lower than 2 Å when Cyscore is smaller than −3.5. It indicates that Cyscore is an indicator for evaluating protein–ligand docking.

2   Materials

The input of Cyscore includes a protein file in PDB format (*see* **Notes 1** and **2**) and a ligand file in SYBYL MOL2 format. The ligand file is obtained from the output of a docking program such as DOCK6. Hydrogen atoms are required for Cyscore calculation. Cyscore package includes Cyscore, CurvatureSurface, RotaBond, and AddH.

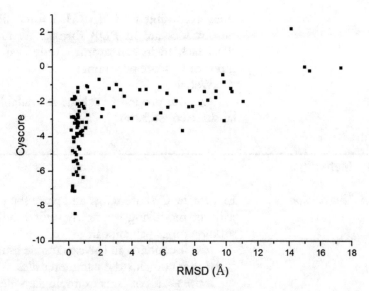

Fig. 1 Cyscore versus RMSD on a 106 protein–ligand docking set

2.1 Programs in the Cyscore Package

Cyscore is an empirical scoring function for protein–ligand binding affinity prediction. It is a combination of hydrophobic free energy, van der Waals interaction energy, hydrogen-bond energy, and the ligand's entropy (*see* **Note 3**). A curvature weighted surface area model was introduced in Cyscore to improve the prediction of hydrophobic free energy. Cyscore is an indicator of the shape complementarity of protein–ligand binding.

CurvatureSurface is used for generating molecular solvent accessible surface grid. It outputs a PDB format file with the grid data in the ATOM records. Their "temperature factor" in standard PDB format is replaced by curvature value at each grid point. The output PDB file can be visualized by molecular visualization software such as Pymol or RasMol. If the surface grid is colored by "B factor" or "temperature factor," the concave regions will be highlighted by warm colors while the other regions will be in cold colors. This tool helps to identify binding pockets and validate the protein–ligand shape complementarity.

RotaBond is used for counting rotatable bonds of ligands, which are defined as any single nonring bond, bounded to nonterminal heavy (i.e., nonhydrogen) atom. The number of rotatable bonds is correlated with the entropy loss upon protein–ligand binding process. It is based on the assumption that each rotor in the unbound state associates with a discrete number of low-energy conformations but 'freezes' into a single conformation upon binding [29–31]. Thus the number of rotatable bonds is proportional to a certain amount of conformational entropy. RotaBond outputs the number of rotatable bonds as well as the list of the atoms that form the bonds.

AddH is a tool for adding hydrogen atoms to a protein. It predicts the coordinates of hydrogen atoms by stereochemical rules according to CHARMM force field [32]. The input and output files are in PDB format. As most protein structures in PDB lack hydrogen atoms, AddH can be used to prepare the input of Cyscore program.

Website

Cyscore program Package is available at the site: http://clab. labshare.cn/software/.

3 Methods

3.1 Installation

Extract the Cyscore.tar.gz and place the folder anywhere in the disk without modifying the newly built subdirectories and files. Three subdirectories will appear:

bin: it contains all the executable binary files of this package.

dat: it contains the parameter files.

example: it contains example data files and the readme file.

Users are allowed to run the software in a different directory by specifying the program path in the command: (<program path>/bin/Cyscore). The program will find the parameter files automatically.

Please note, programs in Cyscore package need to be run on Linux system (*see* **Note 4**).

3.2 Cyscore Program

Usage:

```
Cyscore [input protein PDB file] [input ligand Mol2 file]
```

Cyscore predicts the binding free energy between the query protein and ligand. It requires protein and ligand containing hydrogen atoms. For a protein structures downloaded from Protein Data Bank (PDB), the hydrogen atoms are suggested adding by AddH in this package (*see* **Note 5**). As for ligand, the hydrogen atoms could be added by OpenBabel (http://openbabel.org/wiki/Main_Page), which is a well-established chemical software for searching and converting compounds. Cyscore was fitted on experimentally determined binding affinity data. The score has the dimension of kcal/mol. Therefore the lower score indicates the higher binding affinity.

Example:

Open the terminal and change the directory to the installed subdirectory of "example". Run:

```
$../bin/Cyscore 3nw9_protein.pdb 3nw9_ligand.mol2
```

Then the output is printed on the screen (Shown in Fig. 2). The first line below the title lists names of input files. The following line shows energies of hydrophobic term, van der Waals interaction

```
------------------------------------------------------
Cyscore:  Protein-Ligand Binding Affinity Predictor
          YC  2016 All Rights Reserved.
                    V 2.0.1
          Wed Jun  7 17:45:39 2017
------------------------------------------------------

Protein: 3nw9_protein.pdb    Ligand: 3nw9_ligand.mol2
Hydrophobic -2.3209 Vdw -3.8894 HBond -0.0093 Ent 0.2520
Cyscore= -5.9676
```

Fig. 2 The output of Cyscore prediction

term, hydrogen-bond term, and the ligand's entropy loss term. The first three terms are usually negative. Only if there are strong atomic clashes between the protein and ligand, van der Waals interaction term is positive. If the ligand is not docked on the protein, the first three terms is zero. Cyscore on the last line is the summation of above terms.

3.3 Curvature-Surface Program

Usage:

```
CurvatureSurface [input PDB file or Mol2 file] [output PDB file
for solvent accessible surface grid]
```

CurvatureSurface supports PDB or SYBYL MOL2 format input files. The output file can be visualized by molecular visualization software such as Pymol or RasMol. The detailed information of surface grid, can be browsed by a text editor, such as gedit or vim. Figure 3 illustrates the format of output file. The first line is the remark information such as the creating time and program name of the file. The following ATOM records indicate the index of grid points (2nd column), grid type name (3rd column), grid name (4th column), the index of molecular atoms which form the surface grid (5th column), three-dimensional coordinates (6–8th column), and the curvature data (10th column, highlight in red) of the grid points. The curvature data varies from 1 to 20. The curvature data larger than 10 implies that the grid point is at concave region.

Example:

Open the terminal and change the directory to the installed subdirectory of "example". Run:

```
$ ../bin/CurvatureSurface 3nw9_protein.pdb 3nw9_protein_grid.
pdb
```

The program will generate a new file named 3nw9_protein_-grid.pdb. It can be opened by Pymol, RasMol, or other molecular visualization software. Figure 4a and 4b demonstrate the visualization of grid by Pymol and RasMol respectively. The grid is colored by b-factor or temperature. The warm color region highlights concave surface which could be the binding pocket. The largest

```
REMARK The PDB FILE IS CREATED BY CurvatureSurface AT Tue May 30 17:50:02 2017
ATOM      1  HOH SAS     0      -2.264  22.783  37.175  1.00 |1.68|        H
ATOM      2  HOH SAS     0      -1.564  22.783  37.088  1.00 |1.81|        H
ATOM      3  HOH SAS     0      -2.048  23.449  37.088  1.00 |1.72|        H
ATOM      4  HOH SAS     0      -2.830  23.194  37.088  1.00 |1.61|        H
ATOM      5  HOH SAS     0      -2.830  22.372  37.088  1.00 |1.62|        H
ATOM      6  HOH SAS     0      -2.048  22.117  37.088  1.00 |1.74|        H
ATOM      7  HOH SAS     0      -0.907  22.783  36.831  1.00 |2.04|        H
ATOM      8  HOH SAS     0      -1.089  23.461  36.831  1.00 |2.00|        H
ATOM      9  HOH SAS     0      -1.586  23.958  36.831  1.00 |1.86|        H
ATOM     10  HOH SAS     0      -2.264  24.140  36.831  1.00 |1.74|        H
ATOM     11  HOH SAS     0      -2.942  23.958  36.831  1.00 |1.62|        H
ATOM     12  HOH SAS     0      -3.439  23.461  36.831  1.00 |1.58|        H
ATOM     13  HOH SAS     0      -3.621  22.783  36.831  1.00 |1.56|        H
ATOM     14  HOH SAS     0      -3.439  22.105  36.831  1.00 |1.59|        H
ATOM     15  HOH SAS     0      -2.942  21.608  36.831  1.00 |1.64|        H
ATOM     16  HOH SAS     0      -2.264  21.426  36.831  1.00 |1.76|        H
ATOM     17  HOH SAS     0      -1.586  21.608  36.831  1.00 |1.89|        H
ATOM     18  HOH SAS     0      -1.089  22.105  36.831  1.00 |2.03|        H
ATOM     19  HOH SAS     0      -0.333  22.783  36.421  1.00 |2.42|        H
ATOM     20  HOH SAS     0      -0.464  23.480  36.421  1.00 |2.38|        H
```

Fig. 3 The solvent accessible surface grid file

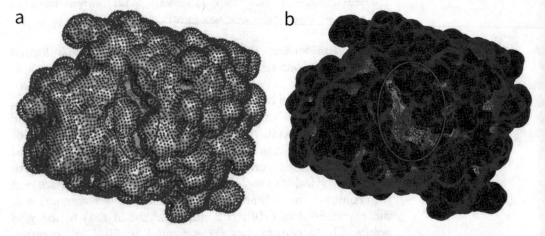

Fig. 4 The solvent accessible surface grid colored by surface curvature. (**a**) 3D visualization by Pymol. (**b**) 3D visualization by RasMol

warm color region in red circle is the active binding site of this protein (Catechol-O-methyltransferase (COMT)).

3.4 RotaBond Program

Usage:

```
RotaBond [input Mol2 file]
```

RotaBond outputs the number of rotatable bonds as well as the list of atoms that form the bonds (*see* **Note 6**).

Example:

Open the terminal and change the directory to the installed subdirectory of "example". Run:

```
--------------------------------------------------------
RotaBond: finding rotatable bonds of small compounds
                Version 1.1  2016
--------------------------------------------------------

    Bond 0 : C6  - C14
    Bond 1 : C15 - C16
    Bond 2 : C16 - N17
    Bond 3 : C18 - C20
    Bond 4 : C22 - C24
    Bond 5 : C1  - N10
    Rotatable Bond Number : 6
```

Fig. 5 The output of RotaBond

```
$ ../bin/RotaBond 3nw9_ligand.mol2
```

Then the output is printed on the screen (Shown in Fig. 5). The atom names forming rotatable bonds are listed in Bond records (Bond 0 to 5). The last line shows the total number of rotatable bonds.

3.5 AddH Program

Usage:

```
AddH [input protein PDB file] [output PDB file]
```

The output PDB file include all the atoms in the input file as well as added hydrogen atoms.

Example.

Open the terminal and change the directory to the installed subdirectory of "example". Run:

```
$ ../bin/AddH 3nw9.pdb 3nw9_protein_h.pdb
```

4 Case Studies

Molecular docking has been widely used in predicting protein–ligand binding conformation. It can provide information about the binding mode, critical residues, binding affinities, etc. which are very helpful to drug discovery and biological study. To evaluate quality of docking prediction, docking result is often visualized by 3D visualization software to inspect the interface complementarity manually. To aid the evaluation, protein–ligand scoring tools could be very helpful. Here we provide a real case for evaluating the docking result of a serine protease and dipeptide inhibitor by using Cyscore.

The protein and ligand structure file (PDB ID: 1BMA, which contains protein PDB file "1bma_protein.pdb" and ligand Mol2 file "1bma_ligand.mol2") were down loaded from PDBbind. We took DOCK6 to predict the docking structure. Following standard DOCK6 protocol, the best docking conformation was generated as 1bma_dock.mol2. Then we employed Cyscore tools, and first add hydrogen atoms to the protein PDB file using AddH as:

```
$ ../bin/AddH 1bma_protein.pdb 1bma_protein_h.pdb
```

Next, we submitted the protein and docking result to Cyscore as:

```
$ ../bin/Cyscore 1bma_protein_h.pdb 1bma_dock.mol2
```

The output showed that Cyscore was −1.7295. According to the above introduction, Cyscore larger than −3.5 implies that the docking result may not be reliable. Then we computed the solvent accessible surface grid to inspect the shape complementarity by:

```
$ ../bin/CurvatureSurface 1bma_protein.pdb 1bma_protein_grid.pdb
```

1bma_protein_grid.pdb and the docking result 1bma_dock.mol2 were visualized by Pymol. The coloring method for 1bma_protein_grid was chosen Color -> spectrum -> b-factor (Shown in Fig. 6). Thus we got the interface image. As shown in Fig. 7a, there were two regions in warm colors (Shown in the black circle), which indicated they are concave surface and good for ligand binding. The lower warm-colored region was partially occupied by a methyl group, while the upper one had no contact with the ligand. Both Cyscore and 3D visualization indicated the docking was unreliable. The true binding structure was shown in Fig. 7b. Obviously the real one is far from the docking structure. It shows highly binding affinity (Cyscore = −5.5216), and occupies both warm-colored regions.

5   Notes

1. If there are missing atoms in the input PDB file, will the programs work?

   Cyscore and CurvatureSurface will output results with warning information in this case. Users should pay attention to the warnings. If any of missing atom reported in the warnings locates at the binding area, it may have impacts on the prediction accuracy. AddH cannot work correctly in this case, because it needs heavy atom's coordinates to add hydrogen atoms.

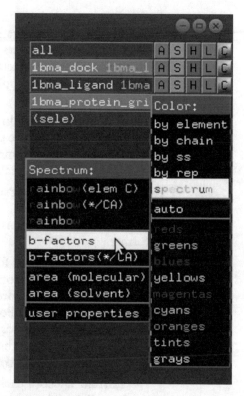

Fig. 6 Coloring methods in Pymol

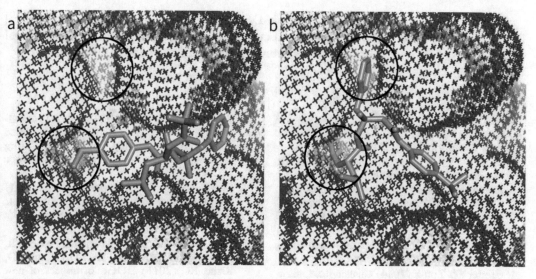

Fig. 7 The location of ligand on the surface grid of 1BMA. Ligand is shown in stick model. (**a**) the docking predicted ligand binding structure. (**b**) the experimentally determined ligand binding structure.

2. Why Cyscore has no term for charge-charge interaction between protein and ligand?

Charge–charge interaction may play a critical role in some of protein–ligand interaction. However, its net effect on binding affinity is very complicated and pH-dependent. Cyscore ignores this term.

3. How do the programs do with HETATM records in PDB file?

Programs in Cyscore package ignore the HETATM records in PDB file. If the head markers of "HETATM" are replaced by "ATOM," they will be taken into account.

4. Can I use other programs to add hydrogen atoms to the protein?

Yes. Cyscore supports any protein file in standard PDB format.

5. What is RotaBond used for?

RotaBond is used for estimating entropy loss of ligand in binding process in Cyscore. In other cases, it is used in lead-like compounds screening. For example, lead-like compounds follow some experience-based rules, such as the rule of three (RO3), which restricts the number of rotatable bonds.

6. Does Cyscore work on Windows system?

Current Cyscore package works on Linux. The Windows version will be released in future.

Acknowledgments

We gratefully thank Dr. Shuang Chen for the help with critical editing of the manuscript. The work was supported by the National Natural Science Foundation of China (#31401130 to Y.C).

References

1. Glaab E (2016) Building a virtual ligand screening pipeline using free software: a survey. Brief Bioinform 17(2):352–366

2. Sousa SF, Ribeiro AJ, Coimbra JT, Neves RP, Martins SA, Moorthy NS, Fernandes PA, Ramos MJ (2013) Protein-ligand docking in the new millennium--a retrospective of 10 years in the field. Curr Med Chem 20 (18):2296–2314

3. Blundell TL (1996) Structure-based drug design. Nature 384(6604 Suppl):23–26

4. Grinter SZ, Zou X (2014) Challenges, applications, and recent advances of protein-ligand docking in structure-based drug design. Molecules 19(7):10150–10176

5. Forli S, Huey R, Pique ME, Sanner MF, Goodsell DS, Olson AJ (2016) Computational protein-ligand docking and virtual drug screening with the AutoDock suite. Nat Protoc 11(5):905–919

6. Li H, Leung KS, Ballester PJ, Wong MH (2014) istar: a web platform for large-scale protein-ligand docking. PLoS One 9(1): e85678

7. Allen WJ, Balius TE, Mukherjee S, Brozell SR, Moustakas DT, Lang PT, Case DA, Kuntz ID, Rizzo RC (2015) DOCK 6: impact of new features and current docking performance. J Comput Chem 36(15):1132–1156

8. Trott O, Olson AJ (2010) AutoDock Vina: improving the speed and accuracy of docking

with a new scoring function, efficient optimization, and multithreading. J Comput Chem 31 (2):455–461

9. Wang C, Zhang Y (2017) Improving scoring-docking-screening powers of protein-ligand scoring functions using random forest. J Comput Chem 38(3):169–177

10. Danishuddin M, Khan AU (2015) Structure based virtual screening to discover putative drug candidates: necessary considerations and successful case studies. Methods 71:135–145

11. Li C, Wang Z, Cao Y, Wang L, Ji J, Chen Z, Deng T, Jiang T, Cheng G, Qin FX-F (2017) Screening for novel small-molecule inhibitors targeting the assembly of influenza virus polymerase complex by a bimolecular luminescence complementation-based reporter system. J Virol 91:e02282-16

12. Humphrey W, Dalke A, Schulten K (1996) VMD: visual molecular dynamics. J Mol Graph 14(1):33–38

13. Pettersen EF, Goddard TD, Huang CC, Couch GS, Greenblatt DM, Meng EC, Ferrin TE (2004) UCSF Chimera–a visualization system for exploratory research and analysis. J Comput Chem 25(13):1605–1612

14. Pencheva T, Soumana OS, Pajeva I, Miteva MA (2010) Post-docking virtual screening of diverse binding pockets: comparative study using DOCK, AMMOS, X-Score and FRED scoring functions. Eur J Med Chem 45 (6):2622–2628

15. Cao Y, Li L (2014) Improved protein-ligand binding affinity prediction by using a curvature-dependent surface-area model. Bioinformatics 30(12):1674–1680

16. Velec HF, Gohlke H, Klebe G (2005) Drug-Score(CSD)-knowledge-based scoring function derived from small molecule crystal data with superior recognition rate of near-native ligand poses and better affinity prediction. J Med Chem 48(20):6296–6303

17. Grinter SZ, Yan C, Huang SY, Jiang L, Zou X (2013) Automated large-scale file preparation, docking, and scoring: evaluation of ITScore and STScore using the 2012 community structure-activity resource benchmark. J Chem Inf Model 53(8):1905–1914

18. Wang R, Lai L, Wang S (2002) Further development and validation of empirical scoring functions for structure-based binding affinity prediction. J Comput Aided Mol Des 16 (1):11–26

19. Li H, Leung KS, Wong MH, Ballester PJ (2014) Substituting random forest for multiple linear regression improves binding affinity prediction of scoring functions: Cyscore as a case study. BMC Bioinformatics 15:291

20. Huang SY, Zou X (2010) Inclusion of solvation and entropy in the knowledge-based scoring function for protein-ligand interactions. J Chem Inf Model 50(2):262–273

21. Wang R, Lu Y, Fang X, Wang S (2004) An extensive test of 14 scoring functions using the PDBbind refined set of 800 protein-ligand complexes. J Chem Inf Comput Sci 44 (6):2114–2125

22. Jackson MB (2016) The hydrophobic effect in solute partitioning and interfacial tension. Sci Rep 6:19265

23. Ball P (2008) Water as an active constituent in cell biology. Chem Rev 108(1):74–108

24. Chandler D (2005) Interfaces and the driving force of hydrophobic assembly. Nature 437 (7059):640–647

25. Tanford C (1979) Interfacial free energy and the hydrophobic effect. Proc Natl Acad Sci U S A 76(9):4175–4176

26. Tolman RC (1949) The effect of droplet size on surface tension. J Chem Phys 3(17):5

27. Nicholls A, Sharp KA, Honig B (1991) Protein folding and association: insights from the interfacial and thermodynamic properties of hydrocarbons. Proteins 11(4):281–296

28. Sharp KA, Nicholls A, Fine RF, Honig B (1991) Reconciling the magnitude of the microscopic and macroscopic hydrophobic effects. Science 252(5002):106–109

29. Bohm HJ (1994) The development of a simple empirical scoring function to estimate the binding constant for a protein-ligand complex of known three-dimensional structure. J Comput Aided Mol Des 8(3):243–256

30. Friesner RA, Banks JL, Murphy RB, Halgren TA, Klicic JJ, Mainz DT, Repasky MP, Knoll EH, Shelley M, Perry JK, Shaw DE, Francis P, Shenkin PS (2004) Glide: a new approach for rapid, accurate docking and scoring. 1. Method and assessment of docking accuracy. J Med Chem 47(7):1739–1749

31. Salaniwal S, Manas ES, Alvarez JC, Unwalla RJ (2007) Critical evaluation of methods to incorporate entropy loss upon binding in high-throughput docking. Proteins 66(2):422–435

32. Vanommeslaeghe K, Hatcher E, Acharya C, Kundu S, Zhong S, Shim J, Darian E, Guvench O, Lopes P, Vorobyov I, Mackerell AD Jr (2010) CHARMM general force field: a force field for drug-like molecules compatible with the CHARMM all-atom additive biological force fields. J Comput Chem 31 (4):671–690

Chapter 13

Molecular Dynamics Simulations of Protein–Drug Complexes: A Computational Protocol for Investigating the Interactions of Small-Molecule Therapeutics with Biological Targets and Biosensors

Jodi A. Hadden and Juan R. Perilla

Abstract

MD simulations provide a powerful tool for the investigation of protein–drug complexes. The following chapter uses the aryl acylamidase–acetaminophen system as an example to describe a general protocol for preparing and running simulations of protein–drug complexes, complete with a step-by-step tutorial. The described approach is broadly applicable toward the study of drug interactions in the context of both biological targets and biosensing enzymes.

Key words Drug development, Drug target, Enzyme biosensors, Force field parameterization, Molecular dynamics simulation, Protein–drug complex

1 Introduction

Molecular dynamics (MD) simulations use principles of classical mechanics to predict the motion of particle-based systems. When applied to the study of biomolecules, particles represent atoms or groups of atoms. Because of their unique ability to provide a high-resolution view of biomolecular behavior, MD simulations are often referred to as the computational microscope [1]. Owing to recent advances in simulation methodology and supercomputing technology, the computational microscope is positioned to play a key role in furthering the field of biomedicine [2].

Small-molecule drugs are a critical aspect of the modern medical approach to managing public health. Drugs are commonly employed as therapeutic interventions to treat pathogenic infection, regulate biological processes that contribute to disease, and provide pain relief, thereby greatly enhancing quality of life. The development of new drug compounds represents a major area of scientific research.

Mohlni Gore and Umesh B. Jagtap (eds.), *Computational Drug Discovery and Design*, Methods in Molecular Biology, vol. 1762, https://doi.org/10.1007/978-1-4939-7756-7_13, © Springer Science+Business Media, LLC, part of Springer Nature 2018

On the other hand, the wide availability and public acceptance of drugs also leads to their misuse. Drug overdose in patients, as well as accumulation of drug compounds in the environment [3], represent a further challenge to human health. The need for methods that allow rapid testing of drug presence and concentration in a sample drives the development of biosensors, which utilize a biological element, such as an enzyme, to facilitate the detection of an analyte [4].

MD simulations provide a powerful tool for the investigation of drug compounds in the context of both biological targets and biosensing enzymes. When performed at the all-atom level of detail, MD simulations can characterize the dynamical interactions of drugs with their protein receptors and capture the subtle structural changes they induce, even in large biomolecular assemblies [5]. The following chapter presents a computational protocol for the study of protein–drug complexes with MD simulations based on an example project and tutorial. The described approach is broadly applicable toward elucidating mechanisms of drug action against biological targets, designing more effective drugs compounds, and engineering improved enzymes for biosensing and bioremediation.

2   Example Project: Aryl Acylamidase–Acetaminophen

Acetaminophen (N-acetyl-p-aminophenol, Fig. 1) is a widely available analgesic drug commonly used to relieve pain and reduce fever. Although it is generally regarded as the safest over the counter analgesic when taken as directed [6, 7], i.e., in therapeutic doses, the misuse of acetaminophen carries serious health risk. Acetaminophen is metabolized by the liver, and high concentration of the drug leads to excessive accumulation of its metabolites, which can cause severe, even fatal liver damage [7]. Acetaminophen toxicity is the leading cause of acute liver failure in the USA [8]. Overdose is often unintentional, the result of misuse of formulations of other drugs that contain acetaminophen as an additive [6]. Successful

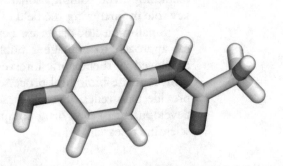

Fig. 1 Chemical structure of the drug acetaminophen

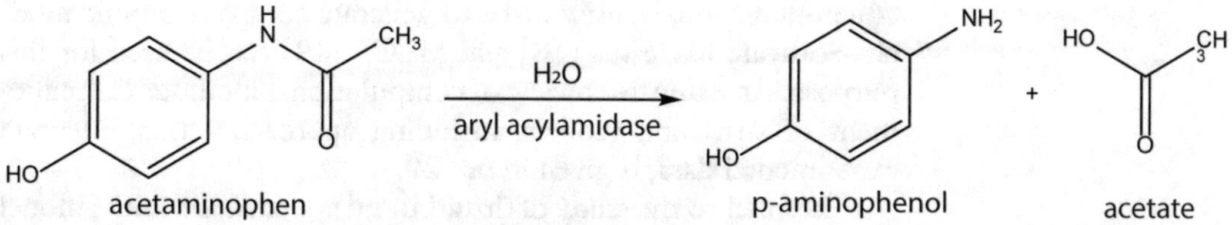

Fig. 2 Schematic of the chemical reaction catalyzed by aryl acylamidase. The enzyme cleaves the amide bond of acetaminophen to yield p-aminophenol and acetate

treatment of hepatotoxicity relies on timely diagnosis via laboratory testing. Diagnostic assays and biosensors designed to quantify the concentration of acetaminophen in a biological sample are often based on aryl acylamidase [9], which cleaves the amide bond of acetaminophen to yield p-aminophenol and acetate (Fig. 2). The concentration of acetaminophen can be inferred from changes in absorbance following reaction of the product p-aminophenol with a color-forming compound [10, 11], or amperometrically following electrochemical oxidation of p-aminophenol [12].

A recent crystallographic structure characterized the binding interaction of a bacterial aryl acylamidase with acetaminophen at atomic detail, revealing key structural features that underlie its enzymatic activity [13]. MD simulations of the crystallographic complex can be used to probe the structure–function relationship of aryl acylamidase, which represents a key component in diagnostic assays and biosensors used to detect acetaminophen toxicity [9]. The following section uses the aryl acylamidase–acetaminophen system as an example to describe a general protocol for preparing and running simulations of protein–drug complexes. Step-by-step instructions are provided for the example project based on using the psfgen plugin from VMD [14] for system setup and the NAMD [15] software for MD simulation.

3 Computational Protocol

3.1 Preparing a Robust Structural Model of the Protein–Drug Complex

The critical prerequisite for any computational study is a robust initial model. In the case of the example project for this chapter, a crystallographic structure is available from the RCSB Protein Data Bank (https://www.rcsb.org) (PDB ID: 4YJI) [13]. Importantly, the structure describes the system at all-atom detail and contains no missing regions (*see* **Note 1**). Experimental structures that are incomplete require computational modeling to fill in missing structural features. Software like Modeller [16] and Rosetta [17] include routines to perform de novo folding of protein loops and terminal domains, regions that are often difficult to resolve experimentally due to their flexible nature. Models based on cryo-electron microscopy or tomography data may require flexible fitting of structural components into density maps to generate complete atomic models. Software like Situs [18] and MDFF [19] can be used for this purpose. An extensive review of computational methods for refinement of structural models, including approaches that integrate experimental data, is given in ref. 20.

Essential to the study of drug-bound systems, the initial model must capture the structural interaction between the target protein and drug molecule (*see* **Note 2**). Ideally, a crystallographic structure will be available for their complex. In the case of the example project for this chapter, the experimental structure already contains atomic coordinates that describe the drug binding mode. When the binding mode is unknown, it may be possible to produce a suitable structural model based on molecular docking. Software like Auto-Dock Vina [21] can be used toward this end; however, experimental validation is recommended to support the predicted binding mode. A review of current molecular docking methodology and comparison of available docking programs is given in ref. 22.

Even when the initial model is based soundly on experimental data, it is important to perform a series of standard structural assessments to verify the model's integrity and to check for subtle issues that may cause serious problems during the simulation phase of the project. One critical test is a check for structural clashes or close contacts within the model. Such deficiencies can exist even in high-resolution crystallographic structures, and if not corrected, may cause the model to distort or blow apart during simulation. Close contacts may also manifest as ring moieties punctured by neighboring functional groups, or valence angles that are extremely small. At minimum, these structural issues may introduce instabilities during simulation, requiring increased equilibration time, so taking care to address them during the model preparation phase of the project is good practice (*see* **Note 3**). In the case of the example project for this chapter, no structural clashes or close contacts within 1 Å are found in the crystallographic structure.

Another structural discrepancy to test for is the presence of *cis* peptides in the protein. Typically, the peptide bonds of the protein backbone adopt a *trans* orientation (Fig. 3a); however, *cis*

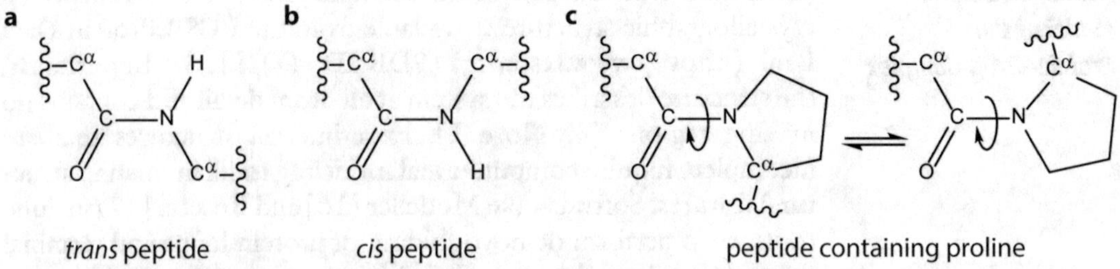

trans peptide   cis peptide   peptide containing proline

Fig. 3 (a) *Trans* orientations of peptide bonds are most common. (b) *Cis* orientations of peptide bonds may be encountered occasionally. (c) Peptides containing proline can readily adopt *trans* or *cis* orientations

orientations are occasionally encountered in experimental structures (Fig. 3b). Sometimes, the *cis* peptide is present in the native form of the molecule and may be biologically important, particularly if the peptide contains proline (Fig. 3c). In other cases, *cis* peptides are introduced during automated refinement of experimental structures, or during computational modeling. In the case of the example project for this chapter, the crystallographic structure contains two *cis* peptides: one between Gly162 and Ser163 and another between Arg212 and Pro213. The former involves a member of the aryl acylamidase's catalytic triad, Lys84-*cis*Ser163-Ser187, and plays a key role in its hydrolysis mechanism [13]. The latter contains a proline, which exhibits similar structural energetics for *trans* and *cis* orientations, and is, thus, considered realistic for the model. In the event that an artifactual *cis* peptide is found, it can be adjusted to the *trans* orientation using a program like cispeptide, available in VMD (*see* **Note 4**).

3.2 Immersing the Protein–Drug Complex in a Realistic Environment

Once the initial structural model has been generated and verified, its surrounding environment must be appropriately accounted for. Careful mimicking of realistic solvent conditions during simulation is key to producing results that are comparable to experiment or have predictive power toward biological questions (*see* **Note 5**).

The first environmental factor to address is pH. For classical simulation methodology, performing a simulation at a given pH means constructing the initial model to represent the likely protonation state at that pH (*see* **Note 6**). This can be achieved by calculating local pKa values and assigning hydrogen atom positions accordingly. Programs like PDB2PQR [23], which performs pKa calculations using PROPKA [24], can be employed to place hydrogen atoms, accounting for both protein protonation states and the likely neutral states of histidine residues, which can carry a hydrogen on either their delta or epsilon nitrogen. The accurate assignment of hydrogen atoms to the system may be critical for reproducing hydrogen bond networks within the higher-order protein structure, as well as between the protein and drug molecule. Further, accounting for differences in these networks as a function of pH is critical to simulation accuracy.

For the example system in this chapter, the protein–drug complex is studied at pH 7. As the project aims to investigate the interaction of an aryl acylamidase with the drug acetaminophen within a biological sample, such as a patient's blood, physiological pH of 7 is appropriate. However, as aryl acylamidases are known experimentally to exhibit optimum enzymatic activity at pH 10 or above [25] and some biosensing approaches recommend increasing system pH to enhance hydrolysis [9], an interesting follow-up study could investigate the system at pH 10 to shed light on the structural origin of increased activity at high pH.

The second environmental factor to address is solvent. Water represents the bulk solvent media in most samples of interest, particularly those of biological origin. Classical simulation methodology can represent solvent either explicitly or implicitly. Explicit solvent uses many copies of discrete water molecules, empirically parameterized to reproduce experimental properties of the pure liquid. Although numerous water models are available, the most widely used is TIP3P [26], which reasonably balances the accurate reproduction of bulk solvent behavior with computational expense. Alternatively, implicit solvent uses a mathematical function to produce a continuum around the solute with the dielectric and hydrophobic properties of water [27]. Implicit solvent is generally more computationally efficient than explicit solvent; however, it is often not the best approach for the study of protein–drug systems. Many drugs interact with their protein receptors through water-mediated hydrogen bonds, an important aspect of binding that only explicit solvent can capture (*see* **Note 7**). Notably, the crystallographic structure for the example system in this chapter exhibits two water-mediated hydrogen bonds, which bridge drug binding with residues Tyr136 and Thr330. To ensure that these and other highly conserved water interactions are in place going into the simulation phase of the project, all crystallographically resolved water molecules should be retained in the initial model (*see* **Note 8**).

With respect to bulk solvent, MD setup packages offer standard routines to immerse the biomolecular system of interest in a box of explicit water molecules, but the user must take care to abide by the minimum image convention and ensure that the box dimensions are large enough to accommodate the system following equilibration of water density. A distance of at least 15 Å between the protein–drug complex and the box edges is recommended (*see* **Note 9**). If the protein–drug complex is likely to tumble during the planned timescale of the simulation, the generated water box should be cubic (*see* **Note 10**).

The third environmental factor to address is salt concentration. Studies intending to investigate systems within a biological context, i.e., interactions of drugs with their receptors within the human body, should use physiological salt concentration of 150 mM NaCl. Studies seeking to investigate systems with the context of an experimental setup, mimicking the conditions of a drug assay or biosensing reaction, should employ a salt concentration that reflects that setup (*see* **Note 11**). For the example system in this chapter, which aims to investigate the interaction of an aryl acylamidase with the drug acetaminophen within a biological sample, such as a patient's blood, physiological salt concentration is used.

MD setup packages offer standard routines to introduce a desired salt concentration, either via a mathematical constant in implicit solvent, or by substituting water molecules for salt ions in explicit solvent. To reduce the equilibration time required for explicit solvent during the simulation phase of the project, a superior approach for introducing ions is to first use a program like CIonize, available in VMD, to place ions around the protein–drug system of interest prior to immersion in a water box. CIonize places ions according to local electrostatic potential of the system, eliminating the additional equilibration time needed to allow randomly placed ions to localize within these energetically favorable regions (*see* **Note 12**). Following placement of ions proximal to the protein–drug system and immersion in explicit water, bulk ions can be added at the desired salt concentration, taking into account the numbers of ions already placed and ensuring the final system charge is neutral (*see* **Note 13**).

3.3 Parameterizing the Protein–Drug System for MD Simulation

Once the initial structural model has been prepared and immersed in a realistic solvent environment, parameterization of the system must be addressed. Biomolecular force fields for describing the protein component of the system are readily available, given that the protein does not contain nonstandard residues. Commonly employed protein force fields include those from the AMBER (http://ambermd.org) and CHARMM (http://mackerell.umaryland.edu/charmm_ff.shtml) families. For the example system in this chapter, CHARMM36 [28, 29] is used (*see* **Note 14**).

Obtaining parameters to describe the drug component of the system is less straightforward. A typical approach is to employ a generalized force field, such as the Generalized AMBER Force Field (GAFF) [30] or the CHARMM General Force Field (CGenFF) [31], which attempts to provide parameter coverage for the numerous chemical substructures commonly encountered in small molecules. Unfortunately, due to the complex structural nature of many drug compounds, generalized force fields do not always contain parameters that reasonably describe all parts of the molecule. Any missing parameters must be derived ab initio, according to the standard protocol of the generalized force field they will be combined with (*see* **Note 15**).

For the example system in this chapter, CGenFF is employed to describe the drug molecule. An online tool is available through ParamChem (https://cgen.paramchem.org) that performs automated atom typing and assignment of parameters and charges available in CGenFF based on analogy of the molecule's structure to the ensemble of substructures covered by the force field [32, 33]. The tool works best when supplied with a MOL2 file, which contains information on connectivity and bond order; the Schrödinger Maestro program [34] is recommended for generating a correctly formatted MOL2.

Importantly, the identification of parameters for the molecule by ParamChem does not necessarily guarantee the suitability of those parameters to accurately reproduce the molecule's dynamical behavior. A penalty score is provided along with each identified parameter to indicate a level of confidence in how well the parameter may be expected to perform. Penalties lower than 10 indicate the parameter analogy is fair; penalties between 10 and 50 mean some basic validation of the parameter within the given molecular context is recommended; penalties higher than 50 indicate poor analogy and mandate extensive validation and/or optimization. Validation of force field parameters against experimental data, such as that from nuclear magnetic resonance or infrared spectroscopy can confirm their ability to accurately describe the drug molecule in question. In the event that parameters with high penalty scores are found unsuitable, they can be optimized using tools such as ffTK [35], which simplifies the workflow required to fit parameters to reproduce quantum mechanical descriptions of small molecules (*see* **Note 16**). For the example system in this chapter, the parameters generated by ParamChem to describe acetaminophen have insignificant penalty scores and may be expected to accurately reproduce the molecule's dynamical behavior.

4   Project Tutorial

Step 1. Download PDB file of aryl acylamidase–acetaminophen complex.

– Visit the RCSB Protein Data Bank (https://www.rcsb.org) and search for PDB ID: 4YJI.

– From the *Download Files* menu, select *PDB Format* and save the file to your working directory (Fig. 4).

Step 2. Load PDB file in VMD and visualize the structure.

– Launch VMD and load the PDB file by clicking *File→New Molecule...* in the *VMD Main* window and selecting 4yji.pdb in the *Molecule File Browser* (Fig. 5).

– Open the *Graphical Representations* window by clicking *Graphics→Representations...* in the *VMD Main* window.

– Create a representation of the protein by entering "protein" in the *Selected Atoms* field and choosing *NewCartoon* from the *Drawing Method* menu.

– Create a representation of the drug molecule by entering "resname TYL" in the *Selected Atoms* field and choosing *Licorice* from the *Drawing Method* menu.

– Create a representation of the crystallographic water molecules by entering "water" in the *Selected Atoms* field and choosing *Licorice* from the *Drawing Method* menu.

– Try creating representations for other structural features of interest, such as the catalytic triad ("resid 84 163 187") or

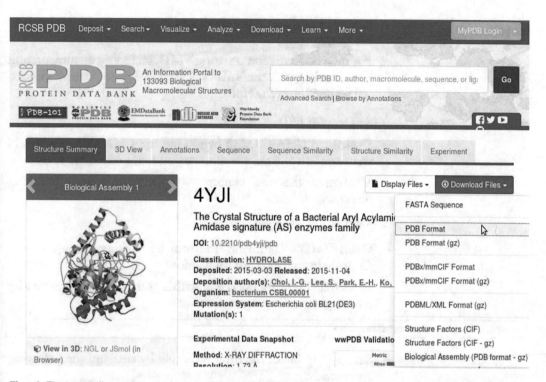

Fig. 4 The crystallographic structure of the aryl acylamidase–acetaminophen complex is available for download through the Protein Data Bank (PDB ID: 4YJI)

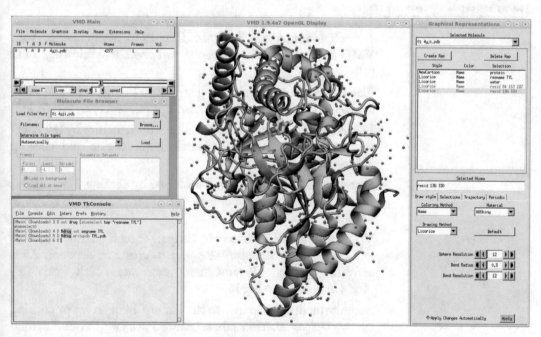

Fig. 5 VMD provides a graphical user interface for biomolecular visualization, as well as a command line tool equipped with numerous functions for MD simulation setup and analysis

residues that form water-mediated hydrogen bonds to the drug molecule ("resid 136 330").

- For more information on using VMD, including documentation and tutorials, visit the VMD software webpage (http://www.ks.uiuc.edu/Research/vmd).

Step 3. Obtain force field files.

- Download CHARMM36 by visiting the CHARMM force field webpage (http://mackerell.umaryland.edu/charmm_ff.shtml).

- Unarchive the file contents (toppar) into your working directory.

Step 4. Obtain drug parameters.

- Open VMD's command line tool by clicking *Extensions→Tk Console* in the *VMD Main* window.

- Ensure that you are operating within your working directory by entering the following command:

```
cd <path to your working directory>
```

- Save a PDB file of the drug molecule by entering the following commands:

```
set drug [atomselect top "resname TYL"] ; # Select drug molecule
$drug set segname TYL ; # Assign segname for psfgen
$drug writepdb TYL.pdb ; # Write segment PDB
```

- Launch Maestro and load the drug PDB file generated with VMD by clicking *File→Import Structures...* and selecting TYL.pdb (Fig. 6).

- Flag double bonds in the drug structure by right clicking them and selecting *Increase Bond Order*. For reference, *see* Fig. 2, left.

- Fill remaining open valencies in the drug structure by left clicking and dragging a box around the molecule and clicking *Edit→Add Hydrogens*.

- Save a MOL2 file of the drug molecule by clicking *File→Export Structures....* Enter the *File name* as "TYL" select *Files of type* as MOL2 (*.mol2).

- Visit the ParamChem server (https://cgenff.paramchem.org) and click on *My Account→Register* to create an account. After activating your ParamChem account, click on *My Account→Login* to log in.

- Submit the drug structure to the ParamChem server by clicking on the *Upload Molecule* tab, selecting *Filename* TYL.mol2, then clicking the *Upload File* button.

- Save the TYL.str file provided under *Output* to your working directory.

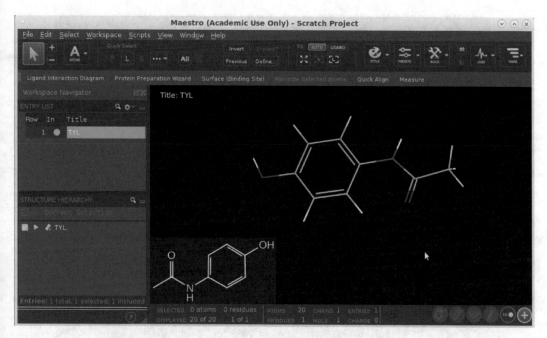

Fig. 6 Maestro is recommended for generating a correctly formatted MOL2 file

- Inspect the parameters in TYL.str, and note that their penalty scores are insignificant.

Step 5. Account for pH of the model.

- Visit the PDB2PQR server (http://nbcr-222.ucsd.edu/ pdb2pqr_2.1.1) and choose the option to *upload a PDB file*, selecting 4yji.pdb from your working directory (Fig. 7).

- Choose CHARMM for the *forcefield* and *output naming scheme* options.

- Also select options to *Ensure that new atoms are not rebuilt too close to existing atoms* and *Optimize the hydrogen bonding network.*

- Under *pKa options*, enter pH 7 and choose the option to *Use PROPKA to assign protonation states at the provided pH.*

- Click the *Submit* button to continue.

- Once the status of the PDB2PQR job updates to complete, download the 4yji.pqr file and save it to your working directory as 4yji_pH7.pqr.

Step 6. Generate PSF/PDB files for the model.

- Return to VMD's command line and run psfgen to generate PSF/PDB files for the model by entering the following commands:

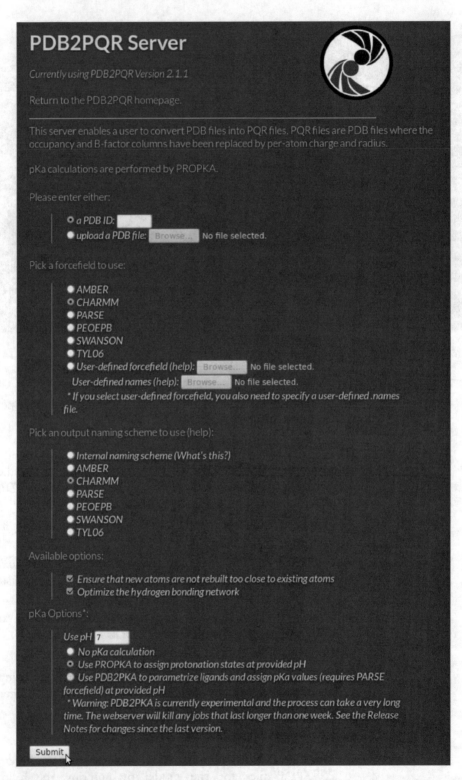

Fig. 7 PDB2PQR assigns hydrogen atoms and protonation states to the model for a given pH based on pKa calculations with PROPKA

```
package require psfgen ; # Load the psfgen plugin


topology toppar/top_all36_prot.rtf ; # Load CHARMM36
topology toppar/top_all36_cgenff.rtf ; # Load CGenFF
topology TYL.str ; # Load drug parameters
topology toppar/toppar_water_ions.str ; # Load TIP3P/ions


pdbalias residue P3M TIP3 ; # Interpret water as TIP3P


mol new TYL.mol2 type mol2 waitfor all ; # Load MOL2
set drug [atomselect top "resname TYL"] ; # Select drug molecule
$drug set segname TYL ; # Assign segname for psfgen
$drug writepdb TYL.pdb ; # Write segment PDB


mol new 4yji_pH7.pqr type pqr waitfor all ; # Load PQR


### PROTEIN
set protein [atomselect top "protein"] ; # Select protein
$protein set segname AAA ; # Assign segname for psfgen
$protein writepdb AAA.pdb ; # Write segment PDB


segment AAA { ; # Build protein segment
        pdb AAA.pdb ; # From segment PDB
        first NTER ; # Patch with Zwitterionic N-terminus
        last CTER } ; # Patch with Zwitterionic C-terminus
regenerate angles dihedrals ; # Critical after patching
coordpdb AAA.pdb ; # Assign coordinates from segment PDB


### DRUG
segment TYL { ; # Build drug segment
        pdb TYL.pdb } ; # From segment PDB
coordpdb TYL.pdb ; # Assign coordinates from segment PDB


### CRYSTALLOGRAPHIC WATER
set water [atomselect top "resname P3M"] ; # Select water
$water set segname W0 ; # Assign segname for psfgen
$water writepdb W0.pdb ; # Write segment PDB


segment W0 { ; # Build water
        pdb W0.pdb } ; # From segment PDB
coordpdb W0.pdb ; # Assign coordinates from segment PDB


writepsf AAA_TYL_pH7.psf ; # Output PSF
writepdb AAA_TYL_pH7.pdb ; # Output PDB
```

Step 7. Perform structural checks for the model.

– Return to VMD's command line and load the PSF/PDB files by entering the following command:

```
mol new AAA_TYL_pH7.psf type psf waitfor all ;# Load PSF
mol addfile AAA_TYL_pH7.pdb type pdb waitfor all ; # Load PDB
```

- Check for close structural contacts and/or clashes in the model by entering the following commands:

```
set complex [atomselect top "protein or resname TYL"] ; # Select atoms in the complex
set clashes [measure contacts 1 $complex] ; # Find atoms within 1 Angstroms of each other
foreach i [lindex $clashes 0] j [lindex $clashes 1] { ; # Report indices of clashing atoms
puts "Atom $i clashes with atom $j" } ; # Indices can be used to visualize clashing atoms
```

- Note that no close contacts are identified for this system.
- Check for *cis* peptides by entering the following commands:

```
package require cispeptide ; # Load cispeptide plugin
cispeptide check -mol top ; # Run cis peptide check
```

- Note that two *cis* peptides are reported for this system, one that is known to be biologically important and one that contains proline and is likely not an artifact.

Step 8. Account for local salt ions.

- Run CIonize to place Na+ and Cl– ions around the model by entering the following commands:

```
package require cionize ; # Load cionize package
namespace import ::cionize::*
# Run with a suffcient number of ions to saturate the model
# This example estimates 3x magnitude of system net charge
set charge [expr {round([vecsum [[atomselect top "all"] get charge]])}] ; # System net charge
set number [expr {abs($charge*3)}] ; # 3x magnitude of system net charge
cionize -mol top -np 1 -mg -ions "{SOD $number 1} {CLA $number -1}"; # Run CIonize
```

- Load the PDB files generated by CIonize by entering the following commands:

```
mol new cionize-ions_1-SOD.pdb type pdb waitfor all ; # Load Na+ PDB
mol new cionize-ions_1-CLA.pdb type pdb waitfor all ; # Load Cl- PDB
```

- Open the *Graphical Representations* window by clicking *Graphics→Representations...* in the *VMD Main* window.
- Create a clear representation of the ions in each PDB file by choosing *VDW* from the *Drawing Method* menu.
- Note that CIonize was run with enough ions to saturate the model, and unneeded ions were placed far away from it, along the edges of a box enclosure (Fig. 8).
- Run psfgen to generate new PSF/PDB files that include local ions by entering the following commands:

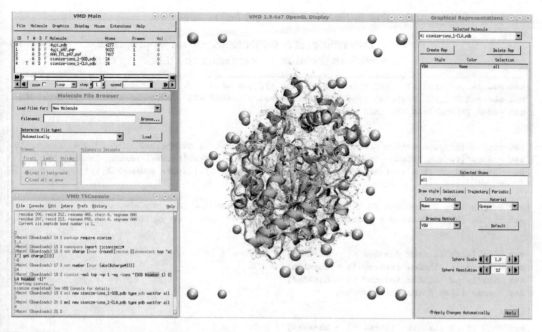

Fig. 8 Clonize places ions around the model according to local electrostatic potential; unneeded ions are placed far away from the model

```
resetpsf ; # Reset psfgen
readpsf AAA_TYL_pH7.psf ; # Read PSF
coordpdb AAA_TYL_pH7.pdb ; # Read PDB


segment SOD { ; # Build Na+ segment
        pdb cionize-ions_1-SOD.pdb } ; # From Cionize PDB
coordpdb cionize-ions_1-SOD.pdb ; # Assign coordinates from PDB


segment CLA { ; # Build Cl- segment
        pdb cionize-ions_1-CLA.pdb } ; # From Cionize PDB
coordpdb cionize-ions_1-CLA.pdb ; # Assign coordinates from PDB


writepsf AAA_TYL_pH7_cionize.psf ; # Output PSF
writepdb AAA_TYL_pH7_cionize.pdb ; # Output PDB


mol new AAA_TYL_pH7_cionize.psf type psf waitfor all; # Load PSF
mol addfile AAA_TYL_pH7_cionize.pdb type pdb waitfor all ; # Load PDB


# Delete ions not within 20 Angstroms of the model based on indices
set bad [atomselect top "(all not within 20 of protein)"]
foreach segid [$bad get segid] resid [$bad get resid] {
delatom $segid $resid }


writepsf AAA_TYL_pH7_ions.psf ; # Output PSF
writepdb AAA_TYL_pH7_ions.pdb ; # Output PDB
```

Step 9. Establish the system box.

– Determine the dimensions of an appropriate cubic box to enclose the model by entering the following commands:

```
mol new AAA_TYL_pH7_ions.psf type psf waitfor all ; # Load PSF
mol new AAA_TYL_pH7_ions.pdb type pdb waitfor all ; # Load PDB
set model [atomselect top "all"] ; # Select model


set center [measure center $model] ; # Measure model center, dimensions, and longest box vector
set dimens [vecsub [lindex [measure minmax $model] 1] [lindex [measure minmax $model] 0]]
set maxvec [expr {max([lindex $dimens 0],[lindex $dimens 1],[lindex $dimens 2])}]


set boxpad 15 ; # At least 15 Angstroms between model and box edge recommended
set boxlen [expr ($maxvec + 2*$boxpad)/2] ; # Length of cubic box vector


set minx [expr [lindex $center 0] - $boxlen] ; # Box min
set miny [expr [lindex $center 1] - $boxlen]
set minz [expr [lindex $center 2] - $boxlen]
set boxmin [list $minx $miny $minz]


set maxx [expr [lindex $center 0] + $boxlen] ; # Box max
set maxy [expr [lindex $center 1] + $boxlen]
set maxz [expr [lindex $center 2] + $boxlen]
set boxmax [list $maxx $maxy $maxz]
```

Step 10. Immerse the model in solvent.

– Generate a cubic water box with the dimensions determined above by entering the following commands:

```
package require solvate ; # Load the solvate plugin
# Run solvate with command as a single line:
solvate AAA_TYL_pH7_ions.psf AAA_TYL_pH7_ions.pdb -minmax [list $boxmin $boxmax] -o
AAA_TYL_pH7_ions_solvent -s W
```

Step 11. Account for salt concentration.

– Neutralize the system and add salt concentration of 150 mM by entering the following commands:

```
package require autoionize ; # Load the autoionize plugin
# Run autoionize with command as a single line:
autoionize -psf AAA_TYL_pH7_ions_solvent.psf -pdb AAA_TYL_pH7_ions_solvent.pdb -cation SOD -
anion CLA -sc 0.150 -o AAA_TYL_pH7_ions_solvent_sc150mM -seg I1
```

– Load the PSF/PDB files for the final model for visualization by entering the following commands:

```
mol new AAA_TYL_pH7_ions_solvent_sc150mM.psf type psf waitfor all ; # Load PSF
mol addfile AAA_TYL_pH7_ions_solvent_sc150mM.pdb type pdb waitfor all ; # Load PDB
```

– The setup phase of the project is now complete. The final model of the protein–drug complex at pH 7, including crystallographic

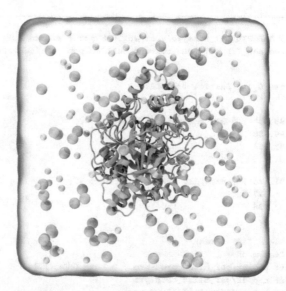

Fig. 9 The final model of the aryl acylamidase–acetaminophen complex within a native solvent environment

water molecules, local ions, solvent, and salt concentration of 150 mM NaCl should resemble Fig. 9.

Step 12. Obtain system box information.

- NAMD requires the dimensions of the initial system box as input. Additionally, the user can specify a box center as the origin for molecule wrapping. Obtain the box dimensions and center of the protein–drug complex by entering the following commands:

```
set all [atomselect top "all"] ; # Select system and measure box dimensions
set dimens [vecsub [lindex [measure minmax $all] 1] [lindex [measure minmax $all] 0]]
set complex [atomselect top "protein or resname TYL"] ; # Select complex and measure center
set center [measure center $complex]
```

- Note that the x-, y-, and z-values of the box dimensions and wrapping center are entered as NAMD inputs in the following section.

Step 13. Minimize potential energy of the system.

- Open a terminal and navigate to your working directory. Make sure that the location of the NAMD executable is contained within your $PATH variable.
- Save the NAMD configuration script given below to your working directory as min.conf.

```
# Input
structure AAA_TYL_pH7_ions_solvent_sc150mM.psf ; # Load PSF
coordinates AAA_TYL_pH7_ions_solvent_sc150mM.pdb ; # Load PDB


temperature 0 ; # Initial temperature


set bx  99.958 ; # Box dimensions (see Step 12)
set by  99.958
set bz  99.958


set cx  31.121 ; # Wrapping center (see Step 12)
set cy   1.777
set cz  -2.136


# Force Field Information
paraTypeCharmm on ; # Use CHARMM
parameters toppar/par_all36_prot.prm ; # Load CHARMM36
parameters toppar/par_all36_carb.prm
parameters toppar/par_all36_lipid.prm
parameters toppar/par_all36_cgenff.prm ; # Load CGenFF
parameters toppar/toppar_water_ions.str ; # Load TIP3P/ions
parameters TYL.str ; # Load drug parameters
exclude scaled1-4 ; # Exclude 1-2s and 1-3s, scale 1-4s
1-4scaling 1.0 ; # 1-4 scaling factor
cutoff 12.0 ; # Cut-off radius for non-bonded interactions
switching on ; # Scale smoothly to zero
switchdist 10.0 ; # Scale smoothly from here to cut-off
pairlistdist 14.0 ; # Pairlist search radius


# Periodic Boundary Conditions
cellBasisVector1 $bx 0    0    ; # Box dimensions
cellBasisVector2 0    $by 0
cellBasisVector3 0    0    $bz
cellOrigin $cx $cy $cz ; # Wrapping center
wrapAll on ; # Wrap coordinates to wrapping center
PME yes ; # PME long-range electrostatics
PMEGridSpacing 1.0 ; # Grid spacing for PME


# Output
outputName min ; # Output file name prefix
binaryOutput yes ; # Output binary files
restartfreq 100 ; # Output frequencies
dcdfreq 100
xstFreq 100
outputEnergies 100


minimize 500 ; # Minimize 500 cycles
```

- Run minimization in NAMD on X processors by entering the following command:

```
namd2 +pX min.conf >& min.log
```

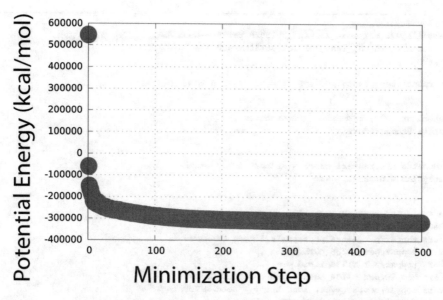

Fig. 10 Potential energy of the system decreases and reaches a plateau during minimization

- Note that energy minimization is essential to resolve any high-energy conformations in the structure that may introduce instabilities during the simulation phase of the project (*see* **Note 17**). Plotting the potential energy of the system versus minimization step produces the plot given in Fig. 10. Note that energy decreases and reaches a plateau, indicating that 500 cycles of minimization is sufficient for the system under study.

- For more information on using NAMD, including documentation and tutorials, visit the NAMD software web page (http://www.ks.uiuc.edu/Research/namd).

Step 14. Set up harmonic restraints for the system.

- Return to VMD's command line and generate a file to impose positional (harmonic) restraints for the protein backbone and drug molecule by entering the following commands:

```
set all [atomselect top "all"] ; # Select system
$all set beta 0 ; # Initialize beta column of PDB
set restraints [atomselect top "(protein and backbone) or resname TYL"] ; # Select restraint atoms
$restraints set beta 5 ; # Set force constant k=5 kcal/mol for restraint atoms
$all writepdb restraints.pdb ; # Write restraints PDB
```

Step 15. Run MD simulation of the system (heat with restraints).

- Open a terminal and navigate to your working directory. Make sure that the location of the NAMD executable is contained within your $PATH variable.

- Save the NAMD configuration script given below to your working directory as heat.conf.

```
# Input
structure AAA_TYL_pH7_ions_solvent_sc150mM.psf ; # Load PSF
coordinates AAA_TYL_pH7_ions_solvent_sc150mM.pdb ; # Load PDB


set restraints restraints.pdb ; # Load restraints PDB


set temperature 50 ; # Initial temperature
temperature $temperature


binCoordinates min.restart.coor; # Restart information
extendedSystem min.restart.xsc


# Force Field Information
paraTypeCharmm on ; # Use CHARMM
parameters toppar/par_all36_prot.prm ; # Load CHARMM36
parameters toppar/par_all36_carb.prm
parameters toppar/par_all36_lipid.prm
parameters toppar/par_all36_cgenff.prm ; # Load CGenFF
parameters toppar/toppar_water_ions.str ; # Load TIP3P/ions
parameters TYL.str ; # Load drug parameters
exclude scaled1-4 ; # Exclude 1-2s and 1-3s, scale 1-4s
1-4scaling 1.0 ; # 1-4 scaling factor
cutoff 12.0 ; # Cut-off radius for non-bonded interactions
switching on ; # Scale smoothly to zero
switchdist 10.0 ; # Scale smoothly from here to cut
pairlistdist 14.0 ; # Pairlist search radius


# Periodic Boundary Conditions
wrapAll on ; # Wrap coordinates
PME yes ; # PME long-range electrostatics
PMEGridSpacing 1.0 ; # Grid spacing for PME
margin 1.5 ; # For box equilibration


# Integrator Parameters
timestep 2.0 ; # Time step
rigidBonds all ; # Constrain bonds to hydrogen
useSettle on ; # Use SETTLE for water molecules
nonbondedFreq 1 ; # Frequency to recalculate nonbonded interactions
fullElectFrequency 2 ; # Frequency to recalculate fullelectrostatics
longSplitting c2 ; # Long/short range splitting method
stepspercycle 20 ; # Pairlist update


# Constant Temperature Control
langevin on ; # Langevin thermostat
langevinTemp $temperature ; # Target temperature
langevinDamping 1.0
langevinHydrogen off
```

```
# Constant Pressure Control
langevinPiston on ; # Nose-Hoover Langevin piston barostat
langevinPistonTarget 1.0 ; # Target pressure
langevinPistonPeriod 200.0
langevinPistonDecay 100.0
langevinPistonTemp $temperature
useFlexibleCell no ; # Isotropic pressure scaling
useGroupPressure yes ; # Required for rigidBonds


# Harmonic restraints
constraints on ; # Restraints active
consexp 2 ; # Exponent for harmonic energy function
consref $restraints ; # File for restraints coords
conskfile $restraints ; # File for restraints k
conskcol B ; # Restraints k in beta column
constraintScaling 1.0 ; # Scaling factor


# Output
outputName heat ; # Output file name prefix
binaryOutput yes ; # Output binary files
restartfreq 500 ; # Output frequencies
dcdfreq 500
xstFreq 500
outputEnergies 500
outputPressure 500


### RUN SCRIPT
# Heat 50 K to 310 K over 500 ps
for {set i 0} {$i < 50} {incr i} {
        run 5000 ; # 10 ps intervals
        incr temperature 5 ; # 5 K increments
        langevinTemp $temperature
        langevinPistonTemp $temperature
}
```

- Run MD in NAMD on X processors by entering the following command:

```
namd2 +pX heat.conf >& heat.log
```

- Note that the target temperature of the system is incremented to 300 K, which represents room temperature. As the example project in this chapter aims to investigate a biosensing reaction within an experimental setup on a laboratory benchtop, room temperature is appropriate. Studies intending to investigate systems within a biological context should use normal human body temperature of 310 K (*see* **Note 18**).

Step 16. Run MD simulation of the system (release restraints).

- Open a terminal and navigate to your working directory. Make sure that the location of the NAMD executable is contained within your $PATH variable.

– Copy the NAMD configuration script heat.conf to a new file release.conf, substituting the ### RUN SCRIPT section with text given below. Also change initial temperature to 300 K, remove the margin command, and update the input (heat) and output (release) file names.

```
### RUN SCRIPT
# Release backbone over 500 ps
for {set i 0} {$i < 10} {incr i} {
        constraintScaling [expr 1.0 - ($i * 0.1)]
        run 25000 ; # 50 ps intervals
}
```

– Run MD in NAMD on X processors by entering the following command:

```
namd2 +pX release.conf >& release.log
```

– Note that the restraints used to maintain the protein fold and drug position during the heating phase of the project are removed gradually to allow the system to slowly adapt to native environmental conditions (*see* **Note 19**).

Step 17. Run MD simulation of the system (equilibrate).

– Open a terminal and navigate to your working directory. Make sure that the location of the NAMD executable is contained within your $PATH variable.

– Copy the NAMD configuration script relase.conf to a new file equil.conf, substituting the ### RUN SCRIPT section with text given below. Also remove the # Harmonic restraints section and update the input (release) and output (equil) file names.

```
### RUN SCRIPT
# Run 5 ns
run 2500000
```

– Run MD in NAMD on X processors by entering the following command:

```
namd2 +pX equil.conf >& equil.log
```

– Note that the system is equilibrated for 5 ns for this example. In a real-world research scenario, the system would be equilibrated until the property of interest for the study has converged (*see* **Note 20**). For a protein–drug complex, the property of interest may be stability of the binding mode.

Step 18. Run MD simulation of the system (collect data).

– Open a terminal and navigate to your working directory. Make sure that the location of the NAMD executable is contained within your $PATH variable.

- Copy the NAMD configuration script equil.conf to a new file prod1.conf and update the input (equil) and output (prod1) file names.

- Run MD in NAMD on X processors by entering the following command:

```
namd2 +pX prod1.conf >& prod1.log
```

- Restart the MD simulation, continuing with NAMD runs for files prod2, prod3, etc., until sufficient sampling of the system is obtained. Given the performance of modern desktop workstations and supercomputers, publication quality MD simulations of protein–ligand complexes commonly explore timescale of hundreds of nanoseconds (*see* **Note 21**).

5 Notes

1. The model should describe the system at all-atom detail and contains no missing regions.

2. The model must capture the chemical interaction between the target protein and drug molecule.

3. The model should be free of structural clashes or close contacts.

4. Any artifactual *cis* peptides in the model should be adjusted to the *trans* orientation.

5. The reproduction of realistic solvent conditions is key to meaningful simulation results.

6. Hydrogen coordinates and protonation states should be assigned to reflect the desired pH of the model's solvent environment.

7. An explicit solvent representation should be employed to capture water-mediated hydrogen bonds between the target protein and drug.

8. Crystallographically resolved water molecules should be retained in the model.

9. A distance of at least 15 Å between the protein–drug complex and the solvent box edges is recommended.

10. A cubic solvent box is most appropriate for long timescale simulations.

11. Salt concentration of the solvent should mimic conditions of the model's realistic environment.

12. Careful placement of local salt ions around the model can reduce equilibration time needed during the simulation phase of the project.

13. The net charge of the final model immersed in its solvent environment should be neutral.

14. Use the latest version of a force field suitable for biological macromolecules to describe the protein component of the system.

15. Use a generalized force field to describe the drug component of the system, deriving any missing parameters by analogy or ab initio, such that they are compatible with the protein force field.

16. Parameters with poor analogy should be validated against experiment, or optimized by fitting to quantum mechanical potentials.

17. Minimizing the potential energy of the system is key to resolving any high energy conformations that may lead to instabilities going into the simulation phase of the project.

18. The simulation should be slowly heated to a target temperature that mimic's the model's realistic environment.

19. Imposing positional (harmonic) restraints to maintain the protein fold and drug binding mode during heating, and gradually releasing those restraints once the target temperature has been reached, allows the system to slowly adjust to its native environmental conditions.

20. Extend the equilibration phase of the project until the property of interest for the study, e.g., drug binding mode, has converged.

21. Extend the production (data collection) phase of the project until sufficient sampling of the system is obtained, e.g., hundreds of nanoseconds at minimum for most protein–drug complexes.

Acknowledgements

The authors acknowledge funding from the University of Delaware and the National Institutes of Health COBRE grant 5P30GM110758-04.

References

1. Lee EH, Hsin J, Sotomayor M, Comellas G, Schulten K (2009) Discovery through the computational microscope. Structure 17:1295–1306

2. Perilla JR, Goh BC, Keith Cassidy C, Bo L, Bernardi RC, Rudack T, Hang Y, Zhe W, Schulten K (2015) Molecular dynamics simulations of large macromolecular complexes. Curr Opin Struct Biol 31:64–74

3. Ebele AJ, Abdallah MA-E, Harrad S (2017) Pharmaceuticals and personal care products (PPCPs) in the freshwater aquatic environment. Emerging Contaminants 3(1):1–16

4. Banica F-G (2012) Chemical sensors and biosensors: fundamentals and applications. John Wiley & Sons, Chichester

5. Perilla JR, Hadden JA, Goh BC, Mayne CG, Schulten K (2016) All-atom molecular dynamics of virus capsids as drug targets. J Phys Chem Lett 7:1836–1844

6. Dart RC, Green JL (2016) The prescription paradox of acetaminophen safety. Pharmacoepidemiol Drug Saf 25(5):599–601

7. Hinson JA, Roberts DW, James LP (2010) Mechanisms of acetaminophen-induced liver necrosis. Handb Exp Pharmacol 196:369–405

8. Yoon E, Babar A, Choudhary M, Kutner M, Pyrsopoulos N (2016) Acetaminophen-induced hepatotoxicity: a comprehensive update. J Clin Transl Hepatol 4(2):131

9. Michael Bulger, Jan Holinsky (2014) Acetaminophen assay. US Patent 8,715,952, 6 May 2014

10. Hammond PM, Scawen MD, Tony Atkinson RSC, Price CP (1984) Development of an enzyme-based assay for acetaminophen. Anal Biochem 143(1):152–157

11. Morris HC, Overton PD, Richard Ramsay J, Stewart Campbell R, Hammond PM, Atkinson T, Price CP (1990) Development and validation of an automated enzyme assay for paracetamol (acetaminophen). Clin Chim Acta 187(2):95–104

12. Vaughan PA, Scott LDL, McAller JF (1991) Amperometric biosensor for the rapid determination of acetaminophen in whole blood. Anal Chim Acta 248(2):361–365

13. Lee S, Park E-H, Ko H-J, Bang WG, Kim H-Y, Kim KH, Choi IG (2015) Crystal structure analysis of a bacterial aryl acylamidase belonging to the amidase signature enzyme family. Biochem Biophys Res Commun 467(2):268–274

14. Humphrey W, Dalke A, Schulten K (1996) VMD–visual molecular dynamics. J Mol Graph 14(1):33–38

15. Phillips JC, Braun R, Wang W, Gumbart J, Tajkhorshid E, Villa E, Chipot C, Skeel RD, Kale L, Schulten K (2005) Scalable molecular dynamics with NAMD. J Comput Chem 26:1781–1802

16. Eswar N, Webb B, Marti-Renom MA, Madhusudhan MS, Eramian D, Shen M-y, Pieper U, Sali A (2006) Comparative protein structure modeling using MODELLER. Cur Protoc Bioinformatics. https://doi.org/10.1002/0471250953.bi0506s15

17. Das R, Baker D (2008) Macromolecular modeling with ROSETTA. Annu Rev Biochem 77:363–382

18. Wriggers W (2010) Using situs for the integration of multi-resolution structures. Biophys Rev 2:21–27

19. Trabuco LG, Villa E, Mitra K, Frank J, Schulten K (2008) Flexible fitting of atomic structures into electron microscopy maps using molecular dynamics. Structure 16:673–683

20. Goh BC, Hadden JA, Bernardi RC, Singharoy A, McGreevy R, Rudack T, Keith Cassidy C, Schulten K (2016) Computational methodologies for real-space structural refinement of large macromolecular complexes. Annu Rev Biophys 45:253–278

21. Trott O, Olson AJ (2010) Autodock vina: improving the speed and accuracy of docking with a new scoring function, efficient optimization, and multithreading. J Comput Chem 31(2):455–461

22. Pagadala NS, Syed K, Tuszynski J (2017) Software for molecular docking: a review. Biophys Rev 9(2):91–102

23. Dolinsky TJ, Czodrowski P, Li H, Nielsen JE, Jensen JH, Klebe G, Baker NA (2007) PDB2PQR: expanding and upgrading automated preparation of biomolecular structures for molecular simulations. Nucleic Acids Res 35(Web Server):W522–W525

24. Søndergaard CR, Olsson MHM, Rostkowski M l, Jensen JH (2011) Improved treatment of ligands and coupling effects in empirical calculation and rationalization of pKa values. J Chem Theory Comput 7(7):2284–2295

25. Ko M, Huang Y, Jankowska AM, Pape UJ, Tahiliani M, Bandukwala HS, An J, Lamperti ED, Koh KP, Ganetzky R, Shirley Liu X, Aravind L, Agarwal S, Maciejewski JP, Rao A (2010) Impaired hydroxylation of 5-methylcytosine in myeloid cancers with mutant TET2. Nature 468:839–843

26. Jorgensen WL, Chandrasekhar J, Madura JD, Impey RW, Klein ML (1983) Comparison of simple potential functions for simulating liquid water. J Chem Phys 79(2):926–935

27. Onufriev A (2008) Implicit solvent models in molecular dynamics simulations: a brief overview. Annu Rep Comput Chem 4:125–137

28. MacKerell AD Jr, Bashford D, Bellott M, Dunbrack RL Jr, Evanseck JD et al (1998) All-atom empirical potential for molecular modeling and dynamics studies of proteins. J Phys Chem B 102:3586–3616

29. MacKerell AD Jr, Feig M, Brooks CL (2004) Improved treatment of the protein backbone in empirical force fields. J Am Chem Soc 126:698–699

30. Wang J, Wolf RM, Caldwell JW, Kollman PA, Case DA (2004) Developing and testing of a

general amber force field. J Comput Chem 25 (9):1157–1174

31. Vanommeslaeghe K, Hatcher E, Acharya C, Kundu S, Zhong S, Shim J, Darian E, Guvench O, Lopes P, Vorobyov I, MacKerell AD Jr (2010) CHARMM general force field: a force field for drug-like molecules compatible with the CHARMM all-atom additive biological force fields. J Comput Chem 31 (4):671–690

32. Vanommeslaeghe K, MacKerell AD Jr (2012) Automation of the CHARMM general force field (CGenFF) I: bond perception and atom typing. J Chem Inf Model 52(12):3144–3154

33. Vanommeslaeghe K, Prabhu Raman E, MacKerell AD Jr (2012) Automation of the CHARMM general force field (CGenFF) II: assignment of bonded parameters and partial atomic charges. J Chem Inf Model 52 (12):3155–3168

34. Maestro Release 2017-2: MacroModel, Schrödinger, LLC, New York, NY, 2017

35. Mayne CG, Saam J, Schulten K, Tajkhorshid E, Gumbart JC (2013) Rapid parameterization of small molecules using the force field toolkit. J Comput Chem 34:2757–2770

Chapter 14

Prediction and Optimization of Pharmacokinetic and Toxicity Properties of the Ligand

Douglas E. V. Pires, Lisa M. Kaminskas, and David B. Ascher

Abstract

A crucial factor for the approval and success of any drug is how it behaves in the body. Many drugs, however, do not reach the market due to poor efficacy or unacceptable side effects. It is therefore important to take these into consideration early in the drug development process, both in the prioritization of potential hits, and optimization of lead compounds. In silico approaches offer a cost and time-effective approach to rapidly screen and optimize pharmacokinetic and toxicity properties. Here we demonstrate the use of the comprehensive analysis system pkCSM, to allow early identification of potential problems, prioritization of hits, and optimization of leads.

Key words ADMET predictions, Computational medicinal chemistry, Drug development, Hit prioritization, Lead optimization, Pharmacokinetics, Toxicity

1 Introduction

Drug development is a fine balance of optimizing drug like properties to maximize efficacy, safety, and pharmacokinetics, with the ultimate goal being to ensure that it can reach the target site in sufficient concentrations to produce the physiological effect safely. Getting this balance right is essential for the successful introduction into the clinic.

The pharmacokinetic profile of a compound defines its absorption, distribution, metabolism, and excretion (ADME) properties, while toxicity describes a compound's safety profile. Small structural modifications can significantly affect the pharmacokinetic and toxicity properties of drug candidates.

Experimental evaluation of small-molecule pharmacokinetic and toxicity properties is both time-consuming and expensive and does not always scale reliably between animal models and humans. To address this, many computational approaches have been developed to guide compound design and selection throughout the drug development process (Fig. 1). These rely upon associations

Mohini Gore and Umesh B. Jagtap (eds.), *Computational Drug Discovery and Design*, Methods in Molecular Biology, vol. 1762, https://doi.org/10.1007/978-1-4939-7756-7_14, © Springer Science+Business Media, LLC, part of Springer Nature 2018

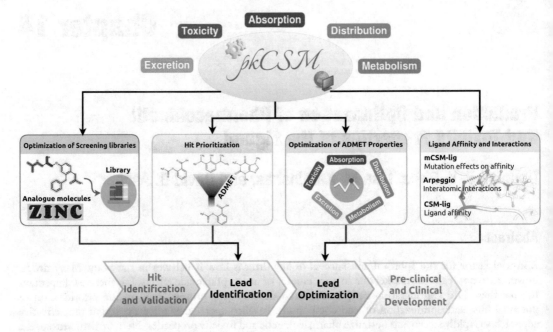

Fig. 1 Screening compound pharmacokinetic and toxicity properties throughout the drug development process using pkCSM as a way to guide and facilitate the drug design process, minimizing risks of failure due to poor ADMET

between the chemical structure of a compound of interest and experimental data for similar structures, and include data-based approaches such as 2D and 3D quantitative structure–activity relationship [1–3], similarity searches [4, 5], and structural-based methods such as ligand–protein docking [6, 7] and pharmacophore modeling [8]. While many of these are unfortunately not freely available, the recent development of pkCSM [9] (http://structure. bioc.cam.ac.uk/pkcsm) has provided a new freely available tool to comprehensively characterize the pharmacokinetic and toxicity properties of your compounds of interest.

pkCSM uses the concept of graph-based structural signatures to study and predict a diverse and complementary range of ADMET properties for novel chemical entities, including the following:

- *Absorption*: Water solubility, Caco2 permeability, human intestinal absorption, and skin permeability, and whether the molecule is a P-glycoprotein substrate or inhibitor.

- *Distribution*: Human volume of distribution, human fraction unbound in plasma, blood–brain barrier and central nervous system permeability.

- *Metabolism*: Whether the molecule is a Cytochrome P450 substrate or inhibitor.

- *Excretion*: Total clearance and whether the molecule is a renal OCT2 substrate.
- *Toxicity*: AMES toxicity, human maximum tolerated dose, oral rat acute and chronic toxicity, hERG inhibition, hepatotoxicity, and skin sensitization.

2 Materials

2.1 Running pkCSM

1. List of compound structures of interest formated as canonical SMILES:

   (a) A SMILES string is a widely used line notation for representing the atomic composition and structure of chemical entities. In short, a SMILES can be generated from a graph representation of a molecule (atoms as nodes and bonds as edges) by executing a depth-first search, generating a spanning tree. Several different SMILES strings can be generated for the same molecule, depending on the search algorithm used. Several algorithms, however, have been developed to generate the SMILES for a given compound in a unique way (Canonical SMILES). Users are advised to use the OpenEye Canonical SMILES as syntax noncompliant molecules might not be processed correctly. Several SMILES strings can be combined into a file for submission to the pkCSM platform to analyse multiple structures at once.

   (b) Molecules of interest can be converted from and to the SMILES format using any of several different open source libraries currently available, including Open Babel [10] and RDKit. There are also several online resources that can generate smiles (e.g., https://cactus.nci.nih.gov/translate/).

2.2 Running CSM-Lig, Arpeggio and mCSM-Lig

Any valid Protein Data Bank (PDB) files are acceptable for running the servers as long as they comply with the format, as defined in http://www.wwpdb.org/documentation/file-format. This way, the servers are capable of handling crystallographic structures as well those generated via molecular docking and homology modeling [11–13] (*see* **Notes 1** and **2**).

1. CSM-lig:

   (a) Structure of the compound bound to the protein target in PDB format; when no experimental structure of the complex is available, molecular docking can be used to model the complex.

   (b) Ligand information;
      - Ligand three-letter code (as used in the PDB file);

  - SMILES string of the ligand bound/docked.

2. mCSM-lig:

  (a) Structure of the compound bound to the protein target in PDB format;

  (b) Mutation information, including:

    - The mutation code, composed by one-letter code of the wild-type residue, residue position, and one-letter code of the mutant residue (e.g., D30N);

    - The chain ID of the wild-type residues;

    - Ligand three-letter code (as used in the PDB file).

  (c) Wild-type affinity in nM. This only needs to be approximate. Experimental data for many molecules can be found in the BRENDA database [14]. Alternatively, the predicted affinity from CSM-lig [7] can be used.

3. Arpeggio:

  (a) Structure of the compound bound to the protein target in PDB format.

  (b) To calculate and visualize interactions being made by the compound, the ligand can be selected from the list of heteroatom groups. Alternatively, the ligand can be specified in the format "/a/b/", where a denotes the chain ID and the compound number, as used in the PDB file. Example: /A/30/will select ligand number 30 of chain A.

3 Methods

3.1 Running pkCSM

1. Open up the pkCSM prediction server on a browser (pkCSM is compatible with most Operating Systems and browsers. We, however, recommend using Google Chrome): http://structure.bioc.cam.ac.uk/pkcsm/prediction;

2. Provide either an input file with a list of molecules in SMILES format (up to a maximum of 100 molecules) or supply a single SMILES string for an individual molecule (Fig. 2a) (*see* **Notes 3** and **4**)

3. Choose the prediction mode, selecting either between the individual ADMET property classes (**A**bsorption, **D**istribution, **M**etabolism, **E**xcretion, and **T**oxicity) by clicking on their corresponding button, or run a systematic evaluation of all predictive models.

4. For single molecules (Fig. 2b), the predictions will be displayed in tabular format, along with a list of calculated molecular properties. The information shown include the ADMET property being predicted, the predictive model name, the actual

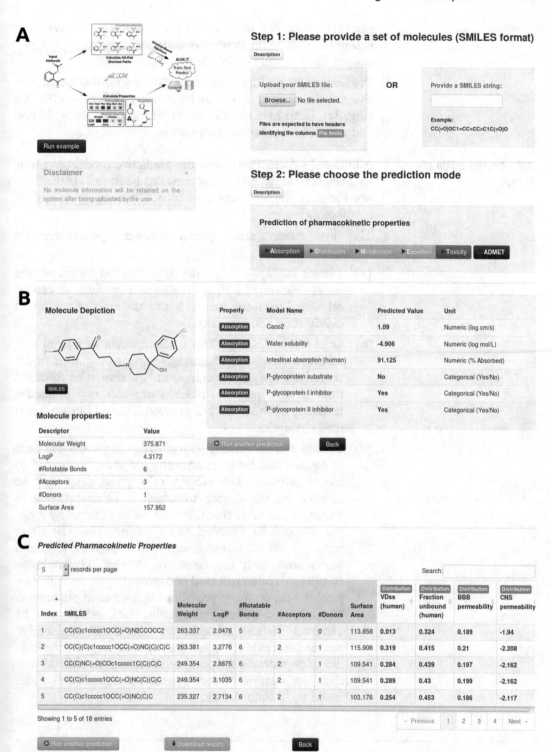

Fig. 2 pkCSM web interface. (**a**) depicts the submission page from pkCSM where users can submit either a single or list of compounds as canonical SMILES to predict their pharmacokinetic and toxicity properties by clicking in the corresponding buttons. A button for calculation of all ADMET properties is also available.

predicted value and whether the prediction is numerical, indicating the unit of the predicted value, or categorical. A depiction of the molecule is also shown.

5. Predictions for multiple molecules will be shown in an interactive tabular format that can be downloaded as a CSV file (Fig. 2c). Users have the option to sort the table by any column and search/filter specific compounds.

3.2 Interpretation of Output

1. Additional information about the predictive models and how to interpret the pkCSM predictions can be found via the Theory menu of the web server at: http://structure.bioc.cam.ac.uk/pkcsm/theory.

2. The five more critical pharmacokinetic parameters are described below.

(a) *Plasma half life*—This is the time required for the plasma concentration of a drug to decrease by 50%. It can be calculated from the natural log of the ratio of volume of distribution and clearance.

(b) *Oral bioavailability*—This is the fraction of a drug that reaches systemic circulation after oral dosing. One of the crucial steps of this is a compound's ability to be absorbed through the intestine. pkCSM provides two predictive measures of this—Caco-2 permeability and human intestinal absorption.

(c) *Plasma protein binding*—Most drugs in plasma will exist in equilibrium between an unbound state, or bound to serum proteins. The efficacy of a given drug may be affected by the degree to which it binds proteins in blood, as the more that is bound the less efficiently it can traverse cellular membranes or diffuse. This can affect renal excretion, blood–brain barrier permeability, and interactions with the target of interest. Hydrophobic compounds often will bind nonspecifically to many hydrophobic sites on many proteins. High-throughput screening often identifies hydrophobic hits, which can be extremely difficult to optimize. Conversely, engineering plasma protein binding has been used to improve the half-life of peptides by reducing renal excretion. pkCSM predicts the fraction of a drug that will remain unbound, based upon human data.

Fig. 2 (continued) (**b**) shows the result page for the predictions of *Absorption* properties for a single molecule. The molecular properties of the ligand are shown on the left hand side of the screen. (**c**) shows the results page for the prediction of *Distribution* properties for multiple molecules. The results can be downloaded as a tab-separated file

(d) *Volume of distribution*—The volume of distribution is the theoretical volume that the total dose of a drug would need to be uniformly distributed across to give the same concentration as in blood plasma. The higher this number, the more the drug distributed in tissues as opposed to plasma. Hydrophilic and negatively charged compounds often have small volumes of distribution, as they do not diffuse effectively into tissues. Compounds that are mostly bound to plasma proteins will also appear to have a small volume of distribution. Hydrophobic and positively charged compounds often have large volumes of distribution as they can readily dissolve in and interact with the negatively charged cell membrane. pkCSM predicts the logarithm of the steady state volume of distribution based upon human clinical data. The ideal volume of distribution depends upon the disease being treated and the targeted half-life. For example, often a large tissue distribution, corresponding to a large volume of distribution is often considered desirable for antibiotics and antivirals targeting intracellular pathogens. By contrast, compounds with a small volume of distribution enable better control of drug plasma levels, important for compounds with small therapeutic windows. Distribution, targeting and clearance of small molecules can also be altered through the use of drug carriers [15].

(e) *Clearance*—This is the rate at which plasma is cleared of the drug. Drug clearance occurs primarily as a combination of hepatic clearance (metabolism in the liver and biliary clearance) and renal clearance (excretion via the kidneys). It is related to bioavailability, and is important for determining dosing rates to achieve steady-state concentrations. pkCSM predicts the total clearance of a drug based upon data from humans.

3. Toxicity measurements are important to consider relative to the concentration of a compound needed to exert a therapeutic effect. This is known as the Therapeutic Index/Window—the ratio of the dose that leads to lethality in 50% of the population (Rat LD50 in pkCSM) divided by the minimum effective dose for 50% of the population. Larger therapeutic indices are preferable since a much larger dose of a drug would need to be administered to reach the toxicity threshold than that needed to elicit the therapeutic effect.

3.3 ADMET Optimization of Screening Libraries

1. When developing a screening library, or identifying analogs to screen, for a particular condition, it is worth tailoring it in order to enrich it for compounds with more favorable properties.

2. Identifying analogues to screen can help expand and develop the initial hit. This is often performed through 2D and 3D

similarity searches of initial hits using databases of compounds from your commercial suppliers (analoging by cataloging) or large databases (such as the ZINC database: http://zinc.doc king.org/search/structure).

3. Compounds should be screened for potential problems including PAINS groups [16], mutagenic groups and groups with known toxicity issues.

4. While maintaining broad chemical diversity, the library can be screened through pkCSM and used to enrich particular ADMET features favorable for the target protein/disease (e.g., BBB permeability for neuroactive compounds [12, 17–19]).

3.4 Modifications to Improve ADMET Properties

1. pkCSM predictions can be used when composing screening libraries, enriching them with compounds that suit the drug target. For example, when screening for neuroactive compounds, it would make sense to enrich your screening libraries for compounds with high blood–brain barrier and central nervous system permeability.

2. However, when a lead compound has been identified, there are chemical modifications that can be performed which may improve the pharmacokinetic and toxicity profile. Small structural modifications can significantly affect the pharmacokinetic and toxicity properties of drug candidates.

3. Using the multiple molecule prediction mode of pkCSM, large libraries of analogues can be screened to identify compounds with promising ADMET profiles. A few common medicinal chemistry strategies used to improve pharmacokinetic profiles are described below. It is always worth bearing in mind how any proposed alterations might affect how the compound binds to the target of interest. While sometimes a successful strategy, there are many times when new cores will need to be explored in order to move away from these unfavorable properties.

   (a) *Improving oral bioavailability*: Oral bioavailability is a function of the proportion of a drug absorbed through the intestine, and the amount that is metabolized in the liver before entering the systemic circulation. Passive intestinal absorption correlates with size, with absorption decreasing as molecules polar surface area increases beyond 60 A^2, with negligible absorption observed beyond 140 A^2. Charged and hydrophilic compounds absorb best when their molecular weight is below 200 Da, and hydrophobic compounds need to be at least partially water soluble.

   (b) *Improving metabolism profile*: High levels of cytochrome P450 metabolism will reduce oral bioavailability and plasma half life [20]. This can be reduced through altering the logP and PSA, and by blocking hydroxylation through fluorination and introduction of heteroatoms at potential sites of hydroxylation.

Other forms of metabolism to watch out for include metabolism by alcohol dehydrogenase, oxidases and reductases, esterases, phosphatases, and proteases; and adduction by strong nucleophiles including glutathione. Alternatively, sometimes metabolic inhibitors can be used to potentiate drug action [21, 22].

(c) *Improving excretion profile*: High levels of renal excretion will lead to lower plasma half lives. Increased levels of protein plasma binding and volume of distribution can reduce renal excretion. Some charged molecules may be actively secreted. Neutral and lipophilic compounds may be resorbed back into plasma.

(d) *Improving permeability*: Blood–brain barrier permeability is linked to small (below 600 Da, polar surface area below 40 A^2), uncharged, lipophilic compounds (log$P$ above 0) with few rotatable bonds. Groups that form hydrogen bonds reduce blood–brain barrier permeability. Blood–-brain barrier permeability may also be decreased through active excretion by P-gp transporters.

(e) *Avoiding toxicity*: Currently, along with lack of efficacy, toxicity issues are the main reason for drug failure. Similar to how the incorporation of ADME screening into the early drug development pipeline drastically reduced failures (in the 80s and 90s pharmacokinetic failures were a leading cause of drug failures), consideration of toxicity issues early in the drug development process can mitigate these issues. Strong electrophiles, and functional groups that are prone to the formation of strong electrophilic metabolites, are often toxic and/or mutagenic. Chromophores such as quinolines may be phototoxic and lead to skin sensitization. Inhibition of human Ether-a-go-go related gene has been linked to the withdrawal of several drugs that led to cardiac complications, and should be avoided.

3.5 Identification of Changes to Affinity

1. Any changes to the drug need to be considered with respect to how they may alter binding to the target. Using a structure of the compounds with the target, these effects can be explored in different ways.

2. *Calculating interatomic interactions between protein and ligand*: A map of important molecular interactions being made by a compound can be generated and visualized using the Arpeggio webserver [23] (http://structure.bioc.cam.ac.uk/arpeggio/). Figure 3a shows the Arpeggio's results pages.

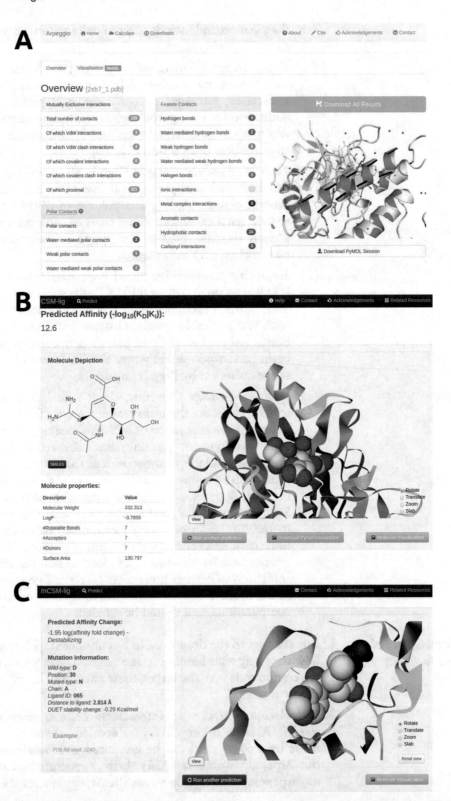

Fig. 3 Assessing different aspects that influence protein–ligand affinity. (**a**) depicts the result page for Arpeggio. A color-coded list of identified interactions and their number is exhibited. (**b**) shows the result

Users have the option to download a Pymol session file to visualize the interactions calculated (*see* **Note 5**).

3. *Calculating protein–ligand affinity and assessing docking poses*: While docking scores have been considered unreliable, a range of new approaches are providing more accurate estimations of binding affinity. For example, the binding affinity of modified compounds can be predicted using CSM-lig [7] (http://structure.bioc.cam.ac.uk/csm_lig/). Figure 3b shows CSM-lig results page. Users have the option to asses either a single protein–ligand complex or submit a compressed file with multiple poses (limited to 50 MB in size) (*see* **Note 6**).

4. *Calculating effects of mutations and identifying resistance mutations*: Potential resistance mutations can be identified using mCSM-lig [24–26] (http://structure.bioc.cam.ac.uk/mcsm_lig/). This can be used to help identify likely resistance mutations early in the drug development process [27], in order to minimize interactions with these resistance hot-spots. When considering possible resistance mutations it is important to consider other affects the mutation might have upon protein stability [28–31] and other interactions [24, 28, 32–37]. The mCSM-lig results page is shown in Fig. 3c (*see* **Note 7**).

4   Notes

1. When uploading a PDB structure generated via homology modeling or docking, make sure a valid chain ID is present. The servers will not accept white spaces as valid chain IDs. You can renumber the chain using a text editor, pymol or web servers (http://www.canoz.com/sdh/renamepdbchain.pl).

2. When using NMR solved structures, it is a good practice to select a single model to be submitted (even though the servers will automatically select the first model).

3. If your compound will not run on pkCSM, make sure that you are using Canonical SMILES.

4. When uploading a file for the servers (e.g., a list of SMILES for pkCSM, a list of mutations for mCSM-lig) make sure that you

---

Fig. 3 (continued) page for CSM-lig. A Pymol session with calculated interactions is available, as well as the calculated ligand properties and its molecule depiction. The predictions are given as the -log(K_D or K_i). (**c**) shows the result page for mCSM-lig. The mutation information is shown and the prediction is given as the log(affinity fold change). Negative values, which will be colored in red, denote mutations reducing ligand affinity

upload a purely textual file, as other formats will now be recognized (e.g., .doc, .xls, and others).

5. If your protein will not run on Arpeggio, mCSM-lig or CSM-lig it is worth checking the PDB structure for nonstandard entities, including:

   • Nonstandard atom groups (e.g., metal atoms such as zinc in capitals ZN);

   • Nonstandard residues;

6. Other possible causes of error while running servers that rely on protein–ligand complexes include:

   (a) Ligand is missing from the structure;

   (b) Ligand information (ID/number/chain) does not match the provided PDB file;

   (c) In the case of mCSM-lig, mutation information is not compatible with PDB file (wild-type residue could not be found in the provided position/chain).

7. Structures with multiple ligands bound might interfere with the predictions (especially if they are in close proximity to the ligand or mutation of interest) since they will be taken into consideration in the calculations.

Acknowledgments

This work was funded by the Jack Brockhoff Foundation (JBF 4186, 2016) and a Newton Fund RCUK-CONFAP Grant awarded by The Medical Research Council (MRC) and Fundação de Amparo à Pesquisa do Estado de Minas Gerais (FAPEMIG) (MR/M026302/1). This research was supported by the Victorian Life Sciences Computation Initiative (VLSCI), an initiative of the Victorian Government, Australia, on its Facility hosted at the University of Melbourne (UOM0017). D.E.V.P. received support from the René Rachou Research Center (CPqRR/FIOCRUZ Minas), Brazil. LMK was supported by a RD Wright Biomedical Career Development Fellowship from the National Health and Medical Research Council of Australia (APP1105383). DBA is supported by a C. J. Martin Research Fellowship from the National Health and Medical Research Council of Australia (APP1072476), and the Department of Biochemistry, University of Melbourne.

References

1. Khan MT (2010) Predictions of the ADMET properties of candidate drug molecules utilizing different QSAR/QSPR modelling approaches. Curr Drug Metab 11(4):285–295

2. Lill MA (2007) Multi-dimensional QSAR in drug discovery. Drug Discov Today 12 (23–24):1013–1017

3. Obrezanova O, Csanyi G, Gola JM, Segall MD (2007) Gaussian processes: a method for automatic QSAR modeling of ADME properties. J Chem Inf Model 47(5):1847–1857

4. Drwal MN, Banerjee P, Dunkel M, Wettig MR, Preissner R (2014) ProTox: a web server for the in silico prediction of rodent oral toxicity. Nucleic Acids Res 42(Web Server issue): W53–W58

5. Fröhlich H, Wegner JK, Sieker F, Zell A (2006) Kernel functions for attributed molecular graphs–a new similarity-based approach to ADME prediction in classification and regression. QSAR Comb Sci 25(4):317–326

6. Moroy G, Martiny VY, Vayer P, Villoutreix BO, Miteva MA (2012) Toward in silico structure-based ADMET prediction in drug discovery. Drug Discov Today 17(1–2):44–55

7. Pires DE, Ascher DB (2016) CSM-lig: a web server for assessing and comparing protein-small molecule affinities. Nucleic Acids Res 44 (W1):W557–W561

8. Guner OF, Bowen JP (2013) Pharmacophore modeling for ADME. Curr Top Med Chem 13 (11):1327–1342

9. Pires DE, Blundell TL, Ascher DB (2015) pkCSM: predicting small-molecule pharmacokinetic and toxicity properties using graph-based signatures. J Med Chem 58 (9):4066–4072

10. O'Boyle NM, Banck M, James CA, Morley C, Vandermeersch T, Hutchison GR (2011) Open babel: an open chemical toolbox. J Cheminform 3:33

11. Sigurdardottir AG, Winter A, Sobkowicz A, Fragai M, Chirgadze D, Ascher DB, Blundell TL, Gherardi E (2015) Exploring the chemical space of the lysine-binding pocket of the first kringle domain of hepatocyte growth factor/scatter factor (HGF/SF) yields a new class of inhibitors of HGF/SF-MET binding. Chem Sci 6(11):6147–6157

12. Albiston AL, Morton CJ, Ng HL, Pham V, Yeatman HR, Ye S, Fernando RN, De Bundel D, Ascher DB, Mendelsohn FA, Parker MW, Chai SY (2008) Identification and characterization of a new cognitive enhancer based on inhibition of insulin-regulated aminopeptidase. FASEB J 22(12):4209–4217

13. Ascher DB, Wielens J, Nero TL, Doughty L, Morton CJ, Parker MW (2014) Potent hepatitis C inhibitors bind directly to NS5A and reduce its affinity for RNA. Sci Rep 4:4765

14. Chang A, Schomburg I, Placzek S, Jeske L, Ulbrich M, Xiao M, Sensen CW, Schomburg D (2015) BRENDA in 2015: exciting developments in its 25th year of existence. Nucleic Acids Res 43(Database issue): D439–D446

15. Kaminskas LM, McLeod VM, Ascher DB, Ryan GM, Jones S, Haynes JM, Trevaskis NL, Chan LJ, Sloan EK, Finnin BA, Williamson M, Velkov T, Williams ED, Kelly BD, Owen DJ, Porter CJ (2015) Methotrexate-conjugated PEGylated dendrimers show differential patterns of deposition and activity in tumor-burdened lymph nodes after intravenous and subcutaneous administration in rats. Mol Pharm 12(2):432–443

16. Baell JB, Holloway GA (2010) New substructure filters for removal of pan assay interference compounds (PAINS) from screening libraries and for their exclusion in bioassays. J Med Chem 53(7):2719–2740

17. Chai SY, Yeatman HR, Parker MW, Ascher DB, Thompson PE, Mulvey HT, Albiston AL (2008) Development of cognitive enhancers based on inhibition of insulin-regulated aminopeptidase. BMC Neurosci 9(Suppl 2):S14

18. Ascher DB, Cromer BA, Morton CJ, Volitakis I, Cherny RA, Albiston AL, Chai SY, Parker MW (2011) Regulation of insulin-regulated membrane aminopeptidase activity by its C-terminal domain. Biochemistry 50 (13):2611–2622

19. Hermans SJ, Ascher DB, Hancock NC, Holien JK, Michell BJ, Chai SY, Morton CJ, Parker MW (2015) Crystal structure of human insulin-regulated aminopeptidase with specificity for cyclic peptides. Protein Sci 24 (2):190–199

20. Silvino AC, Costa GL, Araujo FC, Ascher DB, Pires DE, Fontes CJ, Carvalho LH, Brito CF, Sousa TN (2016) Variation in human cytochrome P-450 drug-metabolism genes: a gateway to the understanding of plasmodium vivax relapses. PLoS One 11(7):e0160172

21. Parker LJ, Italiano LC, Morton CJ, Hancock NC, Ascher DB, Aitken JB, Harris HH, Campomanes P, Rothlisberger U, De Luca A, Lo Bello M, Ang WH, Dyson PJ, Parker MW (2011) Studies of glutathione transferase P1-1 bound to a platinum(IV)-based anticancer compound reveal the molecular basis of its activation. Chemistry 17(28):7806–7816

22. Parker LJ, Bocedi A, Ascher DB, Aitken JB, Harris HH, Lo Bello M, Ricci G, Morton CJ, Parker MW (2017) Glutathione transferase P1-1 as an arsenic drug-sequestering enzyme. Protein Sci 26(2):317–326

23. Jubb HC, Higueruelo AP, Ochoa-Montano B, Pitt WR, Ascher DB, Blundell TL (2017) Arpeggio: a web server for calculating and

visualising interatomic interactions in protein structures. J Mol Biol 429(3):365–371

24. Pires DE, Blundell TL, Ascher DB (2016) mCSM-lig: quantifying the effects of mutations on protein-small molecule affinity in genetic disease and emergence of drug resistance. Sci Rep 6:29575

25. Pires DE, Blundell TL, Ascher DB (2015) Platinum: a database of experimentally measured effects of mutations on structurally defined protein-ligand complexes. Nucleic Acids Res 43(Database issue):D387–D391

26. Phelan J, Coll F, McNerney R, Ascher DB, Pires DE, Furnham N, Coeck N, Hill-Cawthorne GA, Nair MB, Mallard K, Ramsay A, Campino S, Hibberd ML, Pain A, Rigouts L, Clark TG (2016) Mycobacterium tuberculosis whole genome sequencing and protein structure modelling provides insights into anti-tuberculosis drug resistance. BMC Med 14:31

27. Singh V, Donini S, Pacitto A, Sala C, Hartkoorn RC, Dhar N, Keri G, Ascher DB, Mondésert G, Vocat A, Lupien A, Sommer R, Vermet H, Lagrange S, Buechler J, Warner DF, McKinney JD, Pato J, Cole ST, Blundell TL, Rizzi M, Mizrahi V (2016) The inosine monophosphate dehydrogenase, GuaB2, is a vulnerable new bactericidal drug target for tuberculosis. ACS Infect Dis 3(1):5–17. https://doi.org/10.1021/acsinfecdis.6b00102

28. Pires DE, Ascher DB, Blundell TL (2014) mCSM: predicting the effects of mutations in proteins using graph-based signatures. Bioinformatics 30(3):335–342

29. Pires DE, Ascher DB, Blundell TL (2014) DUET: a server for predicting effects of mutations on protein stability using an integrated computational approach. Nucleic Acids Res 42(Web Server issue):W314–W319

30. Pandurangan AP, Ascher DB, Thomas SE, Blundell TL (2017) Genomes, structural biology, and drug discovery: combating the impacts of mutations in genetic disease and antibiotic resistance. Biochem Soc Trans 45(2):303–311

31. Pandurangan AP, Ochoa-Montaño B, Ascher DB, Blundell TL (2017) SDM: a server for predicting effects of mutations on protein stability and malfunction. Nucleic Acids Res 39(Web Server issue):W215–W222. https://doi.org/10.1093/nar/gkx439

32. Pires DE, Chen J, Blundell TL, Ascher DB (2016) In silico functional dissection of saturation mutagenesis: interpreting the relationship between phenotypes and changes in protein stability, interactions and activity. Sci Rep 6:19848

33. Ascher DB, Jubb HC, Pires DEV, Ochi T, Higueruelo A, Blundell TL (2015) Protein-protein interactions: structures and druggability. In: Scapin G, Patel D, Arnold E (eds) Multifaceted roles of crystallography in modern drug discovery. Springer Netherlands, Dordrecht, pp 141–163

34. Jubb H, Blundell TL, Ascher DB (2015) Flexibility and small pockets at protein-protein interfaces: new insights into druggability. Prog Biophys Mol Biol 119(1):2–9

35. Pires DE, Ascher DB (2017) mCSM-NA: predicting the effects of mutations on protein-nucleic acids interactions. Nucleic Acids Res. https://doi.org/10.1093/nar/gkx236

36. Pires DE, Ascher DB (2016) mCSM-AB: a web server for predicting antibody-antigen affinity changes upon mutation with graph-based signatures. Nucleic Acids Res 44(W1):W469–W473

37. Jubb HC, Pandurangan AP, Turner MA, Ochoa-Montano B, Blundell TL, Ascher DB (2017) Mutations at protein-protein interfaces: small changes over big surfaces have large impacts on human health. Prog Biophys Mol Biol 128:3–13. https://doi.org/10.1016/j.pbiomolbio.2016.10.002

Chapter 15

Protein–Protein Docking in Drug Design and Discovery

Agnieszka A. Kaczor, Damian Bartuzi, Tomasz Maciej Stępniewski, Dariusz Matosiuk, and Jana Selent

Abstract

Protein–protein interactions (PPIs) are responsible for a number of key physiological processes in the living cells and underlie the pathomechanism of many diseases. Nowadays, along with the concept of so-called "hot spots" in protein–protein interactions, which are well-defined interface regions responsible for most of the binding energy, these interfaces can be targeted with modulators. In order to apply structure-based design techniques to design PPIs modulators, a three-dimensional structure of protein complex has to be available. In this context in silico approaches, in particular protein–protein docking, are a valuable complement to experimental methods for elucidating 3D structure of protein complexes. Protein–protein docking is easy to use and does not require significant computer resources and time (in contrast to molecular dynamics) and it results in 3D structure of a protein complex (in contrast to sequence-based methods of predicting binding interfaces). However, protein–protein docking cannot address all the aspects of protein dynamics, in particular the global conformational changes during protein complex formation. In spite of this fact, protein–protein docking is widely used to model complexes of water-soluble proteins and less commonly to predict structures of transmembrane protein assemblies, including dimers and oligomers of G protein-coupled receptors (GPCRs). In this chapter we review the principles of protein–protein docking, available algorithms and software and discuss the recent examples, benefits, and drawbacks of protein–protein docking application to water-soluble proteins, membrane anchoring and transmembrane proteins, including GPCRs.

Key words Drug design and discovery, GPCRs, Molecular modeling, Protein–protein docking, Transmembrane proteins, Water-soluble proteins

1 Introduction

Protein–protein interactions (PPIs) are at the heart of most cellular processes as they are involved in a number of cellular phenomena and greatly contribute to the complexity and diversity of living organisms [1]. The human interactome has been estimated to cover about 400,000 PPIs [2]. Protein–protein interactions underlie the very basics of any aspect of life, including protein regulation or signal transmission. Malfunctions of such interaction patterns may result in cancer or immune disorders [1]. Gathering knowledge on interactions of viral or bacterial protein can facilitate the

Mohini Gore and Umesh B. Jagtap (eds.), *Computational Drug Discovery and Design*, Methods in Molecular Biology, vol. 1762, https://doi.org/10.1007/978-1-4939-7756-7_15, © Springer Science+Business Media, LLC, part of Springer Nature 2018

design of vaccines or anti-infective drugs. Protein–protein interactions are thus responsible for various functions of the cell. The nature of those interactions can be better explained by applying three-dimensional structures of protein–protein complexes and binding affinity data [3]. Understanding the physical and structural principles which govern proteins binding is a challenging and only partially resolved problem in structural bioinformatics [4].

Targeting protein–protein interactions by small-molecule modulators has received a considerable attention as a drug design approach, conditioned, however, by the knowledge of 3D structure of a protein complex. [5]. Unfortunately, design of compounds targeting protein complexes has been hampered for a long time by the typical large and flat nature of protein interaction surfaces, often missing clear pockets for potential modulators [2]. The discovery of so-called "hot spots" in PPI interfaces which are well-defined regions responsible for most of the protein–protein binding energy has enabled the design and discovery of small molecule modulators, including orthosteric PPI inhibitors, stabilizers, and allosteric modulators [2].

In order to design PPI modulators, the 3D structure of the protein–protein complex has to be known from experimental or computational studies. As the number of X-ray-resolved protein–protein complexes is limited in available databases, computational approaches are a method of choice [6–8] when obtaining a reliable structure of the complex. In particular, protein–protein docking (PPD), which is not as resource-demanding as molecular dynamics, is commonly used for predicting the structures of protein complexes. While small-molecular docking is one of the most commonly applied molecular modeling methods (starting from the DOCK method published in 1982 by Kuntz et al. [9]), it should be stressed, however, that protein–protein docking is as old method (or even older) as traditional small-molecular docking [8], as the first true example of protein–protein docking originates to as early as 1970s [10]. Unfortunately, PPD is often much more problematic than docking of small molecules. One of the main reasons is the dynamic nature of proteins. While small molecules have a limited number of degrees of freedom, and some of them are rigid and well-defined, a typical protein structure undergoes constant fluctuations to a remarkable degree, and therefore should rather be considered as an ensemble of structures. This raises the problem with generating sufficient ensemble of conformations of docked proteins. Moreover, while a small-molecule orthosteric binding site can be reliably identified with various methods, identification of protein interaction interfaces is a challenging task. In terms of pose sampling, it is a bit easier when at least one of the partner is a membrane-spanning protein, because then it is possible to restrict the search for interaction interfaces to some protein surfaces (transmembrane regions when both partners are membrane-spanning proteins, or extracellular/intracellular when the other protein is soluble). Meanwhile, docking of two soluble proteins has to be careful and well validated.

Despite these difficulties, protein–protein docking is currently a well-established method, albeit not as widely used as small-molecular docking [8]. The number of reports on protein–protein docking applications are growing at an extraordinary rate. It can be explained by the emerging enormous importance of PPIs in many fields. The huge number of reports makes a detailed review impossible to fit in this chapter. However, some of the most recent reports may serve as good examples of various strategies of input data preparation, docking, and analysis of the results.

2 Basic Principles of Protein–Protein Docking

Although it could be expected that the performance of protein–protein docking is far below the one of small-molecular docking [8], an excellent review by Joël Janin [11] clearly does not support this assumption. Moreover, The Critical Assessment of PRedicted Interactions (CAPRI) [10–13], a community-wide initiative established in 2001, regularly reports the considerable progress in protein–protein docking algorithms and more and more reliable protein complexes structure prediction [14]. Among 42 CAPRI protein–protein complexes modeled in 2001–2010 only six have not been successfully modeled.

Docking of two proteins requires appropriate rotational and translational positioning of the binding partners, which can be efficiently solved by fast-Fourier transformation techniques or geometric hashing techniques, both referred to as rigid-body docking [15]. A common assumption of protein–protein docking methods is that protein–protein interaction can be modeled based on shape complementarity and using simplified amino acid models (in a similar fashion as typically used in early day molecular mechanics united-atom force fields) [8]. Rigid-body docking programs usually locate one protein in a fixed position while the other is moved, exploring its rotatranslational space around the first one [16]. The process of docking usually consists of two or three steps [17] which include: (a) the searching stage which involves generation of putative protein–protein complexes, (b) the sampling stage which involves clustering and scoring of complexes obtained in stage (a), and (c) the last stage which includes refinement (optional) and ranking of potential solutions (scoring, filtering) [16]. In the scoring step, the candidate protein complexes are evaluated using scoring functions reflecting the geometric and physicochemical complementarity of the proteins, using measures that describe electrostatics, H-bonding interactions and solvation, and that might include also empirical potentials or database-derived functions [16].

While originally most of the protein–protein docking methods were based on the rigid-docking approach, the majority of the present approaches are able to consider at least protein side-chain flexibility [8]. Flexibility is a critical condition of the quality of protein–protein docking, as in the CAPRI experiment most of the failures are connected with inaccurately predicting protein conformational changes upon protein–protein interaction [8]. One possibility to directly apply computationally efficient rigid docking algorithms is to indirectly consider receptor flexibility by representing the receptor target as an ensemble of structures (e.g., from NMR studies or molecular dynamics simulations) [17]. A limited number of starting configurations (in case of knowledge of the binding sites) can be modeled by combination of docking with molecular dynamics or Monte Carlo simulations which enables full atomic flexibility or flexibility restricted to relevant parts of the proteins during docking [17]. In case of some protein complexes, not only partner adjustment occurs during the process of binding, but also a global conformational change takes place. In such a situation Elastic Network Model (ENM) calculations (based on simple distance-dependent springs between protein atoms) may be successfully used to address the mobility of proteins around a stable state [17]. Another possibility is to apply soft collective normal mode directions as additional variables during docking by energy minimization [17].

3   Algorithms and Software for Protein–Protein Docking

Global docking programs that are used for ab initio docking, sample the relative binding orientations or poses between interacting proteins over all six translational and rotational degrees of freedom without the necessity of knowledge about the binding site [5]. Due to the high cost of the searching stage of docking, an efficient search strategy is critical for good performance of global docking software. In this context, the majority of available global docking programs make use of FFT (Fast Fourier Transform) correlation search algorithms (FTDock, GRAMM, MolFit, DOT, ZDOCK, PIPER), while few global docking programs such as ATTRACT, PatchDock, and SwarmDock are based on other types of search strategies like randomized search or local shape matching over the whole protein [5]. Because of the required computational efficacy, some early docking programs used only simple scoring functions including shape complementarity and/or hydrophobic interactions (e.g., GRAMM or MolFit). More advanced programs, such as PatchDock uses geometric hashing for fast surface patch matching [5]. ZDOCK also employs an advanced pairwise method to use efficiently shape complementarity. Electrostatic interactions contribution was first introduced in Fit-Dock and later became routine in such programs like MolFit, DOT, HEX, and ATTRACT. The desolvation effects are also considered in ZDOCK, FRODOCK, and SDOCK. A summary of main global docking programs is given in Table 1.

Table 1
A summary of global docking programs

Software	Search algorithm	Scoring function	Reference (s)
ATTRACT	Randomized search	LJ-type effective potentials and electrostatics	[18]
PatchDock/ SymmDock	Local shape match	Geometric shape complementarity	[19]
FTDOCK	FFT-based correlation	Shape complementarity and electrostatic interactions	[20]
GRAMM	FFT-based correlation	Shape and hydrophobic match	[21]
GRAMMX	FFT-based correlation	Soft Lennard–Jones potential, evolutionary conservation of predicted interface, statistical residue–residue preference, volume of the minimum, empirical binding free energy and atomic contact energy	[22]
MolFit	FFT-based correlation	Geometric complementarity, hydrophobic complementarity, and electrostatic interactions	[23–25]
DOT	FFT-based correlation	van der Waals and electrostatic energies	[26, 27]
ZDOCK	FFT-based correlation	Shape complementarity, electrostatics, and knowledge-based pair potentials	[28]
PIPER	FFT-based correlation	Shape complementarity, electrostatic interactions, and knowledge-based pair potentials	[29]
SDOCK	FFT-based correlation	van der Waals attractive potential, geometric collision, electrostatic potential, and desolvation energy	[30]
ClusPro	FFT-based correlation	Shape complementarity, electrostatics and desolvation energy	[31, 32]
HEX	SFT-based correlation	Surface complementarity and electrostatics	[33]
FRODOCK	SFT-based correlation	van der Waals, electrostatics, and desolvation	[34]
HADDOCK	Randomization of orientations and rigid body energy minimization followed by semi-rigid simulated annealing in torsion angle space, and finally refinement in Cartesian space with explicit solvent	Sum of intermolecular van der Waals, electrostatic, ambiguous interaction restraint energy, the buried surface area and the desolvation energy	[35, 36]

4   Application of Protein–Protein Docking to Water-Soluble, Membrane-Anchoring, and Integral Membrane Proteins

Most protein–protein docking software was tailored for water-soluble proteins (Fig. 1). There are a number of attempts to evaluate protein–protein docking software for this purpose. In particular, the protein–protein docking benchmark 4.0 by the Weng group [37] was used to evaluate the docking performance of available software. The benchmark has a total of 176 diverse targets including 52 enzyme–inhibitor, 25 antibody–antigen, and 99 cases with other function. Huang et al. [5] performed a comprehensive assessment of the 18 docking/scoring protocols of 14 global docking

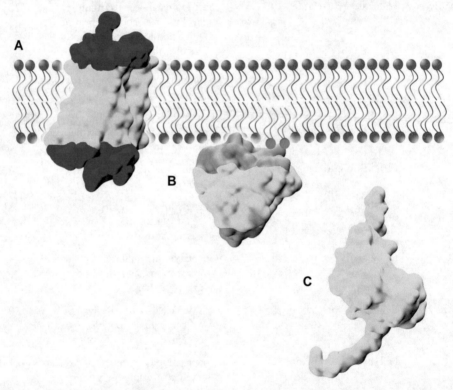

Fig. 1 Example of protein–protein interaction interfaces considered in particular classes of proteins. (**a**) Transmembrane protein dimerization involves only transmembrane domains, which restricts interface search to these regions only (yellow), which can facilitate docking as long as the software allows for appropriate settings. On the other hand, interactions of transmembrane proteins with soluble proteins are likely to involve the solvent-exposed regions only (blue; on the example of a GPCR, discussed farther in the main text, PDB ID: 4dkl). (**b**) Also dimerization of membrane-anchored proteins is to some extent facilitated by supposed restriction of possible dimerization interface localization (yellow; on example of K-Ras protein investigated by Prakash et al., discussed in the text, PDB ID: 4lv6). (**c**) In turn, soluble proteins are surrounded by solvent, and a binding partner can approach from any side (the entire surface can potentially bind proteins, which is indicated by yellow surface; on example of viral capsid protein investigated by Antal et al., which is discussed in the text, PDB ID: 1za7)

programs on the protein docking benchmark 4.0. They demonstrated that the docking performance depends on the target and no program is able to perform well for all the cases of the benchmark, though some algorithms are more robust than others [5]. They concluded that ZDOCK3.0.2, SDOCK, and PIPER resulted in the relatively higher success rates with 30.7%, 22.7%, and 21.0% for top ten predictions. Moreover, ZDOCK3.0.2, ATTRACT, and FRO-DOCK are all good choices if more predictions can be evaluated which is often the case in a postdocking approach [5].

Not only the suitability of the programs but also other factors might affect the docking results. Vajda et al. [38] demonstrated that the success in protein–protein docking experiment depends on three factors: (a) the quantity of conformational changes upon binding, (b) the area of interface surface, and (c) the hydrophobicity of the interface which allows to classify the docking tasks into five groups based on the difficulty of docking [16]. Briefly, Vajda et al. [38] postulated that docking is facilitated by low conformational change upon complex formation (Ca RMSD < 2 Å) (*see* **Note 1**), a large surface interface (700–1000 Å), and high hydrophobicity ($DG_{des} < -4.0$ kcal/mol).

Some of the most recent examples of application of protein–protein docking (PPD) software to water-soluble and membrane-anchoring proteins described below provide a general overview on the potential and importance of the method.

In the field of cancer research Ramatenki et al. focused on the ubiquitin-conjugating enzyme E2D4 and its binding partner, ubiquitin ligase CHIP. They used a range of tools to identify putative binding sites, and dock the ligase with PatchDock server [19]. The resultant complex structure was used for further virtual screening. Unfortunately, the study lacks any experimental validation. However, it is an example of application of protein–protein docking for design of small-molecule ligands.

Selent et al. [39] used protein–protein docking with Patch-Dock to model the survivin/CDK4 complex. Survivin is the smallest known inhibitor of apoptosis protein (IAP) and a valid target for cancer research [39]. Selent et al. also assessed electrostatic complementarity using APBS software and shape complementarity based on fractal approach [40–43]. They performed molecular dynamics simulation to obtain a refined survivin/CDK4 model that can be used for structure-based design of inhibitors modifying its interface recognition (*see* **Note 2**).

Research on viral infections can also take advantage from PPD. A very interesting and promising application was recently reported by Yoshiyuki Suzuki [42]. It focuses on the problem of interspecies transmission of viruses, which poses a potential threat for present medicine. He investigated interactions of a viral protein from measles virus with a transmembrane protein—signaling lymphocyte activation molecule (SLAM). The protein is known to be one of the main players involved in virus entry. Variants of the protein found in various species show different propensity to be targeted by the virus. Suzuki used this fact in his computational study. He prepared models of various variants of SLAM and performed docking of the viral protein with ClusPro. It turned out that the docking score values appropriately ranked SLAM variants with different potential of viral protein binding. Suzuki proposes this approach as a possible method for evaluation of the risk of viral interspecies transmission.

Another valuable application of PPD to understand viral infection mechanisms was reported by Dar et al. [43]. They focused on the problem of the Zika virus infections. The problem is important, since there is an increase in the number of infections, while there is no FDA approved drug for Zika treatment. Dar et al. investigated interactions of Zika non-structural protein 5 (NS5) with targets in human cells, i.e., signal transducer and activator of transcription 2 (STAT2) and seven in absenthia homolog 2 (SIAH2). The study contributes to understanding of how the virus decreases antiviral response in infected individuals. The input was carefully elaborated; for example, the authors prepared the input structures with short molecular dynamics simulations instead of utilizing rough minimized X-ray structures. The docking step was performed with HADDOCK.

While studies of Dar et al. and of Suzuki touch the problem of viral infections, a recent work of Antal et al. utilizes viral proteins for a more general study [44]. They use a viral capsid protein as an example of a protein with multiple interaction surfaces, capable of spontaneous hierarchical oligomerization into capsids. For instance, they use Rosetta and Amber for rescoring the results. Rosetta and ZDOCK were used for blind docking. Their approach allowed for estimation of possible oligomerization order, starting from dimer formation and further to higher-order complexes.

Mechanisms of bacterial infections can also be elucidated with PPD. Such efforts can support design of efficient vaccines. For instance, Hossain et al. recently examined antigenic proteins of *Mycobacterium tuberculosis* [45]. The aim of their study was to find a bacterial protein suitable as a target for potential vaccines. The initial search performed with Vaxign server [46] suggested that the extracellular protein 85B might be a favorable target. Subsequently, the docking simulation with Molsoft ICM pro [47] was used to investigate interactions of the epitope with the major histocompatibility complex proteins (MHC).

MHC is a group of protein complexes responsible for processing of antigens and presenting them to T lymphocytes. Rawal et al. recently investigated an MHC complex called DM, formed by association of DMa and DMb subunits [48]. They used the Computed Atlas of Surface Topography of Protein (CASTp) server [49] to find putative residues participating in the interaction. The identified residues were used as docking restraints in HADDOCK. They generated a large initial population of complexes, and 20% of the top scoring results were subjected to next iteration, refined and scored with HADDOCK score, Z-score and electrostatic energy values. The best cluster of complexes was analyzed with PISA (Protein Interfaces, Surfaces, and Assemblies) [50].

The study of Rawal et al. used PPD as a complement of experimental study, which allowed for better characterization of the investigated complex. The in silico part of the work focused on preparation and examination of a static complex structure. In turn, a recent work of Sinha et al. investigates dynamic behavior of a complex of an enzyme (trypsin) and an enzyme-activated protein (Complement component 4) with PPD and subsequent molecular dynamics simulations [51]. The docking was performed with ClusPro server. The molecular dynamics step was performed with Gromacs. Notably, the trajectory analysis was performed with Principal Component Analysis which is, next to information theory-based methods, one of the best ways of getting insight into underlying mechanisms of protein function. The study provided some insights into activation of complement components.

A recent contribution of Prakash et al. can serve as a great example of a complex study in the field of cancer research, employing protein–protein docking method [52]. It focuses on K-Ras4B. Mutations of this protein are responsible for a significant percent of human cancers. The protein contains a membrane-anchoring fragment, which facilitates rejection of the least probable docking results. The docking was based on previous studies, which provided some insights into possible dimerization interfaces with probe-based molecular dynamics. These putative interfaces were used during docking with RosettaDock. Docking results were grouped in clusters, and cluster representatives were investigated with regular molecular dynamics simulations in membrane. This step allowed for rejection of complexes which dissociated, and the complexes which improved their interaction energy and presented increase in the buried surface area were chosen for further investigation. The computational part of the study allowed for identification of key regions crucial for dimerization. Subsequent mutagenetic study confirmed the role of postulated interactions in dimerization. The work of Prakash et al. demonstrates how the protein–protein docking study, preceded by careful interaction interface prediction and followed by experimental validation can provide valuable insight into protein behavior.

5   Application of Protein–Protein Docking to GPCR Oligomers

G-protein coupled receptors (GPCRs) are a class of receptor proteins that constitute the largest part of transmembrane proteins in the human genome. Currently they are the molecular target of above 30% of marketed drugs [53]. Receptors belonging to this class share a common topology of seven transmembrane helixes, connected by three extracellular and intracellular loops, and an amphipathic helix 8. They react to extracellular stimuli like light or chemical molecules, and in response initiate diverse signaling cascades through binding with intracellular signaling agents. Due to their diversity and ubiquity in the human organism, these receptors are involved in almost every aspect of human physiology and various diseases [54].

The initial understanding of those proteins was that they elicit their signaling response as a consequence of interacting with various ligands in a 1:1 stoichiometry [55]. Currently, overwhelming experimental data suggests that those proteins can form dimers and higher order oligomers with other GPCRs. Intriguingly, those complexes have a different signaling profile than a monomer [56–58], and in fact in C-class receptor, dimer formation is obligatory for canonical function [59]. Moreover, in A-class some signaling pathways cannot be initiated by monomer proteins [60, 61]. It also appears that there exists functional allosteric cross talk between receptors in a dimer, thus activation of one of the receptors through binding of a molecule can have effect on the other (i.e., change its ligand affinity) [62, 63]. Although GPCR dimerization seems to be an established concept, there is still a debate over prevalence of oligomerization and to what extent it impacts signaling [64, 65]. These doubts arise, because observed phenomena can be artifacts derived from protein overexpression [66, 67], and also current methods to study oligomerization describe protein–protein proximity, but not stability of formed oligomers [65].

Alterations in the formation of dimers in GPCRs have been suggested to be involved in many pathological conditions [68, 69]. Since those conditions are related to the dimer, and not one receptor alone, targeting oligomers shows promise for a tailored and effective therapeutic intervention. Such ligands can utilize two strategies (Fig. 2):

- Act through both proteins forming the dimers, thus stabilizing the dimer.
- Bind to the dimer binding site to prevent its formation.

Ligands from the first group (called multivalent or bivalent ligands) consist of pharmacophores, which are able to bind specific receptors forming the oligomer, a spacer connecting them, and two linkers connecting the pharmacophores to the spacer [70]. Ligands from the second group are primarily peptides [71–74].

Obtaining reliable GPCR multimer structures enables further insight into the dynamics of dimer formation, stability, and rational design of ligands targeting dimers (i.e., adjusting the length and flexibility of the spacer in case of bivalent ligands). That being said,

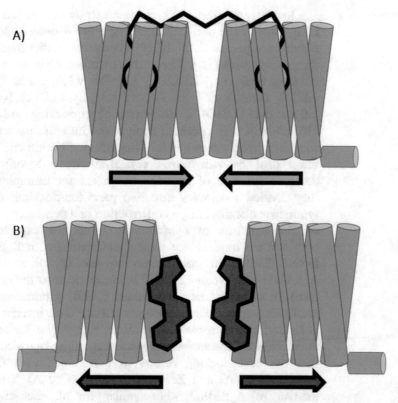

Fig. 2 A schematic representation of two drug design strategies when targeting GPCR dimers: (**a**) Ligands that stabilize and facilitate the formation of dimers; (**b**) ligands that prevent the formation of dimers, by competitively binding to sites involved in GPCR-GPCR binding

it is very hard to obtain experimentally solved structures of GPCR multimers. Currently, the GPCR-OKB database holds information of about 192 distinct GPCR multimers [75]. Among them only a very small fraction has an available experimentally solved crystal structure. Moreover, all of the available structures are homodimers, whereas detailed structural insights into heteromers are completely missing.

Numerous experimentally solved structures of individual proteins forming the multimer (protomers) exist. Furthermore, homology modeling is highly efficient in predicting their structure [76], and thus it is tempting to utilize PPD for obtaining structural insights into the structure of GPCR oligomers.

PPD is not commonly used to model complexes of transmembrane proteins (Fig. 1). The same research group [78] published an extension to the outer membrane phospholipase A protein (OMPLA) of the docking-based protocols previously developed for quaternary structure predictions of transmembrane oligomeric proteins and for estimating mutational effects on the thermodynamics of protein–protein and protein–DNA association.

Recently an extensive benchmark study was carried out, evaluating most of the currently available protein–protein docking protocols in respect to their ability to correctly predict transmembrane dimer structures [16]. The authors studied eight protein–protein docking tools, i.e., ZDOCK, ClusPro v.1.0, HEX, GRAMM-X v.1.2.0, PatchDock (version beta 1.3), SymmDock (version beta 1.0), and HADDOCK. They used blind docking; only in case of HADDOCK they indicated a pair of residues for interaction as only such an option was available. They selected multimeric transmembrane proteins with known crystal structure deposited in PDB database. In case of proteins which are for example pentamers they divided a complex into two parts for docking or applied a symmetric docking, i.e., a construction of a pentamer model based on the structure of a monomer. In all the experiments they obtained ten models that were characterized with B_RMSD (the lowest RMSD in comparison to the crystal structure) and A_RMSD (the average RMSD in comparison to the crystal structure). In addition, they determined CAPRI parameters and structural parameters, such as complex surface area, interface area, and polar and hydrophobic contributions to complex surface area and interface area. The analysis of results regarding B_RMSD indicated that the best docking results were obtained with GRAMM-X (median 0.27 Å) and ZDOCK (median 4.20 Å). The values of median of A_RMSD were similar for all the studied tools (11–13 Å). It can be concluded that best protein–protein docking tools result in a few correct models which need to be separated from a great number of incorrect models. Thus, it is not problematic to obtain a correct model but it is a challenge to select scoring functions for the obtained population of models which place the correct models on the top of the ranking list (*see* **Note 3**). The encouraging results obtained using GRAMM-X may be illustrated by the fact that it was possible to reconstruct 9 of 12 studied complexes using this tool. As a comparison, the next successful tools, i.e., ZDOCK, HADDOCK, ClusPro (symmetric docking), and HEX were able to reconstruct four correct models only. Importantly, only one correct model was obtained with ClusPro using unsymmetrical docking. The main advantage of GRAMM-X over other tools may be connected with the presence of evolutionary conservation score (for interface) in a scoring function in this tool. The authors also analyzed structural features of transmembrane proteins which facilitate or hamper the application of protein–protein docking approach for generating reliable models. As it can be expected, it is easier to model transmembrane protein complexes with a large interface rich in structurally complementary cavities. This explains the lack of success in application of protein–protein docking technique to GPCR dimers. It is also well-known that if the complex formation is accompanied by a significant conformational change, protein–protein docking approach is not able to consider this change in conformation (*see* **Note 2**). The obtained results indicate that protein–protein docking should be used with great care when applied to modeling transmembrane protein complexes. Moreover, the main problem is to select a correct model from a large population of obtained models. It can be facilitated by taking into consideration the degree of evolutionary conservation of the interface and surface roughness.

One of the issues that prohibit protocols optimized for aqueous proteins to be used for GPCRs is scoring. When carrying out protein–protein docking, desolvation energy is an important scoring factor in many PPD methods. However, desolvation energy of aqueous proteins is an estimate of the energetic effect of residues which go out of the aqueous solution when engaging in protein–protein contacts [77]. This parameter is inaccurate for membrane proteins as they mainly desolvate from a hydrophobic membrane environment instead of an aqueous solution (*see* **Note 3**).

Currently there exists a protocol that aims specifically at generating accurate GPCR oligomer structures [79]. The approach generates 144 input structures by rotating each monomer by an increment of 30°, and submits those complexes to docking by Rosetta [80]. Afterward each complex is scored based on an extensive consensus approach tailored toward GPCR proteins that incorporates 11 scoring factors. The protocol provided satisfactory predictions for the structure of GPCR dimers available at the time. This protocol was used to model the dopamine D_2 receptor homodimer [81] resulting in asymmetric dimer model with TM1-TM2-TM4-TM5 interface [82]. To our knowledge, currently there are no other protocols aimed specifically at GPCRs, although in recent years a few other protocols aimed at membrane proteins have been developed.

The membrane-protein version of DOCK/PIERR [83] scores generated poses based on empirically derived residue contact potentials and further rescores them using a membrane protein-specific energy function. The rescoring function employs predicted energy costs of residue transfers between the solute and membrane, obtained from molecular dynamics experiments [84].

Transmembrane protein complexes are often modeled using RosettaDock [5, 17, 80] which is a multiscale docking algorithm based on the Monte Carlo (MC) method. This approach which incorporates both a low resolution, centroid-mode, coarse-grain stage and a high resolution, all-atom refinement stage that optimizes both rigid-body orientation and side-chain conformation [79].

A newly developed Rosetta framework for membrane proteins (Rosetta MP) includes a protocol for protein docking [85]. It consists of a prepacking step to generate a starting structure (in which the proteins are separated by a distance, optimized by rotamer trials of the residues, and moved back together). Next, it samples and scores different interfaces, using a function taking into account membrane score terms.

Memdock is an algorithm developed specifically for α-helical transmembrane proteins [86]. In this approach, the docking poses are generated using rigid docking, with subsequent structure refinement carried out through side-chain rotations and a normal mode analysis-based backbone refinement. In both the steps the proteins complexes are kept in a membrane consistent orientation. The scoring of obtained complexes is carried out using a function that takes into account membrane properties, distinguishing its specific sublayers. The weights for scoring were optimized using a training set of available membrane proteins.

Due to their impressive speed in generating and scoring poses, protein–protein docking methods are an attractive tool, when studying GPCR-GPCR dimerization. Using these methods, it is possible to quickly obtain reliable structures of membrane protein multimers, without having to rely on computationally demanding lengthy molecular dynamics simulations. Currently, the main challenge appears to be optimizing protocols for membrane proteins. First of all, it is necessary to limit the pose generation step, so it takes into account only complexes where both of the proteins are in the membrane. Secondly, the energetic scoring functions need to be adapted to properly score binding events occurring in the hydrophobic environment of the membrane (see Note 3).

The latter point raises the question as to the type of implicit membrane that should be utilized in scoring algorithms as the membrane environment has been shown to impact GPCR-GPCR dimerization [87]. In particular, receptor aggregation is sensitive to the membrane thickness which depends on the composition of the membrane. For instance, membranes with a high content of unsaturated lipids are condensed and thicker, whereas fully saturated lipids yield thinner membranes [88]. While it is easy to address this issue using full-atom simulations, in terms of docking we are still away from a unified algorithm that can take into account membrane diversity.

It is important to mention that docking provides a static snapshot of the interaction between the two proteins. A reliable oligomer model can help rationalize the impact of certain mutations or signaling diversity on the frequency of protein–protein contacts, it can be also used as a tool for the rational design of ligands targeting GPCR multimers, but to observe how formation of such a unit impacts signaling, it is crucial to utilize techniques that have a bigger temporal resolution, and better account for protein fluctuations.

6   Advantages and Disadvantages of Protein–Protein Docking

The examples of PPD studies described above show that the method can be used for various purposes. Nowadays, protein–protein docking is the most useful technique for modeling protein complexes by combining several advantages: (a) It is easy to use; (b) it returns results quickly and does not require significant computer resources (particularly when compared to MD techniques); and (c) it provides a structural model for the complexes (unlike sequence based methods that only highlight interface-forming residues) [16]. As such, it can very quickly provide some clues or initial hypotheses for further investigation. It can also provide several complexes for further testing. It is clearly an advantage over the more accurate, but significantly slower experimental methods like X-ray crystallography. However, it has to be stressed that drawbacks of the method, i.e., difficulty of proper identification of interaction interface, limited possibility of side chain and backbone flexibility consideration (*see* **Note 2**) and uncertainty of scoring (*see* **Note 3**), make the method more suitable as support for experimental methods or to be used together with molecular dynamics simulations rather than an independent experimental tool. Therefore, while application of PPD can significantly reduce the time and cost of a mutagenetic study, any protein–protein docking results should be treated with a limited trust, and can be considered conclusive only if validated.

7   Summary and Perspective

A number of protein–protein docking algorithms are now available to address the problem of protein–protein interactions and to provide 3D structures of protein complexes necessary for application of structure-based design techniques. A considerable progress has been achieved regarding the development of scoring functions based on physical interactions, shape complementarity, geometry, interface water molecules, and the accommodation of protein flexibility [3]. The capabilities of protein–protein docking software can be improved as it can be concluded from CAPRI experiments. The importance of protein–protein docking approaches can increase in future due to the attractive possibility of designing protein–protein interaction modulators. On the other hand, along with the availability of advanced molecular dynamics techniques and progress in computational power and resources, the application of protein–protein docking might become complementary to molecular dynamics simulations.

8 Notes

1. In case of proteins undergoing significant conformational changes upon binding, sampling of available conformational space would be useful. In such cases, molecular dynamics can be used as a source of additional conformations. However, sufficient sampling would require computationally expensive long simulations. Moreover, there would be no guarantee that all obtained conformations would be gathered from one well of potential, restrained by energetic barriers easy to overcome after the other protein binding. Therefore, accelerated molecular dynamics can be a tempting alternative—it is less computationally expensive and can easily overcome energetic barriers. However, it should still be handled with care, especially when applied to transmembrane proteins. Accelerated MD of a transmembrane protein immersed in a simplified, to fluid membrane may result in artifacts. At least, appropriate content of cholesterol should be ensured.

2. PPD methods take into account the flexibility of protein backbones and side chains to a very limited degree. As the formation of oligomers can induce significant structural changes in the participating molecules, it is prudent to refine the obtained complexes using molecular dynamics. Importantly, in the case of membrane proteins the complex should be embedded in a lipid bilayer of a similar composition as the environment where the modeled interaction is occurring. In the first step the simulated system should be equilibrated over the course of around 20 ns in npt conditions, with restraints applied to the backbone of the studied proteins. This step ensures sufficient lipid packing around the studied complex. In the step, the restraint should be gradually released from the complex during 20 ns, to enable the proteins to structurally adapt to each other and the environment. Finally, the complex should be simulated without any restraints until the backbone RMSD is converged.

3. A benchmark of the available PPD methods [16] has shown that most of the methods generate a complex that is highly similar to the experimentally solved structure. The pose is not selected as the best solution, due to the employed scoring methods. Thus when performing PPD of membrane proteins, the scoring method should be carefully considered. The method should not take into account parameters specific for aqueous proteins, like desolvation energy.

Acknowledgments

The chapter was developed using the equipment purchased within the project "The equipment of innovative laboratories doing research on new medicines used in the therapy of civilization and neoplastic diseases" within the Operational Program Development of Eastern Poland 2007–2013, Priority Axis I Modern Economy, operations I.3 Innovation promotion. T.S. and J.S. acknowledge support from Instituto de Salud Carlos III FEDER (CP12/03139 and PI15/00460). A.A.K., T.S. and J.S. participate in the European COST Action CM1207 (GLISTEN). T.S. acknowledges financial support from Hospital del Mar Medical Research Institute.

References

1. Andreani J, Guerois R (2014) Evolution of protein interactions: from interactomes to interfaces. Arch Biochem Biophys 554:65–75. https://doi.org/10.1016/j.abb.2014.05.010

2. Petta I, Lievens S, Libert C et al (2016) Modulation of protein-protein interactions for the development of novel therapeutics. Mol Ther J Am Soc Gene Ther 24:707–718. https://doi.org/10.1038/mt.2015.214

3. Gromiha MM, Yugandhar K, Jemimah S (2016) Protein-protein interactions: scoring schemes and binding affinity. Curr Opin Struct Biol 44:31–38. https://doi.org/10.1016/j.sbi.2016.10.016

4. Moal IH, Moretti R, Baker D, Fernández-Recio J (2013) Scoring functions for protein-protein interactions. Curr Opin Struct Biol 23:862–867. https://doi.org/10.1016/j.sbi.2013.06.017

5. Huang S-Y (2015) Exploring the potential of global protein-protein docking: an overview and critical assessment of current programs for automatic ab initio docking. Drug Discov Today 20:969–977. https://doi.org/10.1016/j.drudis.2015.03.007

6. Rodrigues JPGLM, Bonvin AMJJ (2014) Integrative computational modeling of protein interactions. FEBS J 281:1988–2003. https://doi.org/10.1111/febs.12771

7. Selent J, Kaczor AA (2011) Oligomerization of G protein-coupled receptors: computational methods. Curr Med Chem 18:4588–4605

8. Kaczor AA, Selent J, Poso A (2013) Structure-based molecular modeling approaches to GPCR oligomerization. Methods Cell Biol 117:91–104. https://doi.org/10.1016/B978-0-12-408143-7.00005-0

9. Kuntz ID, Blaney JM, Oatley SJ et al (1982) A geometric approach to macromolecule-ligand interactions. J Mol Biol 161:269–288

10. Wodak SJ, Janin J (1978) Computer analysis of protein-protein interaction. J Mol Biol 124:323–342

11. Janin J (2010) Protein-protein docking tested in blind predictions: the CAPRI experiment. Mol Biosyst 6:2351–2362. https://doi.org/10.1039/c005060c

12. Lensink MF, Wodak SJ (2013) Docking, scoring, and affinity prediction in CAPRI. Proteins 81:2082–2095. https://doi.org/10.1002/prot.24428

13. Lensink MF, Velankar S, Wodak SJ (2017) Modeling protein-protein and protein-peptide complexes: CAPRI 6th edition. Proteins 85:359–377. https://doi.org/10.1002/prot.25215

14. Bohnuud T, Luo L, Wodak SJ et al (2017) A benchmark testing ground for integrating homology modeling and protein docking. Proteins 85:10–16. https://doi.org/10.1002/prot.25063

15. Park H, Lee H, Seok C (2015) High-resolution protein-protein docking by global optimization: recent advances and future challenges. Curr Opin Struct Biol 35:24–31. https://doi.org/10.1016/j.sbi.2015.08.001

16. Kaczor AA, Selent J, Sanz F, Pastor M (2013) Modeling complexes of transmembrane proteins: systematic analysis of protein-protein docking tools. Mol Inform 32:717–733. https://doi.org/10.1002/minf.201200150

17. Zacharias M (2010) Accounting for conformational changes during protein-protein docking. Curr Opin Struct Biol 20:180–186. https://doi.org/10.1016/j.sbi.2010.02.001

18. Zacharias M (2003) Protein-protein docking with a reduced protein model accounting for side-chain flexibility. Protein Sci Publ Protein Soc 12:1271–1282. https://doi.org/10.1110/ps.0239303

19. Schneidman-Duhovny D, Inbar Y, Nussinov R, Wolfson HJ (2005) PatchDock and Symm-Dock: servers for rigid and symmetric docking. Nucleic Acids Res 33:W363–W367. https://doi.org/10.1093/nar/gki481

20. Gabb HA, Jackson RM, Sternberg MJ (1997) Modelling protein docking using shape complementarity, electrostatics and biochemical information. J Mol Biol 272:106–120. https://doi.org/10.1006/jmbi.1997.1203

21. Vakser IA (1997) Evaluation of GRAMM low-resolution docking methodology on the hemagglutinin-antibody complex. Proteins (Suppl 1):226–230

22. Tovchigrechko A, Vakser IA (2006) GRAMM-X public web server for protein-protein docking. Nucleic Acids Res 34:W310–W314. https://doi.org/10.1093/nar/gkl206

23. Katchalski-Katzir E, Shariv I, Eisenstein M et al (1992) Molecular surface recognition: determination of geometric fit between proteins and their ligands by correlation techniques. Proc Natl Acad Sci U S A 89:2195–2199

24. Berchanski A, Shapira B, Eisenstein M (2004) Hydrophobic complementarity in protein-protein docking. Proteins 56:130–142. https://doi.org/10.1002/prot.20145

25. Heifetz A, Katchalski-Katzir E, Eisenstein M (2002) Electrostatics in protein-protein docking. Protein Sci Publ Protein Soc 11:571–587

26. Mandell JG, Roberts VA, Pique ME et al (2001) Protein docking using continuum electrostatics and geometric fit. Protein Eng 14:105–113

27. Roberts VA, Thompson EE, Pique ME et al (2013) DOT2: macromolecular docking with improved biophysical models. J Comput Chem 34:1743–1758. https://doi.org/10.1002/jcc.23304

28. Wiehe K, Pierce B, Mintseris J et al (2005) ZDOCK and RDOCK performance in CAPRI rounds 3, 4, and 5. Proteins 60:207–213. https://doi.org/10.1002/prot.20559

29. Kozakov D, Brenke R, Comeau SR, Vajda S (2006) PIPER: an FFT-based protein docking program with pairwise potentials. Proteins 65:392–406. https://doi.org/10.1002/prot.21117

30. Zhang C, Lai L (2011) SDOCK: a global protein-protein docking program using stepwise force-field potentials. J Comput Chem 32:2598–2612. https://doi.org/10.1002/jcc.21839

31. Comeau SR, Gatchell DW, Vajda S, Camacho CJ (2004) ClusPro: a fully automated algorithm for protein-protein docking. Nucleic Acids Res 32:W96–W99. https://doi.org/10.1093/nar/gkh354

32. Comeau SR, Kozakov D, Brenke R et al (2007) ClusPro: performance in CAPRI rounds 6-11 and the new server. Proteins 69:781–785. https://doi.org/10.1002/prot.21795

33. Ritchie DW (2003) Evaluation of protein docking predictions using Hex 3.1 in CAPRI rounds 1 and 2. Proteins 52:98–106. https://doi.org/10.1002/prot.10379

34. Garzon JI, Lopéz-Blanco JR, Pons C et al (2009) FRODOCK: a new approach for fast rotational protein-protein docking. Bioinformatics 25:2544–2551. https://doi.org/10.1093/bioinformatics/btp447

35. Dominguez C, Boelens R, Bonvin AMJJ (2003) HADDOCK: a protein-protein docking approach based on biochemical or biophysical information. J Am Chem Soc 125:1731–1737. https://doi.org/10.1021/ja026939x

36. de Vries SJ, van Dijk ADJ, Krzeminski M et al (2007) HADDOCK versus HADDOCK: new features and performance of HADDOCK2.0 on the CAPRI targets. Proteins 69:726–733. https://doi.org/10.1002/prot.21723

37. Hwang H, Vreven T, Janin J, Weng Z (2010) Protein-protein docking benchmark version 4.0. Proteins 78:3111–3114. https://doi.org/10.1002/prot.22830

38. Vajda S (2005) Classification of protein complexes based on docking difficulty. Proteins 60:176–180. https://doi.org/10.1002/prot.20554

39. Selent J, Kaczor AA, Guixà-González R et al (2013) Rational design of the survivin/CDK4 complex by combining protein-protein docking and molecular dynamics simulations. J Mol Model 19:1507–1514. https://doi.org/10.1007/s00894-012-1705-8

40. Renthal R (1999) Transmembrane and water-soluble helix bundles display reverse patterns of surface roughness. Biochem Biophys Res Commun 263:714–717. https://doi.org/10.1006/bbrc.1999.1439

41. Kaczor AA, Guixà-González R, Carrió P et al (2012) Fractal dimension as a measure of surface roughness of G protein-coupled receptors: implications for structure and function. J Mol Model 18:4465–4475. https://doi.org/10.1007/s00894-012-1431-2

42. Suzuki Y (2017) Predicting receptor functionality of signaling lymphocyte activation molecule for measles virus hemagglutinin from docking simulation. Microbiol Immunol. https://doi.org/10.1111/1348-0421.12484

43. Dar HA, Zaheer T, Paracha RZ, Ali A (2017) Structural analysis and insight into Zika virus NS5 mediated interferon inhibition. Infect Genet Evol 51:143–152. https://doi.org/10.1016/j.meegid.2017.03.027

44. Antal Z, Szoverfi J, Fejer SN (2017) Predicting the initial steps of salt-stable cowpea chlorotic mottle virus capsid assembly with atomistic force fields. J Chem Inf Model 57:910–917. https://doi.org/10.1021/acs.jcim.7b00078

45. Hossain MS, Azad AK, Chowdhury PA, Wakayama M (2017) Computational identification and characterization of a promiscuous T-cell epitope on the extracellular protein 85B of mycobacterium spp. for peptide-based subunit vaccine design. Biomed Res Int 2017:4826030. https://doi.org/10.1155/2017/4826030

46. He Y, Xiang Z, Mobley HLT (2010) Vaxign: the first web-based vaccine design program for reverse vaccinology and applications for vaccine development. J Biomed Biotechnol 2010:297505. https://doi.org/10.1155/2010/297505

47. Totrov M, Abagyan R (1997) Flexible protein-ligand docking by global energy optimization in internal coordinates. Proteins (Suppl 1):215–220

48. Rawal L, Panwar D, Ali S (2017) Intermolecular interactions between DMα and DMβ proteins in BuLA-DM complex of water buffalo Bubalus bubalis. J Cell Biochem. https://doi.org/10.1002/jcb.26075

49. Dundas J, Ouyang Z, Tseng J et al (2006) CASTp: computed atlas of surface topography of proteins with structural and topographical mapping of functionally annotated residues. Nucleic Acids Res 34:W116–W118. https://doi.org/10.1093/nar/gkl282

50. Krissinel E, Henrick K (2007) Inference of macromolecular assemblies from crystalline state. J Mol Biol 372:774–797. https://doi.org/10.1016/j.jmb.2007.05.022

51. Sinha VK, Sharma OP, Kumar MS (2017) Insight into the intermolecular recognition mechanism involved in complement component 4 activation through serine protease-trypsin. J Biomol Struct Dyn:1–15. https://doi.org/10.1080/07391102.2017.1288658

52. Prakash P, Sayyed-Ahmad A, Cho KJ et al (2017) Computational and biochemical characterization of two partially overlapping interfaces and multiple weak-affinity K-Ras dimers. Sci Rep 7:40109. https://doi.org/10.1038/srep40109

53. Congreve M, Langmead CJ, Mason JS, Marshall FH (2011) Progress in structure based drug design for G protein-coupled receptors. J Med Chem 54:4283–4311. https://doi.org/10.1021/jm200371q

54. Pierce KL, Premont RT, Lefkowitz RJ (2002) Seven-transmembrane receptors. Nat Rev Mol Cell Biol 3:639–650. https://doi.org/10.1038/nrm908

55. Gilman AG (1987) G proteins: transducers of receptor-generated signals. Annu Rev Biochem 56:615–649. https://doi.org/10.1146/annurev.biochem.56.1.615

56. Bouvier M (2001) Oligomerization of G-protein-coupled transmitter receptors. Nat Rev Neurosci 2:274–286. https://doi.org/10.1038/35067575

57. Ferre S, Casado V, Devi LA et al (2014) G protein-coupled receptor oligomerization revisited: functional and pharmacological perspectives. Pharmacol Rev 66:413–434. https://doi.org/10.1124/pr.113.008052

58. González-Maeso J (2011) GPCR oligomers in pharmacology and signaling. Mol Brain 4:20. https://doi.org/10.1186/1756-6606-4-20

59. Kniazeff J, Prézeau L, Rondard P et al (2011) Dimers and beyond: the functional puzzles of class C GPCRs. Pharmacol Ther 130:9–25. https://doi.org/10.1016/j.pharmthera.2011.01.006

60. Bellot M, Galandrin S, Boularan C et al (2015) Dual agonist occupancy of AT1-R-α2C-AR heterodimers results in atypical Gs-PKA signaling. Nat Chem Biol 11:271–279. https://doi.org/10.1038/nchembio.1766

61. Rashid AJ, So CH, Kong MMC et al (2007) D1–D2 dopamine receptor heterooligomers with unique pharmacology are coupled to rapid activation of Gq/11 in the striatum. Proc Natl Acad Sci U S A 104:654–659. https://doi.org/10.1073/pnas.0604049104

62. Han Y, Moreira IS, Urizar E et al (2009) Allosteric communication between protomers of dopamine class A GPCR dimers modulates activation. Nat Chem Biol 5:688–695. https://doi.org/10.1038/nchembio.199

63. Smith NJ, Milligan G (2010) Allostery at G protein-coupled receptor homo- and heteromers: uncharted pharmacological landscapes. Pharmacol Rev 62:701–725. https://doi.org/10.1124/pr.110.002667

64. Bouvier M, Hébert TE (2014) CrossTalk proposal: weighing the evidence for class A GPCR dimers, the evidence favours dimers. J Physiol

304   Agnieszka A. Kaczor et al.

592:2439–2441. https://doi.org/10.1113/jphysiol.2014.272252

65. Lambert NA, Javitch JA (2014) CrossTalk opposing view: weighing the evidence for class A GPCR dimers, the jury is still out. J Physiol 592:2443–2445. https://doi.org/10.1113/jphysiol.2014.272997

66. James JR, Oliveira MI, Carmo AM et al (2006) A rigorous experimental framework for detecting protein oligomerization using bioluminescence resonance energy transfer. Nat Methods 3:1001–1006. https://doi.org/10.1038/nmeth978

67. Meyer BH, Segura J-M, Martinez KL et al (2006) FRET imaging reveals that functional neurokinin-1 receptors are monomeric and reside in membrane microdomains of live cells. Proc Natl Acad Sci U S A 103:2138–2143. https://doi.org/10.1073/pnas.0507686103

68. Gaitonde SA, Gonzá Lez-Maeso J (2017) Contribution of heteromerization to G protein-coupled receptor function. Curr Opin Pharmacol 32:23–31. https://doi.org/10.1016/j.coph.2016.10.006

69. Guidolin D, Agnati LF, Marcoli M et al (2014) G-protein-coupled receptor type A heteromers as an emerging therapeutic target. Expert Opin Ther Targets 8222:1–19. https://doi.org/10.1517/14728222.2014.981155

70. Shonberg J, Scammells PJ, Capuano B (2011) Design strategies for bivalent ligands targeting GPCRs. ChemMedChem 6:963–974. https://doi.org/10.1002/cmdc.201100101

71. Viñals X, Moreno E, Lanfumey L et al (2015) Cognitive impairment induced by delta9-tetrahydrocannabinol occurs through heteromers between cannabinoid CB_1 and serotonin 5-HT2A receptors. PLoS Biol. https://doi.org/10.1371/journal.pbio.1002194

72. Jastrzebska B, Chen Y, Orban T et al (2015) Disruption of rhodopsin dimerization with synthetic peptides targeting an interaction interface. J Biol Chem 290:25728–25744. https://doi.org/10.1074/jbc.M115.662684

73. Wang J, He L, Combs C et al (2006) Dimerization of CXCR4 in living malignant cells: control of cell migration by a synthetic peptide that reduces homologous CXCR4 interactions. Mol Cancer Ther 5:2474–2483. https://doi.org/10.1158/1535-7163.MCT-05-0261

74. Hebert TE, Moffett S, Morello JP et al (1996) A peptide derived from a beta2-adrenergic receptor transmembrane domain inhibits both receptor dimerization and activation. J Biol Chem 271:16384–16392. https://doi.org/10.1074/jbc.271.27.16384

75. Khelashvili G, Dorff K, Shan J et al (2010) GPCR-OKB: the G protein coupled receptor oligomer knowledge base. Bioinformatics 26:1804–1805. https://doi.org/10.1093/bioinformatics/btq264

76. Kufareva I, Katritch V, Participants of GPCR Dock 2013, Stevens RC, Abagyan R (2014) Advances in GPCR modeling evaluated by the GPCR Dock 2013 assessment: meeting new challenges. Structure 22:1120–1139. https://doi.org/10.1016/j.str.2014.06.012

77. Casciari D, Seeber M, Fanelli F (2006) Quaternary structure predictions of transmembrane proteins starting from the monomer: a docking-based approach. BMC Bioinformatics 7:340. https://doi.org/10.1186/1471-2105-7-340

78. Dell'Orco D, Casciari D, Fanelli F (2008) Quaternary structure predictions and estimation of mutational effects on the free energy of dimerization of the OMPLA protein. J Struct Biol 163:155–162. https://doi.org/10.1016/j.jsb.2008.05.006

79. Kaczor AA, Guixà-González R, Carrió P et al (2015) Multi-component protein – protein docking based protocol with external scoring for modeling dimers of g protein-coupled receptors. Mol Inform 34:246–255. https://doi.org/10.1002/minf.201400088

80. Chaudhury S, Berrondo M, Weitzner BD et al (2011) Benchmarking and analysis of protein docking performance in Rosetta v3.2. PLoS One 6:e22477. https://doi.org/10.1371/journal.pone.0022477

81. Jörg M, Kaczor AA, Mak FS et al (2014) Investigation of novel ropinirole analogues: synthesis, pharmacological evaluation and computational analysis of dopamine D2 receptor functionalized congeners and homobivalent ligands. MedChemComm 5:891–898. https://doi.org/10.1039/C4MD00066H

82. Kaczor AA, Jörg M, Capuano B (2016) The dopamine D2 receptor dimer and its interaction with homobivalent antagonists: homology modeling, docking and molecular dynamics. J Mol Model 22:203. https://doi.org/10.1007/s00894-016-3065-2

83. Viswanath S, Dominguez L, Foster LS et al (2015) Extension of a protein docking algorithm to membranes and applications to amyloid precursor protein dimerization. Proteins 83:2170–2185. https://doi.org/10.1002/prot.24934

84. MacCallum JL, Bennett WFD, Tieleman DP (2007) Partitioning of amino acid side chains into lipid bilayers: results from computer simulations and comparison to experiment. J Gen

Physiol 129:371–377. https://doi.org/10.1085/jgp.200709745

85. Alford RF, Koehler Leman J, Weitzner BD et al (2015) An integrated framework advancing membrane protein modeling and design. PLoS Comput Biol. https://doi.org/10.1371/journal.pcbi.1004398

86. Hurwitz N, Schneidman-Duhovny D, Wolfson HJ (2016) Memdock: an α-helical membrane protein docking algorithm. Bioinformatics 32:2444–2450. https://doi.org/10.1093/bioinformatics/btw184

87. Guixà-González R, Javanainen M, Gómez-Soler M et al (2016) Membrane omega-3 fatty acids modulate the oligomerisation kinetics of adenosine A2A and dopamine D2 receptors. Sci Rep 6:19839. https://doi.org/10.1038/srep19839

88. Tusnády GE, Dosztányi Z, Simon I (2005) TMDET: web server for detecting transmembrane regions of proteins by using their 3D coordinates. Bioinformatics 21:1276–1277. https://doi.org/10.1093/bioinformatics/bti121

Chapter 16

Automated Inference of Chemical Discriminants of Biological Activity

Sebastian Raschka, Anne M. Scott, Mar Huertas, Weiming Li, and Leslie A. Kuhn

Abstract

Ligand-based virtual screening has become a standard technique for the efficient discovery of bioactive small molecules. Following assays to determine the activity of compounds selected by virtual screening, or other approaches in which dozens to thousands of molecules have been tested, machine learning techniques make it straightforward to discover the patterns of chemical groups that correlate with the desired biological activity. Defining the chemical features that generate activity can be used to guide the selection of molecules for subsequent rounds of screening and assaying, as well as help design new, more active molecules for organic synthesis.

The quantitative structure–activity relationship machine learning protocols we describe here, using decision trees, random forests, and sequential feature selection, take as input the chemical structure of a single, known active small molecule (e.g., an inhibitor, agonist, or substrate) for comparison with the structure of each tested molecule. Knowledge of the atomic structure of the protein target and its interactions with the active compound are not required. These protocols can be modified and applied to any data set that consists of a series of measured structural, chemical, or other features for each tested molecule, along with the experimentally measured value of the response variable you would like to predict or optimize for your project, for instance, inhibitory activity in a biological assay or $\Delta G_{binding}$. To illustrate the use of different machine learning algorithms, we step through the analysis of a dataset of inhibitor candidates from virtual screening that were tested recently for their ability to inhibit GPCR-mediated signaling in a vertebrate.

Key words Fingerprint analysis, GPCR, Invasive species control, Ligand-based screening, Machine learning, Pharmacophore, Quantitative structure–activity relationship, Random forest, Virtual screening

Abbreviations

2D	Two-dimensional
3D	Three-dimensional
3kPZS	3-keto petromyzonol sulfate
CAS	Chemical Abstracts Service Registry
CSD	Cambridge Structural Database
DKPES	3,12-diketo-4,6-petromyzonene-24-sulfate

Mohini Gore and Umesh B. Jagtap (eds.), *Computational Drug Discovery and Design*, Methods in Molecular Biology, vol. 1762, https://doi.org/10.1007/978-1-4939-7756-7_16, © Springer Science+Business Media, LLC, part of Springer Nature 2018

EOG   Electro-olfactogram
GPCR   G protein-coupled receptor
QSAR   Quantitative structure–activity relationship
SBS   Sequential backward selection
SFS   Sequential feature selection
VS   Virtual screening
ZINC12   Zinc Is Not Commercial database, version 12

1 Introduction

In this chapter, we apply machine learning to analyze the results from a virtual screening (VS) project for discovering inhibitors of GPCR signaling in a vertebrate, to infer the importance of functional groups for their biological activity. Computer-based ligand screening, also known as ligand-based screening, is frequently used in pharmaceutical discovery because it performs robustly in identifying active molecules from the top-scoring set and does not require the availability of an atomic structure of the protein target [1, 2]. Further, it has been shown that ligand-based virtual screening is capable of exploring different active scaffolds, making it a valuable alternative to structure-based methods such as molecular docking, even when atomic structures of the protein target are known [3, 4].

However, scientists typically focus on the most active handful of compounds and test their closest analogs while not making use of the activity data available from all the tested compounds to identify correlations between their chemical groups and activity values. Part of this may be due to the need to establish spatial correspondences between chemical groups in compounds containing different molecular scaffolds (e.g., comparing substituents on a steroid ring system versus a purine nucleotide). This problem has been circumvented in the protocols presented here by considering all molecules as fully flexible 3D structures and determining their optimal overlay based on the volumes and partial charges of the atoms, followed by comparing the chemical identities of neighboring atoms and small organic groups such as $-NH_2$. We will use the term "functional groups" to refer to single or small groups of atoms that are being compared between molecules. This flexible overlay procedure provides a rational and quantitative way of comparing chemical groups between compounds.

The most prominent approaches in the computer-aided discovery of biologically active molecules are *structure-based* screening [5–8] and *ligand-based* screening [1, 2, 9, 10] as well as hybrids thereof [11, 12]. Traditionally, structure-based screening is restricted to applications where an experimentally determined, high-resolution three-dimensional (3D) structure of the ligand's

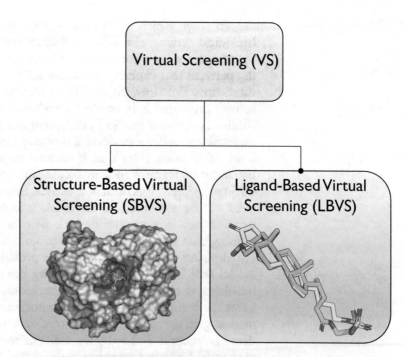

Fig. 1 An illustration of the two broad categories of virtual screening: Structure-based virtual screening involves docking into a binding site to maximize protein–ligand surface complementarity, and ligand-based virtual screening involves evaluating small-molecule similarity with a known ligand

binding partner (usually a protein or nucleic acid) is available from X-ray crystallography or nuclear magnetic resonance experiments.

While ligand-based screening does not require knowledge of the binding target, it assumes that active molecules are likely to share shape and chemical similarities with a known, biologically active ligand. In short, ligand-based screening can be described as a similarity search between a known ligand and the molecules in a database (Fig. 1).

1.1 Using Machine Learning to Identify Functional Groups Associated with Biological Activity

To guide virtual screening, understand biological mechanisms, and aid the design of more potent inhibitors or activators of molecular processes, several different techniques have been developed to analyze datasets of molecular descriptors and measured activity. A common goal in quantitative structure–activity relationship (QSAR) modeling includes the prediction of the in vitro or in vivo activity of molecules given their features. Another common goal is to gain insights into the importance of individual functional groups for binding or chemical activity; such insights are invaluable for the discovery and optimization of potent agonists or inhibitors. More detailed discussions of QSAR can be found in Kubinyi et al. [13] and Verma et al. [14].

To infer which functional groups are most important for biological activity, this chapter focuses on the use of supervised machine learning algorithms to discover functional group matching patterns that explain the relative activity of the tested inhibitor candidates. Primarily, the analysis of the discriminants of biological activity presented here employs tree-based machine learning algorithms. A decision tree [15] that separates active from non-active molecules provides a model that is readily interpretable, resulting in a set of decision rules that if chained together, can explain the hierarchy of features in a molecule that are most important for distinguishing actives from non-actives. Secondly, multiple decision trees will be combined via the random forest method [16]. Each decision tree in a random forest is fit to a random sample of the training data and feature set. This produces an ensemble of different decision trees, which together provide a robust predictive model that is less prone to overfitting the training data than any individual decision tree [16]. Furthermore, a random forest facilitates the computation of feature importance as the average information gain over the individual trees, as will be explained in more detail in section 3. Lastly, we will utilize an implementation of sequential backward selection, a sequential feature selection algorithm that identifies subsets of features to maximize the performance of a given model in a greedy (fastest improvement, rather than exhaustive) fashion [17, 18]. Sequential feature selection algorithms can be combined with any machine learning algorithm, and hence, they provide a flexible, model-agnostic solution for the analysis of combinations of functional groups that explain biological activity.

1.2 Predicting the Essential Features of GPCR Inhibitors: A Real-World Case Study

This chapter presents an automated, machine learning-based approach to infer the discriminants of activity in molecules from assays performed on compounds prioritized by ligand-based screening. To explain the methodology behind this approach, we will consider a novel dataset of 56 molecules that have been prioritized as candidates for inhibiting GPCR-mediated pheromone signaling in an invasive species control project. Readers can access the same data and software and then perform the same analyses and compare their results with ours.

The goal of this invasive species control project is to inhibit a pheromone-induced GPCR olfactory signaling pathway. We hypothesized that the inhibition of pheromone detection by the olfactory system will prevent mature female sea lamprey from reaching mature males at spawning grounds in tributaries of the Laurentian Great Lakes, and thus reduce the invasive sea lamprey population. Controlling the sea lamprey with pesticide applications currently costs millions of dollars per year, with native fish populations and commercial fishing continuing to be impacted by sea lamprey parasitism [19]. The rationale behind the screening side

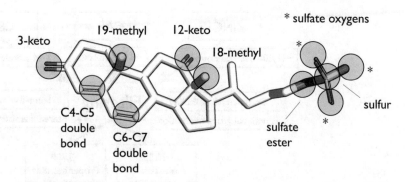

Fig. 2 3D structure of a favorable (low-energy) DKPES conformer, where the functional group features corresponding to the columns in the olfactory response dataset are highlighted with gray circles. White indicates carbon, red indicates oxygen, and yellow indicates sulfur

of this project is based on a recently completed project [10], focusing on inhibiting the GPCR signaling pathway induced by a male sea lamprey mating pheromone, 3-keto petromyzonol sulfate (3kPZS). The successful approach described in this chapter is equally applicable to human drug discovery for GPCRs and other targets.

The dataset analyzed here consists of the chemical structures and assay data for another male sea lamprey mating pheromone, the sulfate-conjugated bile acid, 3,12-diketo-4,6-petromyzonene-24-sulfate (DKPES, Fig. 2). The 56 molecules prioritized by ligand-based screening according to their degree of 3D DKPES similarity were assayed for their ability to block the in vivo sea lamprey olfactory response to DKPES, as measured by an electro-olfactogram assay (EOG). The activity data was then analyzed using machine learning algorithms to uncover structure–function patterns. A brief summary of the virtual screening approach that we used to identify inhibitory mimics of DKPES is provided in Fig. 3.

As a result, 56 candidate molecules were prioritized for biological assays based on the following criteria:

- Steroidal substructure containing molecules with a high degree of shape and charge match to the reference pheromone, DKPES (Fig. 2).

- Four DKPES analogs with oxidized (double bond-containing) rings that are naturally produced by mature male sea lamprey (molecule IDs: ENE 1–4, Fig. 4) [22].

- Diverse compounds to test the hypothesis that compounds with the best charge and shape match will mimic DKPES (without requiring a steroid core or sulfate tail match).

- Non-steroid compounds having 3-keto or 3-hydroxy and 12-keto or 12-hydroxy matches and at least one sulfate oxygen

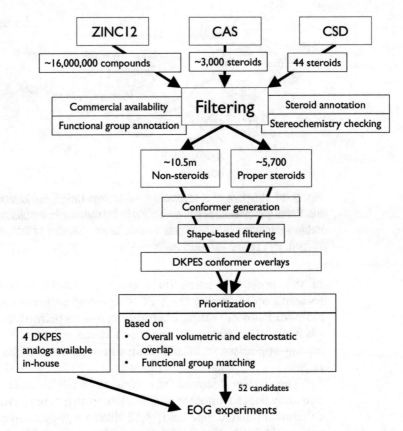

Fig. 3 Summary of the virtual screening workflow to prioritize molecules for electro-olfactogram (EOG) assays. The Screenlamp toolkit [10] (https:/github.com/psa-lab/screenlamp) was used to prepare the virtual screening pipeline, including ROCS v3.2.0.4 (OpenEye Scientific Software, Santa Fe, NM; https:/www.eyesopen.com/rocs), OMEGA v2.4.6 (OpenEye Scientific Software, Santa Fe, NM; https:/www.eyesopen.com/omega), and QUACPAC/molcharge (OpenEye Scientific Software, Santa Fe, NM; https:/docs.eyesopen.com/toolkits/python/quacpactk/molchargetheory.html). The screening databases of small molecules, mostly commercially available, were the drug-like molecules in ZINC12 (http:/zinc.docking.org) [20], steroid structures from Chemical Abstracts Service Registry (CAS; https:/www.cas.org), and steroid structures from the Cambridge Structural Database (CSD; https:/www.ccdc.cam.ac.uk/solutions/csd-system/components/csd/) [21]

match that overlay on the corresponding oxygen atoms in DKPES (Fig. 2).

To measure the biological activity of the 56 DKPES inhibitor candidates selected with the above screening and prioritization criteria, we used an electro-olfactogram (EOG) [10]. The measured EOG response, acting as the target variable in this dataset, was the percentage reduction of the standard DKPES signal when the sea lamprey nose was perfused with a known concentration (10^{-6} M) of inhibitor candidate (computed as the average of 2–5 experimental replicates). Figure 5 shows four of the 56 molecules for illustrative purposes, two actives and two non-actives, with the percent DKPES olfactory inhibition for each. In the context of

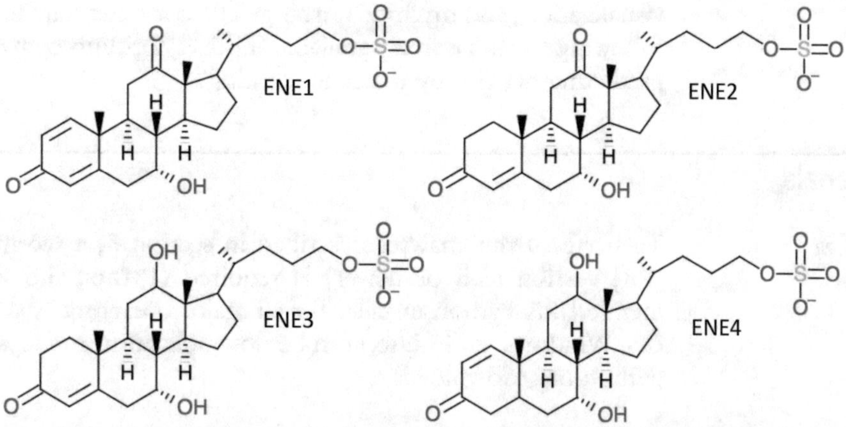

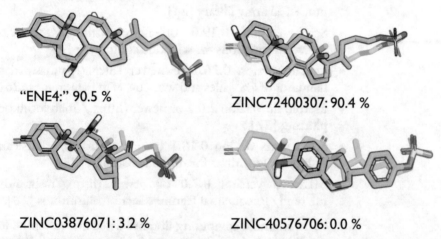

Fig. 4 2D structures of the four DKPES analogs ("ENE" compounds) [22]. ENE1: 7,24-dihydroxy-3,12-diketo-1,4-choladiene-24-sulfate; ENE2: 7,24-dihydroxy-3,12-diketo-4-cholene-24-sulfate; ENE3: 7,12,24-trihydroxy-3-keto-4-cholene-24-sulfate; ENE4: 7,12,24-trihydroxy-3-keto-1-cholene-24-sulfate

"ENE4:" 90.5 %   ZINC72400307: 90.4 %

ZINC03876071: 3.2 %   ZINC40576706: 0.0 %

Fig. 5 3D structures and percent DKPES olfactory inhibition of the two most active molecules (actives, top row) and two low-activity molecules (non-actives, bottom row) from the screening set, shown in green as overlayed with the best-matching DKPES 3D conformer (cyan)

this project, *non-actives* were defined as molecules that block the olfactory response by less than 40% in EOG assays, and molecules that block the signaling response by at least 60% were defined as *actives*.

The DKPES dataset for analysis by machine learning contains the ROCS overlay scores from ligand-based screening (Fig. 3) as well as the functional group matching information provided by Screenlamp in tabular form [10] (https://github.com/psa-lab/screenlamp).

Using the DKPES dataset as a case study, section 3 will explain how to work with such tabular datasets consisting of samples and molecular features using open source libraries for data parsing, visualization, and machine learning. The code and data used in the following section is freely available at https://github.com/psa-lab/predicting-activity-by-machine-learning.

---

2 Materials

2.1 Python Interpreter

To perform the analyses described in section 3, a recent Python [23] version (3.5 or newer) is required (Python 3.6 is recommended). A Python installer for all major operating systems (Mac OS, Windows, and Linux) can be downloaded from https://www.python.org/downloads/.

2.2 Python Libraries for Scientific Computing

The following list specifies the Python libraries used in this chapter, the recommended version number, and a short description of their use:

- NumPy version 1.13.0 or newer (http://www.numpy.org); numerical array library [24].
- SciPy version 0.19.0 or newer (https://www.scipy.org); advanced functions for scientific computing [25].
- Pandas version 0.20.1 or newer (http://pandas.pydata.org); handling of CSV files and working with data frames [26].
- Matplotlib version 2.0.2 or newer (https://matplotlib.org); 2D plotting [27].
- Scikit-learn version 0.18.1 or newer (http://scikit-learn.org/stable/); algorithms for machine learning [28].
- MLxtend version 0.7.0 or newer (http://rasbt.github.io/mlxtend/); sequential feature selection algorithms [18].

The scientific computing libraries listed above can be installed using Python's in-built Pip module (https://pypi.python.org/pypi/pip) by executing the following line of code directly from a Mac OS/Unix, Linux, or Windows MS-DOS terminal command line:

```
pip install numpy scipy pandas matplotlib scikit-learn
pydotplus mlxtend
```

If you encounter problems with version incompatibilities, you can specify the package versions explicitly, as shown in the following terminal command example:

```
pip install numpy==1.13.0 scipy==0.19.0 pandas==0.20.1
matplotlib==2.0.2 scikit-learn==0.18.1 pydotplus==2.0.2
mlxtend==0.7.0
```

2.3 Graph Visualization Software

To visualize the decision trees later in this chapter, an installation of GraphViz is needed. The GraphViz package is freely available at http://www.graphviz.org with the installation and setup instructions.

2.4 Dataset

The datasets used in this chapter, as well as the source files of all the accompanying code, are available online under a permissive open source license at https://github.com/psa-lab/predicting-activity-by-machine-learning.

2.5 Additional Resources

If you are unfamiliar with Python and the Python libraries that you installed in section 2.2, it is highly recommended to familiarize yourself with their basic functionality by reading these freely available resources:

- *Python Beginner Guide*: https://wiki.python.org/moin/BeginnersGuide
- *NumPy Quickstart Tutorial*: https://docs.scipy.org/doc/numpy-dev/user/quickstart.html
- *Introduction to NumPy*: https://sebastianraschka.com/pdf/books/dlb/appendix_f_numpy-intro.pdf
- *10 Minutes to Pandas*: http://pandas.pydata.org/pandas-docs/stable/10min.html
- *Matplotlib Tutorials*: https://matplotlib.org/users/index.html
- *An Introduction to Machine Learning Using Scikit-learn*: http://scikit-learn.org/stable/tutorial/basic/tutorial.html

3 Methods

This section walks through the individual steps involved in a typical analysis pipeline for identifying which functional groups and atoms (or other molecular properties or *features*) are predictive of the measured biological activity of the molecules.

3.1 Loading and Inspecting the Biological Activity Dataset

This section explains how to load a CSV-formatted dataset table (e.g., the DKPES dataset) into a current Python session. A convenient way to parse a dataset from a tabular plaintext format, such as CSV, is to use the `read_csv` function from the Pandas library as shown in the code example in Fig. 6, which loads the DKPES dataset into a Pandas DataFrame object (`df`) for further processing (*see* **Note 1**).

As a result from executing the code shown in Fig. 6, the `df.head(10)` call will display the first ten rows in the dataset, to confirm that the data file has been parsed correctly. The DKPES dataset consists of 56 rows, where each row stores the functional

```
>>> import pandas as pd
>>> df = pd.read_csv('../data/csvs/dkpes.csv')
>>> df.head(10)
```

	index	Signal-inhibition	3-Keto	3-Hydroxy	12-Keto	12-Hydroxy	19-Methyl	18-Methyl	Sulfate-Ester	Sulfate-Oxygens	...
0	ENE4	0.905	1	0	0	1	1	1	1	3	...
1	ZINC72400307	0.904	0	0	0	1	1	1	1	3	...
2	ENE3	0.897	1	0	0	1	1	1	1	3	...
3	ENE1	0.893	1	0	1	0	1	1	1	3	...
4	ENE2	0.845	1	0	1	0	1	1	1	3	...
5	ZINC12494532	0.741	0	0	0	0	0	0	1	3	...
6	ZINC35044325	0.739	0	1	0	0	1	1	0	3	...
7	ZINC04095893	0.722	0	0	0	0	1	1	0	3	...
8	ZINC01532179	0.686	0	0	0	0	0	0	1	3	...
9	ZINC70666191	0.627	0	0	0	1	1	1	0	0	...

Fig. 6 Code for reading the DKPES dataset into a data frame. The characters >>> denote a Python interpreter prompting for a command to enter and execute. The table resulting from the execution of this code example (df.head(10)) shows an excerpt from the DKPES data table sorted by signal inhibition: the ten most active molecules from the EOG experiments and their functional group matching patterns

group matching information for an assayed molecule with the reference molecule DKPES (see **Note 2**).

Please note that this protocol assumes that a tabular dataset containing information on the molecules as well as the assay response has already been collected. However, the analysis approach outlined in this chapter is a general one, and it is not restricted to the specific functional group matching patterns shown in Fig. 6. For more information on how this functional group matching data can be generated from a ligand-based screening, see [10] (https://github.com/psa-lab/screenlamp).

The first column of the DKPES data table (Fig. 6), "index," numbers each molecule. The "Signal Inhibition" column contains the response variable measured by the biological assay, in this case ranging from 0 (non-active) to 1 (highly active, with 100% DKPES signal inhibition). For instance, we can see from the table (Fig. 6) that ENE4 and ZINC72400307 (petromyzonol sulfate) were the most promising candidate inhibitors, as they reduced the olfactory response to DKPES by 90.5% and 90.4%, respectively, when each inhibitor candidate was used at the same equimolar concentration (10^{-6} M) as DKPES. The consequent columns, labeled as 3-Keto, 3-Hydroxy, and so forth, contain information about whether an atom or functional group in the candidate molecule overlayed

```
>>> y = df['Signal-inhibition'].values
>>> fgroup_cols = ['3-Keto', '3-Hydroxy', '12-Keto',
...                  '12-Hydroxy', '19-Methyl', '18-Methyl', 'Sulfate-Ester',
...                  'Sulfate-Oxygens', 'C4-C5-DB', 'C6-C7-DB', 'Sulfur']
>>> X = df[fgroup_cols].values
>>> fig, ax = plt.subplots(1, 2, figsize=(10, 3))
>>> ax[0].hist(y, bins=np.arange(0, 1.1, 0.1))
>>> ax[0].set_ylabel('Molecule count')
>>> ax[0].set_xlabel('Signal inhibition')
>>> ax[1].scatter(y, df['TanimotoCombo'].values)
>>> ax[1].set_ylabel('Tanimoto similarity')
>>> ax[1].set_xlabel('Signal inhibition')
>>> plt.show()
```

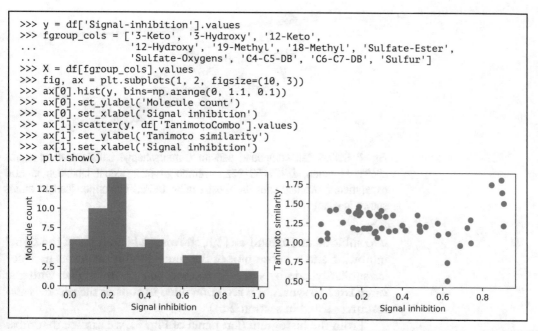

Fig. 7 Code for performing exploratory analysis in Python using the matplotlib library to plot a histogram of the "Signal Inhibition" data and a scatter plot to inspect the relationship between the signal inhibition and overlay scores. In the corresponding programming code, the "Signal Inhibition" column is first assigned to a variable y, and the functional groups of interest are assigned to the variable fgroup_cols, which is then used to create the matrix X that stores the functional groups matching patterns of those functional groups of interest. Next, a figure with two subplots is initialized by calling plt.subplots from matplotlib. The plt.hist function adds the histogram to the first subplot (ax[0]), and the plt.scatter function draws the scatter plot in the subplot to the right (ax[1]). The resulting plots show the DKPES inhibitor activity distribution for the 56 compounds that were assayed (left) and the relationship between activity and overlay similarity from ROCS (right), given as the TanimotoCombo score in the range 0–2, where 2 means that two 3D structures have an identical volume and partial charge distribution

(within 1.3 Å) with the same group in DKPES. This functional group matching data is stored as a binary variable, where 0 indicates "no overlay" and 1 indicates "overlay." In addition, the ROCS shape and chemistry ("color") overlay scores were appended to the dataset. For information on how the overlay scores are computed, the reader is referred to https://docs.eyesopen.com/rocs/shape_theory.html and Hawkins et al. [4]; other molecular similarity measures could be used instead (*see* **Notes 3–5**).

It is always helpful to perform exploratory analyses when working with a new dataset. The following code snippet shown in Fig. 7 will generate the histogram of the signal inhibition values shown, plus the 2D scatter plot comparing the signal inhibition values with the molecular similarity measured in the overlays. First, the signal inhibition data from the data frame (df) is assigned to a variable y, and the functional group columns of interest to a variable X. Next, the code in Fig. 7 demonstrates how to use matplotlib to create

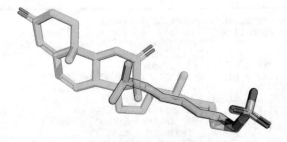

Fig. 8 Sulfate tail compound sodium 6-methylheptyl sulfate (carbon atoms shown in green; ZINC14591952, average of 62% signal inhibition in EOG experiments) overlaid with the most similar DKPES conformer (carbon atoms shown in cyan)

two sublots, `ax[0]` and `ax[1]`, showing a histogram of the signal inhibition and a scatter plot of the signal inhibition versus molecular similarity side by side. (If you are new or unfamiliar with the `matplotlib` syntax, it is recommended to consult the tutorials and resources listed in section 2.5.)

From the histogram (left panel of Fig. 7), we can see that most molecules inhibit the DKPES signal by less than 50% in in vivo EOG assays. The scatter plot in Fig. 7 shows that four out of the five most active molecules have a high overlay similarity value of 1.5 or greater. The *TanimotoCombo* value is the sum of the volumetric and chemical similarity components, where an exact match (two identical molecules in the same conformation) will result in a maximum score of 1 for each, summing to a maximum score of 2. While the top four most active molecules have the highest overlay similarity, no correlation between overlay similarity and signal inhibition can be observed across the remaining 52 molecules. This indicates that more specific determinants of activity are at play, motivating the pattern analysis of functional groups matching DKPES. Interestingly, the outlier with a very low Tanimoto similarity score and a moderately high signal inhibition value of 0.62 is a sulfate tail-containing natural product (ZINC14591952) produced by sea squirts [29], shown in Fig. 8.

From this molecule we can conclude that mimicking the sulfate group in DKPES alone can block the olfactory response of DKPES by approximately 60%, likely by competing with interactions of the similar tail in DKPES with the GPCR ligand binding site.

3.2 Chemical and Functional Groups

This section explains how to visualize the other features in the dataset: the functional group matches with the DKPES reference molecule (Fig. 2). Using the code in Fig. 9, we will plot the functional group matching pattern of the top ten most active and ten least active molecules via two heat maps shown side by side for a visual comparison (*see* **Note 6**).

```
>>> fig, ax = plt.subplots(1, 2, figsize=(10, 3))
>>> ax[0].imshow(X[:10], cmap='binary')
>>> ax[0].set_title('10 most active molecules')
>>> plt.sca(ax[0])
>>> plt.xticks(range(len(fgroup_cols)),
...            fgroup_cols, rotation='vertical')
>>> plt.yticks(range(10), df['index'][:10])
>>> ax[1].imshow(X[-10:], cmap='binary')
>>> ax[1].set_title('10 least active molecules')
>>> plt.sca(ax[1])
>>> plt.xticks(range(len(fgroup_cols)),
...            fgroup_cols, rotation='vertical')
>>> plt.yticks(range(10), df['index'][-10:])
>>> plt.show()
```

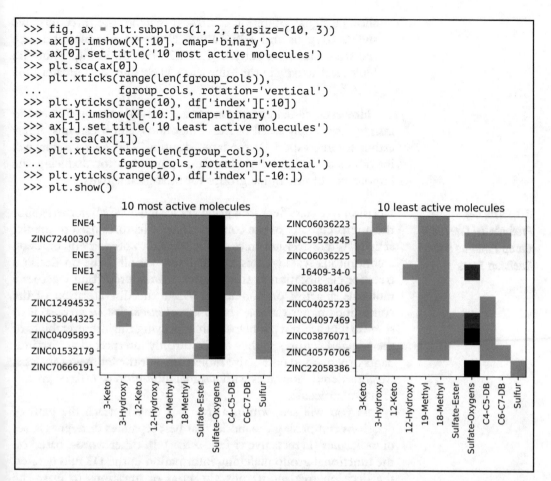

Fig. 9 Code to generate heat maps showing matches of functional groups in DKPES by the ten most active (left) and ten least active (right) molecules tested in EOG assays. Using the `matplotlib.pyplot` function that was imported as `plt` earlier (Fig. 7), we create two subplots stored in the array `ax`. Using `matplotlib.pyplot`'s `imshow`, we plot the functional group patterns of the ten most active molecules (`X[:10]`, the first ten elements in the sorted data array) as a heat map in left subplot (`ax[0]`). Similarly, we plot the ten least active molecules (the last ten molecules in the array, `X[-10:]`) as a heat map in the right subplot (`ax[1]`). As the heat maps show, all features except sulfate-oxygens are encoded as binary variables (0: white cell background, no match; 1: light gray, match). Sulfate-oxygens refers to the three terminal oxygens, excluding the sulfate ester oxygen. This variable has values from 0 to 3 (up to all three terminal oxygens being matched), where black cell backgrounds correspond to three matches, dark gray corresponds to two matches, and light gray to one match, respectively

Looking at the heat maps in Fig. 9, the following conclusions can be drawn:

- The top nine most active molecules have a sulfur match and match three of the oxygen atom in the DKPES sulfate group.
- Sulfur and sulfate oxygen atom matches alone are not sufficient for activity. From the previous scatter plot analysis (Fig. 7), we know that the sulfate tail analog alone (Fig. 8; ZINC14591952)

shows a signal inhibition of 60%. It matches the three terminal sulfate-oxygens and sulfur atom. However, a compound with the same matching pattern (ZINC22058386 in Fig. 9) has no biological activity in the same assay, likely due to its greater bulk (Fig. 5).

However, casual inspection of the data does not always lead to insights that apply to all of the compounds, and it can miss interesting trends, especially for large datasets. The next section will introduce several machine learning approaches for deducing the importance of functional groups for biological activity.

3.3 Tracing Preferential Chemical Group Patterns Using Decision Trees

Decision tree classifiers are a good choice if we are concerned about the interpretability of the combinations of features used to predict activity. While decision trees can be trained to predict outcomes on a continuous scale (regression analysis), we fill focus on decision trees for classification in this chapter, that is, predicting whether a molecule is active or non-active. While the discretization of the continuous target variable (here: *signal inhibition in percent*) is to some extent arbitrary, it helps with improving the interpretability of the selected features as they can be directly interpreted as discriminants of active and non-active molecules. For the following analysis, we considered molecules with a signal inhibition of 60% or greater as active molecules.

As you will see, within a tree it is easy to trace the path of decisions comprising the model that best separates different classes of molecules (here: active vs non-active). In other words, based on the functional group matching information in the DKPES dataset, the decision tree model poses a series of questions to infer the discriminative properties between active and non-active molecules (*see* **Note 7**).

The learning algorithm that is constructing a nonparametric decision tree model from the dataset works as follows. Starting at the tree root, it splits the dataset (the active and non-active molecules) on the feature (e.g., *presence of a sulfur match*) that results in the largest information gain. In other words, the objective function of a decision tree is to learn, at each step, the splitting criterion (or decision rule) that maximizes the information gain upon splitting a parent node into two child nodes. The information gain is computed as the difference between the impurity of a parent node and the sum of its child node impurities. Intuitively, we can say that the lower the impurity of the child nodes, the larger the information gain. The impurity itself is a measure of how diverse the subset of samples is, in terms of the class label proportion, after splitting. For example, after asking the question "does a molecule have a positive sulfur match?" a pure node would only contain either active or non-active molecules when answering this question with a "yes." A node that consisted of 50% non-active and 50% active samples after applying a splitting criterion would be most impure—such a result would indicate that it was not a useful criterion for distinguishing between active and non-active molecules. In the decision tree implementation that we use in this chapter, the metric for computing the impurity of a given node is measured as *Gini impurity* as used in the CART (classification and regression tree) algorithm [15]. Gini impurity is defined as follows:

$$\text{Impurity}(t) = \sum_{i=1}^{c} p(i|t)(1 - p(i|t)) = 1 - \sum_{i=1}^{c} p(i|t)^2$$

Here, t stands for a given node, i is a class label in $c =$ {*active, non-active*}, and $p(i|t)$ is the proportion of the samples that belongs to class i for a particular node t. Looking at the previous equation, it is easy to see that the impurity of a given node is minimal if the node is pure and only contains samples from one class (e.g., actives), since $1 - (1^2 + 0^2) = 0$. Vice versa, if samples at one node are perfectly mixed, the Gini impurity of a node is maximal: $1 - (0.5^2 + 0.5^2) = 0.5$. In an iterative process, the splitting procedure is then repeated at each child node until the leaves of the tree are pure, which means that the samples at each node all belong to the same class (either *active* or *non-active*), or cannot be separated further due to the lack of discriminatory information in the dataset. For more information about decision tree learning, *see* [30, 31].

To build a decision tree classifier (as opposed to a decision tree regressor), we discretize the signal inhibition variable, creating a binary target variable y_binary. Using the code in Fig. 10, active molecules are specified as molecules with signal inhibition of 60% or greater (class 1), and molecules with less than 60% signal inhibition are labeled as non-active (class 0):

As can be seen from computing the sum of values in the y_binary array (np.sum(y_binary), Fig. 10), discretization of the continuous signal inhibition variable resulted in 12 molecules labeled as active; consequently, the remaining 44 molecules in the dataset are now labeled as non-active. In the next step, we will initialize a decision tree classifier from scikit-learn with default values, let it learn the decision rules that discriminate between actives and non-actives from the dataset, and export the model and display it as a decision tree (Fig. 11) (*see* **Note 8**).

```
>>> y_binary = np.where(y >= 0.6, 1, 0)
>>> np.sum(y_binary)
12
```

Fig. 10 Code for discretizing the continuous signal inhibition variable. The np.where function creates a new array, y_binary, where all molecules with more than 60% signal inhibition will be labeled as 1 (active), and all other molecules will be labeled with a 0 (non-active)

```
>>> from sklearn import tree
>>> clf = tree.DecisionTreeClassifier()
>>> clf = clf.fit(X, y_binary)
>>> dot_data = tree.export_graphviz(clf, out_file=None,
...                                 feature_names=fgroup_cols,
...                                 class_names=['non-active', 'active'],
...                                 filled=True, rounded=True)
>>> graph = pydotplus.graph_from_dot_data(dot_data)
>>> graph.write_pdf("tree.pdf")
```

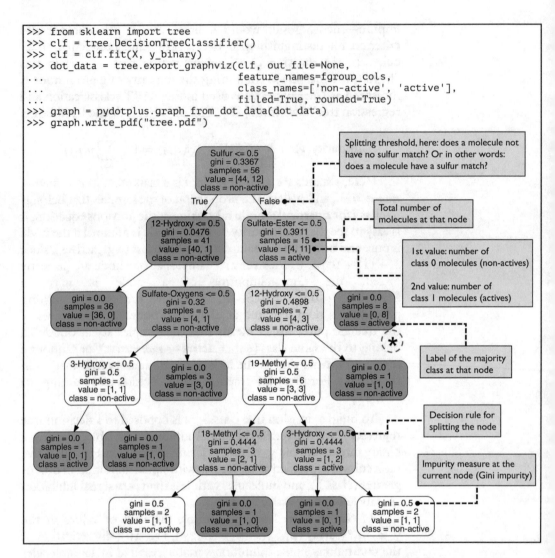

Fig. 11 Binary classification tree separating active from non-active compounds. After importing the tree submodule from the scikit-learn machine learning library, the first line of code initializes a new Decision-TreeClassifier object that is then learning the decision rules from the functional group matching pattern array (X) and the discretized response variable (binary labels of the active and non-active molecules, y_binary) by calling the fit method. The last three lines of code then export the fitted decision tree as a PDF image, which is shown here. The first node at the top of the tree, for example, uses a decision rule asking which molecules in the 56-molecule dataset (44 actives and 12 non-actives) match a sulfur group in DKPES. Note that this question is posed as a conditional (true/false) statement "Molecules do *not* contain a sulfur group match," due to the implementation of the decision tree in scikit-learn. The molecules for which the condition is "False"—that is, molecules that do match the sulfur group in DKPES—are then passed to the child node on the right (here: 4 non-actives and 11 actives), where the next conditional statement is "Molecules do not contain a 'Sulfate-Ester' match." Each node in the tree contains the impurity measure after the split (Gini impurity), reflecting the degree of separation between active and non-active compounds; a Gini impurity value of 0 reflects a set containing purely active or non-active compounds. The number of samples refers to the compounds at each node that pass the filtering criteria. The first value within brackets in the bottom row in each terminal node denotes the number of non-active compounds at that node, and the second number denotes the number of active compounds. Highlighted with an asterisk is the terminal node

We conclude from the binary classification tree (Fig. 11) that a majority of the active inhibitors (8 of 12) share a sulfur atom and a sulfate ester group that overlay with the respective functional groups in DKPES; none of the non-active compounds have these characteristics. With decision trees, the resulting models can offer intuitive insights into the hypothesis space. Specifically, the tree in Fig. 11 indicates that, given a set of molecules initially selected as having high volumetric and chemical similarity with DKPES, the presence of a sulfur atom and sulfate ester group matching those two groups in DKPES predicts the subset of molecules that are active as DKPES inhibitors. Using machine learning to derive decision rules objectively and automatically is convenient and less error-prone in providing insights compared with visual analysis of functional group patterns in a heat map (*see* **Note 9**).

3.4 Deducing the Importance of Chemical Groups via Random Forest

To estimate the relative importance of the different functional groups based on active and non-active labels, we will now construct a random forest model [16], which is an ensemble of multiple decision trees. In the random forest models, the feature importance is measured as the averaged impurity decrease computed from multiple decision trees. In the following code example (Fig. 12), we will use the random forest algorithm implemented in scikit-learn to create an ensemble of 1000 decision trees, which are grown from different bootstrap samples of the molecule dataset and randomly selected subsets of functional group feature variables. (A bootstrap sample is generated by randomly drawing samples from the original dataset with replacement to generate a resampled dataset of the same size as the original one.)

Based on the random forest model, we can infer feature importance by averaging the impurity decrease for each feature split from all 1000 trees in the forest. Conveniently, the random forest implementation in scikit-learn already computes the feature importance upon model fitting, so that we can access this information from the forest, after calling the `fit()` method via its `feature_importances_` attribute. The code in Fig. 13 will create a bar plot of the feature importance values, which are normalized to sum up to 1 for easier interpretation.

As shown by the bar plot in Fig. 13, the feature importance values computed from the 1000 regression trees agree with the conclusions drawn previously in sections 3.3 and 3.4: sulfur, sulfate ester, and sulfate oxygen groups are the most important functional group features for DKPES inhibitor activity (Fig. 11) (*see* **Notes 10** and **11**).

Fig. 11 (continued) (to the center-right of the plot), which contains eight active compounds and no non-active compounds. For visual clarity, containing more non-active molecules than actives are labeled in orange, and nodes that contain more actives than actives are colored in blue. The higher the color intensity, the higher the ratio of active molecules or non-active molecules, respectively

```
>>> from sklearn.ensemble import RandomForestClassifier
>>> forest = RandomForestClassifier(n_estimators=1000,
...                                  random_state=0,
...                                  n_jobs=-1)
>>> forest.fit(X, y_binary)
```

Fig. 12 Similar to fitting a DecisionTreeClassifier (Fig. 11), we first initialize a new `RandomForest-Classifier` object from scikit-learn and fit it to the functional group matching pattern array (`X`) and labels of the active and non-active molecules (`y_binary`). By setting `n_estimators = 1000`, we will use 1000 decision trees for the forest. `n_jobs = −1` means that we are utilizing all processors on our machine to fit those decision trees in parallel to speed up the computation. The `random_state` parameter accepts an arbitrary integer for the bootstrap sampling and feature selection in the decision tree to make the experiment deterministic and reproducible

```
>>> importances = forest.feature_importances_
>>> indices = np.argsort(importances)[::-1]
>>> feature_labels = np.array(fgroup_cols)
>>> plt.bar(range(X.shape[1]),
>>>         importances[indices],
>>>         align='center')
>>> plt.xticks(range(X.shape[1]),
...            feature_labels[indices], rotation=90)
>>> plt.xlim([-1, X.shape[1]])
>>> plt.ylabel('Relative feature importance')
>>> plt.tight_layout()
>>> plt.show()
```

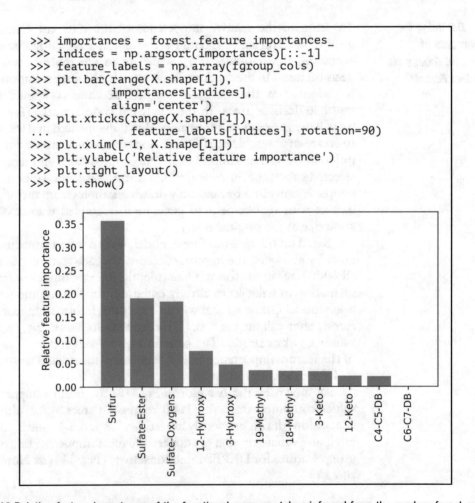

Fig. 13 Relative feature importance of the functional group matches inferred from the random forest model that was trained to discriminate between active and non-active molecules. First, the importances values are sorted from highest to lowest using NumPy's `argsort` function. Next, we summarize the computed feature importance in a bar plot using matplotlib's `pyplot` submodule, which was imported as `plt` earlier

3.5 Sequential Feature Selection with Logistic Regression

As an alternative approach and to probe the robustness of our conclusions, we will apply a Sequential Backward Selection (SBS) algorithm combined with logistic regression [32] for the classification of active versus non-active compounds. SBS is a model-agnostic feature selection algorithm that evaluates different combinations of features, shrinking the subset of features to be considered one by one. Here, model-agnostic refers to the fact that SBS can be combined with any machine learning algorithm for classification or regression.

In general, sequential feature selection algorithms are greedy search algorithms that reduce the d-dimensional feature space to a smaller k-dimensional subspace, where $k < d$. The sequential feature selection approach selects the best-performing feature subsets automatically and can help optimizing two objectives: improving the computational efficiency and reducing the generalization error of a model by getting rid of features that are irrelevant.

The SBS algorithm removes features from the initial feature subset sequentially until a new, reduced feature subspace contains a specified number of features. To determine a feature that is to be removed at each iteration of the SBS algorithm, we need to define a criterion function J, which is to be minimized. For instance, this criterion function is defined as the difference between the performance of the model before and after the feature removal. In other words, at each iteration of the algorithm, the feature that results in the least performance loss (or highest performance gain) is eliminated. This removal of features is repeated in each iteration of the algorithm until the desired, pre-specified size of the feature subset is reached. More formally, we can express the SBS algorithm in the following pseudo-code notation adapted from [30]:

1. Initialize the algorithm with $k = d$, where d is the dimensionality of the full feature space X_d.

2. Determine the feature x^- that maximizes the criterion: $x^- = \text{argmax } J(X_d - x)$, where $x \in X_k$.

3. Remove the feature x^- from the feature set: $X_{k-1} = X_k - x^-$; $k = k - 1$.

4. Terminate if k equals the number of desired features; otherwise, go to **step 2**.

The reason why we chose sequential feature selection to deduce functional group matching patterns that are predictive of active and non-active molecules is that it presents an intuitive method that has been shown to produce accurate and robust results (*see* **Note 12**). For more information on sequential feature selection, please read [17].

Logistic regression is one of the most widely used classification algorithms in academia and industry. One of the reasons why logistic regression is a popular choice for predictive modeling is that it is easy to interpret as a generalized linear model: The output always depends on the sum of the inputs and model parameters. However, note that sequential feature selection can be used with many different machine learning algorithms for supervised learning (classification and regression).

To introduce the main concept behind logistic regression, which is a probabilistic model, we need to introduce the so-called *odds ratio* first. The odds ratio computes the *odds* in favor of a particular event E, which is defined as follows, based on the probability p of a positive outcome (for instance, the probability that a molecule is active):

$$\text{odds} = \frac{p}{(1 - p)}$$

Next, we define the *logit* function, which is the logarithm of the odds ratio:

$$\text{logit}(p) = \log\frac{p}{(1 - p)}$$

The logit function takes values in the range 0–1 (the probability p) and transforms them to real numbers that describe the relationship between the functional group matching patterns, multiplied with weight coefficients (that need to be learned) and the odds that a given molecule is active:

$$\text{logit}(p(y = 1|x)) = w_1 x_1 + w_2 x_2 + \cdots + w_m x_m + b$$

$$= \sum_{i=1}^{m} w_i x_i + b$$

Here, m is an index over the input features (functional group matches, x), w refers to the weight parameters of the parametric logistic regression model, and b refers to the y-axis intercept (typically referred to as *bias* or *bias unit* in literature). The input to the logit function, $p(y = 1| x)$, is the conditional probability that a particular molecule is active, given that its functional group matches x.

However, since we are interested in modeling the probability that a given molecule is active, we need to compute the function inverse ϕ of the logit function, which we can compute as:

$$\phi(z) = \frac{1}{1 + e^{-z}}$$

Here, z is a placeholder variable defined as follows:

$$z = \sum_{i=1}^{m} w_i x_i + b$$

The logistic regression implementation used in this section learns the weights for the parameters (matched chemical features) of the logistic regression model that minimizes the logistic cost function, which is the probability of making a wrong prediction given the number of n active and non-active molecule labels in the set of compounds, where the binary vector y stores the class labels (1 = active, 0 = non-active):

$$l(w) = \sum_{i=1}^{n} \left[y^{(i)} \log\left(\phi\left(z^{(i)}\right)\right) + \left(1 - y^{(i)}\right) \log\left(1 - \phi\left(z^{(i)}\right)\right) \right]$$

For more information about logistic regression, *see* ref. 32.

Now, by combining a logistic regression classifier with a sequential feature selection algorithm, we can identify a fixed-size subset of functional groups that maximizes the probability of correct prediction of which compounds are active.

Since we are interested in comparing feature subsets of different sizes to identify the smallest feature set with the best performance, we can run the SBS algorithm stepwise down to a set with only one feature, allowing it to evaluate feature subsets of all sizes, by using the code shown in Fig. 14. Furthermore, the SBS implementation uses k-fold cross-validation for internal performance validation and selection. In particular, we are going to use fivefold cross-validation.

In fivefold cross-validation, the dataset is randomly split into k nonoverlapping subsets or folds (a molecule cannot be in multiple subsets). From the five splits, four folds are used to fit the logistic regression model, and one fold is used to compute the predictive performance of the model on held-out (test) data. Fivefold cross-validation repeats this splitting procedure five times so that we obtain five models and performance estimates. The model performance is then computed as the arithmetic average of the five performance estimates. For more details about k-fold cross-validation, please see the online article, "Model evaluation, model selection, and algorithm selection in machine learning—Cross-validation and hyperparameter tuning" at https://sebastianraschka. com/blog/2016/model-evaluation-selection-part3.html   (*see* **Note 13**).

As can be seen in Fig. 14, the performance of the classification algorithm does not change significantly across the different feature subset sizes. The feature subsets with size 2–6 have the highest accuracy, indicating that adding more features to the 2-feature subset does not provide additional discrimination between active and non-active molecules. The decline in accuracy after adding a seventh feature to the set is likely due to the curse of dimensionality [33]. In brief, the curse of dimensionality describes the phenomenon that a feature space becomes increasingly sparse if we increase the number of dimensions (e.g., by adding additional functional

```
>>> from mlxtend.feature_selection import SequentialFeatureSelector as SFS
>>> from mlxtend.plotting import plot_sequential_feature_selection as plot_sfs
>>> from sklearn.linear_model import LogisticRegression
>>> classifier = LogisticRegression()
>>> sfs = SFS(classifier,
...           k_features=1,
...           forward=False,
...           floating=False,
...           scoring='accuracy',
...           verbose=0,
...           cv=5)
>>> sfs = sfs.fit(X, y_binary)
>>> fig1 = plot_sfs(sfs.get_metric_dict(), kind='std_err')
>>> plt.ylim([0.5, 1])
>>> plt.ylabel('Accuracy')
>>> plt.xlabel('Number of features in the selected subset')
>>> plt.grid()
>>> plt.show()
```

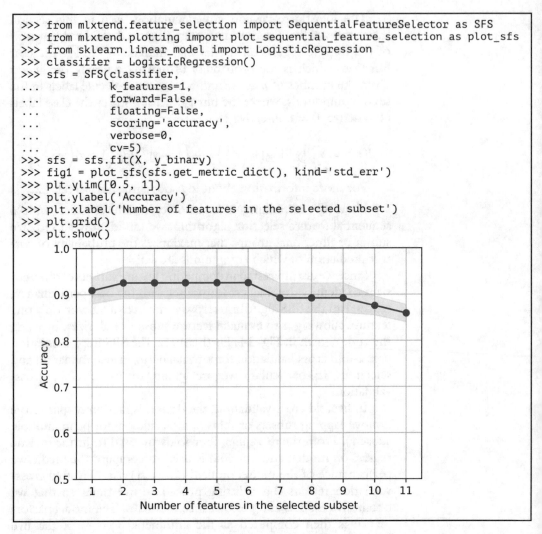

Fig. 14 Performing sequential feature selection using logistic regression to identify features that discriminate between active and non-active molecules. After importing the Python classes for fitting the `LogisticRegression` classifier within the `SequentialFeatureSelector`, by setting `forward = False` and `floating = False`, we specify that the sequential feature selector should perform regular backward selection. Then we use the `plot_sfs` function to visualize the results with matplotlib's `pyplot` submodule. The resulting plot in this figure shows the classification accuracy of the logistic regression models trained on different feature subsets (functional group matching patterns) via sequential backward selection. The prediction accuracy (0 = worst, 1 = best), where 1 corresponds to 100% accuracy in predicting active versus non-active compounds across the input set, was then computed via fivefold cross validation. The plot presents the average prediction accuracy (whether the model can predict held-out active and non-active molecules given their functional group matching patterns) across the five different test sets. The error margin (pale blue region above and below the dark blue average points) shows the standard error of the mean for the fivefold cross validation

```
>>> sfs.subsets_[2]
{'avg_score': 0.92545454545454553,
 'cv_scores': array([ 1., 1., 0.81818182, 0.90909091, 0.9 ]),
 'feature_idx': (10, 6)}
```

Fig. 15 Code to obtain the feature names of the best-performing feature subset from sequential backward selection (Fig. 14). The `subsets_` attribute of the sequential feature selector (sfs) refers to a Python dictionary that stores the feature (functional group match) indices and cross-validation information. By looking up the dictionary entry at index position 2, we can access the feature indices of the 2-feature subset, 10 and 6, and by using `sfs.subsets_[2]` as an index to the `feature_labels` array that we defined earlier (Fig. 13) and reporting the feature labels, we can see that "Sulfur" and "Sulfate-Ester" matches are the most discriminatory features of active and non-active molecules

group matching features) given a fixed number of samples in the training set, which will more likely result in overfitting and less accurate results. While the execution of the code in Fig. 14 provided us with insights regarding the best-performing feature subset sizes via SBS in predicting active or non-active molecules, we have not determined what those features are. Since there is no information gain by going beyond two-feature set (Fig. 14), we will use the following code (Fig. 15) to extract the feature names:

The output from the code executed in Fig. 14 shows that the 2-feature subset consisting of "Sulfur" and "Sulfate-Ester" matches has the most discriminatory information for separating active and non-active molecules as DKPES mimics. This information is consistent with the conclusions drawn from the previous random forest and decision tree analyses.

Now we have shown how to use decision trees, random forest models, and logistic regression to analyze which features can best discriminate between active and inactive compounds, and to assess the relative importance of the different features for discrimination. Such methods provide clearly interpretable information on chemical features important for activity, and concurrence between the methods strengthens the conclusions. In a related pheromone inhibitor project, we used the results of feature importance analysis to drive the selection of compounds in a subsequent round of virtual screening that required fewer compounds to be assayed and resulted in significant enhancement of activity and new knowledge about functional group importance. Those compounds are now being tested by members of our research team for invasive species behavioral modification in the tributaries of the Laurentian Great Lakes under an EPA permit [10]. Analysis of whether the set of features and their relative importance hold equally well for different subsets of assayed compounds (e.g., steroids versus non-steroids) is another valuable direction of inquiry (*see* **Note 14**).

3.6 Conclusion

From the decision tree analysis (section 3.3), random forest feature importance estimation (section 3.4), and sequential feature selection results (section 3.5), we can conclude that the sulfate groups (*Sulfur, Sulfate-Ester,* and *Sulfur-Oxygen* features) are the most discriminatory features for distinguishing active from non-active compounds in DKPES-mediated olfactory responses. From the inspection of heat maps showing the top ten active and ten least active molecules (section 3.2), we also observed that presence of sulfate tails are a consistent determinant of activity. One compound consisting only of a sulfate tail (ZINC14591952, Fig. 8) resulted in 62% signal inhibition, which supports the hypothesis that sulfate groups are a key feature of active molecules. Figure 16 summarizes the results from the random forest feature importance estimation by comparing the importance values to the proportion of functional group matches in active and non-active molecules.

The data in Fig. 16 shows that "Sulfur" and "Sulfur Oxygens" are the most discriminatory features for a random forest to distinguish actives from non-actives, and both features also have a high rate of occurrence in active versus non-active molecules. Features

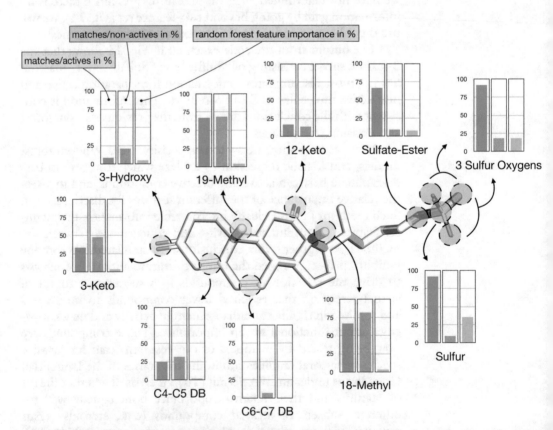

Fig. 16 Proportion of functional group matches across the 12 active and 44 inactive molecules and relative functional group feature importance (from the random forest analysis, Fig. 13) mapped onto the DKPES reference molecule. DB refers to "double bond"

that do not appear substantially more frequently in active molecules than in non-actives (are not discriminatory of activity), for example, 18-methyl, 19-methyl, 3-keto, or the presence of either the C4–C5 or C6–C7 double bond ("DB"), also have a low random forest feature importance. Interestingly, the feature importance of Sulfate-Ester is much less than the feature importance of Sulfur or Sulfur-Oxygens, which may be because it is highly correlated with the sulfur and sulfur oxygen matches in the sulfate group and thereby, to some extent, redundant. An alternative explanation is that the ester oxygen is less highly charged than the terminal sulfate oxygens (causing it to make weaker hydrogen bonds) and is also less accessible for interaction with the receptor.

The machine learning techniques presented in this chapter can be used for *any* kind of data for which a set of feature values across a set of objects is used to predict activity (or any observable value determined by an experimental technique, e.g., solubility, selectivity, and reactivity). We hope this chapter has whetted your appetite for machine learning, which can be used to fit robust models that relate features of interest to molecular activity and other observables. The code provided here and on the corresponding website (https://github. com/psa-lab/predicting-activity-by-machine-learning) makes it possible for you to learn and then use these techniques in your own research. For further information about machine learning, and to carry out further explorations with prepared datasets or your own data, we recommend the following tutorials and references: Raschka and Mirjalili [34], Raschka et al. [35], Friedman et al. [36], Mueller and Guido [37], and the scikit-learn online tutorials (http://scikit-learn.org/stable/tutorial/index.html).

---

4   Notes

1. For this section, we used a CSV file where the features and target variable (signal inhibition) were stored as columns separated by commas. Note that the `read_csv` function does not strictly require this input format. For instance, pandas's `read_csv` function supports any possible column delimiter (e.g., tabs and whitespaces), which can be specified via the delimiter function argument. For more information about the `read_csv` function, please refer to the official documentation at   https://pandas.pydata.org/pandas-docs/stable/generated/pandas.read_csv.html. Furthermore, if you are planning to work with datasets where the features are stored as rows as opposed to columns, you can use the transpose method (`df = df.transpose()`) after loading a dataset to transpose the data frame index and columns.

2. Throughout section 3, we assumed that the data frame of activity data was already sorted by signal inhibition in decreasing order. While sorting the data frame is not essential for fitting the machine learning models in the later section, you may consider sorting your datasets for the heat map visualization, to show the ten molecules with the highest inhibition activity, for example. To sort the data frame `df`, you can use `sort_values` method of a given pandas data frame object. For example, the following code sorts the molecules stored as a data frame df from most active to least active: `df = df.sort_values(Signal-Inhibition', ascending = False)`. More information about this `sort_values` method can be found in the official pandas documentation at https://pandas.pydata.org/pandas-docs/stable/generated/pandas.DataFrame.sort_values.html.

3. While we recommend working with 3D structures because they provide spatial relationships between chemical groups, molecular features can also be derived from 1D string representations of molecules or 2D structural representations. For example, the presence of certain substructures or atom types, using so-called molecular fingerprints, can be computed using the open-source toolkit OpenBabel (https://openbabel.org/docs/dev/Fingerprints/intro.html).

4. To convert a 1D or 2D representation of a molecule into a 3D structure as input for the spatial functional group matching in the DKPES dataset that was done via Screenlamp [10] using ROCS overlays (OpenEye Scientific Software, Santa Fe, NM; https://www.eyesopen.com/rocs), you may find the following tools helpful:

   • The CACTUS online SMILES translator and structure file generator (https://cactus.nci.nih.gov/translate/).

   • OMEGA (OpenEye Scientific Software, Santa Fe, NM; https://www.eyesopen.com/omega), which creates multiple favorable 3D conformers of a given structure from 1D, 2D, or 3D representations [38, 39]. This software is available free for academic researchers upon completion of a license agreement with OpenEye.

5. Further, you may find the BioPandas toolkit [40] helpful (http://rasbt.github.io/biopandas/), which reads 3D structures from the common MOL2 file format into the pandas data frame format. This can be useful if you are working with large MOL2 databases that contain thousands or millions of structures that you want to filter for certain properties prior to generating overlays via ROCS or compute the functional group matching patterns via Screenlamp: https://github.com/psa-lab/screenlamp.

6. We chose a 1.3 Å cutoff between overlayed atoms to identify functional group matches in 3D. If two molecules share the same atom type at a distance greater than 1.3 Å, this was not considered a functional group match. This relatively generous distance cut-off (nearly a covalent bond-length) was chosen to account for minor deviations in the crystal structures and overlays when comparing functional groups between pairs of molecules. Note that changing the distance threshold generally will affect the resulting functional group matching patterns. For instance, the 3-hydroxy group in ZINC72400307 (Fig. 5) does not overlay with the 3-keto group of the DKPES query (Fig. 2) in our analysis since the distance between those two atoms is 1.7 Å. We recommend choosing distance thresholds up to 1.3 Å.

7. While there is technically no minimum number of molecules required for using the techniques outlined in this chapter, we recommend collecting datasets of at least 30 structures for the automatic inference of functional groups that discriminate between active and non-active molecules. Although this is difficult to achieve in practice, an ideal dataset for supervised machine learning would be balanced, that is, with an equal number of positive (active) and negative (non-active) training examples. While there is no indication that class imbalance was in issue for the DKPES dataset, as the results of the decision tree analysis were unambiguous, imbalance may be an issue in other datasets. There are many different techniques for dealing with imbalanced datasets, including several resampling techniques (oversampling of the minority class or undersampling of the majority class), the generation of synthetic training samples, and reweighting the influence of different class labels during the model fitting. A comprehensive review of techniques for working with imbalanced datasets can be found in [34]. For machine learning with scikit-learn, a compatible Python library that has been developed to deal with imbalanced datasets (http://contrib.scikit-learn.org/imbalanced-learn/) [35]. Also note that classifiers in scikit-learn, including the `DecisionTreeClassifier`, accept a `class_weight` argument, which can be used to put more emphasis on a particular class (e.g., active or non-active) during model fitting, thereby preventing that the decision tree algorithm becomes biased toward the most frequent class in the dataset. For more information on how to use the `class_weight` parameter of the `DecisionTreeClassifier`, refer to the documentation at http://scikit-learn.org/stable/modules/generated/sklearn.tree.DecisionTreeClassifier.html.

8. Deep, unpruned decision trees with many decision points are notoriously prone to overfitting. This is analogous to the

overfitting problem in parametric regression, where including more terms with adjustable weights allows better fit to a set of training data, while resulting in complex decision rules that are hard to interpret and do not perform well on held-out or new data. This is why we preferred classification trees over decision trees for regression analysis for the single decision tree and random forest analyses in this chapter.

9. Note that the problem analyzed here as a case study is not a classical example of machine learning, in which a classifier is fit to a training dataset, and then its accuracy of prediction (and generalizability to new data) is estimated on held-out data by using a test set or cross-validation techniques. In this chapter, we are describing general approaches for analyzing the importance of various functional groups for the activity of molecules. Our primary goal is not to build a predictor to classify new molecules as active or non-active, although the models developed in this chapter could indeed be used in such a way.

10. While the feature importance values provide us with a numeric value to quantify the importance of features, these quantities do not provide information about whether the presence or absence of the particular functional group matches are characteristic of the active molecules. However, we can easily determine whether active molecules match a certain functional group by inspecting the heat map visualizations of active and non-active molecules (Fig. 9).

11. Concerning the interpretation of feature importance values from random forests, note that if two or more features are highly correlated, one feature may be ranked much higher than the other feature, or both features may be equally ranked. In other words, the importance or information in the second feature may not be fully captured. The potential bias in interpreting the feature importance from random forest models has been discussed in more detail by Strobl et al. [41]. In general, this issue can be preassessed by measuring the degree to which series of values for two features across a set of compounds are correlated by calculating the Pearson linear correlation coefficient to evaluate if there is a linear relationship between the features' values, or by calculating the Spearman rank correlation coefficient to assess similar ranking of values between the features across a set of compounds (which does not assume colinearity). The Spearman and Pearson correlation coefficients can be computed using the `peasonr` and `spearmanr` functions from the `scipy.stats` package (please refer to the official SciPy documentation at https://docs.scipy.org for more information). While the predictive performance of a random forest is generally not negatively affected by high correlation among feature variables (multicolinearity), it is

recommended to exclude highly correlated features from the dataset for feature importance analysis, for instance, via recursive feature importance pruning [42].

12. Sequential feature selection constitutes just one of many approaches to select feature subsets. Univariate feature selection methods that consider one variable at a time and select features based on univariate statistical tests, for example, percentile thresholds or p-values. A good review of feature selection algorithms can be found in Saeys et al. [43]. However, the main advantage of sequential feature selection over univariate feature selection techniques is that sequential feature selection analyzes the effect of features on the performance of a predictive model considering the features as a synergistic group. Other techniques, related to sequential feature selection, are genetic algorithms, which have been successfully used in biological applications to find optimal feature subsets in high-dimensional datasets as discussed in Raymer et al. [44, 45].

13. We chose fivefold cross-validation to evaluate the logistic regression models in the sequential backward selection, since $k = 5$ it is a commonly used default value in k-fold cross-validation. Generally, small values for k are computationally less expensive than larger values of k (due to the smaller training set sizes and fewer iterations). However, choosing a small value for k increases the pessimistic bias, which means the performance estimate underestimates the true generalization performance of a model. On the other hand, increasing the size of k increases the variance of the estimate. Unfortunately, the No Free Lunch Theorem [46]—stating that there is no algorithm or choice of parameters that is optimal for solving all problems—also applies here (as shown in [47]. For an empirical study of bias, variance, and bias-variance trade-offs in cross-validation, also *see* [48].

14. The chemical features identified as most important by machine learning will depend on the chemical diversity within the set of molecules for which assay results and chemical structures are analyzed. For instance, if only steroid compounds are tested versus only non-steroids, likely the chemical features found to be most important will differ. In our case, for the steroid set, the side groups providing specific interactions were most important (since the steroid scaffold is in common to all of them), whereas for the non-steroids, compounds that mimic and shape and hydrophobic interactions of the steroidal pheromone may also be important. Thus, considering the set of compounds to be analyzed, and testing the generalizability of the features derived is worth some thought. If you have different chemical classes of compounds to analyze, and a significant number of compounds in each, you can carry out the machine

learning analysis of the most important features for each of the groups of compounds separately, as well as all of the compounds together, to discern the extent to which highly ranked features that discriminate between actives and non-actives are shared among compounds based on different chemical scaffolds.

Acknowledgments

This research was supported by funding from the Great Lakes Fishery Commission from 2012 to 2017 (Project ID: 2015_KUH_54031). We gratefully acknowledge OpenEye Scientific Software (Santa Fe, NM) for providing academic licenses for the use of their ROCS, Omega, QUACPAC (molcharge), and OEChem toolkit software. We also wish to express our special appreciation to the open source community for developing and sharing the freely accessible Python libraries for data processing, machine learning, and plotting that were used for the data analysis presented in this chapter.

References

1. Ripphausen P, Nisius B, Bajorath J (2011) State-of-the-art in ligand-based virtual screening. Drug Discov Today 16:372–376

2. Geppert H, Vogt M, Bajorath J (2010) Current trends in ligand-based virtual screening: molecular representations, data mining methods, new application areas, and performance evaluation. J Chem Inf Model 50:205–216

3. Pérez-Nueno VI, Ritchie DW, Rabal O, Pascual R, Borrell JI, Teixidó J (2008) Comparison of ligand-based and receptor-based virtual screening of HIV entry inhibitors for the CXCR4 and CCR5 Receptors using 3D ligand shape matching and ligand-receptor docking. J Chem Inf Model 48:509–533

4. Hawkins PCD, AG S, Nicholls A (2007) Comparison of shape-matching and docking as virtual screening tools. J Med Chem 50:74–82

5. Sukuru SCK, Crepin T, Milev Y, Marsh LC, Hill JB, Anderson RJ, Morris JC, Rohatgi A, O'Mahony G, Grøtli M et al (2006) Discovering new classes of Brugia malayi asparaginyl-tRNA synthetase inhibitors and relating specificity to conformational change. J Comput Aided Mol Des 20:159–178

6. Lyne PD (2002) Structure-based virtual screening: an overview. Drug Discov Today 7:1047–1055

7. Ghosh S, Nie A, An J, Huang Z (2006) Structure-based virtual screening of chemical libraries for drug discovery. Curr Opin Chem Biol 10:194–202

8. Li Q, Shah S (2017) Structure-based virtual screening. Methods Mol. Biol. 1558:111–124

9. Yan X, Liao C, Liu Z, T Hagler A, Gu Q, Xu J (2016) Chemical structure similarity search for ligand-based virtual screening: methods and computational resources. Curr Drug Targets 17:1580–1585

10. Raschka S, Scott AM, Liu N, Gunturu S, Huertas M, Li W, Kuhn LA (2018) Enabling hypothesis-driven prioritization of small molecules in big databases: screenlamp and its application to GPCR inhibitor discovery. J Comput Aided Mol Des 32:415–433

11. Zavodszky MI, Rohatgi A, Van Voorst JR, Yan H, Kuhn LA (2009) Scoring ligand similarity in structure-based virtual screening. J Mol Recognit 22:280–292

12. Buhrow L, Hiser C, Van Voorst JR, Ferguson-Miller S, Kuhn LA (2013) Computational prediction and in vitro analysis of potential physiological ligands of the bile acid binding site in cytochrome c oxidase. Biochemistry 52:6995–7006

13. Kubinyi H, Folkers G, Martin YC (eds) (2006) 3D QSAR in drug design: recent advances. Springer, Berlin

14. Verma J, Khedkar VM, Coutinho EC (2010) 3D-QSAR in drug design-a review. Curr Top Med Chem 10:95–115

15. Breiman L, Friedman J, Stone CJ, Olshen RA (1984) Classification and regression trees. CRC Press, Boca Raton, FL

16. Breiman L (2001) Random forests. Mach Learn 45:5–32

17. Ferri F, Pudil P, Hatef M, Kittler J (1994) Comparative study of techniques for large-scale feature selection. Pattern Recognit Pract IV 1994:403–413

18. Raschka S (2017) rasbt/mlxtend: Version 0.7.0. https://doi.org/10.5281/zenodo.816309

19. Hansen GJA, Jones ML (2008) A rapid assessment approach to prioritizing streams for control of Great Lakes sea lampreys (Petromyzon marinus): a case study in adaptive management. Can J Fish Aquat Sci 65:2471–2484

20. Irwin JJ, Shoichet BK (2005) ZINC—a free database of commercially available compounds for virtual screening. J Chem Inf Model 45:177–182

21. Allen F (2002) The Cambridge Structural Database: a quarter of a million crystal structures and rising. Acta Crystallogr Sect B Struct Sci 58:380–388

22. Johnson NS, Yun S-S, Li W (2014) Investigations of novel unsaturated bile salts of male sea lamprey as potential chemical cues. J Chem Ecol 40:1152–1160

23. Van Rossum G (2007) Python programming language. In: USENIX annual technical conference, p 36

24. Van Der Walt S, Colbert SC, Varoquaux G (2011) The NumPy array: a structure for efficient numerical computation. Comput Sci Eng 13:22–30

25. Jones E, Oliphant T, Peterson P (2001) SciPy: open source scientific tools for Python. http://www.scipy.org/

26. McKinney W, et al. (2010) Data structures for statistical computing in Python. In: Millman J, vand der Walt S (eds) Proceedings of the 9th Python Science conference, pp 51–56

27. Hunter JD (2007) Matplotlib: a 2D graphics environment. Comput Sci Eng 9:90–95

28. Pedregosa F, Varoquaux G, Gramfort A, Michel V, Thirion B, Grisel O, Blondel M, Prettenhofer P, Weiss R, Dubourg V (2011) Scikit-learn: machine learning in Python. J Mach Learn Res 12:2825–2830

29. Aiello A, Carbonelli S, Esposito G, Fattorusso E, Iuvone T, Menna M (2000) Novel bioactive sulfated alkene and alkanes from the Mediterranean ascidian Halocynthia papillosa. J Nat Prod 63:1590–1592

30. Raschka S (2015) Python machine learning, 1st edn. Packt Publishing, Birmingham

31. Louppe G (2014) Understanding random forests: from theory to practice. Ph.D. thesis

32. Walker SH, Duncan DB (1967) Estimation of the probability of an event as a function of several independent variables. Biometrika 54:167–179

33. Hughes G (1968) On the mean accuracy of statistical pattern recognizers. IEEE Trans Inf Theory 14:55–63

34. Raschka S, Mirjalili V (2017) Python machine learning, 2nd edn. Packt Publishing, Birmingham

35. Raschka S, Julian D, Hearty J (2016) Python: deeper insights into machine learning, 1st edn. Packt Publishing, Birmingham

36. Hastie T, Tibshirani R, Friedman J, Hastie T, Tibshirani R (2001) Springer series in statistics. Springer, New York, NY

37. Müller AC, Guido S (2017) Introduction to machine learning with Python: a guide for data scientists. O'Reilly Media, Sebastopol, CA

38. Hawkins PCD, Skillman AG, Warren GL, Ellingson BA, Stahl MT (2010) Conformer generation with OMEGA: algorithm and validation using high quality structures from the Protein Databank and Cambridge Structural Database. J Chem Inf Model 50:572–584

39. Hawkins PCD, Nicholls A (2012) Conformer generation with OMEGA: learning from the data set and the analysis of failures. J Chem Inf Model 52:2919–2936

40. Raschka S (2017) BioPandas: working with molecular structures in pandas DataFrames. J Open Source Softw. doi:10.21105/joss.00279

41. Strobl C, Boulesteix A, Kneib T, Augustin T, Zeileis A (2008) Conditional variable importance for random forests. BMC Bioinformatics 9:307

42. Strobl C, Malley J, Tutz G (2009) An introduction to recursive partitioning: rationale, application, and characteristics of classification and regression trees, bagging, and random forests. Psychol Methods 14:323

43. Saeys Y, Inza I, Larrañaga P (2007) A review of feature selection techniques in bioinformatics. Bioinformatics 23:2507–2517

44. Raymer ML, Punch WF, Goodman ED, Kuhn LA, Jain AK (2000) Dimensionality reduction using genetic algorithms. IEEE Trans Evol Comput 4:164–171

45. Raymer ML, Sanschagrin PC, Punch WF, Venkataraman S, Goodman ED, Kuhn LA (1997) Predicting conserved water-mediated and polar ligand interactions in proteins using a K-nearest-neighbors genetic algorithm. J Mol Biol 265:445–464

46. Wolpert DH (1996) The lack of a priori distinctions between learning algorithms. Neural Comput 8:1341–1390

47. Bengio Y, Grandvalet Y (2004) No unbiased estimator of the variance of k-fold cross-validation. J Mach Learn Res 5:1089–1105

48. Kohavi R (1995) A study of cross-validation and bootstrap for accuracy estimation and model selection. Int Jt Conf Artif Intell 14:1137–1143

Chapter 17

Computational Exploration of Conformational Transitions in Protein Drug Targets

Benjamin P. Cossins, Alastair D. G. Lawson, and Jiye Shi

Abstract

Protein drug targets vary from highly structured to completely disordered; either way dynamics governs function. Hence, understanding the dynamical aspects of how protein targets function can enable improved interventions with drug molecules. Computational approaches offer highly detailed structural models of protein dynamics which are becoming more predictive as model quality and sampling power improve. However, the most advanced and popular models still have errors owing to imperfect parameter sets and often cannot access longer timescales of many crucial biological processes. Experimental approaches offer more certainty but can struggle to detect and measure lightly populated conformations of target proteins and subtle allostery. An emerging solution is to integrate available experimental data into advanced molecular simulations. In the future, molecular simulation in combination with experimental data may be able to offer detailed models of important drug targets such that improved functional mechanisms or selectivity can be accessed.

Key words Molecular dynamics, Protein conformation, Conformational transition, Hidden pocket, Allostery, Drug discovery

1 Nature of Conformational Space of Proteins

1.1 Structural and Dynamical Nature of Proteins

Protein is one of the fundamental materials of living organisms along with RNA and DNA. The seemingly simple amino-acid building blocks hide a stunning complexity of structure and dynamical behavior. Proteins have evolved for particular functions and their structural and dynamical nature reflects these functions.

Some proteins have very stable 3D structures such as crystallins, which have evolved to form the transparent eye lens [1]. Other proteins have no single stable structure but are dynamic ensembles of various different conformations. These dynamic ensembles range from the surprisingly prevalent intrinsically disordered proteins (IDPs) to those with very specific and tightly ordered motions like mechanical machine molecules. The mechanical-like protein motions have been studied in an evolutionary context. These

Mohini Gore and Umesh B. Jagtap (eds.), *Computational Drug Discovery and Design*, Methods in Molecular Biology, vol. 1762, https://doi.org/10.1007/978-1-4939-7756-7_17, © Springer Science+Business Media, LLC, part of Springer Nature 2018

motions have been found to be much conserved in evolution and often repurposed [2, 3]. Proteins also tend to evolve through modular combination of domains with particular functions [4]. Hence, rigid and dynamic or disordered proteins can be combined in a myriad of ways. Also, and importantly, proteins often react to stimuli such as pH, phosphorylation, changes in membrane composition, and molecular recognition of other molecules.

Proteins have many rotatable bonds and their conformational space is hyperdimensional, which makes it intrinsically hard to understand. However, those rigid or machine like proteins, mentioned above, are characterized by small numbers of connected spaces which have relatively low dimensionality, evolved so they can carry out their function efficiently and structured by their native contacts/interactions. The scientific community has started to move towards a view of protein folding defined by intermediates or network hubs with progressively lower dimensionality, rather than the previous folding funnel theories [5–8]. This is a pertinent example of one of the major problems we have in trying to understand the high-dimensional space of proteins. High dimensionality clouds our understanding of protein dynamics; we often project important aspects of conformational space onto a small number [2, 3] of important dimensions. However, many important processes take place in more than three dimensions and this can be difficult to understand and visualize.

Technology to design proteins already exists but thus far only superstable examples have been generated and not the delicately balanced dynamic ensembles found in most evolved proteins [9]. This mastery of protein dynamic ensembles is not close owing to the high complexity. Currently we are still developing the ability to efficiently understand the dynamic ensembles of evolved proteins we may come across in nature.

1.2 What Is a Conformational Transition?

The phrase "conformational transition" is not always entirely clear and can cause confusion. Hence, a clear definition of what we mean by "conformational transition" is important. This requires the definition of what is and what is not a separate conformation. These discussions can, in some situations, revolve around the available structural data for a given protein. For those interested in biomolecular simulations these discussions are more and more related to the "slowest motions" of a system. The slowest motions are, in general, most likely to be important functional motions. Of course, the motions themselves are not necessarily slow, and they may be rapid but rare as events, yielding a slow kinetic rate. However, the so-called faster motions can also be correlated and functionally important. Fast motions can mediate allosteric signals over surprisingly long distances across protein molecules with a conformational change which cannot be detected easily with modern experimental techniques [10]. Given this complexity, there is often a layer of subjectivity over whether a region of conformational space is a separate conformation or a part of a larger major conformation. The current authors believe that it makes sense to understand conformational space with protein function as the primary consideration.

1.3 Energy Surfaces (Sensible Projections of Conformational Space)

The energy surface or landscape concept was first suggested to understand protein folding [11]; it is now often used to understand the space which a protein's conformation moves within. While the energy surface concept is useful for thinking about protein conformational space and folding, it is generally not sensible to attempt to build and visualize an energy surface using all the degrees of freedom of a protein, or even just torsions (*see* **Note 1**).

Many state-of-the-art techniques for studying protein dynamics use free-energy surfaces (FES) as the primary means of calculating and visualizing a protein's conformational space. Hence, we have to try and understand protein conformational space using only a small number of dimensions, and choosing these dimensions (for an energy surface) is difficult but very important (*see* **Note 2**).

1.4 Kinetic Transitions

Another sensible way to describe and analyze the motions of a target protein system is through the kinetics of conformational transitions. This requires some definition of conformational states and in order that the transition probability can be converged between them they should be in a relatively fine discretization. The analysis of time (kinetics) with respect to protein motions, rather than potential energy, is easier to work with and understand, mainly because it is easier to coarse-grain and analyze the temporal hierarchy. A kinetic network model is a sensible way to understand and visualize an average protein drug target.

2 Classification of Computational Models of Protein Transition

The field of modeling protein dynamics has grown along with the development of the two most common approaches, molecular dynamics (MD) and Metropolis Monte-Carlo (MMC) simulations.

MD simulates the dynamics of biomolecules using Newtonian and statistical physics. MD simulations generally start with an experimentally determined structure of a protein that is placed in a box of water molecules. Each atom is assigned a velocity in accordance with the Boltzmann distribution and small time steps are made which modify atom positions using an integration scheme. Time steps must be very small to ensure that the conservation of energy law is adhered to. Hence, the main drawback; standard MD simulations can be computationally expensive and are currently limited to timescales of single digit milliseconds [12] (*see* **Note 3**).

MMC, like MD, is based on statistical physics; but rather than using Newtonian theory to model motions, Monte-Carlo random numbers are used to generate changes to the model which are then filtered with a Metropolis test to ensure sampling from the Boltzmann distribution.

MD and MMC are favored for different types of simulation such as MMC for gas-phase or low-density models or calculations of chemical potential. Generally MD is used for condensed phase systems where collective motions are important. However, there are some areas of overlap such as calculation of binding free-energies. Furthermore, hybrid methods are becoming increasingly popular as they offer great combinations of features [13]. Here we will focus on MD simulations as we are mainly interested in condensed phase simulations of proteins.

3   Fundamental Challenges in Simulations of Conformational Change

The fundamental challenges of using dynamic simulation to explore protein conformational transitions are related to the two interrelated limitations of molecular dynamics.

1. Model quality: It is difficult to produce a dynamic model which is able to capture all aspects of the interactions of proteins yet sufficiently simple such that it can be sampled rapidly.

2. Timescales: The protein conformational transitions of interest often take place on slower timescales than what we are able to sample with a suitable dynamic model.

3.1   Model Resolution

Within the field of biosimulation various resolutions of model are available from quantum mechanical (QM) to coarse-grained.

The QM level is the most detailed representation which includes electronic structure. Dynamical simulations at the QM level is carried out with either Born–Oppenheimer molecular dynamics (BOMD) using the time-independent Schrödinger equation or Car–Parrinello molecular dynamics (CPMD) which explicitly includes the electron dynamics. QM dynamics is normally restricted to small chemical systems (*see* **Note 4**). Well known hybrid models (QM/MM) are also too slow for work on the slow protein transitions of interest in many drug targets, and are generally used for models of enzyme reactions.

In terms of protein model resolution, after QM we have classical mechanics, which for proteins means molecular mechanics (MM). Atomistic MM generally refers to Lifson like models or force fields with van der Waals (VDW) spheres for atoms, point charges and springs controlling bond angles and dihedrals [14] (*see* **Note 5**). In addition, modern atomistic simulations have periodic-boundary conditions and provision for long-range electrostatics.

These atomistic MM models of proteins are, with modern GPU hardware, sufficiently fast to access biologically relevant timescales. They are able to reasonably accurately reproduce many experimental observables including NMR measurements. In addition they are transferable between almost any protein system/model. For these reasons the atomistic MM resolution is by far the most popular and important resolution for protein simulations.

At the other end of the spectrum of protein model resolution, coarse-grained (CG) models offer very large time steps and timescales at the expense of reduced accuracy and detail. Protein conformational change is complex and therefore it is very difficult to produce a transferable CG model which is predictive for conformational change (*see* **Note 6**). While examples of transferable CG models for conformational change exist none are widely used or applicable to large complex systems [15–17].

3.2 Sampling Large Motions with Collective Motions

An interesting protein sampling strategy is to make large collective motions based on Eigen-function calculations or prior knowledge about structure. In general approaches which make large collective motions must use an implicit solvation model owing to the potential clashes with the solvent as a result of the motions introduced. Also these approaches do not generally offer properly weighted dynamic ensembles, but are generally designed to be very efficient for large motions, like hinge bending, within a low dimensional subspace or energy basin.

Normal mode analysis (NMA) is a well-known approach for recovering the motions of a protein using an approximation which assumes the potential energy is harmonic. A normal mode is a "pattern of motion in which all parts of the system move sinusoidally with the same frequency, with a fixed phase relation and is independent from other normal modes." Hence, NMA has been mainly used for understanding the slowest or lowest frequency motion of a protein. This generally means motions whose start and end points are within the same low energy basin or low-dimensional subspace. NMA with a full atomistic molecular mechanics model is considered computationally expensive as it requires a large amount of computer memory (*see* **Note 7**).

Reduced NMA models, namely elastic network models (ENMs), have become popular owing to their simplicity, computational lightness, and remarkable accuracy compared to experiment and more expensive computational approaches. ENMs use simplified potentials which often utilize harmonics with a single force constant between all alpha-carbons [18, 19]. Improved ENMs are common and often focus on generalized plans for adjusting the connections and strengths of the harmonics [20–22] (*see* **Note 8**).

Protein energy landscape exploration (PELE) is a minimized Monte-Carlo basin-hopping method which combines advanced ligand moves with an ENM and side-chain sampling. PELE is able to make large ligand displacements and protein collective motions enabling very efficient ligand migration and protein conformational sampling [23, 24]. PELE is being used in the pharmaceutical industry for highly flexible docking [25]. It is also clear that having some knowledge of important motions can help the ENM capture the correct motions [26].

Natural move Monte-Carlo (NMMC) is another interesting basin-hopping approach utilizing collective motions. The philosophy of NMMC is to produce very large-scale simulations with detailed models (e.g., atomistic or three-particle per residue CG). This is achieved by customizing Monte-Carlo moves such that natural collective motions are made and any backbone breakage is fixed with a clever closure algorithm [27, 28]. A recent study shows how NMMC can be applied to a protein system with customized hierarchical moves [29].

Like PELE, NMMC sampling does not adhere to the condition of detailed balance and therefore does not strictly speaking sample the canonical distribution, although in both cases it could be argued that they are in a regime which is close to the correct distribution. Hence, these basin-hopping approaches attempt to overcome the fundamental limitations of atomistic protein simulations by optimally localizing sampling and approximating the statistical mechanical rules.

3.3 Current Important Classes of Molecular Dynamics Exploration

For exploring protein conformational transitions there are currently two major groups of approaches: biased potential methods like umbrella-sampling, meta-dynamics, or replica-exchange [30–32] and celling approaches like Markov state models [33]. These two groups of approaches can in theory be used for the same problems but in practice tend to be used in different cases. This difference between these two approaches is rooted in the fundamental sampling problem of large energy barriers and large entropic conformational spaces. Biased potential methods are good at scaling large energy barrier while celling approaches struggle as these events happen so rarely. Celling approaches are good at exploring large conformational spaces as they are systematic.

3.3.1 Biased Potential Methods

Umbrella sampling adds a biasing potential (often harmonic) with respect to a predefined collective variable to the Hamiltonian. These calculations are usually broken up into a series of overlapping simulation windows such that simple biases can be used to achieve intensive sampling. The unbiased free-energy profile is then recovered by removing the previously added bias. The most common method for this reweighting is the weighted histogram analysis [34].

Metadynamics conceptually fills a system's energy surface with computational sand. In similarity to umbrella sampling, metadynamics biases a simulation with respect to carefully chosen predefined collective variables (CVs). However, in contrast, meta-dynamics biases in a history-dependent manner by periodically depositing Gaussians to discourage the simulation from revisiting the same region of the CV space. Once the CV space is filled, the free-energy surface can then be recovered by integrating over the added Gaussians. Normally the simulation is stopped when the system is diffusing freely through the CV space. The problem of slow or difficult convergence has been improved through the development of well-tempered metadynamics [35] (*see* **Note 9**).

In general umbrella sampling is almost certain to converge and has fewer parameters than metadynamics. However, as mentioned earlier for both of these approaches the choice of collective variables is crucial and often difficult. It is generally easier to see problems with the chosen biasing variables with metadynamics owing to its diffusivity. Interestingly, other methods like adaptive biasing force MD offer some of the advantages of both umbrella sampling and metadynamics [36].

Replica-exchange uses a set of replicas of the same simulation which have successively improved sampling properties owing to some variables like temperature. The variables are then exchanged between replicas such that conformations from the replicas which sample more rapidly are fed into other replicas with the required distribution. These exchanges are carried out in a way which preserves the correct distribution. Generally this means adhering to detailed balance and using a Metropolis test, although more advanced and efficient arrangements becoming more common [37–39] (*see* **Note 10**).

Recently, easy-to-implement forms of Hamiltonian-exchange have become popular as they offer enhanced sampling of particular regions or interactions at much reduced computational expense compared to temperature replica-exchange [40] (*see* **Note 11**). Even with these highly efficient new methods replica-exchange approaches alone are not sufficient to sample many of the transitions of interest. Hence, it is now increasingly common to combine umbrella sampling or metadynamics with replica-exchange in various arrangements [41–44]. The combination of biasing collective variables along with generalized orthogonal sampling from multiple replicas offers well-converged simulations when reasonable variables can be found (*see* **Note 12**).

3.3.2 Celling Approaches—Markov State Models (MSM)

The most well-known celling approach is Markov state models (MSMs) or kinetic transition networks. MSMs are simplified models defining the regularity of transitions between discretized states (microstates) derived from dynamics data. Since they are based on kinetic information these MSMs provide kinetic data such as transition times and are more readily compared to experimental data of dynamics [45]. MSMs allow the combination of many short simulations into one analysis and hence can be easily parallelized across any size of computer resource.

MSM analyses of very rare events are more difficult as the simulations which provide kinetic data will not sample these events often. One way around this difficulty is to "seed" simulations with data from potential bias methods which explore these rare events more readily. These seeded kinetic analyses have the potential to provide the highest quality biophysics data on rare events of interest with a lower cost [46]. Even in the absence of seed data, adaptive sampling arrangements can be utilized to enhance sampling efficiency [47, 48].

One of the likely difficulties for large scale celling approaches is analyzing the huge amount of MD data produced. D. E. Shaw's research has developed an open-source code for analyzing many terabyte trajectories using highly parallel computation [49]. On-the-fly analysis of data as it is produced such that the best starting points for new trajectories can be used will be critical for exploration with high performance celling approaches (*see* **Note 13**). If a specialized hardware/software solution for an enhanced celling approach could be designed it would be more efficient than the single very long trajectory as the simulation would not spend time exploring space it has already characterized.

4 What Is Useful for Working with Protein Targets in Drug Discovery?

The field of molecular simulation is now being taken more seriously in drug discovery research as projects driven by computational biosimulation have very publically produced valuable candidate compounds [50]. These nice examples have so far used MD to predict small molecule binding affinities allowing the rapid exploration of larger swathes of chemical space.

As have been described by various experts, computational approaches are not yet close to being the first choice technology in the drug discovery process [51]. However, it is the belief of these authors that molecular simulation can offer more to drug discovery research than these examples of binding affinity prediction. A concept for this could be the use of dynamical models to predict target tractability prior to the engagement of experimental approaches like protein production allowing a more developed strategy from the early stages of a therapeutic project [52].

Another concept for the use of molecular dynamics in drug discovery research is exemplified by the approach of D.E. Shaw research (DESRES). Since 2002 David Shaw has focused on building MD technology and applying it to biochemistry and drug discovery. DESRES has built specialized computers for MD which encode the calculation into ASIC (applications specific circuit) hardware and advanced interprocessor networks [53–55] (*see* **Note 14**). Published work shows very long timescale simulations and detailed study of how important drug targets (tyrosine kinases) function [56, 57]. Emphasis for DESRES seems to be on the details of interaction networks and change points in protein dynamics rather than thermodynamic and kinetic details found in similar work from academic groups [58–61]. This emphasis has led to the development of advanced statistical analysis to replace painstaking visual analysis [62, 63].

4.1 Target Tractability

Many of the most valuable activities related to conformational transitions in structure-enabled drug discovery can be classed as target tractability work. This is mainly due to the fact that it is sensible to understand the details of a target's dynamics and function before embarking on a therapeutic project. Of course such understanding is also valuable during lead optimization; however as definition of conformational transitions can be time-consuming, it can be more difficult to impact rapid chemistry cycles at this later stage of a project.

4.2 Searching for Hidden Pockets for New Chemical Entities (NCEs)

An important aspect to NCE target tractability is the presence of a pocket/cavity capable of sustaining strong binding to a small molecule. For many years there have been computational analyses able to find pockets in protein crystal structures; some are physics-based [64] while others are trained on large sets of known (substrate) pockets [65, 66]. Even when a potential pocket is discovered with one of these approaches, there is still much work required to discover a compound which will experimentally validate it as a binding site; additionally generating structural information on the bound complex is even rarer.

There are many important target proteins which do not seem, in available crystal structures, to have a cavity suitable for traditional small molecules. However, there are pockets which only reveal themselves when a compound, generally found only through experimental screening, binds.

It is unclear how numerous these hidden or cryptic pockets might be, however, molecular dynamics-based approaches have been emerging which are able to suggest some of these pockets. The simplest examples of this are studies where a relatively short, normal MD simulation reveals a cavity which is predicted to be ligandable by a prediction algorithm or a subcavity in a known pocket [67–72]. These studies move on from those which analyze static crystal structures to allow for a more realistic representation of the protein target. However, these MD-enabled studies are limited in that they can only hope to discover cavities which emerge on relatively fast timescales, and often an element of chance is involved. Other studies attempt to remove chance and use some form of enhanced sampling to search for useful pockets more thoroughly [73–76].

Currently, the most common application of MD for hidden pockets is the mixed solvent simulations reported in 2009 by a few different groups [77, 78]. By including small chemical probes in simulations of target proteins, pockets can be induced or maintained in an open state once discovered. Recent studies using mixed solvents are being applied to find cryptic pockets in PPIs, build pharmacophores for new pockets, and carry out large scale virtual screening efforts [79–81]. In addition there are now even a few examples of approaches combining enhanced sampling and fragments to maximize both sampling of conformational selection and the ability of probes to induce and maintain pockets [82, 83].

4.3 Understanding Conformational Change and Searching for Hidden Conformations

Many proteins have functionally important conformational states which are lightly populated and hence are often not seen in experimental structural studies; alternatively some conformations are not readily crystallized. Understanding functional motions and conformations of target proteins can allow the targeting of complex allostery or delicate selectivity for elegant therapeutic interventions (*see* **Note 15**).

Capture of functionally interesting conformations with antigen-binding fragment (Fab) of antibody or single domain camelid antibody (VHH) along with crystallography [84–88], NMR [89], and electron microscopy [90] has emerged as a route to valuable structural information. This conformational capture can then directly link structure to function, in some cases enable the understanding of complex allostery [91, 92]. Given this interesting conformation capture work, discussion about the use of these Fab: target complexes for small molecule screening against specifically useful conformations is a logical extension [93] (*see* **Note 16**).

Further to this, biotechnology companies offering this technology have started to emerge. For example, Confo Therapeutics focuses on generating antibody stabilized structural data for structure-based design on GPCRs. Attempting to discover hidden but important conformations using molecular simulation can be very challenging but in some cases can yield crucial structural information and thermodynamic details to complement the conformational capture strategy.

4.3.1 Directed by Experimental Data

It is common that we do have some experimental data about a hidden conformation which has prompted our interest. There are advanced examples of researchers using X-ray crystallography, X-ray scattering (SAX), double electron-electron resonance (DEER), 2D infra-red spectroscopy (2DIR), and nuclear magnetic resonance (NMR) to drive conformational exploration with molecular simulation.

Crystal structure coordinates have been used for many years as a target to drive MD simulations. Fittingly an early approach along these lines is called "targeted MD" [94, 95]. There are many other approaches which drive transitions between crystal structures, but a particularly interesting and automated example, called normal-mode analysis and umbrella sampling molecular dynamics or NUMD, uses an ENM model to build a transition coordinate between structures and then calculates the PMF using umbrella sampling [96].

SAX data is relatively low resolution compared to crystallography but can still be used to drive exploratory biosimulations both with biasing or correction potentials and adaptive sampling of a common classical force-field [97–99].

DEER is a pulse electron paramagnetic resonance (EPR) technique that provides distance distributions which relate to the distances between nitroxide spin labels (probes) introduced into the target protein via site-directed mutagenesis. There are various limitations to the size of the distances and the number of probes which can be used at once, but DEER offers average interspin distributions and so can detect hidden but important conformations [100]. DEER has also been combined with MD to correct easily sampled ensembles which may be inaccurate owing to an imperfect force-field [101, 102].

NMR offers dynamic detail of proteins from experiment at biologically relevant timescales and hence can offer information to drive molecular simulations. Granata et al. have used NMR chemical shifts as a bias-exchange metadynamics collective variable through their camshift metric, which measures the difference between calculated and experimental chemical shifts [103]. This combination provides a considerable speed up for their case of folding a small protein. However, lightly populated conformations cannot be observed with normal NMR spectra. Specialized NMR approaches such as chemical-exchange saturation transfer (CEST), Carr–Purcell–Meiboom–Gill (CPMG) relaxation dispersion, or paramagnetic relaxation enhancement (PRE) are able to find structural information on these transient states, although they are each constrained to particular ranges of timescales [104]. A recent study has been able to measure an interesting transient state in T4 lysozyme and build a NMR restrained MD simulation of the related enzyme catalytic process [105]. Despite some success in finding hidden conformations with NMR, it remains a challenge for routine applications due to difficulties in interpreting NMR data (*see* **Note 17**). In addition, the methods for evaluating consistency between structural conformations and chemical shift data are of limited accuracy [106]. Furthermore, NMR is often not able to generate data for larger proteins or homomultimers, which, along with the time it often takes to assign spectra, is a major limitation for applications in drug discovery [107]. This suggests that NMR-driven MD alone is not the answer to routinely finding hidden conformations.

Two-dimensional infrared spectroscopy (2DIR) is another interesting technique able to probe protein secondary structure elements without protein labeling. While the structural resolution of 2DIR is not particularly high compared to NMR it is able to cover a large array of timescales as the underlying time resolution is in the ps range. Labeling with azides or NO can offer residue level resolution. Thus far combinations with simulation have been at the level of cross-validation to help with assignment of spectra and understanding the timescales of ion-channel and [108, 109]. The use of temperature-jump 2DIR offers more detailed timescale data which can help validate information-rich simulations like MSMs [110]. The emergence of reliable methods for calculating 2DIR spectra from simulation data suggests that a more integrated combination with MD is a possibility [111].

The dream of integrative structural biology is to bring all of these different sources of structural data together in one model, which can be used to guide drug design. Platforms for the integration of any form of structural data into MD simulations have started to emerge and the favored approaches for this are Bayesian inference and the maximum entropy principle. The optimal combination and arrangement of these approaches is not completely clear yet and reviews and perspectives are starting to appear [112–114]. MELD uses a parameter describing the fraction of an experimental data set which is reliable combined with Bayesian inference picking out the most appropriate sets of restraints for each frame in a simulation. MELD is a well-developed platform with published examples of difficult problems like structure prediction but its application is limited to small systems [115]. Metainference is another advanced integrated simulation method implemented in Plumed, the well-known metadynamics plugin. Metainference is able to produce accurate simulations even with reduced models, such as implicit solvation, when combined with NMR chemical shift data [116].

A common use case when searching for hidden conformations is the non-direct use of experimental structural data. Any type of insight or hypothesis can be used to manually build variables for biasing potentials or adaptive sampling; but even with rich structural data, producing the conformational transitions often requires variables which are not obvious. The capture of a hidden conformation with Fab domains and X-ray crystal can suggest the existence of a whole new region of conformational space and be a great aid to MD-based conformational exploration. An interesting example is the antibody captured linear conformation of IgE; a large metadynamics simulation showed that this conformation is likely not stable in solution without the stabilizing Fab domains. Other conformations predicted to be metastable by the simulation were captured by the therapeutic antibody omalizumab [117, 118].

4.3.2 Utilizing Information from Related Proteins Families

Another important case is protein conformations which represent an inactive form. Examples can be found in the kinase and GPCR target classes. In these cases there may be structural data from related proteins allowing the generation of homology models. Additionally with large sets of related sequence data, evolutionary analysis can suggest contacts which may be important in conformational dynamics [119–121]. These coevolution contacts could be used in collective variables to drive molecular dynamics approaches such as metadynamics or adaptive sampling, although there are no successful studies of this so far. An example of coevolution contacts alone being used to predict large open to closed functional motion in the case of the glutamate receptor has been demonstrated by Marcos et al. [122]. In another interesting example, coevolution contacts were used to filter out important conformations proposed by a very coarse and rapid protein sampling method called discrete molecular dynamics [123]. Platforms like MELD have been used to bias all potential contacts in a conformational search [124], which might allow for easy searching based on coevolution contacts.

4.3.3 Working with No Knowledge of a Hidden Conformation

A small number of MD based approaches offer general (i.e., no knowledge of the hidden conformation required), transferable biasing potentials for larger systems. One potential approach is accelerated-MD (aMD) which adds a boost potential to all torsions and/or the potential energy, flattening the free-energy surface and making transitions more likely. Canonical ensemble averages and free-energies can be recovered by reweighting a process made easier with the more recent variant Gaussian-aMD (GaMD) [125]. aMD has been used to find transitions between known active and inactive conformations of Ras [126] and to find hidden conformations of maltose binding protein [127]. These studies have used a fraction of the simulation time of the DESRES studies discussed above, but aMD and GaMD are much more difficult to interpret even if a reweighted free-energy surface can be recovered.

Replica-exchange based approaches have been developing over many years and have been demonstrated in a great many forms, with generalized ensembles over temperature, biasing potentials, interaction scaling, etc. These methods have recently been used to improve orthogonal sampling for simulations where some specific variables are being biased.

There are examples of testing combinations of Hamiltonian exchange with aMD to evaluating its sampling power [128]. Replica-exchange methods were also combined with NMA to raise the temperature of specific modes, which were found by NMA without any prior knowledge [129, 130]. There is a recent example where a variation of replica-exchange called selective integrated tempering sampling (SITS) were applied to analyze global conformational transitions of protein kinases [131] (*see* **Note 18**).

Without any knowledge of potential hidden conformations, a search with molecular simulation can rely on computational brute force, which, despite many recent advances in high performance computing, is still far from sufficient in most cases. DESRES has reported examples where long unbiased simulations attempting to make difficult transitions between known active and inactive conformations have found intermediate states which might be amenable to structure-based design [132, 133]. Seeded adaptive, unbiased sampling has achieved similar feats to DESRES and Anton by exploring known transitions with unbiased dynamics and finding useful conformations and hidden pockets [12, 46, 75].

These authors have been unable to find examples of any enhanced simulation applied to a system with a single known conformation and finding significantly kinetically separated new conformations. While it is likely that these hidden conformations are waiting to be found, current simulation methods may not be sufficiently powerful to find them. Combinations of adaptive celling and potential biasing approaches may hold the key to this type of powerful search routine (*see* **Note 19**).

4.4 Understanding Allostery Without Conformational Change

Allostery without conformational change is a concept which has been discussed for many years [134]. This allostery is not restricted to those systems which are more rigid and ordered but just excludes a significant conformational change in geometry as the allosteric mechanism. The most relevant situation in drug discovery is the discovery of an allosteric compound through experimental screening where comparisons of available crystal structures of actives and non-actives or apo-structures seem the same. Often an allosteric small molecule will need to be optimized, which can be difficult when the molecular mechanism of action is not understood. Understanding the potential for allostery when evaluating target tractability is probably a less common problem, but this is a requirement for evaluation of a target or an allosteric pocket. Understanding transitions or allosteric signals without an obvious or significant geometrical change has many of the same challenges discussed above for transitions with obvious changes. The added difficulty is characterizing the transition even if this has been discovered or sampled as their structures can be very similar.

4.4.1 Challenge of Long Timescales and Hidden Transitions

This difficulty in predescribing cryptic allosteric transitions has caused a dearth of studies investigating these problems with driven simulation methods which use specific CVs. An interesting but rare example of this is the recent study of the KIX domain of CREB-binding protein with metadynamics [135] (*see* **Note 20**). aMD is also a sensible sampling method to sample cryptic allosteric transitions within single geometric conformations [136, 137].

Given the difficulty of sampling long timescale cryptic transitions, less computationally expensive approaches may offer a way forward. NMA methods can access many collective motions and has been used in approaches which look for correlated displacements between pockets [138] or modes which can transmit perturbations made in predicted pockets [139]. NMA approaches have been shown to capture long timescale dynamics of proteins but not the less populated states when compared to the millisecond trajectories of DESRES [140]. However, the lightly populated states were missed by NMA; motions with a low degree of collectively can also be missed.

Evolutionary constraint offers another rapid method for understanding correlated dynamics which may be able to access longer timescale phenomena. Studies to date have applied statistical coupling analysis (SCA) [141] which derives a statistical energy from the probability of a particular amino acid appearing at a given site. A conservation-weighted covariance matrix built with SCA leads to a "correlation entropy" which describes the allosteric coupling between groups of highly coupled residues. This coevolution derived analysis of allostery has been applied to serine proteases, hemoglobin, GPCRs, PDZ domains, PAS domains, SH2 and SH3, identifying functionally important residue sectors and allosteric couplings between them [142–144]. Subsequently, SCA correlation analysis combined with a small molecule pocket search and high-throughput docking has discovered an active compound for cathepsin K which binds at a novel allosteric binding site [145]. If the required sequence data is available, SCA offers detail of allosteric connections at any timescale with minimal computational costs. Although, coevolution approaches cannot account for post-translational modification or ligand binding which can be a problem for many drug targets.

The concepts of local instability relating to functionally important regions and minimal frustration have been described since the early discussions of protein folding [146, 147]. The group of Peter Wolynes evaluates residue frustration mutations or alternate configurations through coarse-grained comparison of energies after mutations and threading of the new sequence to available crystal structures [148, 149]. If the mutated energies are high compared to the wild-type then this position is considered minimally frustrated and vice versa. This approach has been packaged in an algorithm called the frustratometer, which can highlight regions which are likely to be functionally important [150, 151]. While based on approximate methods, prediction of dynamics by the frustratometer has been favorably compared to NMR data for the catabolite activator protein [152]. Another approach called CONTACT models alternate residue configurations into crystallography electron density, scoring potential van der Waals clashes and deriving a score similar to the frustratometer [153]. Pathways of residues which frustrate each other have been show to coincide with NMR data and extensive mutational studies [154].

4.4.2 MD Can Offer
Detailed Models at Shorter
Timescales

Despite the difficulty of accessing long timescales, analysis of relatively short unbiased MD simulations is a very popular approach for understanding cryptic allostery. The diversity of analysis approaches in the literature is very broad, but all attempt to statistically correlate the dynamics of two remote regions of the protein target. Mutual information has emerged as a powerful way to look at the potentially subtle correlations in protein dynamics, as it makes fewer assumptions than other common approaches like covariance analysis. Mutinf applies mutual information to analyze sets of repeated MD trajectories for correlations in dihedral motions [155]. Mutinf compares trajectory replicas and applies bootstrapping to remove predicted correlations which are considered noise. This analysis was qualitatively compared to NMR chemical shifts but has subsequently been used to understand allosteric pockets in kinase systems [156, 157]. In one recent example a previously unknown allosteric site was predicted, and subsequently active compounds were discovered with virtual screening and experimentally validated [158].

Researchers have now moved on from presenting pairwise correlation matrices to considering network community analysis of correlated motions [159]. Community analysis groups highly correlated residues together and scores the size of correlations between blocks. This is an important step, as it allows for simpler understanding and comparison of these highly degenerate networks. A series of studies have applied a mutual information community approach to understand the dynamical correlation network of protein kinase A (PKA) [160]. Calculated communities could be functionally annotated but did not fit with motifs based on sequence or secondary structure and were modified by conformational changes or ligand binding. This analysis of PKA also gave new understanding to known functional mutations which was then investigated with detailed biochemical experiments [161]. Also some of the dynamic correlations of the important hydrophobic spine regions have been validated with methyl-TROSY NMR [162].

A similar approach applied to thrombin has been able to explain how changes in the dynamics of the proteases surface loops on active site occupation lower the entropic penalty for binding an allosteric modulator [136, 137]. Interestingly, the slower dynamics of thrombins surface loops required the application of aMD and the frustratometer for the dynamic models to closely match the NMR data.

4.4.3 Combined
Platforms Maybe
an Optimal Way Forward

Analysis of atomistic MD clearly gives the quality models and detail required to understand how ligand binding and mutations affect the molecular switches which are often drug targets. However, as exemplified by this last set of studies, combining approximate methods like the frustratometer with detailed enhanced MD may bridge the gap to longer timescales. Another effective combination is that of SCA analysis and MD [121, 163]. Platforms for analyses of structures and trajectories have started to emerge [164, 165]. These combined platforms allow for rapid pipelining of combinations of advanced methods to achieve high quality models.

5   Conclusions

Understanding how protein drug targets function is very complex indeed. Many experienced drug hunters opine that there is much serendipity involved in discovering a drug candidate. At the level of drug target molecular mechanisms, the continual progress in molecular dynamics, in terms of timescales and model accuracy, offers a new level of rationality. In the future complex molecular mechanisms might be identified and understood at earlier stages in the drug discovery process, allowing valuable new functional effects and fine-tuned selectivity.

It is clear that atomistic, explicitly solvated molecular dynamics models offer a good balance between sampling speed and transferable accuracy. However, detailed aspects of protein drug targets such as protonation states and metal ion binding are especially important for delicate dynamic transitions, and in some cases require advanced and computationally more expensive models. Also, building models from crystal structures can be challenging even for experienced practitioners. Details about the local environment of the protein such as oxidation, lipids, and glycosylation are often crucial. In many cases mistakes made in initial model building can cause artifactual or misleading simulation data.

Despite the well-known limitations of molecular dynamics models, finite simulation length and underlying model quality, there are now many examples where simulations offer unique understanding of important dynamic transitions in protein drug targets. Crucially, these models are now often validated and sometimes driven by experimental data. Highlights discussed here are for important kinase, GPCR, and protease targets.

Many pharmaceutical companies now have specialists in molecular dynamics simulations within their research departments along with some significant high-performance computing capabilities. However, the majority of these researchers focus on small molecule binding affinity calculations such as those developed by Schrodinger. DESRES is a well-known leader in applying molecular dynamics to conformational transitions of drug targets. Another small company called Accellera is selling a specialist MSM and adaptive sampling platform to the industry along with support and services.

Hence, this activity is growing but currently is not a major focus for the pharma industry in general.

The authors recognize that for computational simulation to impact mainstream drug discovery it has to offer improved generality and speed. Computational simulation is not currently applicable to all targets of interest and can be extremely time consuming. The authors are acutely aware that the traditional pharma approach of high throughput screening has been successful and continues to deliver candidate molecules and successful drugs. Computational design is expensive, and a great deal of screening can be done for equivalent cost. While the authors believe that computational approaches will at least complement and eventually supersede traditional drug discovery approaches, particularly in difficult areas such as targeting protein–protein interactions with small molecule drugs, we are at the early stages of this transition. While intellectually challenging and occasionally satisfying, computational approaches need to be mindful of how successful drugs have been discovered in the past, and respectful of this heritage in order to truly impact drug discovery in real time and to influence the design of candidate molecules.

6 Notes

1. Apart from a small protein system (e.g., 2–3 residues), with current computing infrastructure it is often not possible to successfully calculate free-energies in more than a few dimensions.

2. For some large higher dimensional spaces, optimal projection descriptors for the energy surface (or collective variables) give useful information but at a much lower resolution (i.e., many details are missed) than what could be achieved in lower dimensions [117]. This issue of optimal collective variables or reaction coordinates is important for efficient sampling of protein motions and understanding of protein simulations.

3. With current computing infrastructure, it is often difficult to ensure all important conformations are explored by MD, especially those separated by large energy barriers [166, 167].

4. QM resolution protein simulations are possible although, even at low levels of theory, it is prohibitively computationally slow. A relatively recent GPU based simulation study using BOMD produced an 8.8 ps trajectory [168].

5. These atomistic MM force fields are designed to capture the most important interactions while being computationally inexpensive; hence the use of harmonic potentials rather than more realistic options such as the Morse potential.

6. MARTINI is a widely used CG model but cannot be used for modeling backbone conformational transitions owing to the use of an elastic network model (ENM) to restrain protein secondary structure to its starting conformation [169]. A recent development of MARTINI has been able to fold some protein fragments by replacing the ENM restraints with a contact map [170].

7. To perform NMA on an atomistic protein model a powerful minimization is required (to find the bottom of the approximated harmonic basin) followed by diagonalization of the second derivative of the potential energy ($3N \times 3N$ Hessian matrix).

8. Recent application code libraries such as Bio3D and ProDy offer advanced combinations of ENMs like pathway sampling strategies or correlation analyses, and can be used to build combinations for custom pipelines [164, 165].

9. The Gaussian height is reduced over time such that the simulation is forced to converge as the height tends to zero.

10. There is continual exploration of the optimal arrangements for replica-exchange but generally exchanges are made every 2–10,000 time steps and optimized such that at least 30% of exchanges are accepted [171].

11. Temperature replica-exchange with even moderately sized, explicitly solvated, systems requires many replicas owing to the high heat capacity of water.

12. The experiences of the current authors suggest that biasing over multiple replicas, each with an uncorrelated driven variable, is often able to explore protein conformational space in a very powerful way but can be difficult to converge.

13. There are currently at least five academic codes for managing large adaptive celling calculations [172–177].

14. A single Anton 2 computer can produce a ~115 us simulation per day on the standard industry test system. It should be noted that many important biological processes take place over much longer timescales. Anton 2 has been optimized for simulations of large models (~700,000 atoms), which fits with their aims of "investigating the mechanisms of several pharmaceutically relevant cellular receptors, transport proteins, and enzymes" as some of the suggested systems of study would be very large.

15. For example Morphic Therapeutics focused entirely on a very detailed understanding of the molecular mode of action of the integrin family of proteins to achieve a first in class therapeutic.

16. This screening strategy is likely to work best where the captured conformation is less affected by the bound Fab/VHH domain [178].

17. CPMG data can be difficult to interpret; there are cases where MD simulations found hidden conformations which in turn enabled the understanding of CPMG data through the fitting of a suitable model [179, 180].

18. This is a particularly interesting study, as it uses an approach which requires only a small amount of initial knowledge about the transition.

19. An interesting recent study combines celling with a self-seeding approach which uses the shape of the local energy surface to guess at new conformations to start unbiased simulations from [181]

20. Previous NMR studies offered limited but specific information about which side-chains were involved in this allostery. However, this information is not sufficient to build a CV to correctly sample these invisible states of KIX as the protein must access an excited state seen on a timescale of ~3 ms. In this case a special form of metadynamics, the well-tempered ensemble (WTE), was applied and the potential energy was used as a CV and biased. With the WTE the average energy is the same as seen without bias but the fluctuations are amplified, and the correct distribution can be generated through reweighting. A WTE simulation was able to extensively sample the excited state of KIX, in 100 ns of atomistic biased simulation, allowing a detailed understanding of the allosteric mechanism previously not possible.

References

1. Xia JZ, Wang Q, Tatarkova S et al (1996) Structural basis of eye lens transparency: light scattering by concentrated solutions of bovine alpha-crystallin proteins. Biophys J 71:2815–2822

2. Micheletti C (2013) Comparing proteins by their internal dynamics: exploring structure-function relationships beyond static structural alignments. Phys Life Rev 10:1–26

3. Striegel DA, Wojtowicz D, Przytycka TM et al (2016) Correlated rigid modes in protein families. Phys Biol 13:025003

4. Moore AD, Björklund ÅK, Ekman D et al (2008) Arrangements in the modular evolution of proteins. Trends Biochem Sci 33:444–451

5. McLeish TCB (2005) Protein folding in high-dimensional spaces: hypergutters and the role of nonnative interactions. Biophys J 88:172–183

6. Bowman GR, Pande VS (2010) Protein folded states are kinetic hubs. Proc Natl Acad Sci 107:10890–10895

7. Rimratchada S, McLeish TCB, Radford SE et al (2014) The role of high-dimensional diffusive search, stabilization, and frustration in protein folding. Biophys J 106:1729–1740

8. Wang K, Long S, Tian P (2015) Hierarchical conformational analysis of native lysozyme based on sub-millisecond molecular dynamics simulations. PLoS One 10:e0129846

9. Huang P-S, Boyken SE, Baker D (2016) The coming of age of de novo protein design. Nature 537:320–327

10. Townsend PD, Rodgers TL, Pohl E et al (2015) Global low-frequency motions in

protein allostery: CAP as a model system. Biophys Rev 7:175–182

11. Dinner AR, Šali A, Smith LJ et al (2000) Understanding protein folding via free-energy surfaces from theory and experiment. Trends Biochem Sci 25:331–339

12. Kohlhoff KJ, Shukla D, Lawrenz M et al (2014) Cloud-based simulations on Google Exacycle reveal ligand modulation of GPCR activation pathways. Nat Chem 6:15–21

13. Sweet CR, Hampton SS, Skeel RD et al (2009) A separable shadow Hamiltonian hybrid Monte Carlo method. J Chem Phys 131:174106

14. Levitt M (2001) The birth of computational structural biology. Nat Struct Biol 8:392–393

15. Pasi M, Lavery R, Ceres N (2013) PaLaCe: a coarse-grain protein model for studying mechanical properties. J Chem Theory Comput 9:785–793

16. Kar P, Gopal SM, Cheng Y-M et al (2013) PRIMO: a transferable coarse-grained force field for proteins. J Chem Theory Comput 9:3769–3788

17. Frembgen-Kesner T, Andrews CT, Li S et al (2015) Parametrization of backbone flexibility in a coarse-grained force field for proteins (COFFDROP) derived from all-atom explicit-solvent molecular dynamics simulations of all possible two-residue peptides. J Chem Theory Comput 11:2341–2354

18. Tirion M (1996) Large amplitude elastic motions in proteins from a single-parameter, atomic analysis. Phys Rev Lett 77:1905–1908

19. Atilgan A, Durell S, Jernigan R et al (2001) Anisotropy of fluctuation dynamics of proteins with an elastic network model. Biophys J 80:505–515

20. Orellana L, Rueda M, Ferrer-Costa C et al (2010) Approaching elastic network models to molecular dynamics flexibility. J Chem Theory Comput 6:2910–2923

21. Leioatts N, Romo TD, Grossfield A (2012) Elastic network models are robust to variations in formalism. J Chem Theory Comput 8:2424–2434

22. Xia F, Tong D, Yang L et al (2014) Identifying essential pairwise interactions in elastic network model using the alpha shape theory. J Comput Chem 35:1111–1121

23. Borrelli K, Vitalis A, Alcantra R et al (2005) PELE: protein energy landscape exploration. a novel Monte Carlo based technique. J Chem Theory Comput 1:1304–1311

24. Cossins B, Hosseini A, Guallar V (2012) Exploration of protein conformational change with PELE and meta-dynamics. J Comp Chem 8(3):959–965

25. Edman K, Hosseini A, Bjursell MK et al (2015) Ligand binding mechanism in steroid receptors: from conserved plasticity to differential evolutionary constraints. Structure 23:2280–2290

26. Grebner C, Lecina D, Gil V et al (2017) Exploring binding mechanisms in nuclear hormone receptors by Monte Carlo and X-ray-derived motions. Biophys J 112:1147–1156

27. Minary P, Levitt M (2010) Conformational optimization with natural degrees of freedom: a novel stochastic chain closure algorithm. J Comput Biol 17:993–1010

28. Sim AYL, Levitt M, Minary P (2012) Modeling and design by hierarchical natural moves. Proc Natl Acad Sci 109(8):2890–2895

29. Demharter S, Knapp B, Deane CM et al (2016) Modeling functional motions of biological systems by customized natural moves. Biophys J 111:710–721

30. Torrie G, Valleau J (1977) Nonphysical sampling distributions in Monte Carlo free-energy estimation: umbrella sampling. J Comput Phys 23(2):187–199

31. Sugita Y, Okamoto Y (1999) Replica-exchange molecular dynamics method for protein folding. Chem Phys Lett 314:141–151

32. Barducci A, Bonomi M, Parrinello M (2011) Metadynamics. WIREs Comput Mol Sci 1 (3):826–843

33. Elber R (2016) Perspective: computer simulations of long time dynamics. J Chem Phys 144 (6):060901

34. Kumar S, Bouzida D, Swendsen R et al (1992) The weighted histogram analysis method for free-energy calculations on biomolecules. I: the method. J Comput Chem 13:1011–1021

35. Barducci A, Bussi G, Parrinello M (2008) Well-tempered metadynamics: a smoothly converging and tunable (free-energy) method. Phys Rev Lett 100:020603

36. Comer J, Gumbart JC, Hénin J et al (2015) The adaptive biasing force method: everything you always wanted to know but were afraid to ask. J Phys Chem B 119:1129–1151

37. Brenner P, Sweet CR, VonHandorf D et al (2007) Accelerating the replica exchange method through an efficient all-pairs exchange. J Chem Phys 126:074103

38. Chodera J, Shirts M (2011) Replica exchange and expanded ensemble simulations as Gibbs

sampling: simple improvements for enhanced mixing. J Chem Phys 135(19):194110

39. Yu T-Q, Lu J, Abrams CF et al (2016) Multiscale implementation of infinite-swap replica exchange molecular dynamics. Proc Natl Acad Sci U S A 113:11744–11749

40. Wang L, Friesner RA, Berne BJ (2011) Replica exchange with solute scaling: a more efficient version of replica exchange with solute tempering (REST2). J Phys Chem B 115:9431–9438

41. Piana S, Laio A (2007) A (bias-exchange) approach to protein folding. J Phys Chem B 111:4553–4559

42. Bussi G (2013) Hamiltonian replica-exchange in GROMACS: a flexible implementation. Mol Phys 112:379

43. Sabri Dashti D, Roitberg AE (2013) Optimization of umbrella sampling replica exchange molecular dynamics by replica positioning. J Chem Theory Comput 9:4692–4699

44. Gil-Ley A, Bussi G (2015) Enhanced conformational sampling using replica exchange with collective-variable tempering. J Chem Theory Comput 11:1077–1085

45. Noé F, Doose S, Daidone I et al (2011) Dynamical fingerprints for probing individual relaxation processes in biomolecular dynamics with simulations and kinetic experiments. Proc Natl Acad Sci 108:4822–4827

46. Shukla D, Meng Y, Roux B et al (2014) Activation pathway of Src kinase reveals intermediate states as targets for drug design. Nat Commun 5:4397

47. Bowman GR, Ensign DL, Pande VS (2010) Enhanced modeling via network theory: adaptive sampling of Markov state models. J Chem Theory Comput 6:787–794

48. Doerr S, De Fabritiis G (2014) On-the-fly learning and sampling of ligand binding by high-throughput molecular simulations. J Chem Theory Comput 10:2064–2069

49. T. Tu, C.A. Rendleman, D.W. Borhani, et al. (2008) A scalable parallel framework for analyzing terascale molecular dynamics simulation trajectories. In: 2008 SC – international conference for high performance computing, networking, storage and analysis, pp. 1–12

50. Abel R, Mondal S, Masse C et al (2017) Accelerating drug discovery through tight integration of expert molecular design and predictive scoring. Curr Opin Struct Biol 43:38–44

51. B. Booth four decades of hacking biotech and yet biology still consumes everything. https://www.forbes.com/sites/brucebooth/2017/04/26/four-decades-of-hacking-biotech-and-yet-biology-still-consumes-everything/

52. Cossins BP, Lawson ADG (2015) Small molecule targeting of protein–protein interactions through allosteric modulation of dynamics. Molecules 20:16435–16445

53. Shaw DE, Deneroff MM, Dror RO et al (2007) Anton, a special-purpose machine for molecular dynamics simulation. In: Proceedings of the 34th annual international symposium on computer architecture. ACM, New York, NY, pp 1–12

54. Shaw DE, Grossman JP, J.A. Bank et al (2014) Anton 2: raising the bar for performance and programmability in a special-purpose molecular dynamics supercomputer. In: Proceedings of the international conference for high performance computing, networking, storage and analysis. IEEE Press, Piscataway, NJ, pp 41–53

55. J.P. Grossman, B. Towles, B. Greskamp, et al. (2015) Filtering, reductions and synchronization in the Anton 2 network. In: Parallel and distributed processing symposium (IPDPS), 2015 I.E. international, pp. 860–870

56. Shan Y, Seeliger MA, Eastwood MP et al (2009) A conserved protonation-dependent switch controls drug binding in the Abl kinase. Proc Natl Acad Sci 106:139–144

57. Foda ZH, Shan Y, Kim ET et al (2015) A dynamically coupled allosteric network underlies binding cooperativity in Src kinase. Nat Commun 6:5939

58. Lovera S, Sutto L, Boubeva R et al (2012) The different flexibility of c-Src and c-Abl kinases regulates the accessibility of a druggable inactive conformation. J Am Chem Soc 134:2496–2499

59. Lin Y-L, Meng Y, Jiang W et al (2013) Explaining why Gleevec is a specific and potent inhibitor of Abl kinase. Proc Natl Acad Sci U S A 110:1664–1669

60. Meng Y, Lin Y, Roux B (2015) Computational study of the "DFG-flip" conformational transition in c-Abl and c-Src tyrosine kinases. J Phys Chem B 119:1443–1456

61. Morando MA, Saladino G, D'Amelio N et al (2016) Conformational selection and induced fit mechanisms in the binding of an anticancer drug to the c-Src kinase. Sci Rep 6:srep24439

62. Dror RO, Arlow DH, Maragakis P et al (2011) Activation mechanism of the β2-adrenergic receptor. Proc Natl Acad Sci 108:18684–18689

63. Fan Z, Dror RO, Mildorf TJ et al (2015) Identifying localized changes in large systems: change-point detection for biomolecular

simulations. Proc Natl Acad Sci 112:7454–7459

64. Kozakov D, Grove LE, Hall DR et al (2015) The FTMap family of web servers for determining and characterizing ligand binding hot spots of proteins. Nat Protoc 10:733–755

65. Halgren T (2009) Identifying and characterizing binding sites and assessing druggability. J Chem Inf Model 49:377–389

66. Radoux CJ, Olsson TSG, Pitt WR et al (2016) Identifying interactions that determine fragment binding at protein hotspots. J Med Chem 59:4314–4325

67. Schames JR, Henchman RH, Siegel JS et al (2004) Discovery of a novel binding trench in HIV integrase. J Med Chem 47:1879–1881

68. Frembgen-Kesner T, Elcock AH (2006) Computational sampling of a cryptic drug binding site in a protein receptor: explicit solvent molecular dynamics and inhibitor docking to p38 MAP kinase. J Mol Biol 359:202–214

69. Eyrisch S, Helms V (2007) Transient pockets on protein surfaces involved in protein–protein interaction. J Med Chem 50:3457–3464

70. Tan YS, Śledź P, Lang S et al (2012) Using ligand-mapping simulations to design a ligand selectively targeting a cryptic surface pocket of polo-like kinase 1. Angew Chem Int Ed 51:10078–10081

71. Kunze J, Todoroff N, Schneider P et al (2014) Targeting dynamic pockets of HIV-1 protease by structure-based computational screening for allosteric inhibitors. J Chem Inf Model 54:987–991

72. Pietro OD, Juárez-Jiménez J, Muñoz-Torrero D et al (2017) Unveiling a novel transient druggable pocket in BACE-1 through molecular simulations: conformational analysis and binding mode of multisite inhibitors. PLoS One 12:e0177683

73. Bowman GR, Geissler PL (2012) Equilibrium fluctuations of a single folded protein reveal a multitude of potential cryptic allosteric sites. Proc Natl Acad Sci 109:11681–11686

74. Yang C-Y (2015) Identification of potential small molecule allosteric modulator sites on IL-1R1 ectodomain using accelerated conformational sampling method. PLoS One 10:e0118671

75. Bowman GR, Bolin ER, Hart KM et al (2015) Discovery of multiple hidden allosteric sites by combining Markov state models and experiments. Proc Natl Acad Sci 112:2734–2739

76. Hart KM, Moeder KE, Ho CMW et al (2017) Designing small molecules to target cryptic pockets yields both positive and negative allosteric modulators. PLoS One 12:e0178678

77. Seco J, Luque FJ, Barril X (2009) Binding site detection and druggability index from first principles. J Med Chem 52:2363–2371

78. Guvench O, MacKerell AD (2009) Computational fragment-based binding site identification by ligand competitive saturation. PLoS Comput Biol 5:e1000435

79. Raman EP, Yu W, Lakkaraju SK et al (2013) Inclusion of multiple fragment types in the site identification by ligand competitive saturation (SILCS) approach. J Chem Inf Model 53:3384–3398

80. Alvarez-Garcia D, Barril X (2014) Molecular simulations with solvent competition quantify water displaceability and provide accurate interaction maps of protein binding sites. J Med Chem 57(20):8530–8539

81. Kimura SR, Hu HP, Ruvinsky AM et al (2017) Deciphering cryptic binding sites on proteins by mixed-solvent molecular dynamics. J Chem Inf Model 57:1388–1401

82. Kalenkiewicz A, Grant BJ, Yang C-Y (2015) Enrichment of druggable conformations from apo protein structures using cosolvent-accelerated molecular dynamics. Biology 4:344–366

83. Oleinikovas V, Saladino G, Cossins BP et al (2016) Understanding cryptic pocket formation in protein targets by enhanced sampling simulations. J Am Chem Soc 138:14257–14263

84. Abskharon RNN, Giachin G, Wohlkonig A et al (2014) Probing the N-terminal β-sheet conversion in the crystal structure of the human prion protein bound to a nanobody. J Am Chem Soc 136:937–944

85. Lawson ADG (2014) Antibody fragments defining biologically relevant conformations of target proteins. Antibodies 3:289–302

86. Ghosh E, Kumari P, Jaiman D et al (2015) Methodological advances: the unsung heroes of the GPCR structural revolution. Nat Rev Mol Cell Biol 16:69–81

87. Huang W, Manglik A, Venkatakrishnan AJ et al (2015) Structural insights into μ-opioid receptor activation. Nature 524:315–321

88. Staus DP, Strachan RT, Manglik A et al (2016) Allosteric nanobodies reveal the dynamic range and diverse mechanisms of G-protein-coupled receptor activation. Nature 535:448–452

89. Sounier R, Mas C, Steyaert J et al (2015) Propagation of conformational changes during μ-opioid receptor activation. Nature 524:375–378

90. Westfield GH, Rasmussen SGF, Su M et al (2011) Structural flexibility of the Gαs α-helical domain in the β2-adrenoceptor Gs complex. Proc Natl Acad Sci 108:16086–16091

91. Irannejad R, Tomshine JC, Tomshine JR et al (2013) Conformational biosensors reveal adrenoceptor signalling from endosomes. Nature 495:534–538

92. DeVree BT, Mahoney JP, Vélez-Ruiz GA et al (2016) Allosteric coupling from G protein to the agonist-binding pocket in GPCRs. Nature 535:182–186

93. Lawson ADG (2012) Antibody-enabled small-molecule drug discovery. Nat Rev Drug Discov 11:519–525

94. Schlitter J, Engels M, Krüger P (1994) Targeted molecular dynamics: a new approach for searching pathways of conformational transitions. J Mol Graph 12:84–89

95. Ovchinnikov V, Karplus M (2012) Analysis and elimination of a bias in targeted molecular dynamics simulations of conformational transitions: application to calmodulin. J Phys Chem B 116:8584–8603

96. Wang J, Shao Q, Xu Z et al (2014) Exploring transition pathway and free-energy profile of large-scale protein conformational change by combining normal mode analysis and umbrella sampling molecular dynamics. J Phys Chem B 118:134–143

97. Chen P, Hub JS (2015) Interpretation of solution X-ray scattering by explicit-solvent molecular dynamics. Biophys J 108:2573–2584

98. Kimanius D, Pettersson I, Schluckebier G et al (2015) SAXS-guided metadynamics. J Chem Theory Comput 11:3491–3498

99. Peng J, Zhang Z (2016) Unraveling low-resolution structural data of large biomolecules by constructing atomic models with experiment-targeted parallel cascade selection simulations. Sci Rep 6:29360

100. Carrington B, Myers WK, Horanyi P et al (2017) Natural conformational sampling of human TNFα visualized by double electron-electron resonance. Biophys J 113:371–380

101. Roux B, Islam SM (2013) Restrained-ensemble molecular dynamics simulations based on distance histograms from double electron–electron resonance spectroscopy. J Phys Chem B 117:4733–4739

102. Marinelli F, Faraldo-Gómez JD (2015) Ensemble-biased metadynamics: a molecular simulation method to sample experimental distributions. Biophys J 108:2779–2782

103. Granata D, Camilloni C, Vendruscolo M et al (2013) Characterization of the free-energy landscapes of proteins by NMR-guided metadynamics. Proc Natl Acad Sci U S A 110:6817–6822

104. Sekhar A, Kay LE (2013) NMR paves the way for atomic level descriptions of sparsely populated, transiently formed biomolecular conformers. Proc Natl Acad Sci U S A 110:12867–12874

105. Simone AD, Aprile FA, Dhulesia A et al (2015) Structure of a low-population intermediate state in the release of an enzyme product. elife 4:e02777

106. Han B, Liu Y, Ginzinger SW et al (2011) SHIFTX2: significantly improved protein chemical shift prediction. J Biomol NMR 50:43–57

107. Frueh DP, Goodrich A, Mishra S et al (2013) NMR methods for structural studies of large monomeric and multimeric proteins. Curr Opin Struct Biol 23:734–739

108. Cheng M, Brookes JF, Montfort WR et al (2013) pH-dependent picosecond structural dynamics in the distal pocket of nitrophorin 4 investigated by 2D IR spectroscopy. J Phys Chem B 117:15804–15811

109. Kratochvil HT, Carr JK, Matulef K et al (2016) Instantaneous ion configurations in the K+ ion channel selectivity filter revealed by 2D IR spectroscopy. Science 353:1040–1044

110. Baiz CR, Lin YS, Peng CS et al (2014) A molecular interpretation of 2D IR protein folding experiments with Markov state models. Biophys J 106:1359–1370

111. Husseini FS, Robinson D, Hunt NT et al (2017) Computing infrared spectra of proteins using the exciton model. J Comput Chem 38:1362–1375

112. Boomsma WJ, Ferkinghoff-Borg L-LK (2014) Combining experiments and simulations using the maximum entropy principle. PLoS Comput Biol 10:e1003406

113. Bonomi M, Heller GT, Camilloni C et al (2017) Principles of protein structural ensemble determination. Curr Opin Struct Biol 42:106–116

114. Perez A, Morrone JA, Dill KA (2017) Accelerating physical simulations of proteins by leveraging external knowledge. WIREs Comput Mol Sci 7(5):e1309

115. Perez A, Morrone JA, Brini E et al (2016) Blind protein structure prediction using accelerated free-energy simulations. Sci Adv 2:e1601274

116. Löhr T, Jussupow A, Camilloni C (2017) Metadynamic metainference: convergence towards force field independent structural ensembles of a disordered peptide. J Chem Phys 146:165102

117. Drinkwater N, Cossins BP, Keeble AH et al (2014) Human immunoglobulin E flexes between acutely bent and extended conformations. Nat Struct Mol Biol 21:397–404

118. Davies AM, Allan EG, Keeble AH et al (2017) Allosteric mechanism of action of the therapeutic anti-IgE antibody omalizumab. J Biol Chem 292:9975–9987

119. Sutto L, Marsili S, Valencia A et al (2015) From residue coevolution to protein conformational ensembles and functional dynamics. Proc Natl Acad Sci U S A 112:13567–13572

120. Stetz G, Verkhivker GM (2017) Computational analysis of residue interaction networks and coevolutionary relationships in the Hsp70 chaperones: a community-hopping model of allosteric regulation and communication. PLoS Comput Biol 13:e1005299

121. Lakhani B, Thayer KM, Hingorani MM et al (2017) Evolutionary covariance combined with molecular dynamics predicts a framework for allostery in the MutS DNA mismatch repair protein. J Phys Chem B 121:2049–2061

122. Morcos F, Jana B, Hwa T et al (2013) Coevolutionary signals across protein lineages help capture multiple protein conformations. Proc Natl Acad Sci U S A 110:20533–20538

123. Sfriso P, Duran-Frigola M, Mosca R et al (2016) Residues coevolution guides the systematic identification of alternative functional conformations in proteins. Structure 24:116–126

124. Morrone JA, Perez A, MacCallum J et al (2017) Computed binding of peptides to proteins with MELD-accelerated molecular dynamics. J Chem Theory Comput 13:870–876

125. Miao Y, Feher VA, McCammon JA (2015) Gaussian accelerated molecular dynamics: unconstrained enhanced sampling and free energy calculation. J Chem Theory Comput 11:3584–3595

126. Grant BJ, Gorfe AA, McCammon JA (2009) Ras conformational switching: simulating nucleotide-dependent conformational transitions with accelerated molecular dynamics. PLoS Comput Biol 5:e1000325

127. Bucher D, Grant BJ, Markwick PR et al (2011) Accessing a hidden conformation of the maltose binding protein using accelerated molecular dynamics. PLoS Comput Biol 7: e1002034

128. Roe DR, Bergonzo C, Cheatham TE (2014) Evaluation of enhanced sampling provided by accelerated molecular dynamics with Hamiltonian replica exchange methods. J Phys Chem B 118:3543–3552

129. Kubitzki MB, de Groot BL (2008) The atomistic mechanism of conformational transition in adenylate kinase: a TEE-REX molecular dynamics study. Structure 16:1175–1182

130. Shao Q (2016) Enhanced conformational sampling technique provides an energy landscape view of large-scale protein conformational transitions. Phys Chem Chem Phys 18:29170–29182

131. Shao Q, Xu Z, Wang J et al (2017) Energetics and structural characterization of the "DFG-flip" conformational transition of B-RAF kinase: a SITS molecular dynamics study. Phys Chem Chem Phys 19:1257–1267

132. Dror R, Arlow D, Borhani D et al (2009) Identification of two distinct inactive conformations of the beta 2-adrenergic receptor reconciles structural and biochemical observations. Proc Natl Acad Sci U S A 106:4689–4694

133. Shan Y, Arkhipov A, Kim ET et al (2013) Transitions to catalytically inactive conformations in EGFR kinase. Proc Natl Acad Sci U S A 110:7270–7275

134. Cooper A, Dryden DT (1984) Allostery without conformational change. A plausible model. Eur Biophys J 11:103–109

135. Palazzesi F, Barducci A, Tollinger M et al (2013) The allosteric communication pathways in KIX domain of CBP. Proc Natl Acad Sci U S A 110:14237–14242

136. Gasper PM, Fuglestad B, Komives EA et al (2012) Allosteric networks in thrombin distinguish procoagulant vs. anticoagulant activities. Proc Natl Acad Sci U S A 109:21216–21222

137. Fuglestad B, Gasper PM, McCammon JA et al (2013) correlated motions and residual frustration in thrombin. J Phys Chem B 117:12857–12863

138. Clarke D, Sethi A, Li S et al (2016) Identifying allosteric hotspots with dynamics: application to inter- and intra-species conservation. Structure 24:826–837

139. Greener JG, Sternberg MJ (2015) AlloPred: prediction of allosteric pockets on proteins using normal mode perturbation analysis. BMC Bioinformatics 16:335

140. Gur M, Zomot E, Bahar I (2013) Global motions exhibited by proteins in micro- to

milliseconds simulations concur with aniso-
tropic network model predictions. J Chem
Phys 139:121912

141. Lockless SW, Ranganathan R (1999) Evolutionarily conserved pathways of energetic
connectivity in protein families. Science
286:295–299

142. Süel GM, Lockless SW, Wall MA et al (2003)
Evolutionarily conserved networks of residues
mediate allosteric communication in proteins.
Nat Struct Mol Biol 10:59–69

143. Halabi N, Rivoire O, Leibler S et al (2009)
Protein sectors: evolutionary units of three-
dimensional structure. Cell 138:774–786

144. McLaughlin RN, Poelwijk FJ Jr, Raman A
et al (2012) The spatial architecture of protein
function and adaptation. Nature
491:138–142

145. Novinec M, Korenč M, Caflisch A et al (2014)
A novel allosteric mechanism in the cysteine
peptidase cathepsin K discovered by computational methods. Nat Commun 5:4287

146. Bryngelson JD, Wolynes PG (1987) Spin
glasses and the statistical mechanics of protein
folding. Proc Natl Acad Sci U S A
84:7524–7528

147. Ferreiro DU, Hegler JA, Komives EA et al
(2007) Localizing frustration in native proteins and protein assemblies. Proc Natl Acad
Sci U S A 104:19819–19824

148. Papoian GA, Ulander J, Wolynes PG (2003)
Role of water mediated interactions in pro-
tein–protein recognition landscapes. J Am
Chem Soc 125:9170–9178

149. Davtyan A, Schafer NP, Zheng W et al (2012)
AWSEM-MD: protein structure prediction
using coarse-grained physical potentials and
bioinformatically based local structure biasing. J Phys Chem B 116:8494–8503

150. Jenik M, Parra RG, Radusky LG et al (2012)
Protein frustratometer: a tool to localize ener-
getic frustration in protein molecules. Nucleic
Acids Res 40:W348–W351

151. Parra RG, Schafer NP, Radusky LG et al
(2016) Protein frustratometer 2: a tool to
localize energetic frustration in protein molecules, now with electrostatics. Nucleic Acids
Res 44:W356–W360

152. Ferreiro DU, Hegler JA, Komives EA et al
(2011) On the role of frustration in the
energy landscapes of allosteric proteins. Proc
Natl Acad Sci U S A 108:3499–3503

153. van den Bedem H, Bhabha G, Yang K et al
(2013) Automated identification of functional dynamic networks from X-ray crystallography. Nat Methods 10:896–902

154. Boehr DD, Schnell JR, McElheny D et al
(2013) A distal mutation perturbs dynamic
amino acid networks in dihydrofolate reduc-
tase. Biochemistry 52:4605–4619

155. McClendon CL, Friedland G, Mobley DL
et al (2009) Quantifying correlations between
allosteric sites in thermodynamic ensembles. J
Chem Theory Comput 5:2486–2502

156. Cembran A, Masterson LR, McClendon CL
et al (2012) Conformational equilibrium of
n-myristoylated camp-dependent protein
kinase a by molecular dynamics simulations.
Biochemistry 51:10186–10196

157. Wan X, Ma Y, McClendon CL et al (2013) Ab
Initio modeling and experimental assessment
of Janus Kinase 2 (JAK2) kinase-pseudokinase
complex structure. PLoS Comput Biol 9:
e1003022

158. Meng H, McClendon CL, Dai Z et al (2016)
Discovery of novel 15-lipoxygenase activators
to shift the human arachidonic acid metabolic
network toward inflammation resolution. J
Med Chem 59:4202–4209

159. Sethi A, Eargle J, Black AA et al (2009) Dynamical networks in tRNA: protein complexes.
Proc Natl Acad Sci U S A 106:6620–6625

160. McClendon CL, Kornev AP, Gilson MK et al
(2014) Dynamic architecture of a protein
kinase. Proc Natl Acad Sci U S A 111:
E4623–E4631

161. Ahuja LG, Kornev AP, McClendon CL et al
(2017) Mutation of a kinase allosteric node
uncouples dynamics linked to phosphotrans-
fer. Proc Natl Acad Sci U S A 114:
E931–E940

162. Kim J, Ahuja LG, Chao FA et al (2017) A
dynamic hydrophobic core orchestrates allostery in protein kinases. Sci Adv 3:e1600663

163. Armenta-Medina D, Pérez-Rueda E, Segovia
L (2011) Identification of functional motions
in the adenylate kinase (ADK) protein family
by computational hybrid approaches. Proteins 79:1662–1671

164. Bakan A, Dutta A, Mao W et al (2014) Evol
and ProDy for bridging protein sequence
evolution and structural dynamics. Bioinformatics 30:2681–2683

165. Skjærven L, Yao XQ, Scarabelli G et al (2014)
Integrating protein structural dynamics and
evolutionary analysis with Bio3D. BMC Bioinformatics 15:399

166. Adcock SA, McCammon JA (2006) Molecular dynamics: survey of methods for simulating the activity of proteins. Chem Rev
106:1589–1615

167. Genheden S, Ryde U (2012) Will molecular
dynamics simulations of proteins ever reach

equilibrium? Phys Chem Chem Phys 14:8662–8677

168. Ufimtsev IS, Luehr N, Martinez TJ (2011) Charge transfer and polarization in solvated proteins from ab initio molecular dynamics. J Phys Chem Lett 2:1789–1793

169. Marrink SJ, Peter Tieleman D (2013) Perspective on the Martini model. Chem Soc Rev 42:6801–6822

170. Poma AB, Cieplak M, Theodorakis PE (2017) Combining the MARTINI and structure-based coarse-grained approaches for the molecular dynamics studies of conformational transitions in proteins. J Chem Theory Comput 13:1366–1374

171. Sindhikara D, Emerson D, Roitberg A (2010) Exchange often and properly in replica exchange molecular dynamics. J Chem Theory Comput 6:2804–2808

172. Beauchamp KA, Bowman GR, Lane TJ et al (2011) MSMBuilder2: modeling conformational dynamics on the picosecond to millisecond scale. J Chem Theory Comput 7:3412–3419

173. Doerr S, Harvey MJ, Noé F et al (2016) HTMD: high-throughput molecular dynamics for molecular discovery. J Chem Theory Comput 12:1845–1852

174. Pronk S, Bowman GR, Hess B et al (2011) Copernicus: a new paradigm for parallel adaptive molecular dynamics. In: 2011 international conference for high performance computing, networking, storage and analysis (SC), pp 1–10

175. Abdul-Wahid B, Feng H, Rajan D et al (2014) AWE-WQ: fast-forwarding molecular dynamics using the accelerated weighted ensemble. J Chem Info Model 54:3033–3043

176. Shkurti A, Laughton C, Goni R et al (2015) ExTASY: a python-based extensible toolkit for advanced sampling and analysis in biomolecular simulation. Presented at the EuroSciPy 2015

177. Feng H, Costaouec R, Darve E et al (2015) A comparison of weighted ensemble and Markov state model methodologies. J Chem Phys 142:214113

178. Saleh N, Ibrahim P, Clark T (2017) Differences between G-protein-stabilized agonist–GPCR complexes and their nanobody-stabilized equivalents. Angew Chem Int Ed 56:9008–9012

179. Shaw DE, Maragakis P, Lindorff-Larsen K et al (2010) Atomic-level characterization of the structural dynamics of proteins. Science (New York, NY) 330:341–346

180. Xue Y, Ward JM, Yuwen T et al (2012) Microsecond time-scale conformational exchange in proteins: using long molecular dynamics trajectory to simulate NMR relaxation dispersion data. J Am Chem Soc 134:2555–2562

181. Chiavazzo E, Covino R, Coifman RR et al (2017) Intrinsic map dynamics exploration for uncharted effective free-energy landscapes. Proc Natl Acad Sci 114(28): E5494–E5503

Chapter 18

Applications of the NRGsuite and the Molecular Docking Software FlexAID in Computational Drug Discovery and Design

Louis-Philippe Morency, Francis Gaudreault, and Rafael Najmanovich

Abstract

Docking simulations help us understand molecular interactions. Here we present a hands-on tutorial to utilize FlexAID (*Flex*ible *A*rtificial *I*ntelligence *D*ocking), an open source molecular docking software between ligands such as small molecules or peptides and macromolecules such as proteins and nucleic acids. The tutorial uses the NRGsuite PyMOL plugin graphical user interface to set up and visualize docking simulations in real time as well as detect and refine target cavities. The ease of use of FlexAID and the NRGsuite combined with its superior performance relative to widely used docking software provides nonexperts with an important tool to understand molecular interactions with direct applications in structure-based drug design and virtual high-throughput screening.

Key words Computer-aided drug design, Binding mode prediction, Lead identification, Molecular docking, Molecular flexibility, Molecular recognition, Protein–ligand complex

1 Introduction

All biological processes are fundamentally guided by molecular recognition events. The study of molecular recognition aims at understanding the factors affecting the selectivity and specificity of molecular interactions. Advances in molecular biology, notably in protein identification, expression, purification, and structural determination, gave rise to an abundance of information about the three dimensional structure of macromolecules and their molecular complexes accessible through the Protein Data Bank (PDB) [1]. As a significant portion of molecular interactions may in principle be modulated by exogenous small molecules, the large-scale analysis of ligand–protein interactions helps understand the evolution of ligand binding [2] and paved the way for the development of computational techniques such as molecular docking. Docking is at the core of virtual high-throughput screening and is frequently used together with other computational techniques for a

Mohini Gore and Umesh B. Jagtap (eds.), *Computational Drug Discovery and Design*, Methods in Molecular Biology, vol. 1762, https://doi.org/10.1007/978-1-4939-7756-7_18, © Springer Science+Business Media, LLC, part of Springer Nature 2018

wide range of applications in computer-assisted drug design. Molecular docking gained interest in the early stages of the drug discovery process because of its relatively low computational cost to evaluate many potential compounds [3].

Molecular docking can be used to tackle three different questions in drug design [4]: (1) Binding mode prediction, (2) Virtual high-throughput screening; and (3) Structure-based prediction of binding affinities. Binding mode prediction aims at obtaining the three-dimensional structure of the complex between a ligand of interest and the target. Binding mode prediction is used to understand the underlying interactions involved in the stabilization of the complex and can be used as a guide for structure-based drug design. Virtual high-throughput screening (vHTS) aims at detecting bioactive ligands from large compound databases. vHTS generally relies on binding-mode prediction but often requires the use of rescoring methods to determine the relative order of compounds with respect to their unknown binding affinities. The last task is the estimation of binding free-energy differences from the structure of the complex. Although it is possible to develop regression or machine learning based methods to predict binding-free energies, it is unclear how generalizable their results may be when encountering different ligands or target classes. It is generally assumed that only a structure based approach should be able to predict correctly binding free energies. A fast and accurate method to calculate binding free energy differences has not been found yet. Such a method would replace existing vHTS rescoring methods but would still require the accurate prediction of the three-dimensional structure of the ligand–protein complex.

Generally speaking, binding mode prediction explores in more detail the degrees of freedom that represent molecular flexibility [5] whereas virtual screening uses a faster search and scoring method to process more compounds and the structure-based prediction of affinities requires accurately predicted binding-modes and lengthy statistical-mechanics based calculations. However, the increase in computational power allows the use of slower docking algorithms, especially those focusing on binding mode prediction, in a high-throughput manner [6] with scoring functions precise enough to discriminate bioactive molecules from decoys [7–10]. Hence, binding mode prediction methods are standard in computer-aided drug discovery, either to explain the molecular mechanism behind the formation of a complex or to search for new bioactive ligands from virtual libraries through high-throughput virtual screening.

Recent advances in molecular docking focus on modeling the docking simulation more realistically through for example inclusion of structural water molecules and molecular flexibility [11–13]. In general, molecular flexibility of the target has at most been restricted to side-chain movements. However, attempts are being made at considering additional degrees of freedom accounting for the target flexibility [14, 15] to account for conformational changes that occur upon binding [16], mostly because proteins exist in a multiconformational thermodynamic equilibrium [17]. Indeed, molecular rearrangements in the binding site are common [18] and, in approximately 30% of cases, are critical for ligand binding [19].

The molecular docking software FlexAID (*Flex*ible *A*rtificial *I*ntelligence *D*ocking) [20] has been developed as an open source binding mode prediction software with a focus on modeling molecular flexibility. Among other features, FlexAID searches the conformational landscape with a genetic algorithm, uses a soft and permissive scoring function based on the surface of contact between atoms, fully simulates ligand flexibility, uses a probabilistic rotameric approach to simulate side-chains flexibility in the target, simulates large-scale backbone movements of the target using the normal mode analysis method ENCoM [21], and allows for the simulation of covalent docking. The energy parameters utilized by the FlexAID scoring function were derived from the supervised learning (classification) of a large dataset of low energy false positive decoys (root-mean squared distance, RMSD >2 Å) and true positive decoys (RMSD ≤ 2.0 Å) for over 1300 ligand–protein complexes from the PDBbind database [22]. Notably, FlexAID outperforms many other open source molecular docking methods specialized in binding mode prediction such as Autodock Vina [23], FlexX [24], and rDock [25], particularly when molecular flexibility is crucial [20]. FlexAID is developed in C and C++, is distributed open source, and runs on all major operating systems for personal computers. FlexAID has an interactive PyMOL plugin graphical user interface, the NRGsuite [26] that greatly simplifies its use and permits the visualization in real time of the docking simulation as well as the detection, refinement, and measurement of cavities. In addition to being widely used as an educational tool, FlexAID has also been successfully used in a number of applications. Notably, to explain the binding mode of primary bile acid in a StaR-related lipid transfer domain [27], to target the germination protease and guanine riboswitch of *Clostridium difficile* as novel antibiotic targets, to analyze binding site specificity in the human serine protease Matriptase [28] and discover new bioactive molecules against the human serine protease TMPRSS6 [28], and further validate hypotheses of potential cross-reactivity targets responsible for the side-effects of approved drugs and their repurposing [29].

In the following sections, we demonstrate how to use FlexAID and the NRGsuite to predict the binding mode of a common drug to its molecular target. As an example of binding mode prediction, FlexAID will be used to predict the binding mode of the influenza neuraminidase inhibitor zanamivir (Fig. 1). We encourage the user to repeat the methodology with different ligands and parameters to

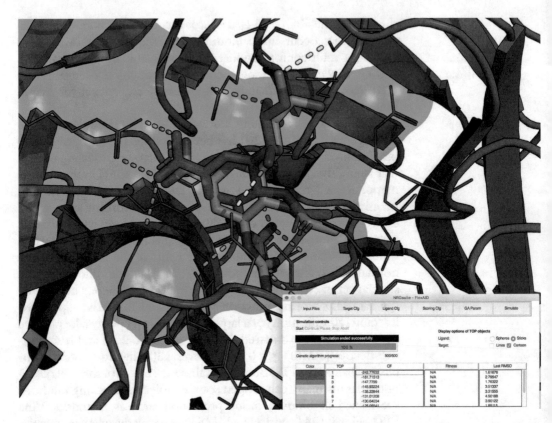

Fig. 1 The binding mode of zanamivir predicted by FlexAID (RESULT_1) is shown in red colored sticks with its predicted hydrogen bonds in yellow dashed lines. The pose of reference is shown in white sticks. By default, however, the target is color-coded using the colors in the table and is shown as "Cartoon." The ligand and other optimized residues (including side-chains) are shown in white as sticks surrounded by its residues shown as lines. FlexAID Simulate tab (shown at the bottom right) displays information in a table format about the coloring scheme of the molecules for different results (column 1), the rank of the results (column 2) an evaluation of their energy of binding (column 3) and the RMSD from the reference (column 5)

compare results. The methodology explained here will allow the user to repeat the experiment with any complex and could easily be adapted for high-throughput applications by more advanced users by means of scripting the use of the input files created with the NRGsuite for a given target.

2   Materials

For this tutorial, it will be necessary to install the molecular visualization system PyMOL (*see* **Note 1**) and the NRGsuite software package that contains every tool to be used in this tutorial (*see* **Note 2**). All the software is available for the major operating systems, i.e., Linux, macOS, and Windows, but it is important to install the appropriate version of the NRGsuite for your system (*see* **Note 3**).

After the installation of both PyMOL and the NRGsuite, the last step required is to open PyMOL and install the NRGsuite as a plugin (*see* **Note 4**).

3 Methods

During this tutorial, the main objective will be to retrieve the experimentally observed binding mode of a drug in complex with its target. Although several experimental methods can now solve high resolution (*see* **Note 5**) tridimensional structures of these complexes, e.g., liquid and solid state nuclear magnetic resonance (NMR) and electron microscopy (EM), X-ray crystallography remains the most popular technique used in structure determination (*see* **Note 6**). The experimental structure of the complex is called the reference, and it will be used as a control to validate the accuracy of the predictions made during the molecular docking simulations (*see* **Note 7**).

The prediction of the binding mode of a drug-like molecule to a biologically relevant target of interest, mostly a chain of amino or nucleic acids (*see* **Note 8**), is entirely performed inside PyMOL and using the graphical user interface NRGsuite for the molecular docking software FlexAID. The following protocol can be executed on any standard personal computer and does not require any specialized hardware.

As a case study during this protocol, we will be interested in the drug zanamivir, commonly distributed under the name Relenza by Gilead Sciences. Zanamivir has been developed as a neuraminidase inhibitor to treat and prevent the transmission of infections by influenza A and B viruses. The neuraminidase enzymes (acylneuraminyl hydrolase, E.C. 3.2.1.18) hydrolyzes the glycosidic bond linking a terminal sialic acid and other sugar molecules located on a host cells' surface and/or on the hemagglutinin [30]. The cleavage of the sialic acid bond, specifically the α-ketosidic linkage between terminal sialic acid and adjacent sugar at the surface of the infected cell, eases the diffusion of viral particles from infected host cells toward new cells, thus facilitating the viral infection [31]. The determination of the tridimensional structure of the glycoprotein neuraminidase [32] in 1983 allowed the structure-based design of antiviral agents targeting the conserved structure of its binding site [33]. Interestingly, computer-aided drug discovery greatly contributed to the development of compounds leading to the FDA approval of zanamivir as a first-in-class neuraminidase inhibitor in 1999 [34].

The first step is to select a structure of zanamivir in complex with its target, the neuraminidase, in the PDB (*see* **Note 9**). The structure that will be used is a crystal of zanamivir bound to the

H1N1 neuraminidase solved by X-ray crystallography at a resolution 1.45 Å (PDB: 3B7E) (*see* **Note 10**).

All the subsequent steps will be performed in PyMOL. Text in italic following the ">" symbol represent commands to be entered in the PyMOL command line interface.

3.1 Preparation of the Work Environment

First, launch the version of PyMOL you installed for your system (*see* **Note 1**) and make sure that the NRGsuite is installed (*see* **Note 2**). The command line below will download the crystal structure of the 1918 H1N1 strain neuraminidase in complex with zanamivir.

> *fetch 3b7e*

1. The influenza virus neuraminidase glycoprotein is a homotetramer with fourfold circular symmetry. The selected PDB entry is a crystal of two monomers assembled into a homodimer. The experiment in this protocol will use a single monomer to model the complex. This command line removes the second monomeric biological assembly found in the chain B of the structure.

> *remove 3b7e and chain B*

2. The complex contains both the target, the neuraminidase, and the reference position of the ligand, i.e., the solution we want to retrieve with molecular docking. The command line below will extract zanamivir, the residue named ZMR, from the complex and create a separate object in PyMOL named ZMR. This object will use as the ligand for docking and as the reference that will be used to evaluate the precision in binding mode prediction.

> *extract ZMR, 3b7e and resn ZMR*

The work environment of the NRGsuite is project-oriented. A project must be activated to access the two main interfaces GetCleft (to detect, refine, and measure the volume of cavities) and FlexAID (to perform the docking simulations). When a project is activated, the objects you work with can only be saved within that active project. Only Target and Ligand object types are automatically saved in your project folder when loaded elsewhere on the computer (*see* **Note 11**). Create a new project for this tutorial by clicking on the *Plugin* menu item in the PyMOL main window (*see* **Note 12**).

Plugin → *NRGsuite* → *New Project...* → 'your_project_name' (*see* **Note 13**).

3.2 Definition of the Target Binding Site with the GetCleft Interface

The definition of the binding site, i.e., the specific area(s) on the surface of the target that will be searched during the optimization process, is an important step to insure the success of a molecular docking experiment. Although it could be possible to use all the accessible surface of the target as a potential binding site for the ligand during a molecular docking simulation, it is highly suggested to refine the conformational search of the ligand to specific areas of interest, hot spots, or, as it will be referred to further, clefts.

GetCleft, one of the two main tools integrated in the NRGsuite, is an algorithm that identifies surface accessible cavities (or clefts) in the target (also internal cavities depending on the parameters used) as potential binding-sites. The GetCleft interface allows you to adjust the parameters of GetCleft as well as to partition existing clefts and calculate their volume. The GetCleft interface contains a menu from where you can save/load clefts. The interface contains three tabs: *Generate*, *Partition*, and *Volume*.

1. Open the GetCleft interface from the Plugin menu found in the main window of PyMOL

   Plugin → NRGsuite → Open GetCleft.... .

2. The *Generate* tab is activated by default upon GetCleft's opening and it allows the generation of clefts for a target, the filtering of the clefts generated and the measurement of their volumes. There are several parameters of interest that can be used here: the minimal and maximal radius of the spheres that will be used to locate and generate the cleft (this parameter controls the general shape of the cleft) (*see* **Note 14**), a given residue that must be included in the cleft (*see* **Note 15**), and the maximal number of clefts desired by the user. For this experiment, there is no need to modify these parameters.

   First, select a target structure from the scrolling list of "PyMOL objects/selections" by clicking on the drop-down menu and selecting 3b7e (*see* **Note 16**). Upon selection of the target, simply click *Start* to retrieve available clefts for the neuraminidase. When clefts are generated, they are automatically loaded into the PyMOL viewer using unique color coded surface representations and unique object names (*see* **Note 17**). Specifically, clefts are in decreasing order of the number of spheres needed to build them, which is somewhat correlated to the volume of the clefts.

3. (*Optional*) Although this section is written as optional for this specific molecular docking experiment, it is important to keep in mind that most other biological targets will require a more precise definition of the binding site to enhance the precision of the predictions.

   The *Partition* tab is used to partition the volume of an existing cleft when it is too large for the need of the user. The process is divided in three distinct steps:

   STEP 1: Select a parent cleft to partition. To partition a cleft, simply select the cleft of interest from the list of clefts. Only objects containing the _sph_ tag are displayed in the list. The selected cleft will flash in the PyMOL viewer. Generally, the largest cleft, numbered 1 and colored red, is the one that will be used for partitioning.

STEP 2: Add one or more sphere(s) to partition. To partition a cleft, you need to add one or multiple partition sphere(s). The cleft volume contained into the volume of the spheres is conserved.

To add a sphere, click the "Add" button. A wizard will activate and a partition sphere will appear centered onto your cleft. The name of the sphere object is SPHERE_X__, where X is a numerical value of the index of the partition spheres inserted.

Once you set the size and location of the partition sphere properly, click the "Done" button in the Wizard (*see* **Note 18**). The partition sphere will appear in the Spheres objects list. If you wish to modify this sphere simply click the "Edit" button. A new wizard will activate. You can also delete partition spheres by clicking the "Delete" button (*see* **Note 19**).

Finally, the greyed-out volume of the cleft represents the volume that will be conserved when the portioned cleft is created.

STEP 3: Name the partitioned child cleft. Click the *Create* button and the partitioned cleft will appear as a new object in the PyMOL viewer with an added suffix "_pt" to its name.

4. (*Optional*) The *Volume* tab of the GetCleft interface calculates the volume of the clefts generated above. It is particularly useful for the user to compare the total available volume of a cleft and the estimated volume of a small molecule as it hints at the relative size of the space to search.

   The clefts that appear are color-coded and are displayed as a list in the volume tab. If your cleft does not appear, try pressing the "Refresh clefts" button at the bottom. A cleft with an uncalculated volume has a null volume (0.0). You can estimate the volume of all clefts ("ALL" button), uncalculated clefts ("Remaining" button) or a selected cleft ("Selected" button). The calculated volume is displayed in $\mathring{A}^3$ upon completion.

5. Clefts are not automatically saved when generated. Thus, the user needs to explicitly save the clefts before importing them into the FlexAID interface. You can save clefts as long as they were generated in the same GetCleft session. If you generate clefts, then close the GetCleft interface without saving and reopen it, the clefts will not be available for saving.

   To save the clefts, click the *Save* menu button in the upper left corner of the GetCleft window and save the files at the default location suggested in the file window. The NRGsuite cannot save a cleft elsewhere than the suggested directory (*see* **Note 20**).

6. Close the GetCleft interface window by clicking on the *Close* button in the lower right corner.

3.3 Configure, Perform, and Analyze the Molecular Docking Experiment with the FlexAID Interface

The FlexAID interface permits users to adjust the parameters of FlexAID in a convenient environment. The basic view of the interface contains four tabs: *Input Files, Target Config, Ligand Config,* and *Simulate.* The functionalities of each tab are reviewed in detail in the following sections. The FlexAID interface contains three menu items in the top left hand corner: *Load* and *Save* sessions (*see* **Note 21**), and *Show,* which turns on the display of two additional tabs: *Scoring Cfg* (scoring function configuration) and *GA Params* (genetic algorithm parameters). These tabs are needed for the *optional* sections of the following protocol.

1. Open the FlexAID interface from the Plugin menu found in the main window of PyMOL.

   Plugin → NRGsuite → Open FlexAID…

2. The *Input* tab is displayed by default upon FlexAID's opening and allows configuration of the target and ligand (*see* **Note 22**). First, select "3b7e" from the PyMOL objects/selection drop-down menu and click "Save as target" (*see* **Note 20**). Then, select "ZMR" from the drop-down menu and click "Save as ligand" (*see* **Note 20**).

3. Click on the *Target Cfg* (target configuration) tab in the Flex-AID interface window to access the parameters of the target (*see* **Note 23**). After selecting a target and a ligand, the definition of the binding site is the third mandatory input to perform a simulation. In the "Binding-site definition" upper box, under "Choose binding-site type," click on "CLEFT" and then click on the button "Import clefts." Select the first cleft which should be named "3b7e_sph_1" (*see* **Note 24**). A new object named "BINDINGSITE_AREA__" will be created in the PyMOL viewer and the red cleft will appear with the mesh, a grid like, representation.

(*Optional*) Although there is no need to consider target flexibility for the docking of zanamivir into the neuraminidase, it is crucial to keep in mind that the docking of any ligand that has not been crystallized with the target might benefit from the defining of key residues on the target in the binding site that interacts with the ligand as flexible. Even when flexibility is not critically needed to retrieve the binding mode of reference, the accuracy of the simulation may improve when highly mobile side chains can change conformations (*see* **Note 25**). There are two options to include flexibility in the target in the "Side-chain flexibility" section of the "Target flexibility" box: (1) the "Add/Delete flexible side-chains" wizard button, which allows the interactive selection of specific side chains by the user in the PyMOL viewer, and (2) the "Residue code" text entry form, which quickly activates the flexibility for a given residue of the target. In our current case, the key residues ARG152A, GLU276A, ARG118A, ARG292A, and ASP151A (*see* **Note 15**) specifically contribute to bind zanamivir (*see* **Note 26**).

4. Click on the *Ligand Cfg* (ligand configuration) tab in the FlexAID interface window to access the parameters of the ligand. The functionalities found in this tab include: the inclusion/exclusion of the ligand's degrees of freedom (rotational, translational, and flexible bonds' dihedrals), the computation of the RMSD compared to the reference's position, and the imposition of geometric constraints between a specific pair of atoms from the target and ligand, which can be useful to simulate covalent docking.

(*Optional*) The "Degrees of freedom" box found on the left side of the interface controls the degrees of freedom that can be introduced for the zanamivir ligand. Ligand translational and rotational degrees of freedom are enabled by default and it allows FlexAID to translate and rotate the ligand anywhere in the binding site where the anchor atom of the ligand can be placed (*see* **Note 27**).

(*Optional*) In the recent version of the NRGsuite, all the rotatable bonds are considered flexible by default. However, the "Ligand flexibility" section includes a "Add/Delete flexible bonds" button that opens a PyMOL Wizard (*see* **Note 18**) that displays all the flexible bonds within the ligand using a ball-and-stick representation: the ones selected as flexible are shown in white while the ones considered rigid are shown in orange (*see* **Notes 28 and 29**).

Check the "RMSD structure" checkbox found next to the right in the interface window (show above) to order FlexAID to compute the RMSD between the position of the atoms of the ligand in the reference (zanamivir position in the 3b7e PDB entry) and its predictions. This measure is used to determine whether FlexAID's predictions are successful or not in cases where the known experimental binding pose is known (*see* **Note 8**).

(*Optional*) The "Constraints" section located directly below the "RMSD structure" box allows FlexAID to specify a desired distance between two atoms to drive the optimization during the genetic algorithm. There are two types of constraints that can be added: intramolecular constraints (the specific distance between two atoms of the ligand itself or two atoms of the target itself) and intermolecular constraints (the specific distance between one atom of the target with one atom of the ligand). This is useful to simulate the covalent binding of an atom of the ligand to an atom of the target with the exact distance of a given bond length. The "Add/Delete constraints" button opens a PyMOL wizard allowing you to select two atoms to constrain. Once two atoms are selected, the distance slider allows the user to set the desired distance for a given constraint. It is possible to sequentially add multiple constraints in the same manner.

5. (*Optional*) The *Scoring Cfg* (scoring function configuration) tab allows you to change the inclusion/exclusion of atoms in the scoring, the inclusion of water molecules, the definition of the solvent, and the permeability of soft-docking. Unless you are interested in including water molecules from the crystal in the simulation, there is no need to modify this section. Including water molecules will tell FlexAID to assign the oxygen atoms in the crystal to the one of water and will include it in its evaluation. Check the "Include water molecules" checkbox of the "HET groups" section to consider water molecules (*see* **Note 30**). The checkbox "Exclude bound molecules" will, once checked, exclude any HET atom that is part of the target structure, which is useful if one wants to remove small organic molecules used during crystallization.

6. (*Optional*) The *GA Params* (genetic algorithm parameters) tab allows you to parametrize the number of energy evaluations (length of simulations), the genetic algorithm operator, and the visual display of the simulation in the PyMOL viewer window. FlexAID uses a genetic algorithm to cover the search space, which uses an initial number of chromosomes in the population that will evolve for several generations. By default, there are 500 chromosomes that will evolve during 500 generations leading to 250,000 energy evaluations. These values can be modified in the "Genetic parameters" section of the *GA Params* tab (*see* **Note 31**).

(*Optional*) It is possible to modify the visual display of real-time docking in the PyMOL viewer with the corresponding section in the *GA Params* tab. The "Number of TOP complexes" indicate the number of complexes that are displayed in the PyMOL viewer. The TOP complexes shown are the ones with the lowest energy according to the scoring function. The "Refresh interval" represents the interval, in number of generations, at which the display of TOP complexes is refreshed. The progress of the genetic algorithm is shown in the Simulate tab (*see* **step 7**). The FlexAID algorithm waits for the NRGsuite to display the TOP complexes before processing the next generation. Thus, we strongly suggest not displaying too many TOP complexes or too short refresh intervals as it may drastically increase the computational runtime for a simulation.

7. Click on the *Simulate* tab to initiate the docking simulation. To start a docking simulation, simply click the "Start" button. Once a simulation has successfully started, you have access to the "Pause," "Stop," and "Abort" buttons. The "Pause"

button allows you to pause the simulation while looking at real-time results in the PyMOL viewer. The "Stop" and "Abort" buttons both end the simulation. However, stopping a simulation generates final results while aborting does not. Stopping a simulation can be particularly useful when the docking optimization has converged already to its minimum energy. FlexAID also offers a way to continue a simulation from previously generated results. When results are activated, the "Continue" button may be clickable depending on the context (*see* **Note 32**). It is possible to see these buttons at the top left corner of the *Simulate* tab of the FlexAID interface.

Click on the "Start" button to initiate the simulation. When the genetic algorithm is under way, FlexAID updates the values of fitness and scoring functions for the best individuals in terms of scoring function. During the simulation, the PyMOL viewer is updated with reserved objects (named TOP_<X>__, where X is the Xth result predicted by FlexAID) displaying the actual best results evaluated by FlexAID. These objects are temporary and color-coded according to the "Color" column shown in the Flex-AID *Simulate* tab (*see* the interface panel at the bottom right of Fig. 1). The NRGsuite offers a quick way of changing the display of TOP_<X>__ complexes objects all at once instead of having to manually update the display for the newly created objects. By default, the target is displayed as "Cartoon" and the ligand as "Sticks." You can change these parameters as you like in the "Display options of TOP objects" in the top right corner of the *Simulate* tab of FlexAID. Whenever a reference is used (*see* **step 4** above), the "Last RMSD" column is updated at every refresh interval (*see* **step 6** above about the *GA Params* tab).

When a simulation is finished, or stopped, the reserved objects RESULT_<X>__ and RESULT_<X>_H_BONDS__ are created in the PyMOL viewer. RESULT_<X>__ are the complex's objects while the RESULT_<X>_H_BONDS__ objects are distances objects displaying the h-bonds for the result. Their according energy value (referenced as CF) and RMSD from the reference (when one is used) of the results are displayed in the table shown at the bottom right of Fig. 1.

In the case where constraints are applied, an extra column, Apparent CF, will appear which is a modified value of the CF to reflect whether the predicted pose respects the desired constraints imposed by the user.

8. *Analysis*—Finally, look at the RESULT__X objects RMSD in the last column of the FlexAID *Simulate* results table. Remember that this docking experiment serves as control with which further docking experiments, e.g., different small molecules, will be compared. FlexAID can retrieve RMSDs below 2.0 Å on

this specific case easily when this protocol is used (*see* **Note 33**). Both the specific interactions (H_BONDS in the PyMOL viewer objects) and the CF score can be used to compare different poses or different ligands (this should be used with caution with ligands of very different in size) during your next experiments.

4   Notes

1. PyMOL is freely distributed as source code or precompiled binaries for academic users at http://pymol.org/educational. For the best results, please make sure to use the latest PyMOL version available for your system.

    (a) As a side note, PyMOL uses its own version of Python to function and the NRGsuite requires at least Python version 2.5 to work properly. Therefore, PyMOL versions 1.0/1.1 are currently unsupported by the NRGsuite.

2. The NRGsuite is available at http://biophys.umontreal.ca/nrg as package installers for Windows and macOS and in the form of an install script for Linux. At the time of this writing, the version of the NRGsuite is *2.48j*, but it is recommended to use the latest version available on our website.

    All software employed in the protocols are free at least for nonprofit users. FlexAID and the NRGsuite are free for everyone and distributed under the GNU General Public License. The NRGsuite is available for Linux (32/64-bit), macOS, and Windows (32/64-bit).

    (a) The suite has been extensively tested on Linux 32/64-bit, Windows 32/64-bit, and macOS 64-bit machines with free-for-academic PyMOL versions 1.2/1.3 as well as PyMOL versions 1.6/1.7/1.8.

3. This is particularly important for operating environments running under Windows, where you need to select either the 32-bit or 64-bit version. It is strongly suggested to install the 64-bit version if you run Windows 7 or any more recent distribution. Here is how to install the NRGsuite for your system:

    Windows
    Double-click the NRGsuite_2.48i_Win<32/64>.exe installer and install. The default location is "C:\Program Files".
    macOS/Mac OS X
    Double-click the NRGsuite_2.48i_MacOSX64.pkg. installer and install the package in its default location. The default location is "/Applications/NRGsuite".

Linux

Open up a terminal and move to the directory in which you downloaded the archive NRGsuite_2.48i_Linux<32/64>.tar, and execute the following commands:

> *tar –xvf NRGsuite_2.48i_Linux<32/64>.tar*
> *sh install.sh NRGsuite.tar.gz*

The default location is "/usr/local/NRGsuite". Therefore, superuser privileges (sudo) are required for installing the NRGsuite. To override the default location, open install_linux. sh with any text editor and change the value of INSTALL_-PATH with the desired location.

4. Open PyMOL and in the upper menu click the following buttons:

Plugin → Manage Plugins → Install...

Browse to the directory in which you installed the NRGsuite on your hard drive (*see* **step A**), and double-click the following file:

NRGsuite → Plugin → NRGsuite.py

Restart PyMOL and the NRGsuite menu should appear in the Plugin menu:

Plugin → NRGsuite

You are now ready to use the NRGsuite.

5. In structural biology, the resolution of a structure is a measure of the quality of the data collected. As the resolution of a structure gets smaller, the confidence in the location of atoms is higher. A resolution of 2.0 Å and below is generally considered as "high resolution" for a structure in that the position of all heavy atoms (i.e., nonhydrogen atoms) is well established.

6. All of the publicly available experimental structures of biological complexes can be parsed and obtained directly from the Protein Data Bank (PDB) at http://rcsb.org. There are multiple ways to parse the PDB and the user can search using specific criteria, e.g., the desired resolution, a specific drug, or the experimental method used to solve the structure. Statistically and historically speaking, the process of drug discovery mostly involved structures solved using X-ray crystallography because of its compatibility with different families of proteins and its better resolution, but structures solved by other methods with high resolution are sometimes available and can be used for molecular docking.

7. In molecular docking, a pose predicted with a root-mean squared distance (RMSD) below 2.0 Å from the experimental pose of reference is considered a success. The resolution of the reference structure has a significant impact on the accuracy of the predictions. For this reason, it is suggested to choose a "high resolution" structure solved at 2.0 Å or lower when it is available.

8. The NRGsuite is developed to allow molecular docking simulations involving any biological target. Although this tutorial will use a protein target to predict the binding mode of the drug of interest, it could be replaced by any other protein or nucleic acid target for which a tridimensional structure is readily available.

9. It is easy to identify all available structures by querying the PDB using the "Zanamivir" keyword and then refining by molecular target and organism. Subsequently, it is possible to sort the structure by resolution in order to choose the best available resolution.

10. The structure information page can be consulted at: http://www.rcsb.org/pdb/explore/explore.do?structureId=3B7E. The PDB file can be found at: http://files.rcsb.org/view/3B7E.pdb.

11. The directory-tree "Documents/NRGsuite" is automatically created in the home folder upon initialization of the NRGsuite plugin in PyMOL. This folder represents the default location in which the different projects of $USER are held (where $USER refers to the currently logged-in user on the system). Depending on the operating system, this folder is located at the following location in your file system:

    Under Windows
    Vista and higher: "C:\Users\$USER\Documents\NRGsuite"
    Older: "C:\Documents and Settings\$USER\Documents\NRGsuite"
    **Do not confuse "Documents" with "My Documents"
    Under macOS or Mac OS X
    "/Users/$USER/Documents/NRGsuite"
    Under Linux
    "/home/$USER/Documents/NRGsuite"

12. PyMOL has two windows: one that is named "PyMOL Molecular Graphics System" and is referred to as the main window. The second window is the "PyMOL Viewer" and will be referred as such.

13. It is preferred to *avoid using whitespaces in any filenames that will be used with the NRGsuite*. Although most of the configurations will allow, it is known to cause bugs on some operating systems, especially for Windows users.

14. GetCleft detects the cavities of a target by introducing spheres between pairs of target atoms and reducing the radii of the spheres until there are no clashes. The radius range can be used to control the volume of generated clefts. By default, the range goes from a Minimum of 1.50 Å to a Maximum 4.00 Å. Reducing the minimum radius allows one to insert spheres in

deeply buried cavities. Thus, clefts generated with a lower minimum are larger.

15. The NRGsuite uses a string representation to identify unique residues by their residue name (written using the three capital letters form), a residue number and the residue chain formatted as *RES1A*. For example, the first methionine, numbered 1, from the chain A will be formatted *MET1A*.

16. The list of PyMOL objects/selections shows every object found in the PyMOL viewer window. If your object does not appear in the list, hit the refresh button on the right.

    Some objects will not be shown in the list, e.g., objects which name contains a double underscore "__" (reserved for Python and PyMOL only) and objects whose names contains an extension "*.*".

17. Each cleft object is named *$TARGET_sph_X* where *$TARGET* is the name of the target (3b7e in this protocol) and X is a numerical value from 1 to the maximum number of clefts desired by the user.

18. Through the FlexAID and GetCleft interfaces, you will eventually need to work with Wizards. Upon activation of a Wizard, the interface that called the Wizard will be locked and you will need to interact with the PyMOL viewer instead. Each Wizard is unique and waits for a different input from the user. The type of input is clearly written on top of the PyMOL viewer.

    To accommodate the different types of input as well as to facilitate working with the Wizard, activating a Wizard may alter:

    - The selection mode ("Selecting")
    - The mouse mode ("Mouse Mode")
    - The PyMOL view
    - The masking of your objects (un-clickable)

    However, these will be reset to your original values once the Wizard turns inactive. The user can also interact with the Wizard menu on the bottom right corner of the PyMOL viewer. The Wizard will remain active until the user clicks the "Done" button in the menu.

19. It is possible to add multiple individual spheres to accurately define the binding site. Whenever a second partition sphere is added, it is also appended to the sphere objects list. To help you distinguish which sphere corresponds to which in the PyMOL viewer, you can refer to the SPHERE_PT_AREA__ object. The object is shown as a transparent violet sphere and refers to the currently selected sphere in the sphere objects list.

20. The NRGsuite has been designed to load and save files in the project directory initially defined by the user upon installation. Therefore, it is best if the user save and load files at the suggested location whenever any file window pops up.

21. A session within the FlexAID interface allows you to store and retrieve the content of all tabs (*see* Subheading 3.3). The content of a session includes:

    - *file references pointing to the target, the ligand*
    - *the binding-site definition*
    - *the target flexibility*
    - *the results of a simulation*
    - *values in each of the tabs*

    Sessions are particularly useful when you want to reproduce a simulation multiple times with the same parameters. **Do not confuse a FlexAID interface session with a PyMOL session (using the file extension *.pse*).

22. There are two ways of importing the target: the first one involves the PyMOL object/selection drop-down menu that allows the selection of an object in PyMOL, while the second allows you to load previously used targets in your project from the Load button located to the right of the "THE TARGET" menu box.

    There are three ways of importing the ligand: the first one involves the drop-down menu that allows the selection of a PyMOL object/selection, the second one uses the *Load* button found to the right of the *"THE LIGAND"* menu box and the last uses the *Input* button to generate a 3D structure of your ligand from a SMILES [35] representation. Please note that the "Generate 3D conformation" checkbox must be checked to generate a 3D structure of your ligand. Finally, the *Anchor* button allows the definition of the anchor atom in a ligand (*see* **Note 27**).

23. When the user activates another tab from the Input tab, the ligand and the target must be processed. This process may take a few seconds to a minute depending on the size of the molecules. This process is necessary to derive (1) the atom types of the molecules, (2) the flexible bonds of the ligand, and (3) to build the necessary input files that are required for executing a docking simulation with FlexAID.

    The processing of the ligand creates a new object called LIGAND__ (reserved name *see* **Note 16**) with newly generated coordinates when generating a 3D structure.

    The processing of the target creates the object TARGET__.

24. There are cases where multiple individual clefts need to be used to define the binding site, e.g., when the active site is

undetermined or when multiple allosteric sites need to be queried altogether. It is possible to import multiple clefts at once by selecting multiple cleft files while holding "Shift" (selects all files from first to last) or "Control" (add the clicked file to the list of currently selected ones) key. Once you have selected your clefts, click the "Open" button to import them. "Delete others" will delete all clefts except for the active cleft.

Once imported, the clefts will appear in the clefts list. The active cleft is highlighted in red in the PyMOL viewer while the others are blue-violet. It is important to note that docking of the ligand will take place in all clefts in the list and not only the active one. You can manipulate the clefts by using the buttons in the "CLEFT" box. "Clear" will delete all clefts in the clefts list. "Delete" will delete the active cleft.

25. The frequency of side-chain rearrangements correlates with their entropy; thus the most entropic side-chains often benefit from flexibility during a docking simulation. Studying the frequency of side-chain rearrangements can help you determine which ones have the greatest probability of changing conformation upon binding [19].

26. A quick way to identify which residues interact with the ligand in the chosen complex is to refer to the "Poseview Image" of the ligand of interest in the PDB (see **Note 6**). This is found in the "Small Molecules" section of a given PDB entry. In the "2D Diagram & Interaction," a visual representation of the ligand is shown along with the residues of the target that contribute to binding.

An alternative method to find these residues for a target that is not found in the PDB, like a homology model, would be to look at the most conserved residues in a multiple sequence alignment of proteins from the same Pfam [36] family.

27. The anchor atom is the first atom to be placed in the binding site and is the only atom that absolutely needs to be inside the volume of the cleft(s) used for the molecular docking experiment.

28. When a ligand is imported, the molecule is considered rigid during docking unless the user explicitly includes ligand flexibility. To include ligand flexibility, click the "Add/Delete flexible bonds" button. Your ligand will appear as the object FLEXIBLE_LIGAND__.

The following objects are also created (do not interact with these PyMOL objects):
POSS_FLEX_BONDS__ (to display the possible flexible bonds of the ligand) SELECTED_BONDS__ (to display the selected flexible bonds of the user).

A wizard will open waiting for you to click on the two atoms that define the flexible bond. Flexible bonds appear in orange. Clicking on the two atoms that define the flexible bond will render this bond as flexible during the docking simulation. The selected bonds of the user appear in white.

Rather than selecting all bonds manually, you can quickly select all flexible bonds by clicking the "Select all flexible bonds" button in the Wizard menu.

The "Clear flexible bonds" button removes all selected flexible bonds.

When the Wizard gets inactivated, the number of selected flexible bonds will be shown in the interface.

29. At the time of the writing, the latest version of PyMOL running on Windows 10 contains an unresolved bug where PyMOL crashes when the user tries to open the "Add/Delete flexible bonds" wizard of the *Ligand Cfg* tab in the FlexAID interface. For this reason, all rotatable bonds of the ligand are now enabled by default in the *Preferences* panel of the NRGsuite found in the *Plugin → NRGsuite → Preferences* menu item of the PyMOL main window. Please note that this bug will be fixed in a future version of the NRGsuite available at our website (*see* **Note 2**).

30. Most of the time, including all water molecules when docking the reference during the control experiment will ease the docking problem because water molecules will fill most of the binding site and the ligand could be fit using geometric criteria. To avoid this, it is suggested to keep only the strongly bound water molecules that directly interact in the binding site. The B-factor column of the PDB file could also be a good indicator of which water molecules must be kept; a low B-factor signifies that this atom is well ordered and there is not a large incertitude on its position. It is suggested to keep the water molecules with the lowest B-factors as well as those who directly interact with the ligand in the reference.

31. The search space is increased when you include additional degrees of freedom in the optimization (e.g., flexible bonds of the ligand flexible and/or flexible side-chains). With these additional degrees of freedom, more energy evaluations are required to converge to a minimum of energy. When the control simulation is not able to retrieve the conformation of reference, you can increase the number of chromosomes and generations by increasing the corresponding values. It is suggested to initially simulate using default ones.

32. You can continue a simulation if and only if the active results were generated with the same parameterization, i.e., the same target and ligand, binding-site definition, flexibility of the molecules, etc. Specifically, the content of the following tabs must be the same: *Input Files*, *Target Cfg*, *Ligand Cfg*, and

Scoring Cfg. You can modify the parameters of the genetic algorithms and still be able to continue a simulation.

33. Docking is an optimization problem and it is possible to have a bad initial population for a simulation (which is randomly generated) or it is also possible that the optimization got stuck in a local minimum of energy. Sometimes, simply repeating the experiment gets you better results.

Acknowledgments

R.J.N. is part of PROTEO (the Québec network for research on protein function, structure, and engineering) and GRASP (Groupe de Recherche Axé sur la Structure des Protéines). The authors would like to thank the users of FlexAID and the NRGsuite for numerous bug reports and feedbacks, thus contributing to their development, and Florence Min for critical reading of the manuscript.

Funding: L.P.M. is the recipient of a Ph.D. fellowship from the Fonds de Recherche du Québec—Nature et Technologies (FRQ-NT).

References

1. Berman HM, Westbrook J, Feng Z, Gilliland G, Bhat TN, Weissig H et al (2000) The Protein Data Bank. Nucleic Acids Res 28:235–242

2. Najmanovich RJ (2017) Evolutionary studies of ligand binding sites in proteins. Curr Opin Struct Biol 45:85–90. https://doi.org/10.1016/j.sbi.2016.11.024

3. Gohlke H, Klebe G (2002) Approaches to the description and prediction of the binding affinity of small-molecule ligands to macromolecular receptors. Angew Chem Int Ed 41:2645–2676

4. Meng X-Y, Zhang H-X, Mezei M, Cui M (2011) Molecular docking: a powerful approach for structure-based drug discovery. CAD 7:146–157. https://doi.org/10.2174/157340911795677602

5. Kitchen DB, Decornez H, Furr JR, Bajorath J (2004) Docking and scoring in virtual screening for drug discovery: methods and applications. Nat Rev Drug Discov 3:935–949. https://doi.org/10.1038/nrd1549

6. Jacob RB, Andersen T, McDougal OM (2012) Accessible high-throughput virtual screening molecular docking software for students and educators. PLoS Comput Biol 8:e1002499.

https://doi.org/10.1371/journal.pcbi.1002499

7. Neudert G, Klebe G (2011) DSX: a knowledge-based scoring function for the assessment of protein-ligand complexes. J Chem Inf Model 51:2731–2745. https://doi.org/10.1021/ci200274q

8. Li Y, Liu Z, Li J, Han L, Liu J, Zhao Z et al (2014) Comparative assessment of scoring functions on an updated benchmark: 1. Compilation of the test set. J Chem Inf Model 54:1700–1716. https://doi.org/10.1021/ci500080q

9. Englebienne P, Moitessier N (2009) Docking ligands into flexible and solvated macromolecules. 4. Are popular scoring functions accurate for this class of proteins? J Chem Inf Model 49:1568–1580. https://doi.org/10.1021/ci8004308

10. Grudinin S, Kadukova M, Eisenbarth A, Marillet S, Cazals F (2016) Predicting binding poses and affinities for protein–ligand complexes in the 2015 D3R Grand Challenge using a physical model with a statistical parameter estimation. J Comput Aided Mol Des 30 (9):791–804. https://doi.org/10.1007/s10822-016-9976-2

11. Mobley DL, Dill KA (2009) Binding of small-molecule ligands to proteins: "what you see" is not always "what you get". Structure 17:489–498. https://doi.org/10.1016/j.str.2009.02.010

12. Wong SE, Lightstone FC (2011) Accounting for water molecules in drug design. Expert Opin Drug Discov 6:65–74. https://doi.org/10.1517/17460441.2011.534452

13. Corbeil CR, Moitessier N (2009) Docking ligands into flexible and solvated macromolecules. 3. Impact of input ligand conformation, protein flexibility, and water molecules on the accuracy of docking programs. J Chem Inf Model 49:997–1009. https://doi.org/10.1021/ci8004176

14. Limongelli V, Marinelli L, Cosconati S, La Motta C, Sartini S, Mugnaini L et al (2012) Sampling protein motion and solvent effect during ligand binding. Proc Natl Acad Sci U S A 109:1467–1472. https://doi.org/10.1073/pnas.1112181108

15. Therrien E, Weill N, Tomberg A, Corbeil CR, Lee D, Moitessier N (2014) Docking ligands into flexible and solvated macromolecules. 7. Impact of protein flexibility and water molecules on docking-based virtual screening accuracy. J Chem Inf Model 54:3198–3210. https://doi.org/10.1021/ci500299h

16. Zhao S, Goodsell DS, Olson AJ (2001) Analysis of a data set of paired uncomplexed protein structures: new metrics for side-chain flexibility and model evaluation. Proteins Struct Funct Genet 43:271–279

17. Boehr DD, Nussinov R, Wright PE (2009) The role of dynamic conformational ensembles in biomolecular recognition. Nat Chem Biol 5:789–796. https://doi.org/10.1038/nchembio.232

18. Najmanovich RJ, Kuttner J, Sobolev V, Edelman M (2000) Side-chain flexibility in proteins upon ligand binding. Proteins Struct Funct Genet 39:261–268

19. Gaudreault F, Chartier M, Najmanovich RJ (2012) Side-chain rotamer changes upon ligand binding: common, crucial, correlate with entropy and rearrange hydrogen bonding. Bioinformatics 28:i423–i430. https://doi.org/10.1093/bioinformatics/bts395

20. Gaudreault F, Najmanovich RJ (2015) FlexAID: revisiting docking on non-native-complex structures. J Chem Inf Model 55:1323–1336. https://doi.org/10.1021/acs.jcim.5b00078

21. Frappier V, Najmanovich RJ (2014) A coarse-grained elastic network atom contact model and its use in the simulation of protein dynamics and the prediction of the effect of mutations. PLoS Comput Biol 10:e1003569. https://doi.org/10.1371/journal.pcbi.1003569

22. Wang R, Fang X, Lu Y, Yang C-Y, Wang S (2005) The PDBbind database: methodologies and updates. J Med Chem 48:4111–4119. https://doi.org/10.1021/jm048957q

23. Trott O, Olson AJ (2010) AutoDock Vina: improving the speed and accuracy of docking with a new scoring function, efficient optimization, and multithreading. J Comput Chem 31:455–461. https://doi.org/10.1002/jcc.21334

24. Rarey M, Kramer B, Lengauer T, Klebe G (1996) A fast flexible docking method using an incremental construction algorithm. J Mol Biol 261:470–489. https://doi.org/10.1006/jmbi.1996.0477

25. Ruiz-Carmona S, Alvarez-Garcia D, Foloppe N, Garmendia-Doval AB, Juhos S, Schmidtke P et al (2014) rDock: a fast, versatile and open source program for docking ligands to proteins and nucleic acids. PLoS Comput Biol 10(4):e1003571. https://doi.org/10.1371/journal.pcbi.1003571

26. Gaudreault F, Morency L-P, Najmanovich RJ (2015) NRGsuite: a PyMOL plugin to perform docking simulations in real time using FlexAID. Bioinformatics 31:3856–3858. https://doi.org/10.1093/bioinformatics/btv458

27. Letourneau D, Lorin A, Lefebvre A, Frappier V, Gaudreault F, Najmanovich R et al (2012) StAR-related lipid transfer domain protein 5 binds primary bile acids. J Lipid Res 53(12):2677–2689. https://doi.org/10.1194/jlr.M031245

28. Duchêne D, Colombo E, Désilets A, Boudreault P-L, Leduc R, Marsault E et al (2014) Analysis of subpocket selectivity and identification of potent selective inhibitors for matriptase and matriptase-2. J Med Chem 57:10198–10204. https://doi.org/10.1021/jm5015633

29. Chartier M, Morency L-P, Zylber MI, Najmanovich RJ (2017) Large-scale detection of drug off-targets: hypotheses for drug repurposing and understanding side-effects. BMC Pharmacol Toxicol 18:1046. https://doi.org/10.1186/s40360-017-0128-7

30. Seto JT, Rott R (1966) Functional significance of sialidose during influenza virus multiplication. Virology 30:731–737

31. Moscona A (2005) Neuraminidase inhibitors for influenza. N Engl J Med 353:1363–1373. https://doi.org/10.1056/NEJMra050740

32. Varghese JN, Laver WG, Colman PM (1983) Structure of the influenza virus glycoprotein antigen neuraminidase at 2.9 Å resolution. Nature 303:35–40. https://doi.org/10.1038/303035a0

33. Itzstein von M, Wu WY, Kok GB, Pegg MS, Dyason JC, Jin B et al (1993) Rational design of potent sialidase-based inhibitors of influenza virus replication. Nature 363:418–423. https://doi.org/10.1038/363418a0

34. Talele T, Khedkar S, Rigby A (2010) Successful applications of computer aided drug discovery: moving drugs from concept to the clinic. Curr Top Med Chem 10:127–141. https://doi.org/10.2174/156802610790232251

35. O'Boyle NM (2012) Towards a universal SMILES representation – a standard method to generate canonical SMILES based on the InChI. J Chem 4:22. https://doi.org/10.1186/1758-2946-4-22

36. Finn RD, Bateman A, Clements J, Coggill P, Eberhardt RY, Eddy SR et al (2014) Pfam: the protein families database. Nucleic Acids Res 42:D222–D230. https://doi.org/10.1093/nar/gkt1223

Chapter 19

Calculation of Thermodynamic Properties of Bound Water Molecules

Ying Yang, Amr H. A. Abdallah, and Markus A. Lill

Abstract

Water molecules in the binding site of a protein significantly influence protein structure and function, for example, by mediating protein–ligand interactions or in form of desolvation as driving force for ligand binding. The knowledge about location and thermodynamic properties of water molecules in the binding site is crucial to the understanding of protein function. This chapter describes the method of calculating the location and thermodynamic properties of bound water molecules from molecular dynamics (MD) simulation trajectories. Thermodynamic profiles of water molecules can be calculated either with or without the presence of a bound ligand based on the scientific problem. The location and thermodynamic profile of hydration sites mediating the protein–ligand interactions is important for understanding protein–ligand binding. The protein desolvation free energy can be estimated for any ligand by summation of the hydration site free energies of the displaced hydration sites. The WATsite program with an easy-to-use graphical user interface (GUI) based on PyMOL was developed for those calculations and is discussed in this chapter. The WATsite program and its PyMOL plugin are available free of charge from http://people.pharmacy.purdue.edu/~mlill/software/watsite/version3.shtml.

Key words Desolvation, Hydration site, Molecular dynamics, Protein desolvation free energy, PyMOL, Solvation, Water thermodynamics, Water models, Water molecule, WATsite

1 Introduction

Water is a crucial participant in virtually all protein functions, e.g., protein folding [1–6] and ligand binding [7–10]. Binding site water contributes significantly to the strength of intermolecular interactions in the aqueous phase by mediating protein–ligand interactions, solvating and desolvating both ligand and protein upon ligand binding and unbinding [9, 11–14].

In structure-based drug design, a ligand is often modified to displace ordered water molecules in the binding site. Due to the inherent entropic contributions, releasing an ordered water molecule from the binding site into the bulk solvent is thought to be favorable for protein–ligand binding. However, in some cases the enthalpic gain from extra water-mediated hydrogen bonds exceeds

Mohini Gore and Umesh B. Jagtap (eds.), *Computational Drug Discovery and Design*, Methods in Molecular Biology, vol. 1762, https://doi.org/10.1007/978-1-4939-7756-7_19, © Springer Science+Business Media, LLC, part of Springer Nature 2018

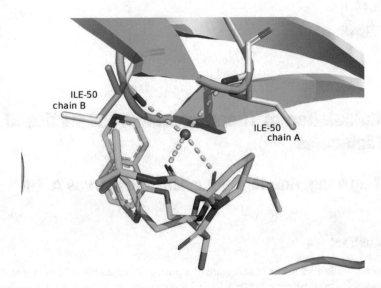

Fig. 1 Example of bound water in HIV-1 protease. Residues Ile-50 and Ile-50′ from two subunits are shown in grey sticks, and inhibitor KNI in green sticks. Water 301 is shown as red sphere, and yellow dashed lines represent hydrogen bonds (PDB ID: 1hpx)

the entropic loss for immobilizing the water involved [10]. Thus, the thermodynamics of water molecules in protein active sites is important for understanding protein–ligand interactions for drug design. A well-known example of water mediated protein–ligand interaction is found among HIV-1 protease inhibitors (Fig. 1) [9, 14]. A conserved water molecule (water 301) is located on the HIV-1 protease symmetry axis. This water molecule forms two hydrogen bonds to residue Ile-50 and Ile-50′ on two subunits and another two hydrogen bonds to the inhibitor. Using the HIV-1 protease as an example, this chapter illustrates the application of WATsite with its PyMOL plugin for calculating the thermodynamic profile of individual water molecules and their potential contribution to ligand binding.

2 Materials

2.1 Prerequisites

The latest version of WATsite utilizes the OpenMM [15] toolkit for GPU-accelerated molecular simulation. A GPU workstation is required as well as OpenMM-WATsite, AmberTools16 [16], and PyMOL [17].

2.2 Installation

The WATsite3.0 package can be downloaded from http://people.pharmacy.purdue.edu/~mlill/software/watsite/version3.shtml. *WATsite.tar.gz* needs to be extracted using "*tar –zxf WATsite.tar.gz*". The file *WATsite_Settings.txt* needs to be copied to your home directory (*$HOME*). WATsite plugin can be installed using "Plugin Manager" under Plugin menu, and choose the file *WATsite.py* under the "Install New Plugin" tab. The WATsite program needs to be compiled on the platform by entering into the WATsite directory and run "*make –f makefile*".

The source code of WATsite compatible with OpenMM is located under "openmm-watsite" and must be compiled with the CUDA platform (*see* **Note 1**).

2.3   Input Data

The inputs for WATsite are a protein structure and a binding site definition both in pdb format. When predicting hydration site at the protein–ligand interface, a ligand file in the mol2 format is required.

2.4   Hydration Site Calculation

Here, we briefly describe the individual computational steps of the WATsite procedure and the associated programs. A detailed description of the WATsite method can be found in previous publications [18]. First, the side-chain conformations of ASN, GLN, HIS, tautomers, and protonation states of HIS protein residues can be adjusted by the Reduce program [19]. The user can also choose to use a protein structure with previously predicted protonation states (*see* **Note 2**). Next, the protein will be solvated in an ortho-rhombic box of user-selected explicit water model (*see* **Note 3**) with a user-specified minimum distance between any protein atom and the faces of the orthorhombic box. Chloride and sodium ions will be added to neutralize the systems. MD simulation will be performed using OpenMM [15] with the user-selected amber force field [20] (*see* **Note 3**). The system will be energy minimized and equilibrated before production run. MD simulations can be performed for a user-specified length (*see* **Note 4**).

After the MD simulation, a 3D grid is placed over the user-defined binding site. The occupancy of the water molecule is distributed onto the 3D grid using all snapshots generated throughout the production run of the MD simulation. The occupancy distribution was then averaged over the production run and a user-specified clustering algorithm (*see* **Note 5**) was used to identify the pronounced peaks that define the hydration site locations. For each identified hydration site, WATsite tools will then be used to compute the enthalpic (ΔH_{hs}) and entropic (ΔS_{hs}) change of transferring a water molecule from the bulk solvent to the hydration site of the protein binding site.

3   Methods and Results

The WATsite PyMOL plugin contains six menu items as shown in Fig. 2a. This section will first describe the steps of using the plugin to (1) modify settings, (2) prepare the system, (3) set parameters for simulation, (4) run simulation with OpenMM, and (5) analyze

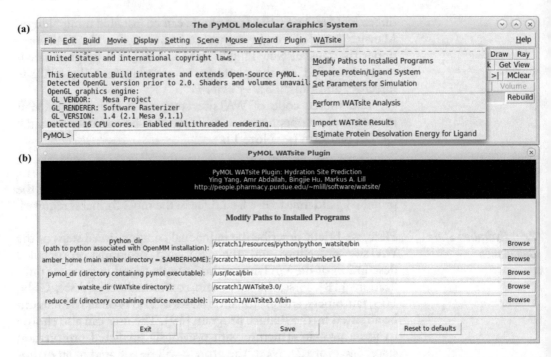

Fig. 2 (**a**) WATsite PyMOL plugin menu, and (**b**) **step 1** to specify the correct paths to the installed program

trajectory with WATsite. Water thermodynamics with (6) and without (7) the presence of ligand can be calculated. We will then explain how to import and analyze those results.

3.1 Modify Settings

The location paths to the required molecular modeling programs need to be correctly specified. Select the menu item "Modify Paths to Installed Programs" from the WATsite menu (Fig. 2b). The users need to specify or modify the paths to the programs according to their installation. For example, the location of WATsite directory should be defined for *watsite_home*, and similarly the python path associated with OpenMM, the path to Amber, PyMOL, and Reduce installations. The settings only need to be modified for the first time, and will be automatically read in subsequent sessions.

3.2 Prepare Protein/ Ligand System

The user can specify a protein structure from a file or a structure already displayed in the current PyMOL session (Fig. 3a). The user can choose to perform protonation site analysis using Reduce [19], or use a structure with previously predicted protonation states (*see* **Note 2**). To define the protein binding site, the user needs to provide a ligand molecule positioned within the binding site or a "pseudo-ligand" using binding site residues. A margin (in Å) will be used to define the binding pocket specifying a box surrounding the ligand/pseudo-ligand. The minimum distance between any ligand heavy atom and the edge of the box equals to the margin value. Hydration sites can be predicted for both ligand-free (apo)

(a)

(b)

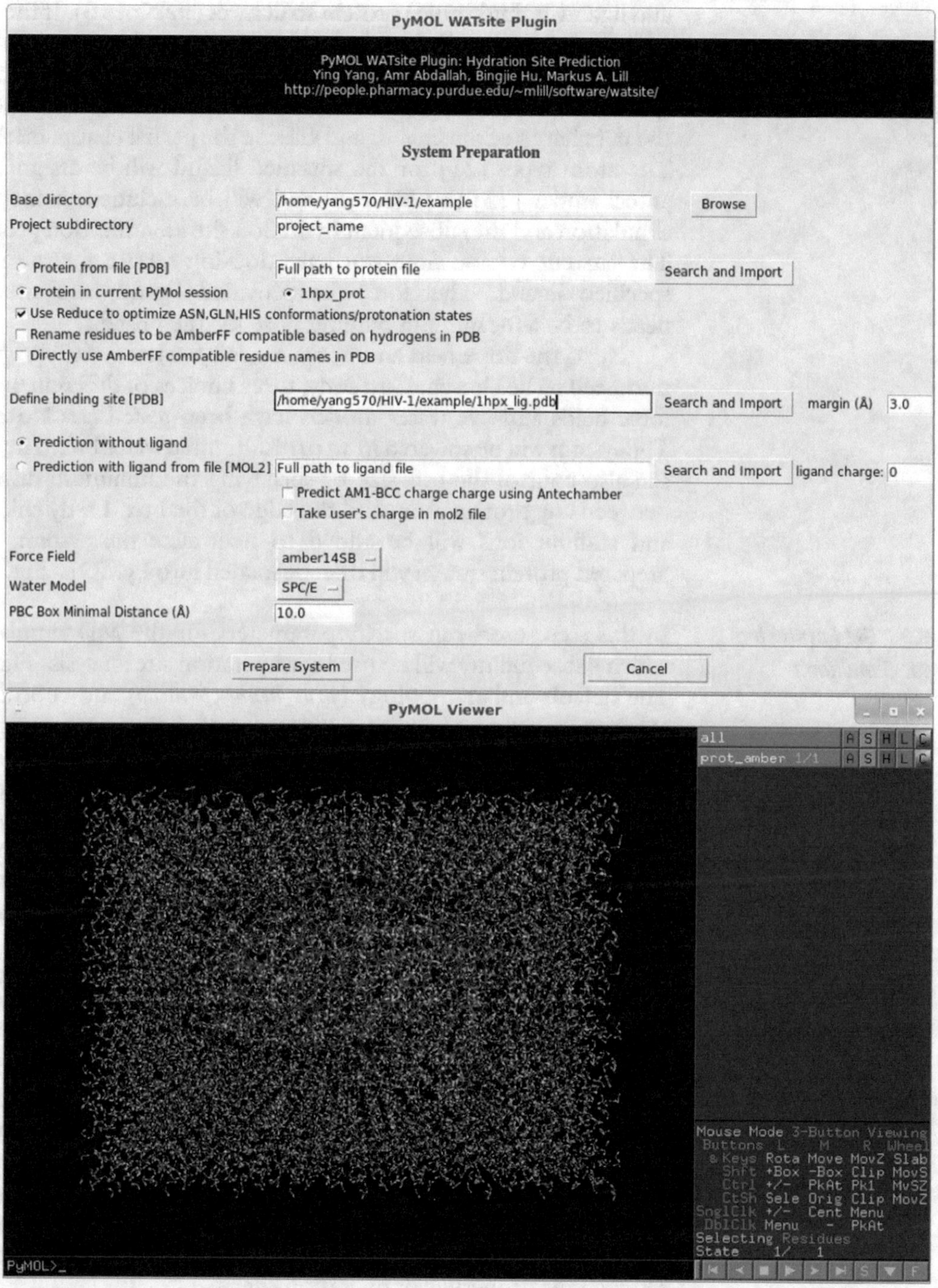

Fig. 3 Step 2 of WATsite procedure to prepare the protein or protein–ligand system

and ligand-bound (holo) protein structures (*see* **Note 6**). If the user intends to predict hydration sites at the interface between the protein and the ligand, the file location of the bound ligand is specified within the PyMOL plugin. The user also needs to specify the net charge of the ligand, and choose the partial charge method. The atom types [21] for the specified ligand will be assigned by antechamber [22] (*see* **Note 6**) and will be included in the MD simulation and the subsequent hydration site identification process. The current version does not have docking service for the user-specified ligand. Therefore, the provided ligand conformation needs to be a meaningful binding pose for the protein.

Next, the force field and water models for the system preparation need to be chosen. Currently, three choices of different amber force fields and five water models have been tested (*see* **Note 3**). The system will be solvated in an orthorhombic water box. The user can also control the box size by specifying the minimum distance between any protein atom and the edge of the box. Lastly chloride and sodium ions will be added to neutralize the system. The prepared protein system will then be loaded into PyMOL (Fig. 3b).

3.3 Set Parameters for Simulation

In this step, users can specify parameters for the MD simulation which subsequently will be used for hydration site analysis (Fig. 4). The default amber topology (*prot_amber.prmtop*) and coordinate (*prot_amber.inpcrd*) files are generated during the system preparation step. The users may also choose amber files from their own preparation. The CUDA device index (*see* **Note 1**) needs to be specified based on the user's workstation CUDA device availability. Long-range electrostatic interactions can be treated using one of three methods (*PME*, *Ewald*, or *NoCutoff*) with direct electrostatic calculations for atom pairs within a specified cutoff distance. If *NoCutoff* is chosen, the cutoff distance will be ignored.

By default, we apply constraints on the length of all bonds involving a hydrogen atom, and make water molecules rigid. This will allow us to run simulations with an integration timestep of 2 fs. However, the user can disable the constraints and rigid water settings by unchecking the box, and change to a smaller timestep accordingly. Temperature and number of steps for the equilibration and production run can also be modified (*see* **Note 4**). For the choice of equilibration and production simulation length, our previous studies [23] showed that at least a 4 ns production simulation is required to obtain reliable prediction of the locations and thermodynamic properties of hydration sites.

3.4 Run Simulation

Once the preparation has been finished the user will change into the project directory and start the OpenMM simulation:

nohup. /run_openmm.sh &

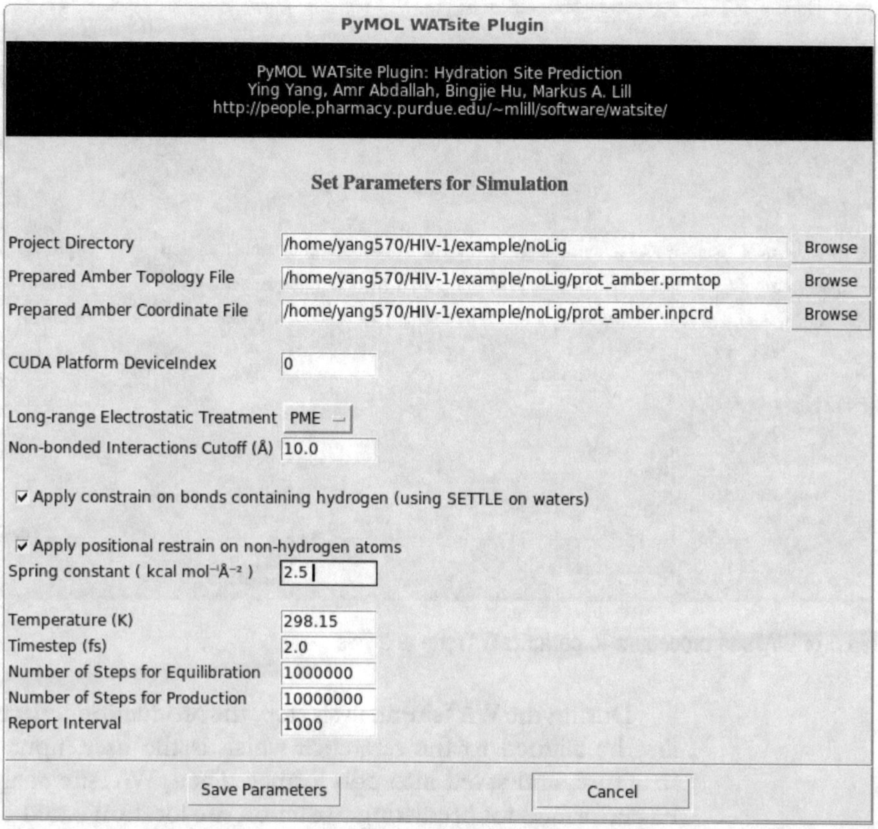

Fig. 4 Step 3 of WATsite procedure to specify parameters for running the MD simulations via OpenMM

Using the default settings for the simulation, the system will first be energy minimized until convergence with a tolerance of 10 kJ/mol. Then the system will be heated to the user's specified temperature using Langevin integrator, and the density will be adjusted using pressure coupling to 1 bar. Equilibration and production simulations will be performed for the user's specified number of steps, and the coordinates will be saved in constant intervals (as specified by user) into the trajectory file (netcdf format). All protein heavy atoms and ligand heavy atoms (if present) are harmonically restrained (spring constant is user-defined).

3.5 Perform WATsite Analysis

In this step, we will perform WATsite analysis on the trajectory file generated in the previous step (Fig. 5). The amber topology (*prot_amber.prmtop*) and coordinate (*prot_amber.inpcrd*) files generated in **step 2**, as well as the trajectory (*sys_md.nc*) file generated in **step 4** should be specified correctly.

The number of steps and water model used for WATsite analysis need to be identical to those used during the production simulation. Clustering algorithm used to predict hydration site locations from water density can also be chosen (*see* **Note 5**).

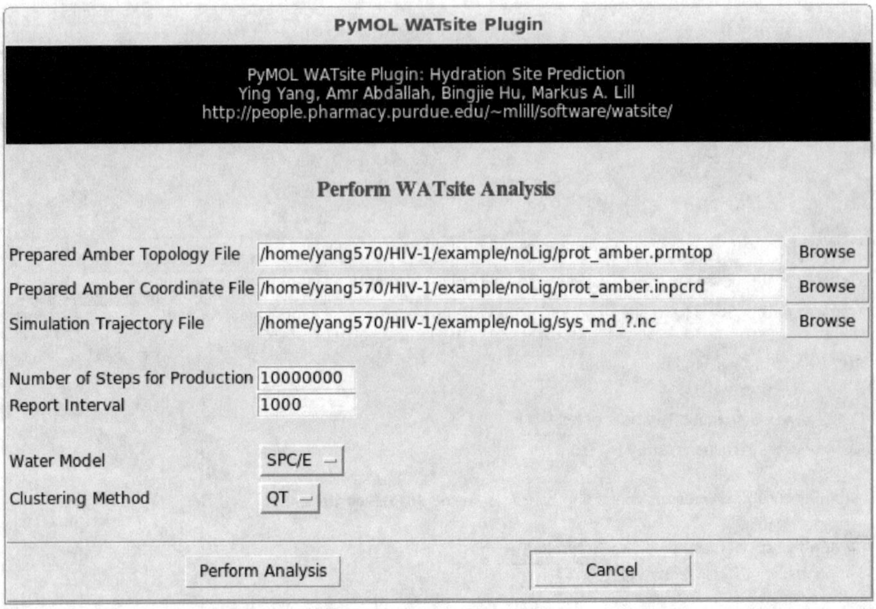

Fig. 5 Step 5 of WATsite procedure to perform WATsite analysis

During the WATsite analysis step, the production trajectory will first be aligned to the reference which is the user input protein structure, and saved into pdb format. Then, WATsite analysis will be performed for predicting hydration site location based on water density analysis, calculating entropy and enthalpy.

3.6 Hydration Site Prediction with Ligand: Water at Binding Interface

In the first example, we performed hydration site prediction with the presence of a bound inhibitor (KNI) for HIV-1 protease discussed in the introduction (PDB: 1HPX). After completion of WATsite analysis, we can import the results through the "Import WATsite Results" command under the WATsite menu, and select the "*WATsite.out*" file which stores the directory to the location of the prediction results (Fig. 6a). Here, we want to investigate water molecules at the binding interface between protein and ligand, so we select "*Protein*," "*Ligand*," and "*Hydration Site*" to load into PyMOL. The results of the example case of HIV-1 protease are shown in Fig. 6b. The crystal waters are all predicted, and the interfacial water mediating the protein–ligand interaction via hydrogen bonding is selected in Fig. 6b.

The PyMOL viewer window shows the predicted hydration sites in the protein binding site. The hydration sites are shown as spheres and colored in this example based on their ΔG values in a blue–white–red spectrum where blue indicates relatively low ΔG values and red indicates relatively high ΔG values. A hydration site with a more positive ΔG value (darker red) indicates an unfavorable environment of the water molecule in the binding site. Therefore, a

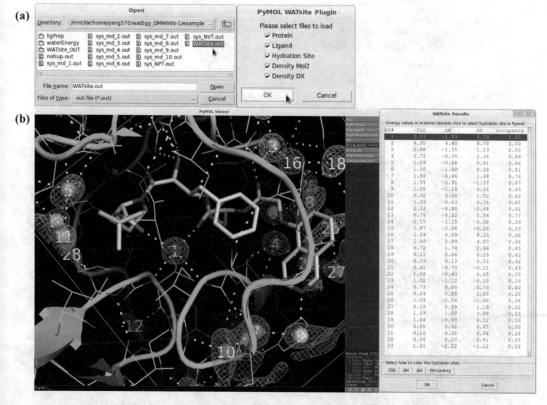

Fig. 6 (**a**) Hydration site results predicted with the presence of ligand. Choose the "WATsite.out" file and select all options to load the results. (**b**) The results of example case of HIV-1 protease with bound ligand. The interfacial water molecules are selected

gain in free energy of binding can be expected if the water in that hydration site is replaced by a ligand. The "occupancy" values indicate the probability a water molecule is observed in the given hydration site during the MD simulation. The "*WATsite results*" window listing the estimated desolvation free energy (ΔG), enthalpy (ΔH), entropy ($-T\Delta S$), and occupancy for each hydration site. The user can also choose according to which descriptor the hydration sites are colored by clicking the corresponding "ΔG", "ΔH", "$-T\Delta S$", or "*Occupancy*" button.

3.7 Hydration Sites Prediction Without Ligand: Water for Protein Desolvation Free Energy Estimation

The user can perform hydration site prediction with the ligand removed from the protein binding site. This method can be useful to compare and evaluate the different protein desolvation free energies from a congeneric series of ligands.

We did the ligand-free prediction for the HIV-1 protease example, and imported the WATsite results as in the previous step. Next, the directory containing all ligands of interest as well as the radius/cutoff used to select the displaced hydration sites need to be specified (Fig. 7a). For each ligand in the directory, the free energies of

(a)

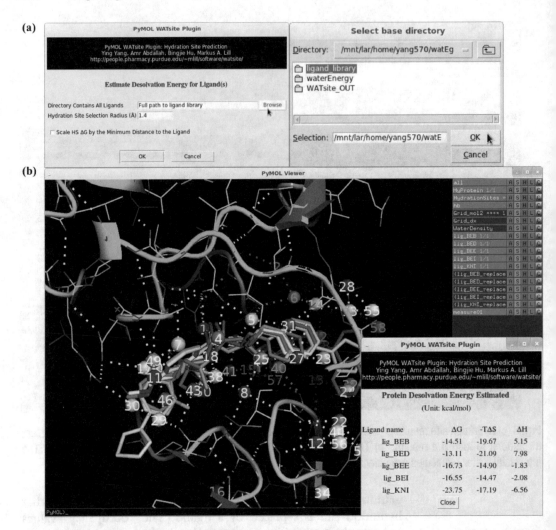

(b)

Fig. 7 (a) Hydration site results predicted without the ligand. (b) The result of example case of HIV-1 protease with bound ligand. The interfacial water molecules are selected

hydration sites that are within the user-specified distance to any of the ligand's heavy atoms are added up to estimate its protein desolvation free energy. A more positive value means a more favorable contribution to the protein–ligand binding free energy. The predicted desolvation energies (ΔG, $-T\Delta S$, and ΔH) are displayed in a new window, and the selection of displaced hydration sites is highlighted in the PyMOL viewer (Fig. 7b).

Binding site water displacement is a significant contribution, if not the driving force, of protein–ligand binding. When a lead compound is already known for a specific target, WATsite can be useful in suggesting ligand modification in order to improve affinity due to the displacement of hydration sites with unfavorable free energies (*see* **Note 7**).

4   Notes

1. CUDA platform on GPU workstation—This latest version of WATsite relies on OpenMM accelerated MD simulation, but a previous version, WATsite2.0, based on Gromacs simulations is available in case a GPU workstation is not available. The WATsite-compatible OpenMM has to be compiled in order to perform MD simulation and generate water interaction energies for later analysis. The source code is located in the *openmm-watsite* folder, and the user can follow the standard OpenMM compilation steps. Here, we will briefly list the steps.

   (a) Download CUDA 8.0 and install both the drivers and CUDA toolkit. Set the environment variable accordingly before compilation. We provide an example below:

   export PATH=$PATH:/usr/local/cuda-8.0/bin/
   export LD_LIBRARY_PATH=/usr/local/cuda-8.0/lib64:
   $LD_LIBRARY_PATH
   export CUDA_HOME=/usr/local/cuda-8.0/
   export   OPENMM_CUDA_COMPILER=/usr/local/
   cuda-8.0/bin/nvcc

   (b) Go to the Openmm-watsite directory, make a new directory and change into the directory.

   (c) Configure with ccmake:
   ccmake ../

   (d) Configure *("c")*.

   (e) Set the variable CMAKE_INSTALL_PREFIX to the location where you want to install OpenMM.

   (f) Set the variable PYTHON_EXECUTABLE to the Python interpreter you plan to use OpenMM with.

   (g) Configure (press "c") again.

   (h) Generate ("g") the Makefile.

   (i) Start the installation by the following command: (if the location of installation is not a system area, sudo is not required)
   (sudo) make install && (sudo) make PythonInstall

   (j) Verify your installation by the following command:
   python -m simtk.testInstallation

   Before starting the OpenMM simulation in **step 4**, the user needs to make sure the environment variables for CUDA in (a) are set correctly. Depending on the number of GPU cards available, the user can spread multiple jobs by specifying the device index in **step 3**.

2. Protonation states —Protonation states for ionizable residues in the protein binding site may significantly affect the

thermodynamics of water molecules. We provide the option for the user to use the Reduce [19] program to adjust the protonation state for HIS based on the local environment, and ASN and GLN side chains may be flipped to optimize the hydrogen-bond network. The user may also use other tools, such as protein preparation wizard in maestro [24], for the protonation states prediction. The hydrogens in ASP, GLU, HIS, and LYS will be evaluated to give appropriate residue names compatible with amber force field.

3. Selection of force field and water model—The current version allows choosing from three different amber force fields. Amber14SB [20] is the recommended choice in the latest amber manual. Two other force fields, Amber99SB [25] and Amber99SBildn [26], can also be chosen depending on the user's interest. Five water models with associated atomic ions have been tested and implemented in the current version of WATsite. TIP3P and SPC/E are three-site water models, and the SPC/E model adds an average polarization correction to the potential energy function [27]. TIP4P and TIP4P-Ew are four-site water models which have four interaction points by adding one dummy atom near the oxygen along the bisector of the HOH angle. The TIP4P-Ew model was reparameterized for use with Ewald summation methods [28]. OPC is a new four-site and three-charge rigid water model which has quite different point charges and charge–charge distances [29].

4. Timestep and number of steps of simulation—Bond stretching is a fast motion which determines the size of the MD timestep. With bond length constraints applied on the bonds involving hydrogen atoms, a timestep of 2 fs can be used. A time step of equal or less than 1 fs is required if constraints are not applied. With a 2 fs timestep, at least 2,000,000 steps for the production simulation are required based on previous analysis [23]. Hydration sites locations and free energies converged over the 4 ns trajectory since all protein heavy atoms and potentially present ligand heavy atoms were harmonically restrained (spring constants are user-specified).

5. Clustering method—To identify locations of hydration sites in high water density regions, a clustering method is used in WATsite analysis. Currently, two clustering algorithms have been implemented: quality threshold (QT) [30] and density-based spatial clustering of applications with noise (DBSCAN) [31]. QT clustering method is superior in identifying hydration sites with a large occupancy value during the simulation, whereas DBSCAN clustering method is advantageous in identifying more hydration sites with lower occupancy throughout the simulation.

6. Hydration site prediction with and without the presence of bound ligand—The ligand-free (apo) protein structure should be used to predict hydration sites for the purpose of computing protein desolvation free energy. WATsite also allows for hydration sites prediction at the protein and ligand binding interface. Partial charge of ligand may significantly influence the outcome of desolvation free energy. The user can predict partial charges in the mol2 file for the ligand with other tools, such as RESP [32] charge by using QM packages. Otherwise, the partial charges are computed via AM1-BCC [33] method using antechamber [22].

7. Protein desolvation free energy—It is worth noting that the estimated desolvation free energy for a ligand only represents the energy of releasing the water molecules from the protein binding site into the bulk solvent. It cannot be used for a direct comparison of the ligands' free energies of binding. The ligand's free energy of binding includes other important contributions such as the direct protein–ligand interaction energy or desolvation energy of the ligand. The predicted protein desolvation free energy, however, can guide further optimization of a lead compound rationally stabilizing or replacing additional water molecules in the binding site.

Acknowledgment

We thank Andrew McNutt for testing the program and critical reading. The authors gratefully acknowledge a grant from the NIH (GM092855) for partially supporting this research.

References

1. Cheung MS, Garcia AE, Onuchic JN (2002) Protein folding mediated by solvation: water expulsion and formation of the hydrophobic core occur after the structural collapse. Proc Natl Acad Sci U S A 99(2):685–690

2. Gao M, Zhu H, Yao XQ, She ZS (2010) Water dynamics clue to key residues in protein folding. Biochem Biophys Res Commun 392 (1):95–99

3. Kovacs IA, Szalay MS, Csermely P (2005) Water and molecular chaperones act as weak links of protein folding networks: energy landscape and punctuated equilibrium changes point towards a game theory of proteins. FEBS Lett 579(11):2254–2260

4. Sessions RB, Thomas GL, Parker MJ (2004) Water as a conformational editor in protein folding. J Mol Biol 343(4):1125–1133

5. Vajda T, Perczel A (2014) Role of water in protein folding, oligomerization, amyloidosis and miniprotein. J Pept Sci 20(10):747–759

6. Zuo GH, Hu J, Fang H (2009) Effect of the ordered water on protein folding: an off-lattice go-like model study. Phys Rev E Stat Nonlinear Soft Matter Phys 79(3 Pt 1):031925

7. Biela A, Betz M, Heine A, Klebe G (2012) Water makes the difference: rearrangement of water solvation layer triggers non-additivity of functional group contributions in protein-ligand binding. ChemMedChem 7 (8):1423–1434

8. Breiten B, Lockett M, Sherman W et al (2013) Water networks contribute to enthalpy/entropy compensation in protein-ligand binding. J Am Chem Soc 135(41):15579–15584

9. Li Z, Lazaridis T (2006) Thermodynamics of buried water clusters at a protein-ligand binding interface. J Phys Chem B 110 (3):1464–1475

10. Michel J, Tirado-Rives J, Jorgensen WL (2009) Energetics of displacing water molecules from protein binding sites: consequences for ligand optimization. J Am Chem Soc 131 (42):15403–15411

11. Baron R, Setny P, McCammon JA (2010) Water in cavity-ligand recognition. J Am Chem Soc 132(34):12091–12097

12. Bortolato A, Tehan BG, Bodnarchuk MS, Essex JW, Mason JS (2013) Water network perturbation in ligand binding: adenosine A (2A) antagonists as a case study. J Chem Inf Model 53(7):1700–1713

13. Hummer G (2010) Molecular binding: under water's influence. Nat Chem 2(11):906–907

14. Ladbury JE (1996) Just add water! The effect of water on the specificity of protein-ligand binding sites and its potential application to drug design. Chem Biol 3(12):973–980

15. Eastman P, Pande VS (2015) OpenMM: a hardware independent framework for molecular simulations. Comput Sci Eng 12(4):34–39

16. Case DA, Cerutti DS, Cheatham TE et al (2017) AMBER 16. University of California, San Francisco

17. The PyMOL Molecular Graphics System, version 1.8, Schrödinger, LLC

18. Hu B, Lill MA (2014) Watsite: hydration site prediction program with Pymol interface. J Comput Chem 35(16):1255–1260

19. Word JM, Lovell SC, Richardson JS et al (1999) Asparagine and glutamine: using hydrogen atom contacts in the choice of side-chain amide orientation. J Mol Biol 285 (4):1735–1747

20. Maier JA, Martinez C, Kasavajhala K et al (2015) ff14SB: improving the accuracy of protein side chain and backbone parameters from ff99SB. J Chem Theory Comput 11 (8):3696–3713

21. Wang J, Wolf RM, Caldwell JW et al (2004) Development and testing of a general amber force field. J Comput Chem 25(9):1157–1174

22. Wang J, Wang W, Kollman PA, Case DA (2006) Automatic atom type and bond type perception in molecular mechanical calculations. J Mol Graph Model 25(2):247–260

23. Yang Y, Hu B, Lill MA (2014) Analysis of factors influencing hydration site prediction based on molecular dynamics simulations. J Chem Inf Model 54(10):2987–2995

24. Sastry GM, Adzhiqirey M, Day T et al (2013) Protein and ligand preparation: parameters, protocols, and influence on virtual screening enrichments. J Comput Aided Mol Des 27 (3):221–234

25. Hornak V, Abel R, Okur A et al (2006) Comparison of multiple Amber force fields and development of improved protein backbone parameters. Proteins 65(3):712–725

26. Lindorff-Larsen K, Piana S, Palmo K et al (2010) Improved side-chain torsion potentials for the Amber ff99SB protein force field. Proteins 78(8):1950–1958

27. Zielkiewicz J (2005) Structural properties of water: comparison of the SPC, SPCE, TIP4P, and TIP5P models of water. J Chem Phys 123 (10):104501

28. Horn HW, Swope WC, Pitera JW (2004) Development of an improved four-site water model for biomolecular simulations: TIP4P-Ew. J Chem Phys 120(20):9665–9678

29. Izadi S, Anandakrishnan R, Onufriev AV (2014) Building water models: a different approach. J Phys Chem Lett 5(21):3863–3871

30. Heyer LJ, Kruglyak S, Yooseph S (1999) Exploring expression data: identification and analysis of coexpressed genes. Genome Res 9 (11):1106–1115

31. Ester M, Kriegel HP, Sander J, Xu X (1996) A density-based algorithm for discovering clusters in large spatial databases with noise. In: Proceedings of the second international conference on knowledge discovery and data mining (KDD-96). AAAI Press, CA

32. Bayly CI, Cieplak P, Cornell W, Kollman PA (1993) A well-behaved electrostatic potential based method using charge restraints for deriving atomic charges: the RESP model. J Phys Chem 97:10269–10280

33. Jakalian A, Jack DB, Bayly CI (2002) Fast, efficient generation of high-quality atomic charges. AM1-BCC model: II. Parameterization and validation. J Comput Chem 23(16):1623–1641

Chapter 20

Enhanced Molecular Dynamics Methods Applied to Drug Design Projects

Sonia Ziada, Abdennour Braka, Julien Diharce, Samia Aci-Sèche, and Pascal Bonnet

Abstract

Nobel Laureate Richard P. Feynman stated: "[…] everything that living things do can be understood in terms of jiggling and wiggling of atoms […]." The importance of computer simulations of macromolecules, which use classical mechanics principles to describe atom behavior, is widely acknowledged and nowadays, they are applied in many fields such as material sciences and drug discovery. With the increase of computing power, molecular dynamics simulations can be applied to understand biological mechanisms at realistic timescales. In this chapter, we share our computational experience providing a global view of two of the widely used enhanced molecular dynamics methods to study protein structure and dynamics through the description of their characteristics, limits and we provide some examples of their applications in drug design. We also discuss the appropriate choice of software and hardware. In a detailed practical procedure, we describe how to set up, run, and analyze two main molecular dynamics methods, the umbrella sampling (US) and the accelerated molecular dynamics (aMD) methods.

Key words Conformational sampling, Enhanced molecular dynamics, Free energy, Ligand (un) binding

1 Introduction

Proteins are versatile organic macromolecules, which have specific functions (transporter, reaction catalyzer, etc.) within living organisms. Small molecules binding to the considered entity can control this specific functionality. The formation of a drug–target complex is the basis of action of most drugs. The lock-and-key model of the early twentieth century, first formulated by Emil Fischer, gives a static point of view of drug–target interactions. In this paradigm, the binding is driven by shape complementarity between the ligand, in one conformation, and the frozen binding site. Since this model has been proposed, numerous evidences have revealed that proteins

---

Author contributed equally with all other contributors.Sonia Ziada and Abdennour Braka

Mohini Gore and Umesh B. Jagtap (eds.), *Computational Drug Discovery and Design*, Methods in Molecular Biology, vol. 1762, https://doi.org/10.1007/978-1-4939-7756-7_20, © Springer Science+Business Media, LLC, part of Springer Nature 2018

show a remarkable flexibility upon ligand binding, making this simple model inadequate to describe correctly the association and dissociation process of high-affinity drugs. It appears that proteins need to change their conformation, essentially near the pocket region, during compound binding [1–3]. Proteins are dynamic entities that are in constant motion and their structural dynamics are dependent on the amino acid composition and folding. Their conformations depend on physiological factors like temperature, pH, but also on direct factors, such as interactions with other entities (proteins, peptides, DNA, membrane, molecules, hormone, etc.). This ability of conformation changing in response to its environment is a key step in biological processes such as protein–ligand interactions, enzyme catalysis, protein–protein interaction, protein transport, and signal transduction. The inherent flexibility of proteins could involve important part of the 3D structure, or just few amino acids side chains, which results in large-scale movement through transition intermediates [4, 5]. A complete understanding of the protein function necessarily implies a structural description and an energetic quantification of the dynamic events of interest. The consideration of these structural mechanisms is very important for the design and development of new drugs and constitutes a fundamental step in our knowledge of key biological processes.

Protein flexibility is an important biological phenomenon that must be taken into account in structure-based drug design (SBDD) strategies. The structural and dynamics events occurring during the process of drug–receptor complex formation and dissociation considerably affect the binding kinetics, thermodynamics and affinity of the drug. This binding kinetics, especially the dissociation kinetic (directly associated to drug residence time) has acquired over a period of 10 years, a considerable importance in drug design [6, 7], because of its significant impact on drug in vivo efficacy [8, 9]. Understanding these structural changes related to transition state(s) formation along the association and/or dissociation pathway is crucial and can provide considerable insights for further optimization of drugs.

Beyond traditional approaches (such as X-ray crystallography and nuclear magnetic resonance (NMR) spectroscopy), considerable efforts were made in the development of new experimental methods to investigate the dynamics and flexibility of biomolecules. Time-resolved studies, solution X-ray scattering, and new detectors for cryo-electron microscopy have pushed the limits of structural investigation of flexible systems but still remain expensive and time consuming. In addition, they could be used only on a limited set of protein conformers and are not always applicable to the biological system of interest [10]. Moreover, the increasing complexity of the studied biomolecule including, for example, large transient protein assemblies and transmembrane proteins makes the consideration of the flexibility role more difficult to apprehend.

From the theoretical point of view, classical molecular dynamics (cMD) simulation method is nowadays an appropriate way to study the dynamics behavior of biological entities, even for large macromolecular systems. Starting from an experimentally determined structure or from a computationally built model (comparative modeling protocol), cMD simulations predict atomic motions of a molecular system as a function of time. Due to the presence of high energetic barriers on the potential energy surface of the system, and the random nature of molecular dynamics simulation, biological processes are stochastic events that usually occur on the microsecond to millisecond or even longer timescales. Even with a great improvement in computing hardware, cMD simulations are limited to timescales of about several hundreds of nanoseconds, making it unsuitable to simulate these "slow" biological processes. To improve the efficiency of conformational sampling, enhanced MD sampling techniques have been developed. Thus, these new methodologies, combined with efficient computing hardware, allow the study of biological processes from a structural, thermodynamic and kinetic point of view in the most appropriate biological environment [11, 12].

In this chapter, we present an overview of the main enhanced MD methods used currently in drug design. We expose the characteristics and limits of each MD method and examples of applications. We also discuss the appropriate choice of software and hardware. We specially focus on two widely used methods, umbrella sampling (US), a reaction coordinate (RC)-dependent method with which the free energy profile can be computed; and accelerated molecular dynamics (aMD), a nondependent RC method that improves the conformational sampling by overcoming high energy barriers. We give a technical, methodological, and detailed guideline to set up, run, and analyze US and aMD simulations. Finally, we highlight important critical points to be analyzed for the relevance and rigor of the study.

2   Materials

To perform an MD simulation, we first need suitable hardware for performing calculations, second a software package with MD capabilities, and finally the initial spatial coordinates of the system of interest. Choices of each of these three aspects are mutually dependent since not all MD methodologies are implemented in all software and not all softwares are compatible with all computer hardware technologies. Therefore we summarize in Table 1 the software in which they are implemented and the supported technology for each MD method.

Table 1
Various molecular dynamics methods, software implementation, hardware support

MD method	Software implementation	Hardware support
Conventional MD (cMD)	AMBER [13], CHARMM[14], NAMD [15], Gromacs [16], Desmond [17], ACEMD [18]	CPU/GPU
Accelerated MD (aMD)	AMBER, NAMD	CPU/GPU
Scaled MD	AMBER, BiKi [19]	CPU/GPU
Random accelerated MD (RAMD)	AMBER, CHARMM, NAMD	CPU
Steered MD (SMD)	AMBER, CHARMM, NAMD, Gromacs Desmond	CPU/GPU CPU
Targeted MD (TMD)	AMBER, CHARMM, NAMD	CPU
Metadynamics (MTD)	AMBER, CHARMM, NAMD, Gromacs, Desmond	CPU/GPU
Replica Exchange MD (REMD)	AMBER, CHARMM, NAMD, Gromacs, Desmond	CPU/GPU
Simulating Annealing (SA)	AMBER, CHARMM, NAMD, Gromacs, Desmond	CPU/GPU

2.1 Hardware

To enhance the computing power, one of the means is to increase the number of central processing units (CPUs) used for the calculation. Several possibilities exist, from Desktop station, containing about 4–16 CPUs, to supercomputer with thousands of CPUs [20]. Nowadays, the arrival in the market of the graphics processing unit (GPU), a very accessible computing technology mainly designed for gaming performances, has revolutionized the field of computational sciences and especially numerical simulations. GPU cards have accelerated calculations by several orders of magnitude compared to CPU and have similar performances to supercomputer [21]. Moreover, several CPU cluster nodes can be replaced by one GPU card, which allows for extensive and parallel calculations, and has the advantage to decrease power consumption compared to CPUs. Desktop workstations equipped with a GPU card have become a useful tool to carry out molecular dynamics simulations, and clusters containing GPUs (allowing multiple GPUs to carry out parallel calculations) open the way toward the simulation of larger biomolecular systems. However, an additional effort should be made in writing the code of the software in specific programing language for GPU cards, called CUDA. A very recent new Intel hardware, called the Xeon Phi, which is a Many-Integrated-Core [MIC] in a single chip, has been recently proposed. These multicore processors have the advantage to perform calculations just like the main CPU on a laptop/desktop but with higher computing performance [22].

The choice of the MD software and the simulation method should be done in relation to hardware recommendations and benchmarks. For AMBER software, the links for recommendations and benchmarks are at http://ambermd.org/gpus/ recommended_hardware.htm and http://ambermd.org/gpus/ benchmarks.htm respectively.

2.2 Software

As presented in Table 1, a large number of software packages are available for MD simulations. For the examples mentioned below, we used AMBER suite as MD simulation software which is distributed in two parts: AMBER, a proprietary software which contains the codes of molecular dynamics calculations for CPUs and GPUs (sander, pmemd, pmemd.cuda) and AmberTools, an open source package that contains tools to parameterize organic molecules and metal centers (antechamber), to prepare the system (tleap, parmed), and to analyze trajectories (cpptraj, pytraj, MMPBSA.py). Other indispensable tools can be found online, for example to choose the number of replicas in the Temperature-REMD simulation (http://folding.bmc.uu.se/remd/) or to predict protonation states of the biological system of interest at the desired pH (PROPKA, http://propka.org/). These recommendations are generally given in the online tutorials that we strongly advise to follow before launching a simulation (http://ambermd. org/tutorials/). To visually display, analyze, and animate trajectories, VMD is one of the appropriate programs, distributed free of charge.

2.3 Studied Biological System

For the two proposed protocols, we chose the human p38α (MAPK14) kinase domain as a case study. The crystallographic structure (pdb code: 3S3I), containing the biaryl-triazolopyridine scaffold derivative in the ATP binding site, was chosen as a starting structure for the simulations. The choice was based on the best resolution of the p38α crystallographic structures available in the RCSB database [23] and the absence of sequence gaps in the 3D structure.

3   Methods

3.1 System Preparation

All the scripts used in the simulations and analysis will be provided in the supporting information. A molecular dynamics simulation protocol always begins with the preparation of the system, which consists of several steps:

1. Cap protein termini with ACE and NME residues if the protein is not fully resolved at the extremities (*see* **Note 1**). Then, save the protein with the ligand for the unbinding simulation using the US and without ligand for conformational sampling with aMD.

2. Predict and assign the protonation states of protein residues at pH = 7 using the PROPKA program (http://propka.org/).

3. Calculate automatic charges and generate mol2 file for the ligand using Antechamber program in AmberTools package. Next, construct additional frcmod file for the ligand with parmchk2.

4. With tleap program in AmberTools, we protonate, solvate, and create the topology and coordinate files using ff14SB and Gaff force fields to describe respectively the protein and the ligand. The TIP3P model of water is used to represent explicit water molecules as solvent. Na^+ and Cl^- are chosen as counterions to neutralize system.

At the end of these steps, we obtain the system topology file (.prmtop) describing the parameters and the topology of the molecules in the system, and the initial molecular coordinates of the system (.rst7).

3.2 System Minimization and Equilibration

Now that the system parameters have been set, a preliminary protocol has to be carried out before running MD simulations. This protocol, constituting of both minimization and equilibration steps, allows the relaxation of the 3D structure of the protein and the equilibration of water molecules around the system. Most of the time, the equilibration begins with a thermalization step, in which the system reaches the thermal equilibrium at the desired temperature. Our equilibration protocol was carried out in five steps (*see* **Note 2**):

1. Minimization of experimentally structure to find a stable state (a minimum) on the potential energy surface from which to begin the simulation. The minimization was performed in two steps: first we minimize the solvent box and second we minimize all the system (protein/ligand/solvent box).

2. Thermal equilibration: the system is incrementally thermalized from 0 to 300 K for 10 ps.

3. Density equilibration: equilibrate the density of the system (NPT) with weak harmonic restraints on the complex during 200 ps.

4. Relaxation of the system in the NVT ensemble by gradually decreasing the harmonic restraints during 600 ps.

5. cMD production with the complete relaxation of the system (no harmonic restraint) during 50 ns.

All the simulations were performed using the SHAKE algorithm on hydrogen atoms, a 2 fs time step and Langevin dynamics for temperature control.

3.3 Enhanced Molecular Dynamics Methods

Once the system is prepared, minimized, and equilibrated, several molecular dynamics methods can be applied and the choice depends on the objective of the study (Table 2). In theory, cMD simulations can be envisaged to describe important biological processes at atomic level such as the binding of the kinase inhibitor PP1 that reaches its binding site and finally reproduces the crystallographic binding pose in 15 μs [24] and the millisecond-order simulation of the reversible folding unfolding process of ubiquitin [25]. However, such simulations require very powerful, specific computer in order to be achieved in an acceptable time frame. To overcome this limitation, a number of enhanced MD methods have been developed where a bias is introduced into the simulation to enhance the sampling of all the system, or along a phenomenon of interest. A large number of biased methods, with a wide diversity of possible bias have been developed during the past 30 years (*see* **Notes 3–5**). Among them, the most used methods are temperature replica exchange molecular dynamics [26], umbrella sampling [27, 28], metadynamics [29, 30], scaled MD [31], and accelerated molecular dynamics simulations [32, 33]. We can classify these methods in two groups depending on whether the bias is added along a reaction coordinate or not. In this case, the bias associated to the reaction coordinate must represent the proper evolution of the biological process of interest. Some methods such as REMD and Simulated Annealing by their implemented algorithm produce a simulation that is not time dependent but rather sampling method, based on a Metropolis–Hastings algorithm.

3.4 Accelerated Molecular Dynamics Method

3.4.1 Boost Potential

Accelerated molecular dynamics (aMD) method improves the conformational sampling by reducing energy barriers separating different conformational states of a system. A boost potential is added to bring up potential energy wells below a certain threshold level (E_{thr}) without modifying those that are above [32]. As a result, the magnitude of energy barriers is reduced, allowing the system to sample conformational space that cannot be easily accessed by cMD simulations [34]. It should be noted that the underlying shape of the real potential is conserved so that the distribution of sampling of different structures is still related to the original potential energy distribution and can be recovered by a reweighing procedure.

When the potential condition is below the chosen threshold E_{thr}, a boost potential, $\Delta V_{boost}(r)$, is added to the original potential energy, $V_0(r)$ where r is the atomic positions. The new modified potential energy $V(r)^*$ is defined as follows (*see* **Note 6**):

Table 2
Description of various molecular dynamics methods: characteristics, limits and applications

	Linear time dependance?	Reaction coordinate dependance?	Methods to bias the system	Characteristics	Limits	Examples of application
cMD	Yes	No	–	No bias introduced	Need long simulation time to cross high energy barrier	• Conformational sampling • Study of Binding/unbinding process • Characterization of open/close state of protein state and opening/closing channels
Scaled MD & aMD			Modification of potential energy surface	• Sampling is not directed • Add of a modified potential energy to the original potential energy	Long simulations often lead to greater statistical errors	• Conformational sampling • Characterization of open/close state of protein state and opening/closing channels • Estimation of free energy
US & SMD		Yes		• Sampling along a geometrical reaction coordinate (distance, angle, etc) • Add an harmonic potential energy to the original potential energy	• Choice of reaction coordinate • Bias parametrization is very system dependent	• Conformational sampling • Study of Binding/unbinding process • Study of unfolding/folding process
TMD				• Sampling along the RMSD as reaction coordinate • Add an harmonic potential energy to the original potential energy		• Characterization of open/close state of protein and opening/closing channels • Estimation of free energy of studied events
MTD				• Sampling along collective variables defined as one or a combination of geometrical reaction coordinate • Add a Gaussian potential energy to the original potential energy	Choice of CVs	
REMD	No		Multicopy searching and sampling	• Sampling is not directed • Several variants of REMD: T-REMD, R-REMD, H-REMD, M-REMD etc.	• No time evolution of structural events • Number of replicas dependent on size system	Conformational sampling
SA	No		Temperature scaling	• Sampling is not directed • Sampling equivalent to the unbiased system	No time evolution of structural events	

$$V(r)^* = V_0(r) + \Delta V_{\text{boost}}(r)$$

Depending on the type of the boost potential ($\Delta V_{\text{boost}}(r)$), we distinguish three methods of aMD.

1. Boosting only the dihedral potential energy by $\Delta V_{\text{d}}(r)$:

$$\Delta V_{\text{d}}(r) = \frac{(E_{\text{thr}}d - V_{\text{d}}(r))^2}{(\alpha D + E_{\text{thr}}d - V_{\text{d}}(r))}$$

where $V_{\text{d}}(r)$, $E_{\text{thr}}d$, and αD are respectively the dihedral energy, the dihedral energy threshold, and the boost factor for the dihedral energy.

In this case, the boost is applied when $V_{\text{d}}(r) < E_{\text{thr}}d$

2. Boosting the total potential energy by $\Delta V_{\text{T}}(r)$:

$$\Delta V_{\text{T}}(r) = \frac{(E_{\text{thr}}p - V(r))^2}{(\alpha P + E_{\text{thr}}p - V(r))}$$

where $V(r) = V_0(r) + \Delta V_{\text{d}}(r)$ and $E_{\text{thr}}p$, αP are respectively the total potential energy threshold and the boost factor for the total potential energy.

3. The dual boost aMD by $\Delta V_{\text{Td}}(r)$ [35], in which the boost is added on the total potential energy in addition of an extra boost on the dihedral energy:

$$\Delta V_{\text{Td}}(r) = \Delta V_{\text{T}}(r) + \Delta V_{\text{d}}(r)$$

In these last two cases ($\Delta V_{\text{T}}(r)$ and $\Delta V_{\text{Td}}(r)$), the boost is applied when $V(r) < E_{\text{thr}}p$.

In our simulations, we use the dual boost aMD to study the improvement of the sampling of the conformational space of the protein structure compared to the cMD (*see* **Note 7**).

3.4.2 Parametrization of aMD Simulation

The parameters that have to be specified by the user and that directly impact the acceleration of the molecular dynamics simulation are: the total potential energy threshold ($E_{\text{thr}}p$), the dihedral energy threshold ($E_{\text{thr}}d$), the boost factors αP and αD. Note that αP and αD are inversely proportional to the strength of the applied acceleration. The bigger is E_{thr} ($E_{\text{thr}}p$ or $E_{\text{thr}}d$), the greater is the region of the potential energy surface affected by the boost, whereas the smaller is α (αP or αD), the more flattened is the energy barrier, which will be easier to cross (Fig. 1) (*see* **Note 8**).

As it was suggested in previous aMD studies [36, 37], it is recommended to calculate these parameters from the estimated average of total potential and dihedral energies ($\langle Ep(\text{tot}) \rangle$ and

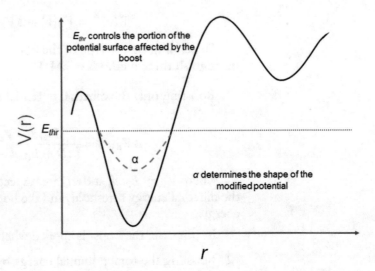

Fig. 1 Schematic representation of the biased potential, the threshold boost energy E_{thr} and the normal potential

$\langle Ed \rangle$) of a precomputed step of equilibration (cMD). From these estimations, we calculate the values of $E_{thr}p$ and $E_{thr}d$ by adding a quantity of energy per degree of freedom to the preestimated average potentials in the form of multiples of alpha as described in the following section.

From the 50 ns precomputed relaxation of the system we obtained:

(a) Average total potential energy $\langle Ep(\text{tot}) \rangle = -165576.6800$ kcal/mol.

(b) Average dihedral energy $\langle Ed \rangle = 4508.4797$ kcal/mol.

(c) Total number of atoms (Nbr Atoms) = 54,126 atoms.

(d) Number of protein residues (Nbr residues) = 351 residues.

Approximate energy contribution per degree of freedom:

(a) $\alpha P = 0.16$ kcal/mol/atom $\times$ Nbr Atoms (*see* **Note 9**)

$= 0.16 * 54126 = 8660.16$ kcal/mol.

(b) $E_{thr}p = \langle Ep(\text{tot}) \rangle + (0.16$ kcal/mol/atom $\times$ Nbr Atoms)

$= -165576.6800 + (0.16 \times 54,126) = -156916.52$ kcal/mol.

(c) $\alpha D = 0.2 \times (4$ kcal/mol/residues $\times$ Nbr residues) (*see* **Note 9**)

$= 0.2 \times (4 \times 351) = 280.8$ kcal/mol.

(d) $E_{thr}d = \langle Ed \rangle + (4$ kcal/mol/residues $\times$ Nbr residues)

$= 4508.4797 + (4 \times 351) = 5912.4797$ kcal/mol.

Once the aMD parameters are defined, we run 200 ns of aMD production with the same conditions of cMD. In addition to the boost of the aMD, we use the power of GPUs to significantly increase the conformational sampling in an acceptable total simulation time. Additional aMD productions can be launched from the output of the previous run.

When using a biased molecular dynamics method to enhance the conformational sampling of a protein, one important analysis step is to assess whether the obtained conformational ensemble is a consistent and robust representation of the accessible conformations of the protein. This implies to identify the largest motions in the protein, more precisely the protein regions whose movements contribute the most to explain the conformational diversity. From a mathematical point of view, a trajectory can be viewed as a matrix of atomic coordinates where each line corresponds to a conformation (snapshot) of the system at a time t (the individuals) and each column corresponds to the considered xyz coordinates of protein atoms (the variables). Extracting the variables that contribute to the largest motions in protein (variance) over a long timescale (number of individuals) and spatial scale (number of variables) is a common task in multivariate statistical analysis. For this purpose, dimensionality reduction methods are particularly suited to achieve a reduction in the number of variables. Among them, the principal component analysis (PCA) is a linear dimensionality reduction technique that linearly combines the set of variables into a reduced number of uncorrelated variables called principal components (PCs), consisting of five major steps:

1. Calculation of the covariance matrix: from the atomic coordinate matrix of the trajectory, a variance-covariance matrix is calculated.

2. Diagonalization of the covariance matrix: in order to de-correlate variables, we seek to minimize the covariance between variables that is the off-diagonal entries of the covariance matrix. Conversely, the diagonal entries, corresponding to the variance, shall be maximized since they correspond to interesting dynamics in the system. Note that the variance is a special case of covariance when the two variables are identical. Since minimizing the covariance consists in being as close to zero as possible, we are then looking to diagonalize the covariance matrix.

3. Extraction of the principal components: the columns of the transformation matrix, that is the matrix having served to diagonalize the covariance matrix, are the eigenvectors of the new basis. These eigenvectors are the principal components of the PCA space.

4. Extraction of the principal components of interest: an eigenvalue is associated with each eigenvector and the eigenvectors in the transformation matrix are sorted in descending order according to their respective eigenvalue. By this way, the first eigenvector of the transformation matrix, that is, the first principal component, corresponds to the direction of largest variance (largest-amplitude fluctuations), the second to the direction of second largest variance, and so on.

5. Dimensionality reduction: the latest components that are the less significant are not considered.

6. Calculation of the new coordinate matrix: the original matrix of atomic coordinates is projected onto the PCA space and the new matrix of atomic coordinates is derived.

In our example, we use the PCA to compare the efficiency of the conformational sampling of the aMD to cMD and its ability to retrieve the experimental crystal structures available in the PDB database.

Trajectory Preparation

Using the module cpptraj of AMBER we:

1. Create a new trajectory by concatenating the trajectory of the 200 ns aMD with that of the 200 ns cMD and all DFG-in structures of p38 without gaps available in the RCSB database.

2. Remove water molecules and counterions from the trajectory. During the analysis, we also remove hydrogens to reduce the size of the trajectory to avoid memory saturation.

3. Align the conformations of the trajectory on the C alpha atoms of the backbone to get all the frames (snapshots) in the same referential.

4. Export the new aligned trajectory and a single frame (or snapshot) as pdb format to use it as information of topology for the next analysis.

Principal Component Analysis of the Trajectory

In PCA, a set of atoms is selected to describe the conformation of the protein during the trajectory. Here, the atoms of the backbone are selected to describe residue positions and the corresponding trajectory constitutes the initial matrix of atomic coordinates (*see* **Note 10**). The PCA was performed with the Bio3D package in R (*see* **Note 11**) [38]. The topology is read from the pdb file. The trajectory can be read in DCD format (format used by CHARMM, NAMD, and X-PLOR) or NetCDF AMBER format after installing the ncdf4 package. Since the trajectory has been previously aligned on the backbone, PCA is directly applied on the initial matrix of atomic coordinates.

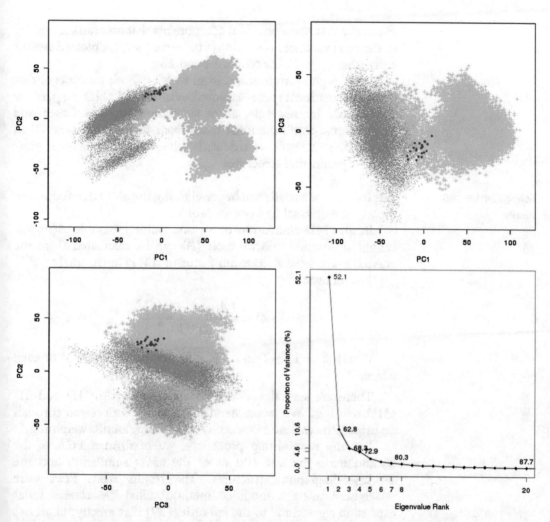

Fig. 2 PCA results for p38α conformational sampling. Individual maps: in green the 200 ns aMD trajectory, in orange the 200 ns cMD trajectory and in blue the experimental structures. Scree plot: cumulative variance as a function of the number of components

Analysis

From the results of PCA, the conformational sampling is analyzed on a 2D principal component plot as depicted in Fig. 2.

Each point represents one conformation of the trajectory at a time t. In general, only the first principal components (PC1, PC2, and PC3) that account for approximately 60–70% of the total variance of atom positional fluctuations, are analyzed. Indeed, these first components capture the most significant global movements, that is, the fluctuations of highest amplitude that are generally biologically relevant motions. On a 2D principal component plot, the larger the cumulative variance on the two considered principal components, the more meaningful is the distance between the points. It means that similar conformations will be grouped while diverse conformations will be separated on the 2D PCA plot.

Here, the first three principal components that accounts for 68.3% of the total variance, as shown on the scree plot, are plotted against each other (Fig. 2) (*see* **Notes 12** and **13**).

After aligning trajectories from each method, we observe that the conformational spaces explored by cMD and aMD are partially overlapped. Interestingly, aMD simulation explores larger and more distant conformational space from the starting point than the cMD. This result is particularly relevant since it includes most of the experimental structures.

Reweighting the aMD Results

The last step of analysis will be reweighting the aMD distribution to recover the original free energy profile.

In an aMD simulation of an observable ensemble $A(r)$, the canonical ensemble distribution $\langle A \rangle$ can be calculated from the ensemble-averaged Boltzmann factor of $\Delta V(r)$ in the aMD ($\langle e^{\beta \Delta V(r)} \rangle *$) as follows:

$$\langle A \rangle = \frac{\langle A(r) \times e^{\beta \Delta V(r)} \rangle^*}{\langle e^{\beta \Delta V(r)} \rangle^*}$$

Where $\beta = 1/k_B T$ and $\Delta V(r)$ is the boost potential of each frame.

There are several available scripts that perform 1D and 2D aMD reweight. We recommend the available scripts and tutorials at: https://mccammon.ucsd.edu/computing/amdReweighting/.

For the reweighting procedure, we perform a PCA of the backbone on the last 100 ns of the aMD simulation and the 22 crystallographic structures. The results from PCA were reweighted using a modified method called "Maclaurin series expansion algorithm" to the kth order [39] that greatly suppresses the energetic noise. In this algorithm, the reweighting factor $\langle e^{\beta \Delta V} \rangle$ is approximated by summation of the Maclaurin series to the tenth order as follows:

$$\langle e^{\beta \Delta V} \rangle = \sum_{k=0}^{\infty} \frac{\beta^k}{k!} \langle \Delta V^k \rangle$$

The results of the reweighting were projected on PC1–PC2 plot (Fig. 3) (*see* **Note 14**).

The projection of the crystallographic structures on the 2D free energy surface shows that the crystal structures are located in low-energy region but not in the lowest ones.

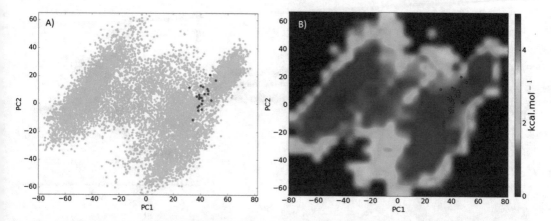

Fig. 3 PC1–PC2 plots of the backbone calculated from the last 100 ns of the aMD simulation in green and the crystallographic structures in red. (**a**) Before reweighting. (**b**) Two-dimensional free energy profile projection (kcal mol^{-1}) after reweighting using Maclaurin series to the tenth order

3.5 Umbrella Sampling (US) Protocol for Unbinding Process

3.5.1 Bias and Parameter Set

In this methodology, the main idea is to force the sampling of the system in a particular direction, with the aim to sample an event of interest. To do this, the system is constrained through the addition of a harmonic potential energy (E_{bias}) to the energy of the system (E_{Sys}) (*see* **Note 15**). ζ is the restrained variable along which the bias is applied and can be of different nature (distance, angle, dihedral, geometrical combination, etc.) depending on the studied biological event. Along ζ several windows are defined. One window is associated to a specific value of the constrained variable (ζ_{th}), and each window consists in a short molecular dynamic simulation with E_{bias} defined with to the considered value of ζ_{th}. The energy of the system is then defined by:

$$E_{US} = E_{Sys} + E_{bias}$$

$$\text{with } E_{bias} = \frac{k}{2} (\zeta - \zeta_{th})^2$$

ζ represents the value of the restrained variable sampled in the current system state, k is the force constant of the harmonic potential, and ζ_{th} is the fixed value of the constrained variable in the considered window. For each window, the value of ζ_{th} is different. The main advantage of this type of protocol is the possibility to unbias the simulation, in order to get the variation of energy associated to the event that was sampled, called the Potential of Mean Force (PMF) [40]. This PMF can be associated to a free energy variation when the convergence of each window is reached, meaning that the system is equilibrated around the corresponding value of ζ_{th}. The sampling of ζ in each window has to be extracted from these simulations, and the Weighted Histogram Analysis Method (WHAM) [41] is used to unbias the simulation and to

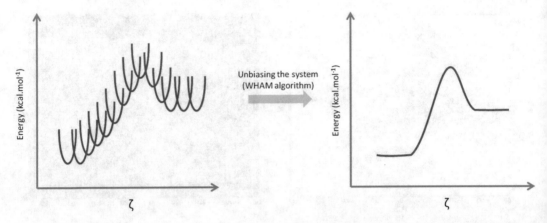

Fig. 4 Scheme of the US principle. Left: Representation of the evolution of the energy along the restrained variable ζ. Each window is centered on a fixed value of ζ_{th}. Right: potential of mean force (PMF) obtained with the use of the WHAM algorithm. The sampling distributions obtained for each window are transformed into free energy profile

construct the PMF (Fig. 4). US protocol has become a routine method for the study of events involving nonequilibrium states, such as conformational changes, binding/unbinding processes, or even chemical reactions when coupled with QM/MM hybrid methods.

In this guideline, we used US method in order to study the unbinding process of the biaryl-triazolopyridine derivative bound to p38 crystal structure. While we provide a detailed description of the methodology, the proposed parameters of this particular study are not necessarily the optimized ones. To make sure that the calculation will provide useful and coherent results, the different parameters of US calculations have to be verified first:

1. The choice of the restrained variable ζ is the crucial step for the preparation of US calculation. The nature of the restrained variable (distance, angle, dihedral, or linear combination of them, etc.) has to be carefully chosen, to represent in the best manner the event to sample. In this example, on p38 kinase in complex with an inhibitor, the distance between one residue of the Hinge region (THR104) and the ligand has been considered as the restrained variable ζ for the unbinding process. This distance is measured between two points: for the threonine residue, the center of mass of the three atoms of the backbone is chosen. Indeed, the backbone of the protein is less flexible than its side chains. The second center of mass is calculated using the two six-membered rings of the inhibitor. The oscillator strength related to the bias is also a parameter to consider and is dependent of the event to study and the nature of ligand–receptor interactions. In this case, the strength is arbitrarily fixed to 20 kcal/mol (*see* **Note 16**).

2. The US calculation consists to simulate several windows along the chosen restrained variable ζ, in order to correctly sample and explore the conformational space of every system state during the unbinding event. To make sure that the potential of mean force (PMF) obtained is correct, the sampling of each window must overlap their neighboring sampling distribution. This is very important when the system is sampling energy states, such as transition states and/or energetic barriers. This overlap allows the validation of sampling exhaustiveness along the path, and then continuity of the free energy profile.

3. Another parameter of importance in this protocol is the step size between windows. As described earlier, the sampling along the restrained variable ζ is made with the definition of several windows, centered on specific values of the bias. In order to have a good overlap between windows, the step size, and consequently the number of windows, must be well defined (see **Note 17**). In our case, the first value of the constrained distance, calculated from the cMD, is about 6.2 Å, but a smaller initial distance (beginning the calculation at a distance of $\zeta_{th} = 5.2$ Å) is chosen in order to correctly sample the global minimum of the PMF. We will consider that the inhibitor is totally separated from the protein once it is surrounded by two water shells, corresponding in this case to a constrained distance of 36.2 Å, and the step between each window is set to 0.5 Å, representing a total number of 62 windows.

4. The last parameter to consider is the simulation time in each window. The simulation time must be long enough to equilibrate the system around each new fixed value ζ_{th} from the current ζ. An equilibration step needs to be performed at the beginning of each window, to allow the system and thus ζ to sample around ζ_{th}. In our example, for each window, 200 ps of equilibration are considered, followed by 2 ns of production. The total simulation time for the 62 windows is 136.5 ns.

3.5.2 Results for the Unbinding Process of p38—Biaryl-Triazolopyridine Ligand

1. Calculations were performed on a Quadro K5000 GPU unit from a standard workstation, with AMBER14 program compiled with CUDA v6.0. Performance is estimated to 20 ns/day, meaning that the whole calculation take about 6.5 days. After the end of the calculation, cpptraj analysis module of Amber-Tools has been used to center, align, and analyze the trajectory. RMSD analysis, combined with distance measurement and solvation estimation, could thus be performed to check the stability of the protein kinase domain and estimate the progress of the unbinding event. Then, the trajectory could be checked with the VMD visualization software in order to verify if the process is complete, meaning that the ligand is positioned in the solvent, with no interactions left with the protein kinase.

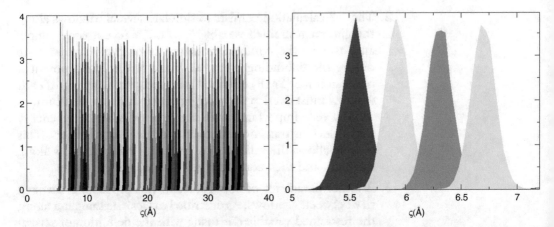

Fig. 5 Left: Sampling distribution, for all windows, of the restrained variable ζ along the whole simulation of the unbinding process. One distribution is associated to one window. Right: Focus on the first four distribution of the simulation. The overlap between windows is quite satisfying, and the distribution shape is the one expected in all cases

2. With the AMBER suite, Umbrella Sampling calculation generates a dump file, in which all the values of the restrained variable ζ along the simulation of the unbinding process are stored. A preprocess step is needed to split the large file into multiple files, one for each window. These files can be viewed and analyzed with, for example, xmgrace (http://plasma-gate. weizmann.ac.il/Grace/), by converting each file into a histogram plot. This analysis is essential to verify the shape of the distribution (each window must have a Gaussian-type distribution, according to Boltzmann law) and an overlap of each window with their neighborhoods all along the unbinding process. In our case, one can see on Fig. 5 that the overlap between all windows during the simulation is reasonable. All distributions of each window have a Gaussian-like shape meaning that the system has reached an equilibrium point and they overlap with their neighborhoods. This protocol is important for the relevance of the potential of mean force (PMF), created in the next step.

From these files, the WHAM (Weighted Histogram Analysis Method) algorithm is used to obtain the potential of mean force (PMF) associated to the evolution of the bias. Information, description of the methodology, and software sources are available at (http://membrane.urmc.rochester.edu/content/wham). Briefly, the WHAM protocol allows for the conversion of sampling distribution of ζ into free energy, by comparison of the distribution center to the expected value ζ_{th} for a single window. This conversion is made for each window in order to build the PMF profile. If the system is equilibrated enough in each window, the PMF profile could be associated to the free

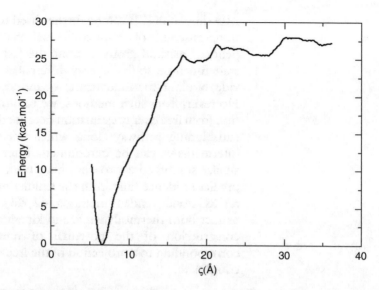

Fig. 6 Potential of mean force obtained for the unbinding process of the inhibitor with p38α MAP kinase

energy variation of the dissociation of the complex. The obtained profile in our case is shown on Fig. 6.

The estimated energetic barrier needed to leave the active site is estimated to be 27.5 kcal/mol, obtained for a distance value of about 30 Å between THR104 and the ligand. The global minimum of the profile, corresponding to the crystallographic position of the ligand in the cavity, is characterized at a distance of 6.5 Å. At the end of the simulation, the PMF profile has reached a plateau meaning that the ligand does not interact anymore with the receptor, and progress in the bulk solvent. This profile could be used to extract thermodynamic and kinetic properties of the molecule of interest, but some replicas of US simulation are required in order to make definitive conclusions on the pathway and on the energetic values.

Umbrella Sampling is one of the state-of-the-art methods to predict free energy variation associated to a rare event, as unbinding and binding process of compounds or catalytic reactions of enzymes (in combination with QM/MM hybrid method). However, it requires a correct representation of the reaction coordinate related to the considered event, and it is less suitable to very complex biological events such as protein folding and protein–protein interaction disruption.

From these two examples, we aimed at illustrating a RC non-dependent method (aMD) and RC dependent method (US). The aMD simulation has been used here to generate an ensemble of protein conformations to enrich the limited conformational space determined by experimental structures and explored by classical

MD simulations. It can be further used to populate the conformational ensemble of a multiconformational docking. The RC nondependent method group exploits the fact that the free energy is a state function, so free energy differences can be calculated to provide binding thermodynamic quantities regardless of the path. However, from such methods, we cannot extract kinetic information from free energy estimation because they need the definition of (un)binding pathway along which energy barriers and possible intermediates can be determined. Interestingly, scaled MD and similar smoothed approaches have been successfully employed to predict residence time from the simulation time, even though they are RC nondependent methods [42, 43]. The US is convenient to extract both thermodynamic and kinetic information through the construction of the potential of mean force (PMF, Fig.6) corresponding to a projection of the free energy along the reaction coordinate.

4 Notes

1. In the absence of crystallographic structure or presence of gaps in the structure, homology modeling can be envisaged.

2. There is no universal protocol for thermal equilibration. The proposed five-step protocol can be modified depending on the system.

3. The choice of the method depends on what we want to simulate but also on what we planned to analyze. For example, if we want to generate several diverse conformations of the protein as we did in our example using aMD, then a method using a reaction coordinate is not appropriate. We can use aMD simulation, REMD simulation, simulating annealing calculation (Table 2) or Monte-Carlo methods. However, if the purpose is to analyze the stability of the conformations through the estimation of their free energy then aMD simulation is more suitable. Now, if the purpose is to sample the conformations of a protein between two states, then methods using reaction coordinate are more suitable because it allows guiding the sampling.

4. When several methods are possible for a given study, an important reflex to have is to compare the performance of the methods and the supported hardware.

5. When using an enhanced molecular dynamics method, important preliminary analyzes must be made to ensure that the bias is not too strong and does not damage the system at the considered physiological temperature. We recommend to always assess the protein structure stability and fold analysis

during the simulation through classical analyzes such as the root mean square deviation, the root mean square fluctuation, and radius of gyration. Moreover, it is also important to analyze the bias per se over the simulation. For example, for the methods that add a potential energy to the original potential energy, an important point is to analyze the evolution of the added restraint potential energy over time and to compare the values with respect to the literature. With a poorly parameterized bias, the simulation can produce improbable processes.

6. In the current aMD implementation, the modified potential is added to all the system, with no possibility to be limited to some dihedrals.

7. It is recommended to use the dual boost if the solvent is described explicitly and only on the torsion terms in the case of implicit solvent.

8. α cannot be set to zero. When $\alpha = 0$, the modified potential is flat and the system experiences a random walk.

9. As it was observed in previous studies of aMD, the value of 0.2 for αD and 0.16 for αP seems to work well for proteins. Following the suggestions, for lower boost, value between 0.15 and 0.19 can be used instead of 0.2 for αD.

10. Instead of considering the protein backbone of the trajectory, alpha carbons or atoms of the binding site constitute an alternative that can be also used for PCA depending on the studied problem.

11. Many statistical packages provide PCA. Bio3D package in R has been employed here for its practicality since it supports both the PCA and diverse relevant graphic plot for PCA result analysis. The cpptraj module supports the PCA but supposes to make the graphic plots with another software. An example of cpptraj script is given in the reweighting section of the supporting information.

12. In the literature, several criteria have been developed to determine the number of principal components to be analyzed. Experience shows that 3–5 dimensions are often sufficient to capture over 60–70% of the total variance; but it is not always the case, especially when the two first components do not express a high percentage of variance, which leads to consider a relatively important number of components. The Cattell scree criterion involves plotting the scree plot as in Fig. 2 and considers the number of meaningful principal components as to be the inflection point between the steep slope and a leveling off. In our case, this number is 3. It is recommended to select the number of component to be analyzed. The famous Kaiser criterion, which considers all principal components having an eigenvalue larger than 1, is not applicable when using a

covariance matrix (only with a correlation matrix in the case of a normalized PCA).

13. In addition to the 2D principal component plots, other types of graphic plot are of interest and provide for example an insight on protein regions whose movements contribute the most to explain the conformational diversity along each principal component (residue wise loadings plot). All these analyses are well described in the section PCA of the online tutorial using bio3d R package at http://thegrantlab.org/bio3d/tutorials/trajectory-analysis.

14. It should be taken into account that the energy used by reweight script is in kT units. In Amber 14 the energy unit is kcal/mol and must be converted.

15. One has to be sure that the considered system has reached its equilibrium state before introducing a bias in the simulation. Indeed, if the system is not equilibrated enough, the estimated free energy variation could be the combination of the nonequilibrated part of the system and the bias introduced.

16. The greater the force constant k, the smaller the region explored by the system. This results in narrower distributions of ζ and therefore a smaller overlap between two successive windows. On the contrary, the lower the force constant k, the greater the region explored by the system. This can have the effect of exploring several stable states and therefore obtaining non-Gaussian multimodal distributions of ζ.

17. The smaller the step size between windows, the greater the sampling. However the number of windows strongly impacts the amount of computing resources needed.

Acknowledgments

This work was supported by the Institut de Recherche Servier and the French National Research Agency (ANR-13-JSV5-0001 and ANR-15-CE20-0015). The authors wish to thank the Région Centre Val de Loire and the Ligue contre le Cancer for financial supports and the Orléans-Tours CaSciModOT at the Centre de Calcul Scientique de la Région Centre Val de Loire and the Centre Régional Informatique et d'Applications Numériques de Normandie (CRIANN) for providing computer facilities.

References

1. Du X, Li Y, Xia Y-L et al (2016) Insights into protein–ligand interactions: mechanisms, models, and methods. Int J Mol Sci 17:144. https://doi.org/10.3390/ijms17020144

2. Changeux JP, Edelstein S (2011) Conformational selection or induced fit? 50 years of debate resolved. F1000 Biol Rep. https://doi.org/10.3410/B3-19

3. Copeland RA (2011) Conformational adaptation in drug-target interactions and residence time. Future Med Chem 3:1491–1501. https://doi.org/10.4155/fmc.11.112

4. Teilum K, Olsen JG, Kragelund BB (2009) Functional aspects of protein flexibility. Cell Mol Life Sci 66:2231–2247. https://doi.org/10.1007/s00018-009-0014-6

5. Antunes DA, Devaurs D, Kavraki LE (2015) Understanding the challenges of protein flexibility in drug design. Expert Opin Drug Discov 10:1301–1313. https://doi.org/10.1517/17460441.2015.1094458

6. Copeland RA, Pompliano DL, Meek TD (2006) Drug-target residence time and its implications for lead optimization. Nat Rev Drug Discov 5:730–739. https://doi.org/10.1038/nrd2082

7. Swinney DC (2004) Biochemical mechanisms of drug action: what does it take for success? Nat Rev Drug Discov 3:801–808. https://doi.org/10.1038/nrd1500

8. Copeland RA (2016) The drug-target residence time model: a 10-year retrospective. Nat Rev Drug Discov 15:87–95. https://doi.org/10.1038/nrd.2015.18

9. Schuetz DA, de Witte WEA, Wong YC et al (2017) Kinetics for drug discovery: an industry-driven effort to target drug residence time. Drug Discov Today 22:896–911. https://doi.org/10.1016/j.drudis.2017.02.002

10. Palamini M, Canciani A, Forneris F (2016) Identifying and visualizing macromolecular flexibility in structural biology. Front Mol Biosci 3:47. https://doi.org/10.3389/fmolb.2016.00047

11. Aci-Sèche S, Ziada S, Braka A et al (2016) Advanced molecular dynamics simulation methods for kinase drug discovery. Future Med Chem 8:545–566. https://doi.org/10.4155/fmc.16.9

12. De Vivo M, Masetti M, Bottegoni G, Cavalli A (2016) Role of molecular dynamics and related methods in drug discovery. J Med Chem 59:4035–4061. https://doi.org/10.1021/acs.jmedchem.5b01684

13. Case DA, Cerutti DS, Cheatham TE et al (2017) AMBER 2017. University of California, San Francisco

14. Brooks BR, Brooks CL, Mackerell AD et al (2009) CHARMM: the biomolecular simulation program. J Comput Chem 30:1545–1614. https://doi.org/10.1002/jcc.21287

15. Phillips JC, Braun R, Wang W et al (2005) Scalable molecular dynamics with NAMD. J Comput Chem 26:1781–1802. https://doi.org/10.1002/jcc.20289

16. Kumari R, Kumar R, Lynn A (2014) g_mmpbsa-A GROMACS tool for high-throughput MM-PBSA calculations. J Chem Inf Model 54:1951–1962. https://doi.org/10.1021/ci500020m

17. Bowers KJ, Chow E, Xu H et al (2006) Scalable algorithms for molecular dynamics simulations on commodity clusters. In: Proceedings of the 2006 ACM/IEEE conference on supercomputing. ACM, New York, NY, USA

18. Harvey MJ, Giupponi G, Fabritiis GD (2009) ACEMD: accelerating biomolecular dynamics in the microsecond time scale. J Chem Theory Comput 5:1632–1639. https://doi.org/10.1021/ct9000685

19. BiKi Technologies s.r.l., Via XX Settembre, 33/10, I-16121 Genova, Italy

20. Shaw DE, Deneroff MM, Dror RO et al (2007) Anton, a special-purpose machine for molecular dynamics simulation. In: Proceedings of the 34th annual international symposium on computer architecture. ACM, New York, NY, USA, pp 1–12

21. Loukatou S, Papageorgiou L, Fakourelis P et al (2014) Molecular dynamics simulations through GPU video games technologies. J Mol Biochem 3:64–71

22. Teodoro G, Kurc T, Kong J et al (2014) Comparative performance analysis of Intel Xeon Phi, GPU, and CPU: a case study from microscopy image analysis. IEEE Trans Parallel Distrib Syst 2014:1063–1072. https://doi.org/10.1109/IPDPS.2014.111

23. RCSB Protein Data Bank – RCSB PDB. https://www.rcsb.org/pdb/home/home.do. Accessed 25 July 2017

24. Shan Y, Kim ET, Eastwood MP et al (2011) How does a drug molecule find its target binding site? J Am Chem Soc 133:9181–9183. https://doi.org/10.1021/ja202726y

25. Piana S, Lindorff-Larsen K, Shaw DE (2013) Atomic-level description of ubiquitin folding. Proc Natl Acad Sci U S A 110:5915–5920. https://doi.org/10.1073/pnas.1218321110

26. Sugita Y, Okamoto Y (1999) Replica-exchange molecular dynamics method for protein folding. Chem Phys Lett 314:141–151. https://doi.org/10.1016/S0009-2614(99)01123-9

27. Torrie GM, Valleau JP (1974) Monte Carlo free energy estimates using non-Boltzmann sampling: application to the sub-critical Lennard-Jones fluid. Chem Phys Lett 28:578–581. https://doi.org/10.1016/0009-2614(74)80109-0

28. Torrie GM, Valleau JP (1977) Nonphysical sampling distributions in Monte Carlo free-energy estimation: umbrella sampling. J Comput Phys 23:187–199. https://doi.org/10.1016/0021-9991(77)90121-8

29. Laio A, Parrinello M (2002) Escaping free-energy minima. Proc Natl Acad Sci U S A 99:12562–12566. https://doi.org/10.1073/pnas.202427399

30. Barducci A, Bonomi M, Parrinello M (2011) Metadynamics. WIREs Comput Mol Sci 1:826–843. https://doi.org/10.1002/wcms.31

31. Sinko W, Miao Y, de Oliveira CAF, McCammon JA (2013) Population based reweighting of scaled molecular dynamics. J Phys Chem B 117:12759–12768. https://doi.org/10.1021/jp401587e

32. Hamelberg D, Mongan J, McCammon JA (2004) Accelerated molecular dynamics: a promising and efficient simulation method for biomolecules. J Chem Phys 120:11919–11929. https://doi.org/10.1063/1.1755656

33. Markwick PRL, McCammon JA (2011) Studying functional dynamics in bio-molecules using accelerated molecular dynamics. Phys Chem Chem Phys 13:20053–20065. https://doi.org/10.1039/c1cp22100k

34. Pierce LCT, Salomon-Ferrer R, de Oliveira CAF et al (2012) Routine access to millisecond time scale events with accelerated molecular dynamics. J Chem Theory Comput 8:2997–3002. https://doi.org/10.1021/ct300284c

35. Hamelberg D, de Oliveira CAF, McCammon JA (2007) Sampling of slow diffusive conformational transitions with accelerated molecular dynamics. J Chem Phys 127:155102. https://doi.org/10.1063/1.2789432

36. de Oliveira CAF, Grant BJ, Zhou M, McCammon JA (2011) Large-scale conformational changes of Trypanosoma cruzi proline racemase predicted by accelerated molecular dynamics simulation. PLoS Comput Biol 7:e1002178. https://doi.org/10.1371/journal.pcbi.1002178

37. Grant BJ, Gorfe AA, McCammon JA (2009) Ras conformational switching: simulating nucleotide-dependent conformational transitions with accelerated molecular dynamics. PLoS Comput Biol 5:e1000325. https://doi.org/10.1371/journal.pcbi.1000325

38. Skjærven L, Yao X-Q, Scarabelli G, Grant BJ (2014) Integrating protein structural dynamics and evolutionary analysis with Bio3D. BMC Bioinformatics. https://doi.org/10.1186/s12859-014-0399-6

39. Miao Y, Sinko W, Pierce L et al (2014) Improved reweighting of accelerated molecular dynamics simulations for free energy calculation. J Chem Theory Comput 10:2677–2689. https://doi.org/10.1021/ct500090q

40. Roux B (1995) The calculation of the potential of mean force using computer simulations. Comput Phys Commun 91:275–282. https://doi.org/10.1016/0010-4655(95)00053-I

41. Kumar S, Rosenberg JM, Bouzida D et al (1992) THE weighted histogram analysis method for free-energy calculations on biomolecules. I. The method. J Comput Chem 13:1011–1021. https://doi.org/10.1002/jcc.540130812

42. Mollica L, Decherchi S, Zia SR et al (2015) Kinetics of protein-ligand unbinding via smoothed potential molecular dynamics simulations. Sci Rep 5:11539. https://doi.org/10.1038/srep11539

43. Mollica L, Theret I, Antoine M et al (2016) Molecular dynamics simulations and kinetic measurements to estimate and predict protein–ligand residence times. J Med Chem 59:7167–7176. https://doi.org/10.1021/acs.jmedchem.6b00632

Chapter 21

AGGRESCAN3D: Toward the Prediction of the Aggregation Propensities of Protein Structures

Jordi Pujols, Samuel Peña-Díaz, and Salvador Ventura

Abstract

Protein aggregation is responsible for the onset and spread of many human diseases, ranging from neurodegenerative disorders to cancer and diabetes. Moreover, it is one of the major bottlenecks for the production of protein-based therapeutics such as antibodies or enzymes. AGGRESCAN3D (A3D) is a web server aimed to identify and evaluate structural aggregation prone regions, overcoming the limitations of sequence-based algorithms in the prediction of the aggregation propensity of globular proteins. A3D allows the redesign of protein solubility by predicting in silico the impact of mutations and protein conformational fluctuations on the aggregation of native polypeptides.

Key words AGGRESCAN3D, Bioinformatics, 3D structure, Protein aggregation, Protein misfolding, Protein production, Protein solubility

1 Introduction

Protein aggregation is currently considered to be a generic property of the vast majority of existing polypeptides [1, 2]. It is triggered by the permanent or transient exposure of specific clusters of amino acids, named Aggregation Prone Regions (APR) or "hot spots", mainly composed by hydrophobic residues. These clusters are able to form non native intermolecular contacts that promote protein self-assembly and deposition into insoluble proteinaceous aggregates [3, 4]. Remarkably, these threatening stretches are present and somehow conserved across all phylogenetic kingdoms, constituting a paradox in protein evolution and biochemistry. It is assumed that they cannot be purged from protein sequences due to a shocking overlap between the physicochemical principles underlying these type of aberrant intermolecular contacts and those that govern native interactions, protein interfaces and structure compaction [1, 5–7]. Accordingly, cellular proteomes have developed orthogonal protecting strategies, best illustrated by the chaperone-proteasome machinery, to prevent an imbalance

Mohini Gore and Umesh B. Jagtap (eds.), *Computational Drug Discovery and Design*, Methods in Molecular Biology, vol. 1762, https://doi.org/10.1007/978-1-4939-7756-7_21, © Springer Science+Business Media, LLC, part of Springer Nature 2018

of the fragile equilibrium between protein solubility and aggregation by energetically favoring the native conformations of targeted proteins and degrading sticky misfolded species [8–10]. Unfortunately, under certain conditions, such as cellular stress, aging, downregulation of proteostasis and/or specific genetic mutations, certain proteins manage to overcome the quality control and consequently aggregate, compromising cell fitness [1, 11, 12]. For this reason, it is not surprising that, protein aggregation is closely related to the onset of more than 40 severe human disorders, including the well-known and devastating neurodegenerative Alzheimer's and Parkinson's diseases [1, 13–16]. In addition, protein aggregation represents one of the major restrictions for pharmaceutical and biotechnology manufacturing of protein-based therapies. Proteins can aggregate during synthesis, purification or storage into visible or subvisible particles with significant immunogenicity [17–21]. Thus, protein aggregation not only limits the disposal of active molecules in the formulation, but can convert a beneficial drug into a deadly agent. Last but not the least, the development of new bioinspired nanomaterials with self-assembling features is significantly constrained by our present understanding of the molecular mechanisms behind protein aggregation and the mechanical and chemical properties of these insoluble structures [22–26].

One classical strategy to overcome the aggregation phenomenon has been the rational design of vulnerable protein regions followed by protein engineering [27–30]. However, the subsequent expression and purification of recombinant proteins and the experimental assessment of their solubility is time-consuming and precludes a high-throughput analysis of a significant number of variants. This limitations pushed the development of a series of predictive algorithms that allow to anticipate the aggregation propensity of protein sequences and to virtually screen for solubilizing mutations. To date, more than twenty 1st generation prediction algorithms are available as on-line servers or packages. They are known as linear predictors, since they use the amino acidic sequence of the protein as an input, and their generic architecture involves a variable-in-length window, which slides over the amino acidic sequence and averages, using different functions, theoretical aggregation propensities of those residues inclosed in the sequence frame. In spite of their pipeline similarity, each predictor take into account different variables when assessing theoretical values of aggregation for a given amino acid. Specifically, this include experimentally obtained data, theoretical physicochemical properties, or a combination of these. Nonetheless, although their performance is notable when predicting over disordered polypeptides or unfolded regions of a protein, they tend to overestimate the aggregation propensities of globular and compact proteins [31]. These regions usually emerge from the spatial approximation in the folded state of amino acids that are originally distant in the sequence. In folded conformations, these potentially dangerous regions are buried and protected inside the tertiary and/or quaternary structure, conforming protein cores, establishing protein–protein interactions or assembling (macro)complexes [2, 32], in such a way that the formation of non native intermolecular contacts is minimized. However, in solution, globular proteins might experiment misfolding and/or structural fluctuations that can transiently expose these hydrophobic regions and trigger aggregation. In a nutshell, the structural context and dynamics of a globular protein requires a new set of algorithms that consider their three dimensional scenario to accomplish reliable predictions of aggregation.

AGGRESCAN3D (A3D) [33] is one of the last generation structural predictors conceived to overcome the limitations of linear predictors when forecasting the aggregation propensity of globular proteins. A3D is based on AGGRESCAN [34], a sequential algorithm that relies on empirical data to build a scale of intrinsic aggregation values for the 20 natural amino acids. Nevertheless, A3D takes profit of the atomistic 3D coordinates of protein structures to correct the aggregation propensity of each amino acid according to the neighboring structural context. Therefore, both the residue exposure to solvent and the influence of other residues in the structural vicinity are also computed for each amino acid according to a multifactorial equation. Using the A3D server, the identified aggregation-prone residues can be mutated in situ to design variants with increased solubility, or to model the impact of pathogenic mutations in disease-linked proteins. Additionally, A3D server enables to take into account the dynamic fluctuations of protein structures in solution, which may significantly modulate the structural intrinsic aggregation propensity, by using fast simulations of the protein backbone with the high-resolution coarse-grained molecular modeling approach CABS-flex [35]. In this way, A3D assembles in a single application the prediction and modeling of different features that are highly relevant for the aggregation of globular states; namely, the modulation of this propensity by the structural context, the assessment of the impact of clinical or synthetic mutations on solubility and the role of conformational fluctuations. The A3D server can be accessed at http://biocomp.chem.uw.edu.pl/A3D/.

2   Materials

2.1   Algorithm

Inspired by AGGRESCAN, A3D benefits from the intrinsic aggregation propensity scale obtained experimentally by De groot et al. (2006) and allocates intrinsic aggregation tendencies (Agg) to each single residue for a given structure. However, in this case, Agg values are subsequently modified by the amino acid exposure

Central Residue Contribution   Structural Neighbouring Residues Contribution

$$A3D_{score} = Agg_i \times (\alpha \times e^{\beta \times RSAi}) + \sum [Agg_e \times (\alpha \times e^{\beta \times RSAe}) \times (\gamma \times e^{-\delta \times dist})]$$

| Intrinsic propensity | Residue Exposure to Solvent | Intrinsic propensity | Residue Exposure to Solvent | Residue Distance from Center |

Fig. 1 Algorithm components. Agg_i and Agg_e are the intrinsic aggregation propensities for the central amino acid i under study and those amino acids e within the sphere, respectively; α and β are numeric parameters of the exponential function referring to amino acid exposure; RSA_i and RSA_e are the relative surface area for the central amino acid i under study and those amino acids e within the sphere, respectively; δ and γ are numeric parameters of the exponential function referring to the amino acid distance to the sphere center; $dist$ is the distance between the Cα Carbons of the sphere center residue and other residues encompassed in the sphere

to solvent, approximated as the relative surface area (RSA) using the Lee and Richards method implemented in the Naccess server http://www.bioinf.manchester.ac.uk/naccess/nac_intro.html (*see* **Note 1**) [36]. The impact of the exposition to solvent is modeled with an exponential function in which the amino acids with: (1) more than 55% RSA have a weight of 1 and contribute as fully exposed; (2) less than 10% RSA have a weight of 0 and are considered as buried; (3) intermediate values of RSA (10–55%) have a weight ranging from 0.1 to 0.99 and contribute as partially exposed residues. In order to obtain a structurally corrected A3D$_{score}$, the algorithm takes into account the corrected aggregation propensities of the amino acid under evaluation "i" plus the sum of those residues "e" included inside a projected sphere of 10 or 5 Å centered on its alpha carbon (Cα_i) (Fig. 1). Besides, the specific distance between the sphere center and the alpha carbon of other residues within the vicinity (Cα_e) is measured in Å and is used to modulate an inverse exponential function to calculate their contribution to the A3D$_{score}$. Accordingly, those amino acids at: (1) shorter distances than 1 Å, receive a weight of 1 and are predicted as strong influencers; (2) larger distances than the sphere radius, receive a weight of 0 and are considered as distant and non influencing residues; (3) distances between the sphere limit and 1 Å receive a weight ranging from 0.1 to 0.99 and are considered as modulators. As a result of this computational scheme, the A3D algorithm provides a value for each single protein residue, which will be positive or negative depending on whether this residue is predicted to contribute more to aggregation or to solubility, respectively, or 0 if the amino acid is not predicted to play a significant role.

2.2 A3D Pipeline   Prior to the aggregation prediction, A3D exploits FoldX algorithm to minimize the energy of the input structure in order to remove unfavorable energies arising from improper torsion angles, steric hindrance between amino acid side chains and suboptimal rotamer configurations of residues in close vicinity [37]. Then, the server starts to calculate the aggregation propensity of the repaired static structure. A3D incorporates the possibility to forecast the impact of structure fluctuations on the aggregation propensity of polypeptides by implementing the CABS-flex protocol [35]. CABS-flex is a high-resolution modeling approach that generates a collection of derived structures, covering the most representative backbone fluctuations. The dynamic mode of A3D calculates the structurally corrected aggregation propensity upon each conformer and only gives as an output the most aggregation prone as a proxy of the conformation that will likely drive the aggregation reaction in solution.

2.3 Input

As an input, A3D only accepts 3D structures obtained from X-ray diffraction, solution NMR, or modeling approaches in PDB format (*see* **Notes 2–4**). A3D has different input requirements depending on the run mode.

- For the standard **static mode**, which represents the vast majority of A3D runs, files containing both monomeric or multimeric protein structures are suitable; however, the A3D server is capped to .pdb files built from a maximum of 20,000 atoms, approximately 1000 amino acids (*see* **Note 5**). The system accepts entries with missing amino acids and sequence gaps (*see* **Note 6**).

- A3D **dynamic mode** is more restrictive in terms of input requirements since multimeric and incomplete structures are no longer accepted, due to incompatibilities with the implemented CABS-Flex algorithm version. Thus, structures must consist of a single and continuous chain containing the complete set of backbone atoms (N, Cα, C, and O). The sequence length is restricted to a maximum of 400 amino acids.

3 Methods

3.1 Front Page and Protein Input

A3D webserver has a clear and friendly display front page (Fig. 2). By using the top-side toolbar links, the user can check the properties of the implemented algorithm ("*About*" tab) and anticipate troubles while running the server ("*tutorial*" tab). It is possible to check the status of submitted predictions and to review previous runs on-line ("*queue*" tab). On the right side, is the submission box, where the user can load the targeted structure and select some optional run settings.

A3D is linked to the Protein Data Bank (PDB) and entries can be introduced by just writing the PDB code inside the "*PDB code*" window. Alternatively, local .pdb files can be uploaded manually using the "*Browse*" button.

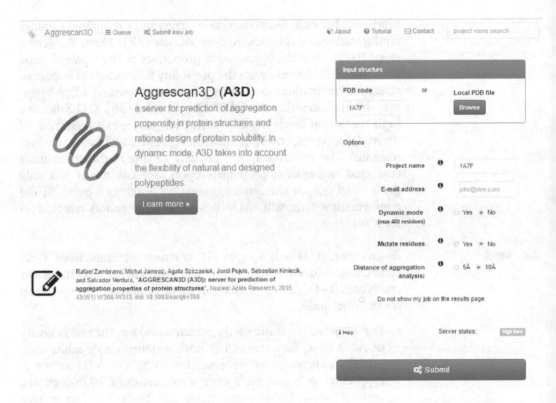

Fig. 2 Front page. Schematic view of the different options the user can select for an A3D calculation

3.2 Run Options

In the lower panel of the submission box named **'options'** the user can name the project and introduce an e-mail address in order to be notified immediately after A3D ends the prediction (*see* **Note 6**). If needed, due to confidentiality issues, it is possible to hide a project from the queue list by ticking the option "*do not show my job on the results page*" (*see* **Note 7**). There are different possibilities to run A3D and the user should use those that are more appropriate for the protein under investigation.

- **Static/dynamic**: By default, A3D operates in static mode, which is more tolerant in terms of input properties. In addition, the absence of simulations provides the static mode with a remarkable speed as compared to the dynamic version of A3D (approximately 15 min vs 2 h for each run). However, in certain occasions, the prediction of structural APRs requires dynamic simulations in order to be biologically/biotechnologically relevant (*see* **Note 8**). Chose "*Yes*" on *Dynamic Mode* in those situations.

- **Mutate**: A3D integrates a useful tool which can be exploited to virtually mutate any amino acid of the protein structure into a different natural residue, select "*Yes*" on *mutate residues*. After submission, this will open a new interactive window entitled *"which residue to mutate?"* where the amino acids from the 3D structure are displayed by chains using one-letter code and its specific chemical structure scheme on the right side (*see* **Note 9**). By clicking each amino acid tab, a small popping window will permit to select the desired amino acid from a scrollable list, set alphabetically. Press *"Save changes and submit"* button to finish the project submission and start the run; or *"undo"* button to restore the *wild type* sequence (*see* **Note 10**).

- **Distance**: Two resolutions, named *"distance of aggregation analysis,"* can be used to run A3D. Maintain the default 10 Å distance to disclose aggregation prone clusters on a structural region. Change to 5 Å when dissecting the specific contribution of each amino acid to an individual aggregation prone region or inspecting the local impact of one residue (*wild type* or mutated) to close surroundings.

3.3 Submitting and Queueing

Press *"Submit"* button to start A3D calculations. The project will be immediately moved to the queue list, accessible from the toolbar *"queue"* tab, and the user will be redirected to a new page with the project details and status (*see* **Note 11**). The status of the user project can be tracked in the queue list or in the project window where it will change from: *"pending"* (orange) to *"queue"* (light blue) and *"running"* (dark blue). If A3D encounters any incompatibility, it will be marked as *"error"* (red) and the developers will be warned. As soon as the server would finish the task, the project will be tagged as *"done"* (green) and A3D will inform through a mail notification (optional). Only then, the user can access to the full report of the prediction.

3.4 Output and Evaluation of the Prediction

The A3D output consists of a set of four different interfaces. Aggregation propensities are presented in a comprehensive manner, incorporating the possibility to download data for a more accurate evaluation of the results.

3.4.1 Aggrescan3D Plot

Probably the most extended and accepted representation of predicted aggregation propensities, where A3D$_{scores}$ are plotted as a function of the amino acidic sequential position (Fig. 3a). It can be downloaded as a .png or .svg image file by opening *"Download plot"* dropping window. By default, only the residues with A3D$_{score}$ different from 0 are included; however, there is also the possibility to show those residues even though they are predicted as non relevant for aggregation. Finally, the interface allows the user to choose which chain of the submitted structure, if several, is charted.

3.4.2 Aggrescan3D Score

The score-table interface displays the numeric values of A3D calculations (Fig. 3b), which can also be downloaded as .csc or .txt files.

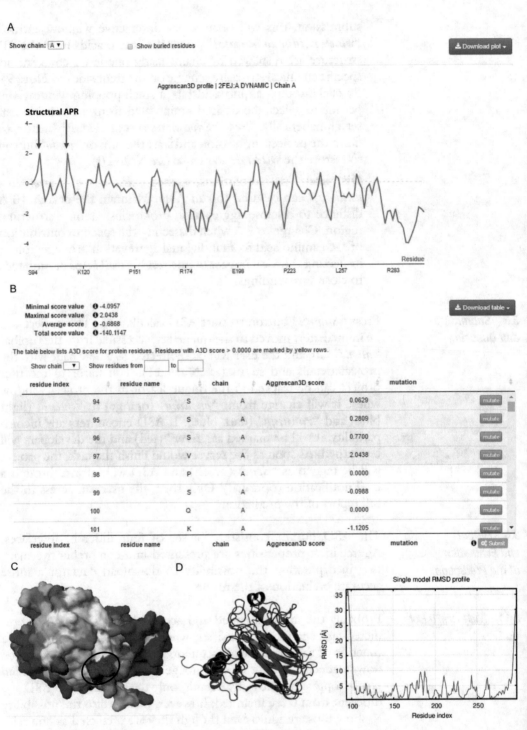

Fig. 3 Output and evaluation. Ensemble of A3D output results obtained after a Dynamic run using the PDB code 2FEJ:A, no mutation, radius = 10 Å. (**a**) A3D-Plot interface, where the A3D scores (*Y* axis) are plotted as a function of the amino acidic position (*X* axis). A structural APR is highlighted with red arrows. (**b**) A3D score-table interface. (**c**) Protein structure representation with JSmol interface. Residue surfaces are painted following a

The user is able to obtain global scores accounting for the overall protein propensity as well as for each specific amino acid (*see* **Note 12**). As in the A3D-plot, there exists the possibility to select individual chains and specific sequence fragments. The central region of the page is a scrollable table, which agglutinates the scores calculated for each amino acid and some extra information, such as the residue number, the 1-letter residue code and the protein chain where the specific amino acid is placed. Besides, the table can be resorted, by clicking the top cell of the column. The amino acids with positive values are colored in clear-yellow, and in this case buried residues are displayed with an $A3D_{score} = 0$. Usefully, at this point there exists the possibility to mutate an amino acid or remutate those changed previously, by clicking the green button "*mutate*" and following the instructions mentioned in Subheading 3.2 (*see* **Note 13**).

3.4.3 Structure

It is the most visual interface of A3D (Fig. 3c). It projects the propensity of each individual amino acid upon the 3D protein surface according to a color code in which blue encodes for solubility and red represents aggregation proneness. The structure is presented in a 2 s looped motion picture, in which the protein rotates 360° through the vertical axis. Both the 3D coordinates of the resulting structure and the video can be downloaded as a .pdb file and in .ogv, .mp4, or .webm formats, respectively (*see* **Note 14**). If needed, A3D also incorporates the option to manually rotate the output structure by clicking the "*JSmol*" button.

3.4.4 Dynamic Mode Details

Only accessible if the A3D run includes dynamic mode simulations (Fig. 3d), two main objects are displayed; on the one hand, 3D structures accounting for the initial input structure (blue) and the most aggregation prone conformation (red) are superposed; on the other hand, the root mean square deviation (RMSD) of the relative distances between reciprocal amino acids of the aligned structures is plotted as a function of the residue number. Both the 3D-structures and the RMSD values can be downloaded as a .pdb and .csv files, respectively.

←——————————————————————————————————————

Fig. 3 (continued) color code as a function of the A3D score, where red is linked to aggregation and blue to solubility. The black circle highlights the equivalent structural APR from (**a**). (**d**) Dynamic details interface. On the left side, superposition of both the initial (blue) and the most aggregation prone structures (red). On the right side, the Single Model RMSD profile, in which in the distance between relative amino acids (*Y* axis) is plotted in function of the residue sequence (*X* axis)

3.5 Evaluating the A3D Output

The evaluation of A3D predictions and the subsequent identification of relevant APRs would benefit from a transversal handling of the four outputs provided by A3D. This would allow the user from a generic landscape of amino acidic propensities to the identification of genuine specific structural APRs. There are five crucial issues that the user should be warned about before evaluating any A3D run:

1. Maximum knowledge of the protein under study is critical to attain a reliable interpretation of the A3D output.

2. The A3D threshold is equal to 0. Thus, a positive $A3D_{score}$ implies aggregation prone residues and structures, and vice versa.

3. Buried residues are considered as noninfluencing aggregation under native conditions, therefore, they are assigned with an $A3D_{score}$ of 0.

4. Positive scores of A3D do not necessarily reflect deleterious APR, these regions might be functional in a biological context.

5. A3D-plot and score-table interfaces are represented on the amino acidic sequence basis, but they reflect structural propensities (*see* **Note 15**).

When predicting APRs over a specific structure in static or dynamic mode, the user should first identify the A3D positive amino acids or regions on the protein sequence. The A3D-plot and score-table combination (Fig. 3a) allow identifying rapidly those putative regions that exceed the threshold. By taking advantage of the *JSmol* tool, those preselected regions can be mapped on the protein surface (red color if positive, blue if negative). A visual inspection of the spatial vicinity—the *JSmol* interface provides the identities of selected amino acids- which would allow to find the neighboring residues contributing to a given structural APR, since, usually, these amino acids are not consecutive in sequence (Fig. 3a and c). The dynamic interface of A3D provides information on the global plasticity of the protein of interest, regions with high flexibility displaying higher RMSDs (*see* **Note 16**). Thus, when an identified APR colocalizes with regions exhibiting high RMSDs values is indicative that this aggregation-prone cluster is being exposed due to conformational fluctuations. On the contrary, positive residues colocalizing with stable nondynamic regions of the protein are always likely to be aggregation-prone and exposed to the solvent.

On the other side, when handling large amounts of data, the user should take advantage of the global numeric parameters from the table-score, dissected in **Note 12**. In particular, the *average score* is the best parameter to compare different proteins, and the *total score* is optimal to scrutinize the effect of mutations over a defined protein.

3.6 Dissecting A3D Performance and Applicability

When compared with intrinsically disordered proteins or short peptides, which are assumed to be highly exposed to solvent, the aggregation propensity of a globular protein is difficult to approximate, because the specific contribution of each amino does not depend exclusively of its sequential neighbors. In fact, globular proteins exhibit diverse structural environments that should be taken into account for a confident prediction; for example, protein cores, which are mainly composed of hydrophobic amino acids and represent regions with the potential to trigger protein aggregation if exposed. From another point of view, protein interfaces involved in protein–protein interactions and oligomerization are established by the same type of contacts than those conforming protein cores. Indeed, it has been demonstrated that in some disease-related proteins such as transthyretin, destabilization and consequent disassembly of the tetrameric form, induce their aggregation and spread of the amyloid disorder [15]. As a consequence, it is not surprising that these regions represent one of the major origin of lineal predictors' failure, because they assume that they are disordered and unprotected, whereas in reality they are protected and contribute little to the aggregation of properly folded globular proteins. The structural-based correction of the A3D algorithm allows to discriminate between buried and exposed APRs, increasing one order of magnitude the ratio between true positive and false positive predictions [33]. To illustrate this, we present the 3D structure of the oligomerization domain of the *human* p53 protein, colored with the A3D scale; in its monomeric state (Fig. 4a), where it exhibits a clear APR; and its tetrameric state (Fig. 4b), where the formation of the oligomeric state masks the threatening region and turns it undetectable for A3D.

Apart, from discarding the contribution of sequential APRs when they are buried, A3D correctly predicts structural aggregation prone regions that are not evident from the linear sequence (Fig. 3a and c) [38–40] because in globular proteins close residues in the sequence are not necessarily contiguous in space and indeed they are usually amino acids from distant regions that coalesce to build up a structural APR.

In solution, globular proteins are not frozen in terms of structure, but fluctuating between different conformations. It has been reported that even for highly stable proteins, transient conformers might expose APRs for a time that is enough to trigger their aggregation [41–43]. Consequently, for those cases in which the static run does not unveil a significant structural APR, it is worth using the dynamic A3D approach, in order to uncover novel potential aggregation prone regions derived from protein fluctuations [44]. This is the case of the DNA-binding domain of *human* p53; whereas the static version of A3D does detect any significant structural APR (Fig. 4c), the dynamic mode brings to light several of them (Fig. 4d).

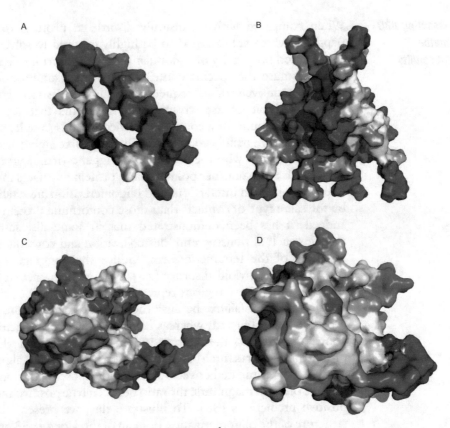

Fig. 4 A3D performance. (**a**, **b**) A3D static run at 10 Å of the oligomerization domain of p53 corresponding to the 3SAK pdb code. Monomeric chain (**a**) and tetrameric structure (**b**). Residues are colored following the A3D scale in which blue means solubility and red aggregation. (**c**) and (**d**) runs at 10 Å of the DNA-binding domain of p53 corresponding to the 2FEJ pdb code. Static mode (**c**) and dynamic mode (**d**). Residues are colored as in (**a**) and (**b**)

The capacity A3D to quickly generate mutated versions of a given structure with the mutation tool is according to our records the most used feature of this algorithm. As commented before, genetically encoded amino acidic changes are linked to the outbreak of several conformational diseases and associated with the severity of their symptoms [1]. Hence, A3D represents a useful tool to model aggressive protein mutations to further redesign them, in order to extend our knowledge about their implications in disease, and, eventually, generate lead therapeutic compounds using this structural knowledge. In the same way, A3D mutation modeling can be used to enhance the solubility of proteins with biotechnological interest, such as antibodies [45], or any protein with biologic or biomedical relevance [46, 47]. A3D can be also used for the screening and evaluation of large mutational protein data sets [33] or as an alternative to phage display-like experimental approaches.

In conclusion, A3D is an extremely versatile tool which aims to approximate protein aggregation propensities in physiological-like environments, where proteins are folded into globular structures, able to oligomerize and can fluctuate between several conformations, thus reshaping the protein aggregation prediction scenario.

4 Notes

1. Naccess server, accessible at http://www.bioinf.manchester.ac.uk/naccess/nac_intro.html, obtains a Surface Accessible Area (SAA) as a spheric probe of 1.4 Å radius, equivalent to a water molecule that rolls over the Van der Waals surface of the molecule. The contour traced by the probe center is the SAA value, which is then normalized for an amino acid X considering the extended tripeptide Ala-X-Ala as SAA_{max}. A3D uses normalized values of Naccess for its algorithm, named RSA (relative surface area).

2. In the best case, the user will use a high quality 3D structure obtained experimentally. Unfortunately, for some proteins or even domains, this crucial information is not available. In these situations, 3D modeling of protein structures represents a suitable alternative approach to estimate the final structure. A3D accept most of the models, if they fulfil the input requirements.

3. The user should take note that, when running A3D upon a solution NMR structure, the algorithm will consider the average structure.

4. If the targeted protein does not have either a well-defined structure or a good quality 3D-model or it simply behaves as an unfolded protein, the user should redirect the aggregation propensity predictions to first generation tools, in which the aggregation prone region is forecasted upon the primary sequence. Examples of useful and powerful predictors are: AGGRESCAN [34], Zyggregator [48], PASTA 2.0 [49], FoldAmyloid [50], and TANGO [51].

5. A significant number of X-ray solved structures in the PDB display artificial multimeric structures due to polypeptide repetitions in the asymmetric unit of the protein crystal. In these cases, the user should select only one of them by writing the letter of the specific sequence after the PDB code. Example: for the PDB XXXX sequence A, XXXX:A.

6. A3D will not take into account for the mathematical calculations residues or atoms missing on the 3D structure. As a consequence, the exposure of certain amino acids could be wrongly estimated by the algorithm. In such a way: (1) apolar

buried regions may become reexposed and overestimated; (2) apolar stretches that were protected by nearby structural gatekeepers could be overestimated; (3) vanishing of a key apolar amino acid that determines an aggregation prone region would cause underestimation. As a conclusion, the probability to predict nondesired artifacts increases as the number of sequence gaps increases. It is the user responsibility to evaluate if the missing region of the protein structure is crucial for the prediction of protein aggregation and if, accordingly, it can lead to wrong A3D score values.

7. If the project has no associated name, A3D will automatically label them using an internal standard code. When performing predictions with large data sets or a large number of mutations it is highly recommended to name the different projects individually.

8. When deciding between the static and dynamic modes of A3D the user should gather as much information as possible on the target protein to balance the benefits and disadvantages that might result from running the protein in any of the two modes.

9. Amino acids without 3D coordinates in the PDB file are not taken into account in predictions and are not visible in the mutation tool of A3D.

10. A3D tolerates as many mutations as the user considers appropriate to scrutinize. However, it has to be taken into account that an excess of mutations might promote the attainment of nonnative conformations and this effect is not considered by the algorithm in its present form.

11. It is important to save the URL or bookmark the project window if we have chosen the option "*do not show my job on the results page.*" Even though the introduction of a user e-mail address is not mandatory, it is highly recommended for those projects that are not visible in the queue list. When the run finishes, the system sends a link that redirects the user to the specific job page, where the results are available. Skipping this step might result in the user not being able to access the prediction results.

12. "*Total score value,*" absolute value resulting of the sum of all A3D$_{score}$; "*Average score,*" results from dividing the total score value for the number of total amino acids in the protein. It also takes into account those buried residues with A3D$_{score}$ = 0; "*Minimal score value,*" amino acid with higher predicted solubility within the structure and "*Maximal score value,*" amino acid with higher aggregation propensity within the structure.

13. Usage of the score-table to mutate residues is recommended when comparing a point mutation to the *wild type* version of the protein, since the energetic correction performed by FoldX

might result into slight differences between initial entries and introduce a bias on the predictions. When a mutation is modeled on top of an output A3D structure, the structures will have the same starting background.

14. After download, .pdb files can be opened with specific any software for 3D protein visualization, although we recommend the use of PyMOL.

15. Despite the sequential plot and the score-table to gather a general idea of the protein aggregation propensity landscape, it has to be taken into account that propensities are not estimated based on the primary sequence. Moreover, for globular proteins most of the A3D detected APRs are built from amino acids occurring in sequentially distant regions of the protein. For this reason, A3D plots usually show profiles in which several aggregation prone regions seem to be isolated on the sequence, whereas in reality they are constituents of structural APRs (Fig. 3a).

16. RMSD values of the dynamic output should be taken with caution since they only account for one of the multiple structures generated during backbone simulations. As a consequence, the relative distances displayed in the interface are not the average values for the protein, but serve as a frozen-picture of the most aggregation-prone conformation.

References

1. Chiti F, Dobson C (2017) Amyloid formation, protein homeostasis, and human disease: a summary of progress over the last decade. Annu Rev Biochem 86:1–42

2. Linding R, Schymkowitz J, Rousseau F, Diella F, Serrano L (2004) A comparative study of the relationship between protein structure and b-aggregation in globular and intrinsically disordered proteins. J Mol Biol 342:345–353

3. Ventura S, Zurdo J, Narayanan S, Aviles FX et al (2004) Short amino acid stretches can mediate amyloid formation in globular proteins: the Src homology 3 (SH3) case. Proc Natl Acad Sci U S A 101:7258–7263

4. Ivanova MI, Sawaya MR, Gingery M, Attinger A, Eisenberg D (2004) An amyloid-forming segment of beta2-microglobulin suggests a molecular model for the fibril. Proc Natl Acad Sci U S A 101:10584–10589

5. Cheon M, Chang I, Mohanty S, Luheshi LM, Dobson CM, Vendruscolo M, Favrin G (2007) Structural reorganisation and potential toxicity of oligomeric species formed during the assembly of amyloid fibrils. PLoS Comput Biol 3:1727–1738

6. Monsellier E, Ramazzotti M, Taddei N, Chiti F (2008) Aggregation propensity of the human proteome. PLoS Comput Biol 4(10): e1000199

7. Pechmann S, Levy ED, Tartaglia GG, Vendruscolo M (2009) Physicochemical principles that regulate the competition between functional and dysfunctional association of proteins. Proc Natl Acad Sci U S A 106:10159–10164

8. Hartl FU, Bracher A, Hayer-Hartl M (2011) Molecular chaperones in protein folding and proteostasis. Nature 475:324–332

9. Kim YE, Hipp MS, Bracher A, Hayer-Hartl M, Ulrich Hartl F (2013) Molecular chaperone functions in protein folding and proteostasis. Annu Rev Biochem 82:323–355

10. Balchin D, Hayer-Hartl M, Hartl FU (2016) In vivo aspects of protein folding and quality control. Science 353:4354–4354

11. Labbadia J, Morimoto RI (2015) The biology of proteostasis in aging and disease. Annu Rev Biochem 84:435–464

12. Mckinnon C, Tabrizi SJ (2014) The ubiquitin-proteasome system in neurodegeneration. Antioxid Redox Signal 5:1–61

13. Wang G, Fersht AR (2017) Multisite aggregation of p53 and implications for drug rescue. Proc Natl Acad Sci U S A 114 (13):2634–2643

14. Mathias Jucker LCW (2013) Self-propagation of pathogenic aggregates in neurodegenerative diseases. Nature 501:45–51

15. Johnson SM, Connelly S, Fearns C, Powers ET, Kelly JW (2012) The transthyretin amyloidoses: from delineating the molecular mechanism of aggregation linked to pathology to a regulatory agency approved drug. J Mol Biol 421:185–203

16. Gallardo R, Ramakers M, De Smet F et al (2016) De novo design of a biologically active amyloid. Science 354:720–730

17. Walsh G (2014) Biopharmaceutical benchmarks 2014. Nat Biotechnol 32:992–1000

18. Hamrang Z, Rattray NJW, Pluen A (2013) Proteins behaving badly: emerging technologies in profiling biopharmaceutical aggregation. Trends Biotechnol 31:448–458

19. Kumar S, Singh SK, Wang X, Rup B, Gill D (2011) Coupling of aggregation and immunogenicity in biotherapeutics: T- and B-cell immune epitopes may contain aggregation-prone regions. Pharm Res 28:949–961

20. Wang W, Singh SK, Li N, Toler MR, King KR, Nema S (2012) Immunogenicity of protein aggregates – concerns and realities. Int J Pharm 431:1–11

21. Roberts CJ (2008) Protein aggregation and its impact on product quality. Curr Opin Biotechnol 23:1–7

22. Knowles TP, Fitzpatrick AW, Meehan S, Mott HR, Vendruscolo M, Dobson CM, Welland ME (2007) Role of intermolecular forces in defining material properties of protein nanofibrils. Science 318:1900–1903

23. Li D, Jones EM, Sawaya MR et al (2014) Structure-based design of functional amyloid materials. J Am Chem Soc 136:18044–18051

24. Hauser CAE, Maurer-Stroh S, Martins IC (2014) Amyloid-based nanosensors and nanodevices. Chem Soc Rev 43:5326–5345

25. Shimanovich U, Efimov I, TO M et al (2014) Protein microgels from amyloid fibril networks. ACS Nano 9:43–51

26. Kamada A, Mittal N, Söderberg LD, Ingverud T, Ohm W, Roth SV, Lundell F, Lendel C (2017) Flow-assisted assembly of nanostructured protein microfibers. Proc Natl Acad Sci U S A 114:1232–1237

27. Lee CC, Perchiacca JM, Tessier PM (2013) Toward aggregation-resistant antibodies by design. Trends Biotechnol 31:612–620

28. Dudgeon K, Rouet R, Kokmeijer I, Schofield P, Stolp J, Langley D, Stock D, Christ D (2012) General strategy for the generation of human antibody variable domains with increased aggregation resistance. Proc Natl Acad Sci U S A 109:10879–10884

29. Perchiacca JM, Tessier PM (2012) Engineering aggregation-resistant antibodies. Annu Rev Chem Biomol Eng 3:263–286

30. Van der Kant R, Karow-Zwick AR, Van Durme J et al (2017) Prediction and reduction of the aggregation of monoclonal antibodies. J Mol Biol 429:1244–1261

31. Belli M, Ramazzotti M, Chiti F (2011) Prediction of amyloid aggregation in vivo. EMBO Rep 12:657–663

32. Buck PM, Kumar S, Singh SK (2013) On the role of aggregation prone regions in protein evolution, stability, and enzymatic catalysis: insights from diverse analyses. PLoS Comput Biol 9:e1003291

33. Zambrano R, Jamroz M, Szczasiuk A, Pujols J, Kmiecik S, Ventura S (2015) AGGRESCAN3D (A3D): server for prediction of aggregation properties of protein structures. Nucleic Acids Res 43:w306–w313

34. Conchillo-Solé O, de Groot NS, Avilés FX, Vendrell J, Daura X, Ventura S (2007) AGGRESCAN: a server for the prediction and evaluation of 'hot spots' of aggregation in polypeptides. BMC Bioinformatics 8:65

35. Jamroz M, Kolinski A, Kmiecik S (2013) CABS-flex: server for fast simulation of protein structure fluctuations. Nucleic Acids Res 41:427–431

36. Lee B, Richards FM (1971) The interpretation of protein structures: estimation of static accessibility. J Mol Biol 55:379–400

37. Schymkowitz J, Borg J, Stricher F, Nys R, Rousseau F, Serrano L (2005) The FoldX web server: an online force field. Nucleic Acids Res 33:382–388

38. Dutta SR, Gauri SS, Ghosh T, Halder SK, Das-Mohapatra PK, Mondal KC, Ghosh AK (2017) Elucidation of structural and functional integration of a novel antimicrobial peptide from Antheraea mylitta. Bioorg Med Chem Lett 27:1686–1692

39. Polo A, Colonna G, Guariniello S, Ciliberto G, Costantini S (2016) Deducing the functional characteristics of the human selenoprotein SELK from the structural properties of its intrinsically disordered C-terminal domain. Mol Biosyst 12(3):758–772

40. Pulido P, Llamas E, Llorente B, Ventura S, Wright LP, Rodríguez-Concepción M (2016) Specific Hsp100 chaperones determine the fate of the first enzyme of the plastidial isoprenoid pathway for either refolding or degradation by the stromal Clp protease in Arabidopsis. PLoS Genet 12:1–19

41. Chiti F, Dobson CM (2009) Amyloid formation by globular proteins under native conditions. Nat Chem Biol 5:15–22

42. Canet D, Last AM, Tito P, Sunde M, Spencer A, Archer DB, Redfield C, Robinson CV, Dobson CM (2002) Local cooperativity in the unfolding of an amyloidogenic variant of human lysozyme. Nat Struct Biol 9:308–315

43. Eakin CM, Berman AJ, Miranker AD (2006) A native to amyloidogenic transition regulated by a backbone trigger. Nat Struct Mol Biol 13:202–208

44. Davies HA, Rigden DJ, Phelan MM, Madine J (2017) Probing medin monomer structure and its amyloid nucleation using 13C-direct detection NMR in combination with structural bioinformatics. Sci Rep 7:45224

45. Soler MA, de Marco A, Fortuna S (2016) Molecular dynamics simulations and docking enable to explore the biophysical factors controlling the yields of engineered nanobodies. Sci Rep 6:34869

46. Pulido D, Arranz-Trullén J, Prats-Ejarque G, Velázquez D, Torrent M, Moussaoui M, Boix E (2016) Insights into the antimicrobial mechanism of action of human RNase6: structural determinants for bacterial cell agglutination and membrane permeation. Int J Mol Sci 17:552

47. Xia X, Kumru OS, Blaber SI, Middaugh CR, Li L, David M, Sutherland MA, Tenorio CA, Blaber M (2017) Factor-1 for 'second generation' therapeutic application. J Pharm Sci 105:1444–1453

48. Tartaglia GG, Pawar AP, Campioni S, Dobson CM, Chiti F, Vendruscolo M (2008) Prediction of aggregation-prone regions in structured proteins. J Mol Biol 380:425–436

49. Walsh I, Seno F, Tosatto SCE, Trovato A (2014) PASTA 2.0: an improved server for protein aggregation prediction. Nucleic Acids Res 42:301–307

50. Garbuzynskiy SO, Lobanov MY, Galzitskaya OV (2009) FoldAmyloid: a method of prediction of amyloidogenic regions from protein sequence. Bioinformatics 26:326–332

51. Fernandez-Escamilla AM, Rousseau F, Schymkowitz J, Serrano L (2004) Prediction of sequence-dependent and mutational effects on the aggregation of peptides and proteins. Nat Biotechnol 22:1302–1306

Chapter 22

Computational Analysis of Solvent Inclusion in Docking Studies of Protein–Glycosaminoglycan Systems

Sergey A. Samsonov

Abstract

Glycosaminoglycans (GAGs) are a class of anionic linear periodic polysaccharides, which play a key role in many cell signaling related processes via interactions with their protein targets. In silico analysis and, in particular, application of molecular docking approaches to these systems still experience many challenges including the need of proper treatment of solvent, which is crucial for protein–GAG interactions. Here, we describe two methods which we developed, to include solvent in the docking studies of protein–GAG systems: the first one allows to de novo predict favorable positions of water molecules as a part of a rigid receptor to be used for further molecular docking; the second one utilizes targeted molecular dynamics in explicit solvent for molecular docking.

Key words Atomic probes, Electrostatics-driven interactions, Explicit solvent, Free energy calculations, Glycosaminoglycans, Molecular docking, Solvent displacement, Targeted molecular dynamics

1 Introduction

Glycosaminoglycans (GAGs) represent a particular class of anionic linear periodic polysaccharides made up repetitive disaccharide units [1], interactions with their protein targets in the extracellular matrix of the cell can crucially affect many important biological processes such as cellular signaling, adhesion, and intercellular communication [2]. These molecules are challenging for computational analysis using standard tools because of their various sulfation patterns [3], high flexibility, extensive conformational space they access [4], and, as a consequence of their highly charged nature, importance and abundance of electrostatics-driven [5, 6] and, in particular, solvent-mediated interactions in the complexes with their protein targets [7]. The amount of water molecules observed in available experimental structures from the PDB for protein–GAG interfaces is about one order higher than in protein–protein interfaces [8]. Although taking into account explicit water molecules into molecular docking approaches was shown to

Mohini Gore and Umesh B. Jagtap (eds.), *Computational Drug Discovery and Design*, Methods in Molecular Biology, vol. 1762, https://doi.org/10.1007/978-1-4939-7756-7_22, © Springer Science+Business Media, LLC, part of Springer Nature 2018

improve their performance [9–11], there is a persisting challenge to predict proper positions of water molecules on the surface of the unbound receptor, which is required when its crystal structure with a ligand is unknown. Even if the structure of unbound receptor is available from X-ray scattering experiments with a high resolution, some of the observed water molecules present in the unbound receptor could be displaced upon binding of a ligand. Moreover, X-ray data represent only a structural snapshot of the receptor molecule which reveals a highly dynamic behavior, therefore rendering the data on solvent positions ambiguous and incomplete [12]. In this chapter, we present methodological details on two methods we developed to include explicit solvent into molecular docking studies: (1) we use atomic probes to de novo predict energetically favorable positions of water molecules on the receptor surface and, furthermore, to exclude water molecules that are supposed to be displaced upon ligand binding [13]; (2) We use fully flexible receptor and ligand in explicit solvent to carry out docking experiments applying targeted molecular dynamics (MD) techniques [14].

Both methods yielded promising results when applied to representative datasets of protein–GAG systems. Here, we discuss their particular features and describe their applicability and limitations one should be aware of.

2 Methods

2.1 De Novo Placement of Explicit Water Molecules on the Protein Surface in the Putative Binding Site Prior to Docking

Application of this method allows to explicitly account for solvent as a part of the receptor in molecular docking considering both water molecules which occupy the same hydration sites in unbound and bound protein receptor and the ones potentially displaced upon ligand binding.

1. The starting structure of the protein receptor in one of the standard molecular formats (pdb, mol2, mol, etc.) could be of experimental origin and downloaded from the PDB or a modeled structure.

2. In case it is an experimental structure obtained by X-ray scattering, all experimental water molecules should be removed from the receptor structure (see **Note 1**).

3. Ligands and ions should be removed from the protein surface/binding site where the predictions are to be carried out (see **Note 2**).

4. A complete receptor molecule (for global docking) or receptor residues in the binding site (for local docking) should be energy minimized (see **Note 3**). In our original study [13], we used the AMBER 99 force field as implemented in MOE (combination

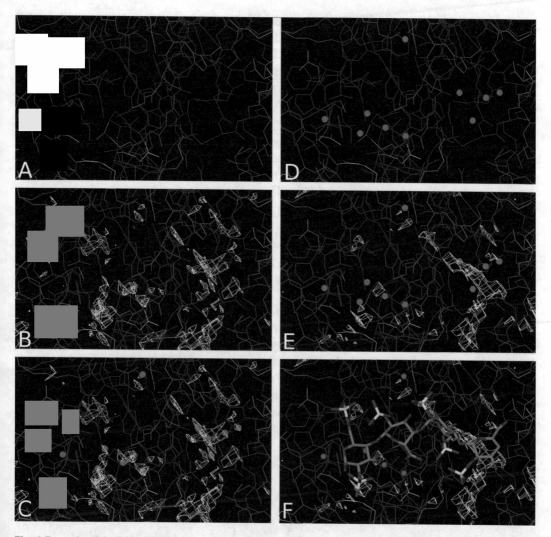

Fig. 1 Example of the Method I pipeline used to de novo predict positions of water molecules on the surface of the protein receptor prior to docking a GAG molecule: the complex of 3-O-sulfotransferase-3 and heparin tetrasaccharide (PDB ID 1T8U, 1.95 Å). (**a**) Minimized protein receptor structure (in stick representation); (**b**) Isosurfaces confining the volumes corresponding to favorable potential energies for water oxygen atomic probe calculated by GRID (in yellow, in wireframe representation); (**c, d**) Water molecules (oxygen atoms) placed into the grid points corresponding to the energy minima for water molecular probe (in red, in ball representation) with and without the corresponding isosurfaces, respectively. (**e**) Isosurfaces confining the volumes corresponding to favorable potential energies for water exclusion sp3-carbone atomic probe calculated by GRID (in white, in wireframe representation); (**f**) Overlap of the exclusion probe isosurfaces with the experimentally obtained structure of the bound ligand (in thick sticks colored by element)

of steepest descent, conjugate gradient, and truncated Newton methods using 0.01 Å RMSD for convergence criteria) [15] (*see* **Note 4**).

5. The obtained structure (Fig. 1a) is used by a GRID run with default parameters for the water oxygen probe [16] to generate a grid corresponding to this probe (Fig. 1b).

The most energetically favorable positions based on the visual inspection of GRID-calculated isosurfaces are used to place water molecules (Fig. 1c and d; *see* **Note 5**).

6. Another GRID run should be carried out on the same initial receptor structure using the carbon sp^3 probe as an approximation to account for solvent exclusion upon ligand binding (Fig. 1e).

7. After overlapping the obtained isosurfaces for the carbon sp^3 probe with the predicted water molecules, the water molecules within 1.5 Å to the minima of the carbon sp^3 energy grid are discarded (Fig. 1f; *see* **Note 6**).

8. The receptor structure together with the de novo placed water molecules can be used for molecular docking experiments (*see* **Note 7**).

2.2 Dynamic Molecular Docking (DMD): Targeted MD-Based Docking Approach Accounting for Explicit Solvent and the Complete Flexibility of Receptor and Ligand

This method exploits an MD approach to perform a local molecular docking experiment (*see* **Note 8**). In the first step, the ligand, which is placed at a certain distance from the receptor, is moved slowly toward a putative binding site on the surface of the receptor as a consequence of the application of an additional harmonic potential (Fig. 2). In the second step, an MD simulation of the complex obtained in the first step is carried out without additional potentials. During both steps, the system is solvated explicitly, therefore, accounting for solvent-mediated interactions. DMD runs are repeated to obtain a statistical ensemble of docking solutions.

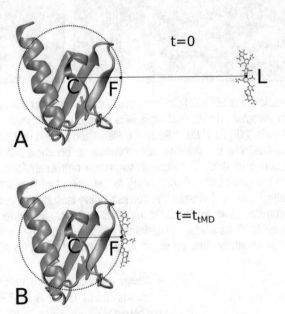

Fig. 2 Schematic representation of DMD procedure from Method II: (**a**) Receptor (in cartoon) and ligand (in stick representation) are at the initial distance, $t = 0$; (**b**) Docked complex after the targeted MD step, $t = t_{tMD}$. *C*, *F*, and *L* points are core, focus, and ligand center atoms

1. To set up a DMD experiment structures of the receptor and the ligand in one of the standard molecular formats are required. In addition, the data about the receptor binding region is needed to define the targeted region for the ligand in this local docking approach (*see* **Note 8**). Such data can be obtained from mutagenesis, mass spectroscopy, NMR experiments, etc.

2. Ligand is placed at a distance of the receptor so that (1) the distance between the closest atoms in the receptor and ligand is several times higher than the cutoff for the nonbonded interactions in the used MD simulations (*see* **Note 9**); (2) the shortest pathway from the ligand to the receptor is roughly directed into the geometrical center of the predefined binding region on the receptor surface. The structure of the ligand should be previously minimized and can be put in a different random orientation for an individual DMD run (*see* **Note 10**).

3. One of the central atoms of the ligand is chosen as a *ligand central atom L*.

4. One of the atoms in the core of the receptor is chosen as *a core atom C* (*see* **Note 11**). The vector connecting L and C define the focus point F on the surface (Fig. 2a).

5. The system then is read into Leap module of AMBER [17], standard counter ions and an octahedral solvent box are added with the minimum distance from solute atoms to the box boundaries of 4 Å (*see* **Note 12**). Standard protein force fields as FF99SB for parameterization of the protein part of the system and GLYCAM 06 [18] for the GAG part are used.

6. An equilibration of the system is carried out, which includes minimization of the solvent with the restrained solute (10 kcal/(mol Å^2)), minimization of the solute, short (10–50 ps) heating of the system to 300 K in NVT canonical ensemble with Langevin thermostat with the restraints on the solvent. Then, 500 ps MD are carried out with Langevin thermostat and Berendsen barostat in NPT ensemble. In all MD simulations, the integration step was chosen as 2 fs, SHAKE algorithm for bonds including hydrogen atoms and Particle Mesh Ewald methods (with the cutoff of 8 Å) are used. Dihedral angles NMR restraints (10 kcal/(mol Å^2)) are applied to GAG sugar rings to keep them in required conformations (as suggested by literature or experimental data) because sufficient sampling of ring conformations is not achieved at the time scales of the MD simulations used in this protocol [4].

7. The distances between L, F, and C should be calculated after the minimization and MD equilibration steps. The changing with the time NMR distance restraint is defined as $||L - C||$ at initial moment of targeted MD, $t = 0$, and as $||F - C||$ at the final moment of targeted MD, $t = t_{tMD}$ (Fig. 2b). The strength

of the restraint is constant, and the restraint is applied to the distance between C and L atoms. Beside this additional restraint, the conditions in the targeted MD step are the same as in the last part of the above-described equilibration step. The restraint force constant k used is 200 kcal/(mol Å^2) and the length of the targeted MD step t_{tMD} is 4 ns (*see* **Note 13**).

8. The complex obtained in the previous step is simulated further without any restraints under the same conditions for 10 ns (*see* **Note 14**).

9. Such procedure is repeated 100 times (*see* **Note 15**).

10. One hundred frames from the last 200 ps of each free MD trajectory are taken for MM-PBSA/MM-GBSA analysis yielding docking poses final scores and single residue energy decomposition. Averaged from repeated DMD runs single residue energy decomposition defines the anchoring residues in the whole ensemble of docking solutions. The poses with MM-PBSA $\Delta G > -1$ kcal/mol are considered not to represent binding and, therefore, are excluded from the further analysis.

11. DBSCAN algorithm [19] is used for clustering the obtained docking solutions. Instead of RMSD as a metric for clustering, we use a distance metric as the root-mean-square of pairwise atomic distances while pairing up the spatially closest atoms of the same type. This distance metric accounts for periodicity of GAGs and so allows avoiding periodicity-related artifacts obtained when classical RMSD is used.

3   Notes

1. After the complete water placement procedure is carried out, these molecules can be used for comparison with the obtained predicted water molecules, which could give an idea about the reproducibility of the experimental data (if the receptor is not energy minimized prior to the water placement) or about the changes in the hydration pattern associated with the energy minimization of the receptor structure (in case the receptor is minimized). Note that although there are water molecules explicitly obtained in X-ray structures, in most of the cases the information about the hydration is far from being complete.

2. This step should be done carefully: some divalent ions, for example, could be crucial for the local protein structure and its hydration properties and, therefore, substantially affect further docking results obtained using this receptor structure. In case there is direct literature evidence for this, such ions should be taken into account either being included into water

placement predictions or returned "in place" after the water placement is accomplished. Then, the water molecules overlapping with the ions should be discarded.

3. If an initial structure includes a ligand in the binding site of interest, the unbound receptor structure should be minimized after discarding the ligand to avoid the bias of using a prebound crystal structure, which could otherwise be a source of bias/error both for water placement and consequent docking performance.

4. Instead any other protocol for energy minimization as, for example, an open source energy minimization implementation in Open Babel [20] can be used.

5. Depending on electrostatic properties of a particular receptor, absolute values of the displayed isosurfaces corresponding to similar-sized confined volumes could be very different making the decision about the number of water molecules to place arbitrary and ambiguous. Therefore, such a decision should be qualitatively based on previous experimental data on the average amount of water molecules in the protein–ligand interfaces of similar sizes/geometry/composition and on sizes of the volumes corresponding to the chosen isovalues that should be big enough to cover at least one water molecule.

6. As in **Note 5**, this step should be carried out manually and cannot be strictly defined qualitatively a priori. Calibration studies on the experimental structures of the complexes similar to the studied one should be carried out in order to gain qualitative insights about how hydrophobic/hydrophilic are the interactions in this particular class of protein–ligand interfaces.

7. Due to the qualitative nature of such predictions, it is recommended to carry out molecular docking both with and without water molecules included into the structure of the receptor and to compare the results rigorously to find out the putative role of the particular water molecules in the interface. Consequent application of MD simulations to the obtained complexes could also help to understand how properly the positions of water molecules are predicted.

8. In case no information about the binding region is available, protein surface can be split into several parts, for each of which an independent DMD study could be carried out. Then, the docking poses obtained for these parts should be compared in terms of scoring to derive the best candidates for binding poses. Since such a division of the protein surface in several segments is not unique, several combinations of segmentation (for example, obtained by shifting the segments representing putative

binding regions) are required in order not to neglect the solutions located on the borders of the chosen segments.

9. Normally, a cutoff used was 8 Å, whereas such a distance between the receptor and the ligand was defined as 20–30 Å. Such difference is needed to provide the ligand enough time to sample its conformational space when targeting to the receptor without perceiving any influence of the receptor on this sampling.

10. Although normally there is enough time for a ligand to be relaxed during the targeted MD step of a DMD run, for consistency we recommend to use the same force field for the minimization of the ligand as the one used in the DMD run. In the original paper [14], we propose several initial orientations of the ligand for different DMD runs. However, for each ligand type and size, dependence of the results on the initial orientation can be different and, therefore, should be investigated. According to our experience, the docking results obtained by DMD using the protocol presented here do not depend on ligand's initial orientation for ligand of the size up to octameric oligosaccharide. However, if this dependence is observed, either several initial random orientations of ligand or a longer targeted MD step should be used to avoid the bias originated from a particular initial orientation of the ligand.

11. The C atom should be chosen based on the following criteria: (1) this atom should not essentially fluctuate in the MD simulation (this information could either be obtained from the previously run MD simulations of the receptor or could be proposed based on the chemical type of the atom and its belonging to secondary structure elements. In particular, the backbone atoms from α-helices and β-sheets in a protein core can be used since they are usually not too mobile); (2) the vector drawn between L and C atoms should be roughly perpendicular to the surface comprising the predefined binding region; (3) the surface of the sphere around C atom with the radius equal to the distance from C to the point of the surface of the protein defined by this vector should have significant overlap with the surface in the predefined binding region. The last criterion is usually fulfilled for most global proteins unless dramatic peculiarities of their surface geometry are observed.

12. Although 4 Å seem to be quite a short distance and a potential source of artifacts, the ligand is targeted toward the receptor, going "into" the octahedral solvated box. Therefore, this initial distance to the solvent box boundaries does not affect the results. Moreover, because of the big size of the box due to the long initial distance between the receptor and the ligand, an increase of the box size would lead to undesirable

computational expenses and to slowing down the performance substantially.

13. These values of k and t_{tMD} were calibrated for GAGs of length up to heptasaccharide [14]. An increase of k and a decrease of t_{tMD} could lead to the insufficient conformational sampling of the ligand during the targeted MD step. On the contrary, a decrease of k and an elongation of the targeted MD step would lead to the scenario when many ligands are not properly targeted to the receptor but would be uniformly distributed on the sphere defined by a distance restraint, which would lead to the need of many more repetitions of the procedure to obtain a statistical ensemble of docking solutions suitable for further analysis. These values of k and t_{tMD} for significantly longer ligands, however, should be calibrated in terms of translational and rotational freedom by comparing their RMSD in an MD simulation with the RMSD expected from the targeting through the shortest possible path.

14. In order to substantially decrease the invested computational time, it is practically convenient to remove all waters and counterions from the structure of the obtained complex, to add them again and to use the equilibration protocol described in Subheading 2.2 (**steps 5** and **6**) before the free MD step. In this case the minimum distance from solute atoms to the box boundaries could be increased to 8–9 Å to avoid possible artifacts related to the insufficient treatment of system's hydration.

15. Some runs can end up with the ligand in an unbound state after the tMD step or the ligand can unbind during the free MD step. Depending on how many events like this are observed, 100 repeated procedures could be enough or not. We recommend obtaining at least 80–90 bound docking poses for the further analysis. In case of longer GAG ligands this number can be increased to obtain higher statistical significance of the results.

Acknowledgments

This work was supported by National Science Center of Poland (Narodowy Centrum Nauki, grant UMO-2016/21/P/ST4/03995). This project received funding from the European Union's Horizon 2020 research and innovation programme under the Marie Skłodowska-Curie grant agreement No. 665778.

References

1. Esko JD, Kimata K, Lindahl U (2009) Proteoglycans and sulfated glycosaminoglycans. In: Varki A, Cummings RD, Esko JD et al (eds) Essentials of glycobiology, 2nd edn. Cold Spring Harbor Laboratory Press, New York

2. Perrimon N, Bernfield M (2000) Specificities of heparan sulphate proteoglycans in developmental processes. Nature 404:725–728

3. Habuchi H, Habuchi O, Kimata K (2004) Sulfation pattern in glycosaminoglycan: does it have a code? Glycoconj J 21:47–52

4. Sattelle B, Hansen S, Gardiner J et al (2010) Free energy landscapes of iduronic acid and related monosaccharides. J Am Chem Soc 132:13132–13134

5. Imberty A, Lortat-Jacob H, Pérez S (2007) Structural view of glycosaminoglycan–protein interactions. Carbohydr Res 342:430–439

6. Samsonov SA, Pisabarro MT (2016) Computational analysis of interactions in structurally available protein-glycosaminoglycan complexes. Glycobiology 26:850–861

7. Sepuru KM, Nagarajan B, Desai U et al (2016) Molecular basis of chemokine CXCL5-glycosaminoglycan interactions. J Biol Chem. https://doi.org/10.1074/jbc.M116.745265

8. Teyra J, Samsonov SA, Schreiber S et al (2011) SCOWLP update: 3D classification of protein-protein, -peptide, -saccharide and -nucleic acid interactions, and structure-based binding inferences across folds. BMC Bioinformatics 12:398

9. Roberts B, Mancera R (2008) Ligand-protein docking with water molecules. J Chem Inf Model 48:397–408

10. Thilagavathi R, Mancera R (2010) Ligand-protein cross-docking with water molecules. J Chem Inf Model 50:415–421

11. van Dijk A, Bonvin A (2006) Solvated docking: introducing water into the modelling of biomolecular complexes. Bioinformatics 22:2340–2347

12. Samsonov S, Teyra J, Pisabarro MT (2008) A molecular dynamics approach to study the importance of solvent in protein interactions. Proteins 73:515–525

13. Samsonov S, Teyra J, Pisabarro MT (2011) Docking glycosaminoglycans to proteins: analysis of solvent inclusion. J Comput Aided Mol Des 25:477–489

14. Samsonov S, Gehrcke JP, Pisabarro MT (2014) Flexibility and explicit solvent in molecular dynamics-based docking of protein-glycosaminoglycan systems. J Chem Inf Model 54:582–592

15. Molecular Operating Environment (MOE), 2013.08; Chemical Computing Group Inc., 1010 Sherbooke St. West, Suite #910, Montreal, QC, Canada, H3A 2R7, 2016

16. Goodford P (1985) A computational procedure for determining energetically favorable binding sites on biologically important macromolecules. J Med Chem 28:849–857

17. Case DA, Berryman JT, Betz RM et al (2015) AMBER 14. University of California, San Francisco

18. Kirschner K, Yongye A, Tschampel S et al (2008) GLYCAM06: a generalizable biomolecular force field. carbohydrates. J Comput Chem 29:622–655

19. Ester M, Kriegel HP, Sander J et al (1996) A density-based algorithm for discovering clusters in large spatial databases with noise. In: Proceedings of 2nd international conference on knowledge discovery and data mining (KDD-96). American Association for Artificial Intelligence, Menlo Park, CA

20. O'Boyle NM, Banck M, James CA et al (2011) Open babel: an open chemical toolbox. J Cheminform 3:33

Understanding G Protein-Coupled Receptor Allostery via Molecular Dynamics Simulations: Implications for Drug Discovery

Shaherin Basith, Yoonji Lee, and Sun Choi

Abstract

Unraveling the mystery of protein allostery has been one of the greatest challenges in both structural and computational biology. However, recent advances in computational methods, particularly molecular dynamics (MD) simulations, have led to its utility as a powerful and popular tool for the study of protein allostery. By capturing the motions of a protein's constituent atoms, simulations can enable the discovery of allosteric hot spots and the determination of the mechanistic basis for allostery. These structural and dynamic studies can provide a foundation for a wide range of applications, including rational drug design and protein engineering. In our laboratory, the use of MD simulations and network analysis assisted in the elucidation of the allosteric hotspots and intracellular signal transduction of G protein-coupled receptors (GPCRs), primarily on one of the adenosine receptor subtypes, A_{2A} adenosine receptor ($A_{2A}AR$). In this chapter, we describe a method for calculating the map of allosteric signal flow in different GPCR conformational states and illustrate how these concepts have been utilized in understanding the mechanism of GPCR allostery. These structural studies will provide valuable insights into the allosteric and orthosteric modulations that would be of great help to design novel drugs targeting GPCRs in pathological states.

Key words Allostery, G protein-coupled receptor, Hotspots, Molecular dynamics simulation, Network model, Structural ensembles

1 Introduction

For more than five decades, researchers have been involved in understanding the mechanism for signal transmission across long distances in biologically active macromolecules, which forms the basis for allostery. Protein allostery is a biophysical phenomenon which explains the ability of interactions occurring at one site to modulate interactions at a spatially distinct binding site in a reciprocal manner [1]. Thus, studying the mechanistic interplay between active and allosteric sites is crucial to better understand

Author contributed equally with all other contributors. Shaherin Basith and Yoonji Lee

Mohini Gore and Umesh B. Jagtap (eds.), *Computational Drug Discovery and Design*, Methods in Molecular Biology, vol. 1762, https://doi.org/10.1007/978-1-4939-7756-7_23, © Springer Science+Business Media, LLC, part of Springer Nature 2018

the functional role of biomolecules. One of the transmembrane (TM) proteins, such as G protein-coupled receptors (GPCRs), provides an exemplary paradigm for allosteric proteins whose basic functioning units are the communications between the two poles of the seven TM helical bundle.

GPCRs are unarguably the most well-known pharmaceutical target. They act as both gate-keepers and molecular messengers of the cell converting extracellular signals to cellular activities. Structurally, this receptor consists of a seven α-helical membrane spanning domain (TM1–TM7) which connects the extracellular environment to the cell interior, and thus, they are also known as seven-transmembrane (7TM or heptahelical) receptors [2, 3]. GPCRs respond to the binding of extracellular ligands inducing a conformational change in the orthosteric binding site, and this change extends via the 7TM scaffold into their intracellular domain, subsequently leading to the binding and activation of G-proteins or arrestins [4, 5]. Identifying the allosteric mechanism of proteins is important not only for understanding their functional role but also as a base for structure-based drug design.

The mechanisms of protein allostery are difficult to be revealed from the static snapshots provided by the X-ray crystallographic structures. Therefore, molecular dynamics (MD) simulation has emerged as a valuable tool in the study of allostery, because they can capture the protein's motion in full atomic detail. This method has a unique strength of presenting the atomistic details of a protein's dynamic behavior on several timescales ranging from femtosecond to seconds, thus acting as a "computational microscope" [6]. However, even with the atomistic details of three-dimensional (3D) structure at hand, determining the structural basis for allostery often proves challenging. Currently, several methods are available to reveal networks or paths of communication in protein ensembles (collected by MD simulation technique). Recent studies have addressed the microscopic mechanism of protein allostery by applying the strategies of network or community analysis in conjunction with MD simulation on model systems [7–9].

When a complex system is simplified into a network (graph), which is represented as "nodes" (vertices) and "edges" (links), the architecture of the network allows one to extract the key properties of the entire system and its individual elements [10]. The network analysis method was first developed for analyzing social phenomena, but now is popularly used in several research areas, including statistical physics, particle physics, computer science, and economics. Recently, it has also been applied in several fields of biology for the investigation of protein–protein interactions, metabolic networks, disease networks, drug–target networks, etc. [10–12]. The 3D structures of proteins can also be represented as networks, where amino acid residues are considered as nodes and their interactions as edges [13]. This residue interaction network has been utilized to explore various aspects of proteins, such as protein structure plasticity, domain folding, identification of key residues for protein folding and function, and residue fluctuation [13–19]. Particularly, the network analysis of protein structures and their wiring diagram can be extended further to identify key residues responsible for allostery.

Several computational methods present the opportunity to explore allosteric events at scales inaccessible for experimental studies. Most of the in silico methods are focused on the identification of allosteric binding sites and their signaling propagation pathway [20]. In our previous work, we studied the link between allosteric signal transduction and functional dynamics in S-adenosyl-homocysteine (SAH) hydrolase using multifaceted computational approaches [21]. In this chapter, we describe a simple, but powerful approach to glean the mechanism of receptor regulation and identify the allosteric hotspots for signal transductions and their pathways. This method has been implemented in our previous study using A_{2A} adenosine receptor ($A_{2A}AR$) and other class A GPCRs, such as $\beta1$ adrenergic receptor, $\beta2$ adrenergic receptor, chemokine CXCR4 receptor, dopamine D3 receptor, histamine H1 receptor, and rhodopsin as model systems [22]. Based on the structural ensemble derived from MD simulations, we revealed the allosteric hotspots and signaling pathway of $A_{2A}AR$ by utilizing betweenness centrality (C_B)-based network analysis, glycine scanning analysis, and cross-correlation analysis. The intramolecular network analysis was applied to identify the key residues responsible for GPCR allostery. The residues with high betweenness centralities constitute physically connected sparse network linking the ligand binding site to the G-protein binding site. These residues also included several highly conserved microswitch residues which are deemed important for GPCR function. Compared to other conventional methods that utilize the information of sequence coevolution or variants of normal mode analysis (NMA), our C_B-based network analysis approach is proven to be quite powerful in elucidating the allosteric hotspots, and the results are in strong correlation with the biochemical studies.

2 Methods

In the following section, we describe the primary steps involved in the mapping of the allosteric signal flow by adopting $A_{2A}AR$ as a model system (Fig. 1).

2.1 Molecular Dynamics Simulations of Membrane Proteins

MD simulation has become a popular tool in the investigation of the dynamics of proteins, membrane proteins, and more complex systems, providing insights into the biological processes at atomistic level which are inaccessible via experiments. MD simulations generate successive configurations of the system by integrating

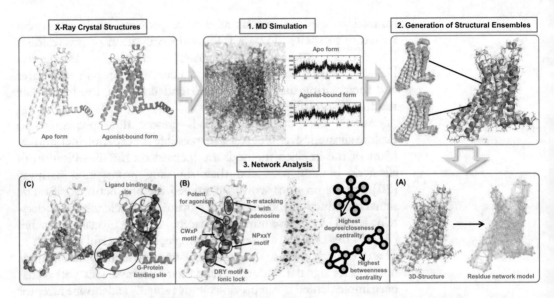

Fig. 1 Overview of our methodology for the identification of allosteric hot spot residues and pathways of signal flow in A$_{2A}$AR signaling. The three major protocols implemented in our method include: (1) MD simulations of the apo (gray) and agonist-bound (cyan) forms of A$_{2A}$AR for 300 ns each; (2) Generation of the conformational ensembles; and (3) Residue interaction network construction and centrality analysis for the receptor's 3D structures. The allosteric hot spots and signaling pathways of A$_{2A}$AR were elucidated using the measure of betweenness centrality (C_B) for each residue in the network, glycine scanning analysis, and cross-correlation analysis. The figures in the bottom from right to left (**A–C**) denote network analysis of the A$_{2A}$AR structure. (**A**) Network representation of A$_{2A}$AR apo form. The residue interaction network was constructed using a cutoff distance of 7 Å; (**B**) Centrality is the most common concept in network analysis. The characteristics of a node or the whole network can be deduced via this centrality analysis. The concepts of the three most popular centrality measures, namely, degree, closeness, and betweenness, have already been detailed (refer to Subheading 2). In the minimal energy structure, the key residues with high betweenness centralities ($C_B \geq 0.05$) were identified as the microswitch residues, which are important for agonistic signal flow or ligand binding. In addition, the residues with high betweenness centralities create physically connected networks; (**C**) Cross-correlation analysis is based on the network analysis for the structural ensembles derived from MD simulation. The highly correlated, but physically distant residue pairs were extracted to quantify long-range coupling. The represented apo- and agonist-bound structures of A$_{2A}$AR show the minimum paths between the cross-correlated residues. Long-range cross-correlations between the extracellular ligand binding site and cytoplasmic G-protein binding site are detected for the agonist-bound structure

Newton's second law of motion. The output is a trajectory which describes the positions and velocities of the particles in the system throughout the simulation as a function of time (*see* **Note 1**). In the following subsections, we describe the MD simulation steps for membrane proteins, particularly focusing on the 7TM model system (i.e., GPCRs).

2.1.1 Preparation of the System

An all-atom MD simulation for a typical membrane protein system consists of a membrane protein, ligand, surrounding lipid bilayer, and water bath with ions. Prior to MD simulations, the ligand and membrane protein structures should be prepared (for details, *see*

Refs. [22, 23]). We performed MD simulation using NAMDv2.8 package with the CHARMM22/CMAP biomolecular force-field [24, 25]. The topology and parameter files for the ligand were generated using SwissParam web server, which provides topologies and parameters based on the Merck molecular force field (MMFF) and is compatible with the CHARMM force field [26]. Apo form of $A_{2A}AR$ was obtained by minimizing the inactive $A_{2A}AR$ structure after the removal of the bound antagonist. The water layer was prepared using the Helmut Grubmuller's SOLVATE 1.0 program, followed by the merging of protein and water layer. Subsequently, the water molecules surrounding the TM-regions were removed. Since GPCRs are embedded in a lipid bilayer system, it is essential to mimic native-like conditions, which remain a crucial aspect in membrane simulations. We implemented the POPC membrane building procedure using a plug-in available at http://www.ks. uiuc.edu/Research/vmd/plugins/membrane/ to do the entire process in VMD [27]. Some groups have made few preequilibrated membrane systems available (Table 1), which may speed up the process of membrane building protocol. To construct an explicit membrane-protein system, the TM region of $A_{2A}AR$ was predicted based on the Orientations of Proteins in Membranes (OPM)

Table 1
List of various software packages/webservers for membrane building.

Program/Server	Output compatibility with simulation packages	Source
Automated Topology Builder (ATB)	GROMACS, GROMOS, LAMMPS	https://atb.uq.edu.au/
CHARMM-GUI Membrane Builder	CHARMM, GROMACS, AMBER, GENESIS, OPENMM, CHARMM/ OPENMM	http://www.charmm-gui. org/?doc=input/membrane
ChemSite Pro®	Information N/A	ChemSW®
CELLmicrocosmos 2.2 MembraneEditor (CmME)	GROMACS	http://www.cellmicrocosmos. org/index.php/cm2-project
MemBuilder II (Beta Ver.)	CHARMM, GROMACS, AMBER	http://bioinf.modares.ac.ir/ software/mb2/builder.php
MemGen	Not restricted	http://memgen.uni- goettingen.de/
Packmol	AMBER, GROMACS, MOLDY	http://www.ime.unicamp.br/ ~martinez/packmol
VMD Membrane-Plugin	CHARMM	http://www.ks.uiuc.edu/ Research/vmd/plugins/ membrane/

database and hydrophobicity of the protein. The prepared receptor was aligned and oriented to the proper position in the POPC lipid bilayer (length: 88 Å in x-axis and 91 Å in y-axis) and the overlapping lipids and water molecules were removed. Removal of the overlapping lipid molecules may result in a vacuum between the receptor and lipid molecules. However, this problem could be circumvented during the first stage of equilibrium, where the vacuum tends to disappear as the lipid molecules relax around the protein. Subsequently, the receptor in the membrane system was solvated with explicit water molecules and ionized with 150 mM KCl salt condition.

2.1.2 Molecular Dynamics Simulation Steps

Before running MD simulation, preparation of the system, topology and force field files are necessary to start the process. The topology file contains all the data about the input structure and connectivity of the atoms in the system. The force field file contains data about the interactions existing between each of the atoms or a group of atoms connected in the initial structure. After setup, the systems for the simulation need to be relaxed in a controlled manner. In our MD protocol, the whole system was energy-minimized using conjugate-gradient method in the order of lipid membranes, water molecules, and entire molecules. Subsequently, gradual heating of the system from 0 to 300 K using a 0.1 K interval at each step was performed. Generally, equilibration of the system is often carried out in two stages: first, the system is simulated under NVT ensemble, where the number of molecules, volume, and temperature are kept constant, followed by NPT ensemble (i.e., to couple a barostat to the simulation and maintain a constant pressure) to more closely resemble the experimental conditions. In our protocol, equilibration was carried out for 50 ns under NVT ensemble at 300 K followed by the production runs for 300 ns under NPT ensemble ($T = 300$ K; $P = 1$ atm).

2.1.3 Quantitative Quality Assurance of the Simulation

Regarding the quality of the simulation, it is necessary to perform additional checks to test for the convergence of thermodynamic parameters, such as temperature, pressure, energy (potential and kinetic energies of the system), volume, density, and root mean square deviation (RMSD). If any of the thermodynamic parameters has not converged sufficiently, it is necessary to extend the required simulation steps (*see* **Note 2**). Particularly, in the case of membrane protein simulation, it is crucial to check the stability of both protein and lipid bilayer. The widely used metrics for checking the stability of the protein is calculating the RMSD of Cα-atoms with respect to the initial structure. However, in the case of lipids, it is essential to measure the mean surface area per lipid, which acts as a reliable indicator for molecular packing and membrane fluidity, and make a direct comparison with the available experimental data. Other details, such as formation of unexpected pores in the membrane system, separation of the lipid leaflets, lipid bilayer thickness, deuterium order parameters, lateral diffusion coefficients of lipids, ion aggregation on the protein surface, and loss of protein secondary structure, should be assessed. If any of these properties calculated during simulation steps is inaccurate, it may lead to major simulation artifacts.

2.1.4 Generation of Conformational Ensemble and Representative Protein Structures

Selecting a representative structure from the MD trajectory frames for analysis is one of the biggest challenges in the utilization of large structural ensembles. The choice of the selection criteria may vary depending on the goal of the subsequent analysis. The representative structure could be selected based on the RMSD, conformational energy, or certain known conformational changes which may be crucial for protein function. In our protocol, the trajectories of the MD production run for each system were monitored based on the total conformational energy, TM6 tilt angle, and RMSD relative to the initial structure. We used an integration time step of 2 fs, and for the analysis, simulated trajectories were saved for every 2 ps and sampled every 300 ps. Thus, each system consists of a conformational ensemble of 1000 structures for a total production run of 300 ns. The minimal energy conformation structures obtained from the conformational ensembles were selected as the representative protein structures for the apo and agonist-bound forms of $A_{2A}AR$, which were subsequently subjected to network analysis.

2.2 Elucidation of GPCR Allostery Using Network Analysis

2.2.1 Sequence Conservation Free Energy

Sequence information of a protein family provides insight into their functional mechanism [28]. In order to compare the conservation pattern in class A GPCR and its specific subtype family, i.e., adenosine receptor (AR), we computed $\Delta G(GPCR)/k_B T^*$ and $\Delta G(AR)/k_B T^*$, each of which is evaluated using different multiple sequence alignment (MSA). Sequences of AR family (219 sequences) and class A GPCR family (26,655 sequences) were collected from UniProtKB and Pfam databases, respectively. After removal of redundant sequences, 208 and 24,507 sequences were considered for AR and GPCR families, respectively. For GPCR family, sequence clustering was performed using a sequence identity of at least 40% to reduce the sequence space size, resulting in 2471 sequences. For a given MSA of a protein family, we quantified the extent of sequence conservation by using the following statistical free energy-like function scaled by an arbitrary energy scale $k_B T^*$ [21, 29]:

$$\Delta G_i/k_B T^* = \sqrt{\frac{1}{C_i} \sum_{\alpha=1}^{20} \left[p_i^\alpha \log\left(p_i^\alpha / p_\alpha \right) \right]^2} \qquad (1)$$

where C_i is the number of amino acid types at position i along the sequence, α denotes amino acid species, p_i^α is the frequency of an amino acid α at the position i, and p_α is the frequency of an amino acid α in the full MSA, which serves as the background frequency. The quantity $S = \sum_{\alpha=1}^{20} p_i^{\alpha} \log(p_i^{\alpha}/p_{\alpha})$ can be regarded as the relative entropy, and $S = 0$ if p_i^{α} is no different than p_{α} for all α. Note that larger values of ΔG_i denote better sequence conservation at position i. In class A GPCR family, the conserved residues are mainly located at the cytoplasmic region, where G-proteins may bind. On the contrary, the residues at the extracellular ligand binding site in AR family are highly conserved affecting ligand binding selectivity. Especially, in $A_{2A}AR$, 15 out of 18 microswitches (except for P189, S281, and E228) are highly conserved, satisfying $\Delta G(GPCR)/k_B T^* \geq 0.2$.

2.2.2 Construction of the Residue-Interaction Network Model

By using 3D structures of proteins, we constructed the 3D-network where each amino acid residue was represented as a single node. To take into account the effect of side chain, we considered two coarse-grained centers per residue, i.e., the alpha carbon (C_α) for backbone and a farthest heavy atom from C_α for the side chain (SC). The mutual distance between residue A and residue B was assumed by the shortest distance among the ones between C_α(residue A) $-$ C_α(residue B), C_α(A) $-$ SC(B), SC(A) $-$ C_α(B), and SC(A) $-$ SC(B). By doing so, we incorporated the cases of backbone–backbone, backbone–side chain, and side chain–side chain contacts. In our network model, a link was established between two residues (C_α), where any pair of backbone and side chain distance is less than 7 Å [30]. Thus, the side chain effects were implicitly included in our network analysis.

2.2.3 Centrality Analysis

Measuring centrality, which is the most studied concept in social network analysis, can be a practical way of selecting essential nodes in the network [11, 31, 32] (*see* **Note 3**). This centrality calculation was successfully applied in identifying functional residues, such as in the active site or metal binding site of proteins [13, 16]. Also, this method is considered to be useful in the investigation of allosteric communications in protein structures [14, 15, 33]. For example, allosteric propagation was modeled by considering all possible signaling routes in a monomeric structure [33]. There are three most popular centrality measures, i.e., degree, closeness, and betweenness [11, 31]:

1. The degree centrality, $C_D(v)$, measures the total number of edges linked to a node v. This value is identical to the number of contacts with its neighboring residues.

$$C_D(v) = \deg(v) \qquad (2)$$

2. The closeness centrality, $C_C(v)$, is an inverse of the mean geodesic distance (shortest path length) from all other nodes to the node v. It measures how fast a signal from the node v can be transmitted to other nodes.

$$C_C(v) = \left(\sum_{i=1}^{N} d(i,v)/(N-1) \right)^{-1} \tag{3}$$

where $d(i,v)$ is the minimal number of edges that bridge the nodes i and v. For a given network topology, $d(i,j)$ can be calculated by using Dijkstra's algorithm [34].

3. The betweenness centrality, $C_B(v)$, measures the extent to which a node has control over transmission of information between the nodes in the network [35].

$$C_B(v) = \frac{2}{(N-1)(N-2)} \sum_{s=1}^{N-1} \sum_{t=s+1}^{N} \frac{\sigma_{st}(v)}{\sigma_{st}} \tag{4}$$

where $s \neq t \neq v$. In the above definition, σ_{st} is the number of shortest paths linking the nodes s and t, and $\sigma_{st}(v)$ is the number of shortest paths linking the nodes s and t via the node v. The factor $(N-1)(N-2)/2$ is the normalization constant. To reduce the computational cost of Eq. 4, we used Brandes algorithm [36], which exploits the sparse nature of typical real-world graphs, and computes the betweenness centrality score for all vertices in the graph in a very short time.

By surmising that allosteric hotspots are the mediators of information flow in a network topology of a given protein structure, we adopted betweenness centrality concept in identifying hotspot residues which can modulate the signal transduction in GPCRs (*see* **Note 4**). Since the betweenness centrality calculates the extent to which a particular node lies between other nodes in the network [31, 36, 37], a member with high betweenness may act as a gatekeeper or broker in the network for either smooth communication or flow of information [37]. Using the minimum energy structures generated by the MD simulation, the residue interaction network was constructed with a cutoff distance of 7 Å. Subsequently, the betweenness centrality was calculated to measure each residue's importance for the flux of information in the residue interaction network (*see* **Note 5**).

2.2.4 Network Vulnerability Analysis (Glycine Scanning)

When a network is attacked by a certain perturbation, it may or may not collapse depending on the importance of the attacked site [38]. The rate at which the network is affected by perturbation could be regarded as a network's tolerance to an error or vulnerability to an attack, and a member with high vulnerability can be considered to have a crucial role in the stable formation or integrity of the network [39]. In the theory of complex network, this vulnerability is evaluated using a relative change in the average network centrality when a node x is removed, which can be written as follows [39]:

$$\Gamma_\xi^x = \frac{\langle C_\xi \rangle - \langle C_\xi^x \rangle}{\langle C_\xi \rangle} \qquad (5)$$

where $\langle C_\xi \rangle \left(\equiv \sum_{i=1}^{N} C_\xi(i)/N \right)$ is the average network centrality, and $\langle C_\xi^x \rangle$ is a value evaluated for a newly constructed network when the node x is removed from the original network.

The idea of network vulnerability is similar to point mutagenesis assay, which measures the effect of mutations up to the degree where proteins can retain their activity. Adopting this vulnerability concept, we performed in silico glycine scanning experiments of the constructed residue interaction network of A$_{2A}$AR. As straightforwardly implicated by the term "glycine scanning," the side chain of each residue was deleted systematically, and the corresponding residue interaction network was reconstructed. Then, we compared the original residue interaction network to the reconstructed one to measure how much the centralities of whole network was changed when the side chain of specific amino acid was deleted. The main difference between our in silico glycine scanning analysis and the previous studies applying network analysis [38, 40] is that only side chain atoms were deleted, rather than the extraction of entire node in the network. Therefore, our method could be considered more realistic as it mimics changes similar to the experimental mutation studies.

We assessed the effect of deleting side chains by calculating the changes in average betweenness centralities ($\langle C_B \rangle$). In our case, readjustment of local environment due to the removal of side chain is not considered. The primary aim of this analysis is to quantitatively assess the role of a specific residue side chain in the original residue interaction network. The greater the role played by the deleted side chain in maintaining the network structure, the more significant the response of average network centrality would be to the removal of that particular residue. Interestingly, the residues with high network vulnerabilities included the regions around NPxxY motif in TM7 and proline kink in TM6, which were reported as important residues providing structural constraints in GPCRs [41, 42]. Along with our analysis, these regions seem to be potent for maintaining the integrity of whole residue interaction network modulating the entire activation process.

2.2.5 Cross-Correlation Between Regions Based on the Structural Ensembles

In the active form of GPCR structure, the ligand binding site in the extracellular side and the intracellular G-protein binding region are functionally coupled, and this coupling is mediated by a structural reorganization of 7TM helices. To quantify such long-range coupling in the dynamics of A$_{2A}$AR, we calculated cross-correlation between residues (CC_{ij}) in terms of C_B (Eq. 4) by using the conformational ensembles generated from the MD simulated trajectories.

$$CC_{ij} = \frac{\langle C_B(i) \cdot C_B(j) \rangle - \langle C_B(i) \rangle \langle C_B(j) \rangle}{\sqrt{\langle (\delta C_B(i))^2 \rangle} \cdot \sqrt{\langle (\delta C_B(j))^2 \rangle}} \qquad (6)$$

where $\langle \ldots \rangle$ indicates an ensemble average, thus $\langle C_B(i) \rangle$ refers to the average betweenness centrality for the residue i. The cross-correlation matrices for the apo and agonist-bound forms showed that the signatures of correlation between residues are scattered all over the structure. In this map, high signal residue pairs indicate that the two residues are linked to each other either via direct contact or long-range communication. In order to identify the residue pairs with long-range cross-correlation, the pairs which showed high cross-correlation values ($CC_{ij} \geq 0.5$) but far from each other, i.e., which have minimum path over six edges ($d_{ij} > 6$), were extracted.

Surprisingly, in the agonist-bound form, there are significant long-range cross-correlations between the extracellular ligand binding site and cytoplasmic G-protein binding site. Between the correlated residues, minimum path seems to pass through the residues with high betweenness centralities, including the important microswitches. The results correlate well with the function of GPCRs, i.e., coordinated domain coupling [43]: an agonist binding induces a significant conformational change in the region where G-protein may bind. On the contrary, such long-range cross-correlation was not observed in the simulated trajectories of the apo structure. The long-range coupling between the ligand binding site and G-protein binding site for the agonist-bound form is also grasped by computing the mean square fluctuation using structural ensembles. In a recent review, Unal et al. proposed that the intrinsically flexible extracellular and intracellular regions are functionally coupled and this coupling is mediated by TM helix structures [44]. It is assumed that when a domain engages a ligand, the intrinsic disorder of receptor structure is decreased, and it cooperatively influences the conformation of the neighboring domain [44]. Our computational analysis gave a more detailed picture of this model, which could be valuable in drug discovery (see **Note 6**).

3 Conclusions

We have presented a computational protocol for the mapping of allosteric signal flow in GPCRs using conventional MD simulations and network analysis. Through network analysis, we identified the hotspots accountable for agonistic activity of $A_{2A}AR$ and the cross-correlation between the agonist- and G-protein binding sites were visualized using their pathways. Compared to other existing methods, our approach proved quite powerful in the identification of allosteric hotspot residues in GPCR signaling pathway, and correlated well with the existing biochemical studies. Additionally, rotameric microswitches, which are deemed critical for Class A GPCR signaling, were located accurately. The strong signals for long-range TM communications were observed only in agonist-bound $A_{2A}AR$ model system. Our method provides valuable information on both GPCR allosteric modulation and orthosteric signaling pathway. This simple approach could not only be extended to other proteins but also to study the allostery of several protein–protein or protein–DNA/RNA complexes that are of biological and pharmaceutical interest.

4 Notes

1. In our protocol, we carried out MD simulations of the model systems through a single trajectory. However, in order to avoid incomplete sampling of larger proteins, it is preferable to use a multicopy approach, through which a series of simulations with different initial velocities could be performed.

2. Insufficient conformational sampling limits the application of traditional all-atom MD simulation technique. However, there are several enhanced MD simulation techniques (Table 2) available to address sampling problems and generate more diverse structural ensembles.

3. An exemplary graph in Fig. 2 nicely represented the significance of betweenness centrality. The node x has a greater connectivity ($C_D = 6$) to other nodes, however, the removal of x from the network does not destroy the communication among other nodes. In contrast, removal of node y, which has less connectivity ($C_D = 4$) than x, would split the whole network into three pieces. With respect to communication or the flow of information, node y could be the most critical one. Node y has the highest betweenness centrality which evaluates the importance of each node based on the amount of traffic or the amount of internode communication. Betweenness could be one of the most ideal measures to identify allosteric hotspots for a given protein structure.

4. In our analysis, there was no significant correlation between the residues' centrality values in the network and sequence conservation. The key residues identified from the network analysis method were not necessarily identical to the entire set of well-conserved residues, but to a subset of them.

Table 2
List of various enhanced sampling methods in molecular dynamics (MD) simulation

Enhanced MD technique	Methodology	Applications
Accelerated MD	Adds a positive boost potential to the system's potential energy (PE) when it drops below a certain threshold, thus decreasing the energy barriers and accelerating the transitions between low energy conformational states	Protein–ligand binding and protein folding mechanisms
Adaptive biasing force (ABF) simulation	Adds a continuously updated biasing force to the equations of motion, such that in the long-time limit a Hamiltonian devoid of an average force acting along the transition coordinate of interest is added	Free-energy calculations along a reaction coordinate, potentials of mean force (PMF) profile estimation
Biased/Steered molecular dynamics (SMD)	A dummy atom is attached to the center of mass (COM) of the ligand through a virtual spring with a spring constant (k), which is later pulled with a constant velocity (v) along a predefined direction for the unbinding of ligand	Free energy calculations, binding/unbinding mechanisms of biomolecular systems, PMF profile estimation
Conformational flooding	Adds a flooding potential to the systems's PE that destabilizes the initial conformation, thus lowering free-energy barriers of structural transitions and accelerating the transitions	Protein structure prediction/conformational search, check protein models stability, predict functional motions, improve thermodynamic quantities like free energies and entropies for proteins
Dynamic importance sampling (DIMS)/self-guided Langevin dynamics	Employs a bias with correction approach to improve the sampling efficiency of rare events	Transition pathways
Local elevation (LE)	Adds a bias term (i.e., sum of repulsive functions) to the PE function	Low-energy structure search
Metadynamics	The location of the system is calculated based on the collective variables. A positive Gaussian potential is subsequently added to the energy landscape to drive the simulation back to its previous location	Folding of small proteins, protein switches, ligand dissociation pathways, and ion-induced diffusion of small molecules in channels or cavities

(continued)

Table 2
(continued)

Enhanced MD technique	Methodology	Applications
Multicanonical ensemble	A constant temperature MD on a deformed PE surface, which provides a multicanonical ensemble with a flat energy distribution The multicanonical ensemble is subsequently converted into a canonical ensemble by reweighting the formula of Ferrenberg and Swendsen	Larger conformational space sampling
Random acceleration molecular dynamics (RAMD)	Applies a force in a random direction to COM of the ligand in addition to its forcefield Allow ligands to explore possible dissociation pathways in an unbiased manner	Ligand dissociation pathways
Replica exchange molecular dynamics (REMD)/Parallel tempering	Run multiple MD simulations with different values of a specific exchange variable, i.e., temperature Based on Metropolis criterion, the systems states are exchanged between neighboring simulations at regular intervals	Free energy landscape, protein protonation states, and peptide/protein folding mechanism
Umbrella sampling (US)	Employs collective variables The restraint bias potential (quadratic or harmonic form) forces the collective variables in a window to remain close to the COM The sets of collective variables must allow slight overlapping of windows	Ligand binding mechanism, and ion-induced diffusion in membrane proteins

5. Elastic network model (ENM) is one of the methods which characterize a protein based on its residue interaction network, and ENM-based NMA was successfully applied to investigate functional dynamics or global motion of proteins [21, 45, 46]. Several methods have been proposed to identify hot spot residues or allosteric communication network for protein function. Statistical coupling analysis (SCA), which adopts sequence covariation analysis based on MSA, has gained growing popularity [29, 47, 48]. Perturbative study based on ENM, known as structural perturbation method (SPM), has also been proposed and provides deep insights into the critical residues for maintaining the functional dynamics of an enzyme [49]. Although each method can predict few key protein residues based on its own concept or algorithm, there are still

(A)

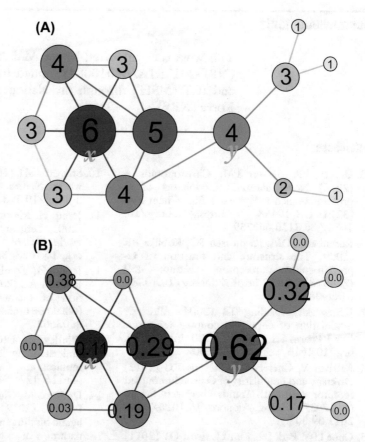

Fig. 2 An exemplary graph showing the importance of betweenness centrality. (a) Degree centrality and (b) betweeness centrality values calculated for each node are shown

limitations linked with the identification of specific key residues for protein function. For example, SPM can only identify residues which affect the global motion of proteins, while SCA is not suitable for highly conserved residues. Therefore, instead of searching for some other methods to predict hot spot residues with a different approach than previous in silico methods, we assume that network analysis of the 3D structures is quite suitable for the identification of allosteric hot spots in the target proteins.

6. With the reliable format of representing network (nodes and their connectivity), the centrality values can also be calculated using Gephi [50], an open source software for exploring and manipulating networks. The residue interaction graph in 2D can be visualized with Force Atlas layout implemented in Gephi.

470   Shaherin Basith et al.

Acknowledgments

This work was supported by the Mid-career Researcher Program (NRF-2017R1A2B4010084) funded by the Ministry of Science and ICT (MSIT) through the National Research Foundation of Korea (NRF).

References

1. Gentry PR, Sexton PM, Christopoulos A (2015) Novel allosteric modulators of G protein-coupled receptors. J Biol Chem 290 (32):19478–19488. https://doi.org/10.1074/jbc.R115.662759

2. Rosenbaum DM, Rasmussen SG, Kobilka BK (2009) The structure and function of G-protein-coupled receptors. Nature 459 (7245):356–363. https://doi.org/10.1038/nature08144

3. Jensen AA, Spalding TA (2004) Allosteric modulation of G-protein coupled receptors. Eur J Pharm Sci 21(4):407–420. https://doi.org/10.1016/j.ejps.2003.11.007

4. Katritch V, Cherezov V, Stevens RC (2012) Diversity and modularity of G protein-coupled receptor structures. Trends Pharmacol Sci 33 (1):17–27. https://doi.org/10.1016/j.tips.2011.09.003

5. Choe HW, Park JH, Kim YJ, Ernst OP (2011) Transmembrane signaling by GPCRs: insight from rhodopsin and opsin structures. Neuropharmacology 60(1):52–57. https://doi.org/10.1016/j.neuropharm.2010.07.018

6. Dror RO, Dirks RM, Grossman JP, Xu H, Shaw DE (2012) Biomolecular simulation: a computational microscope for molecular biology. Annu Rev Biophys 41:429–452. https://doi.org/10.1146/annurev-biophys-042910-155245

7. Sethi A, Eargle J, Black AA, Luthey-Schulten Z (2009) Dynamical networks in tRNA:protein complexes. Proc Natl Acad Sci U S A 106 (16):6620–6625. https://doi.org/10.1073/pnas.0810961106

8. Yao XQ, Grant BJ (2013) Domain-opening and dynamic coupling in the alpha-subunit of heterotrimeric G proteins. Biophys J 105(2): L08–L10. https://doi.org/10.1016/j.bpj.2013.06.006

9. Miao Y, Nichols SE, Gasper PM, Metzger VT, McCammon JA (2013) Activation and dynamic network of the M2 muscarinic receptor. Proc Natl Acad Sci U S A 110 (27):10982–10987. https://doi.org/10.1073/pnas.1309755110

10. Strogatz SH (2001) Exploring complex networks. Nature 410(6825):268–276. https://doi.org/10.1038/35065725

11. Jeong H, Mason SP, Barabasi AL, Oltvai ZN (2001) Lethality and centrality in protein networks. Nature 411(6833):41–42. https://doi.org/10.1038/35075138

12. Jeong H, Tombor B, Albert R, Oltvai ZN, Barabasi AL (2000) The large-scale organization of metabolic networks. Nature 407 (6804):651–654. https://doi.org/10.1038/35036627

13. Whitley MJ, Lee AL (2009) Frameworks for understanding long-range intra-protein communication. Curr Protein Pept Sci 10 (2):116–127

14. De Ruvo M, Giuliani A, Paci P, Santoni D, Di Paola L (2012) Shedding light on protein-ligand binding by graph theory: the topological nature of allostery. Biophys Chem 165–166:21–29. https://doi.org/10.1016/j.bpc.2012.03.001

15. Atilgan AR, Akan P, Baysal C (2004) Small-world communication of residues and significance for protein dynamics. Biophys J 86(1 Pt 1):85–91. https://doi.org/10.1016/S0006-3495(04)74086-2

16. Amitai G, Shemesh A, Sitbon E, Shklar M, Netanely D, Venger I, Pietrokovski S (2004) Network analysis of protein structures identifies functional residues. J Mol Biol 344 (4):1135–1146. https://doi.org/10.1016/j.jmb.2004.10.055

17. Bagler G, Sinha S (2007) Assortative mixing in protein contact networks and protein folding kinetics. Bioinformatics 23(14):1760–1767. https://doi.org/10.1093/bioinformatics/btm257

18. Brinda KV, Vishveshwara S (2005) A network representation of protein structures: implications for protein stability. Biophys J 89 (6):4159–4170. https://doi.org/10.1529/biophysj.105.064485

19. Dokholyan NV, Li L, Ding F, Shakhnovich EI (2002) Topological determinants of protein folding. Proc Natl Acad Sci U S A 99

(13):8637–8641. https://doi.org/10.1073/pnas.122076099

20. Kaczor AA, Rutkowska E, Bartuzi D, Targowska-Duda KM, Matosiuk D, Selent J (2016) Computational methods for studying G protein-coupled receptors (GPCRs). Methods Cell Biol 132:359–399. https://doi.org/10.1016/bs.mcb.2015.11.002

21. Lee Y, Jeong LS, Choi S, Hyeon C (2011) Link between allosteric signal transduction and functional dynamics in a multisubunit enzyme: S-adenosylhomocysteine hydrolase. J Am Chem Soc 133(49):19807–19815. https://doi.org/10.1021/ja2066175

22. Lee Y, Choi S, Hyeon C (2014) Mapping the intramolecular signal transduction of G-protein coupled receptors. Proteins 82 (5):727–743. https://doi.org/10.1002/prot.24451

23. Lee Y, Choi S, Hyeon C (2015) Communication over the network of binary switches regulates the activation of A2A adenosine receptor. PLoS Comput Biol 11(2):e1004044. https://doi.org/10.1371/journal.pcbi.1004044

24. Buck M, Bouguet-Bonnet S, Pastor RW, AD MK Jr (2006) Importance of the CMAP correction to the CHARMM22 protein force field: dynamics of hen lysozyme. Biophys J 90(4):L36–L38. https://doi.org/10.1529/biophysj.105.078154

25. Phillips JC, Braun R, Wang W, Gumbart J, Tajkhorshid E, Villa E, Chipot C, Skeel RD, Kale L, Schulten K (2005) Scalable molecular dynamics with NAMD. J Comput Chem 26 (16):1781–1802. https://doi.org/10.1002/jcc.20289

26. Zoete V, Cuendet MA, Grosdidier A, Michielin O (2011) SwissParam: a fast force field generation tool for small organic molecules. J Comput Chem 32(11):2359–2368. https://doi.org/10.1002/jcc.21816

27. Humphrey W, Dalke A, Schulten K (1996) VMD: visual molecular dynamics. J Mol Graph 14(1):33–38. 27–38

28. Bjarnadottir TK, Gloriam DE, Hellstrand SH, Kristiansson H, Fredriksson R, Schioth HB (2006) Comprehensive repertoire and phylogenetic analysis of the G protein-coupled receptors in human and mouse. Genomics 88 (3):263–273. https://doi.org/10.1016/j.ygeno.2006.04.001

29. Dima RI, Thirumalai D (2006) Determination of network of residues that regulate allostery in protein families using sequence analysis. Protein Sci 15(2):258–268. https://doi.org/10.1110/ps.051767306

30. da Silveira CH, Pires DE, Minardi RC, Ribeiro C, Veloso CJ, Lopes JC, Meira W Jr, Neshich G, Ramos CH, Habesch R, Santoro MM (2009) Protein cutoff scanning: a comparative analysis of cutoff dependent and cutoff free methods for prospecting contacts in proteins. Proteins 74(3):727–743. https://doi.org/10.1002/prot.22187

31. Freeman LC (1978) Centrality in social networks conceptual clarification. Soc Networks 1(79):215–239

32. Borgatti SP (2005) Centrality and network flow. Soc Networks 27:55–71. https://doi.org/10.1016/j.socnet.2004.11.008

33. Park K, Kim D (2011) Modeling allosteric signal propagation using protein structure networks. BMC Bioinformatics 12(Suppl 1):S23. https://doi.org/10.1186/1471-2105-12-S1-S23

34. Dijkstra EW (1959) A note on two problems in connexion with graphs. Numerische Math 1 (1):269–271. https://doi.org/10.1007/bf01386390

35. Newman MEJ (2005) A measure of betweenness centrality based on random walks. Soc Networks 27(1):39–54. https://doi.org/10.1016/j.socnet.2004.11.009

36. Brandes U (2001) A faster algorithm for betweenness centrality. J Math Sociol 25 (2):163–177

37. Qin J, Xu JJ, Hu D, Sageman M, Chen H (2005) Analyzing terrorist networks: a case study of the global salafi jihad network. Lect Notes Comput Sci 3495:287–304

38. Singer Y (2006) Dynamic measure of network robustness. In: IEEE 24th convention of electrical and electronics engineers, Israel, 2006, pp 366–370. https://doi.org/10.1109/EEEI.2006.321105

39. Albert R, Jeong H, Barabasi AL (2000) Error and attack tolerance of complex networks. Nature 406(6794):378–382. https://doi.org/10.1038/35019019

40. del Sol A, Fujihashi H, Amoros D, Nussinov R (2006) Residues crucial for maintaining short paths in network communication mediate signaling in proteins. Mol Syst Biol 2:2006.0019. https://doi.org/10.1038/msb4100063

41. Fritze O, Filipek S, Kuksa V, Palczewski K, Hofmann KP, Ernst OP (2003) Role of the conserved NPxxY(x)5,6F motif in the rhodopsin ground state and during activation. Proc Natl Acad Sci U S A 100(5):2290–2295. https://doi.org/10.1073/pnas.0435715100

42. Shi L, Liapakis G, Xu R, Guarnieri F, Ballesteros JA, Javitch JA (2002) Beta2 adrenergic receptor activation. Modulation of the proline

kink in transmembrane 6 by a rotamer toggle switch. J Biol Chem 277(43):40989–40996. https://doi.org/10.1074/jbc.M206801200

43. Trzaskowski B, Latek D, Yuan S, Ghoshdastider U, Debinski A, Filipek S (2012) Action of molecular switches in GPCRs – theoretical and experimental studies. Curr Med Chem 19(8):1090–1109

44. Unal H, Karnik SS (2012) Domain coupling in GPCRs: the engine for induced conformational changes. Trends Pharmacol Sci 33 (2):79–88. https://doi.org/10.1016/j.tips. 2011.09.007

45. Bahar I, Lezon TR, Bakan A, Shrivastava IH (2010) Normal mode analysis of biomolecular structures: functional mechanisms of membrane proteins. Chem Rev 110 (3):1463–1497. https://doi.org/10.1021/ Cr900095e

46. Thirumuruganandham SP, Urbassek HM (2009) Low-frequency vibrational modes and infrared absorbance of red, blue and green opsin. J Mol Model 15(8):959–969. https:// doi.org/10.1007/s00894-008-0446-1

47. Suel GM, Lockless SW, Wall MA, Ranganathan R (2003) Evolutionarily conserved networks of residues mediate allosteric communication in proteins. Nat Struct Biol 10(1):59–69. https://doi.org/10.1038/nsb881

48. Lockless SW, Ranganathan R (1999) Evolutionarily conserved pathways of energetic connectivity in protein families. Science 286 (5438):295–299

49. Zheng W, Brooks BR, Doniach S, Thirumalai D (2005) Network of dynamically important residues in the open/closed transition in polymerases is strongly conserved. Structure 13 (4):565–577. https://doi.org/10.1016/j.str. 2005.01.017

50. Bastian M, Heymann S, Jacomy M (2009) Gephi: an open source software for exploring and manipulating networks. In: Third international AAAI conference on weblogs and social media, San Jose, CA, May 2009. pp 361–362

Chapter 24

Identification of Potential MicroRNA Biomarkers by Meta-analysis

Hongmei Zhu and Siu-wai Leung

Abstract

Meta-analysis statistically assesses the results (e.g., effect sizes) across independent studies that are conducted in accordance with similar protocols and objectives. Current genomic meta-analysis studies do not perform extensive re-analysis on raw data because full data access would not be commonplace, although the best practice of open research for sharing well-formed data have been actively advocated. This chapter describes a simple and easy-to-follow method for conducting meta-analysis of multiple studies without using raw data. Examples for meta-analysis of microRNAs (miRNAs) are provided to illustrate the method. MiRNAs are potential biomarkers for early diagnosis and epigenetic monitoring of diseases. A number of miRNAs have been identified to be differentially expressed, i.e., overexpressed or underexpressed, under diseased states but only a small fraction would be highly effective biomarkers or therapeutic targets of diseases. The meta-analysis method as described in this chapter aims to identify the miRNAs that are consistently found dysregulated across independent studies as biomarkers.

Key words microRNA, Noncoding RNAs, Meta-analysis, Quality assessment, Biomarkers, Differential expression, Early diagnosis

1 Introduction

Meta-analysis is a statistical method for systematically synthesizing the scientific reports and quantifying an overall results such as effect size from multiple independent studies by weighing each one by its reliability and credibility [1, 2]. Meta-analysis has been widely used in synthesizing the evidence for efficacy of medical treatments and performance of diagnostic tests. It is increasingly used in many other fields of research, such as education, psychology, criminology, ecology, and molecular biology [3, 4]. Depending on the types of the included studies and the information provided therein, their outcome measures should be comparable for a meta-analysis.

Electronic supplementary material: The online version of this chapter (https://doi.org/10.1007/978-1-4939-7756-7_24) contains supplementary material, which is available to authorized users.

Mohini Gore and Umesh B. Jagtap (eds.), *Computational Drug Discovery and Design*, Methods in Molecular Biology, vol. 1762, https://doi.org/10.1007/978-1-4939-7756-7_24, © Springer Science+Business Media, LLC, part of Springer Nature 2018

Common outcome measures include relative risk, odds ratio, correlation coefficient, risk difference, and (standardized) mean difference [5]. Since most of gene expression studies have small sample sizes [6], meta-analysis is useful to increase statistical power by combining multiple gene expression studies. A recent academic literature review discussed pros and cons of genomic meta-analysis for biomedical sciences, particularly on the identification of differentially expressed genes, analysis of pathways/networks and predictive models [6]. It is noticed that most of the genomic meta-analysis methods are designed for those studies published with the raw data. However, many of such genomic studies still do not make their raw data readily accessible to the public. For this reason, this chapter describes a proper statistical meta-analysis method (instead of the simple vote-counting that was misused in many genomic meta-analyses) that is widely used in evidence-based medicine [7] and applicable to the situations with or without raw data. This chapter also covers the quality assessment (which are missing from many genomic meta-analysis) of studies in accordance with the evidence-based research guidelines including the PRISMA [8] and MIAME [9]. Here, meta-analysis of microRNA (miRNA) differential expression studies on type 2 diabetes (T2D) is taken as an example.

Type 2 diabetes is a complex metabolic disorder characterized by insulin resistance [10] that is often undetected until hyperglycemia is observed [11]. The pathogenesis of T2D involves genetic, environmental, and lifestyle factors. Over time, multiple organ damages can occur, especially to the heart, blood vessels, eyes, kidneys, and nerves [12]. According to the International Diabetes Federation (IDF) [13], 415 million adults were estimated to live with diabetes with 46.5% undiagnosed in 2014. By 2040, this figure will rise to 642 million. High prevalence and no cure available make achieving and maintaining glycemic control as the primary goal of an initial pharmacological treatment to prevent progressive deterioration, which can be markedly improved by identifying novel early biomarkers and therapeutics for diabetes. MiRNAs are likely candidates of the early biomarkers of T2D for detecting and monitoring of the disease [14]. Meta-analysis may help to screen the miRNA-related biomarkers of highest potential for experimental and clinical validation.

MiRNAs are a class of small (approximately 22 nucleotides), endogenous, noncoding, highly stable RNAs that regulate gene and protein expression. Generally, precursors of miRNAs are co-transcribed with their hosting gene in mammal [15] by RNA polymerase II, which contain a characteristic stem-loop structure [16]. The pri-miRNAs are subsequently cleaved by the nuclear ribonuclease III (RNase III) enzyme Drosha to produce pre-miRNAs of 70–100 nucleotides that are transported by Exportin-5 into cytoplasm. Following the transportation, a further

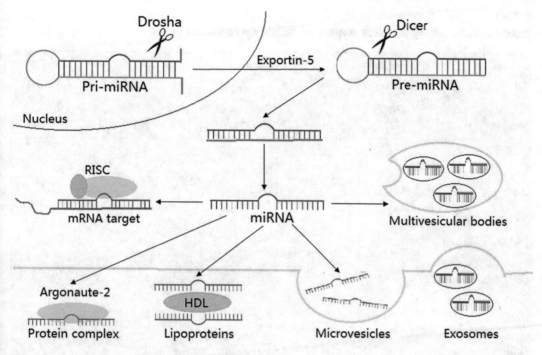

Fig. 1 Biogenesis and release of miRNAs

cleavage occurs via the endoribonuclease Dicer to generate the mature miRNAs [17]. Mature miRNAs can associate with one of Argonaute (AGO) proteins to form an RNA-induced silencing complex (RISC) and guide translational repression of fully or partially complementary target mRNAs [18]. Mature miRNAs can also be released by the cells after binding to proteins such as Argonaute-2 [19] or lipoproteins [20] or loading in the microvesicles [21] formed by plasma membrane blebbing. Alternatively, miRNAs can be associated with exosomes that are released by exocytosis [21]. Figure 1 shows the biogenesis and release of miRNAs.

MiRNAs are involved in many biological processes, including cellular differentiation, metabolism, and cancer development [22, 23]. Their modes of dysregulation are related to many diseases [24]. In attempts to identify novel early biomarkers of T2D, most of the miRNA expression profiling studies were performed in cultured cells, blood, or solid tissue samples [25–28]. A large number of miRNAs were identified to be differentially expressed, either overexpressed or underexpressed, while only a small number would be important signatures or therapeutic targets. It is, therefore, challenging to determine which miRNAs are potential biomarkers; which miRNAs are tissue-specific; whether circulating miRNAs make the best biomarkers; and whether animal models are sufficient for pilot studies. The results from these studies are, however, subject to rigorous evaluation for consistency and reproducibility by meta-analysis. Academic laboratories provide only

Table 1
Inconsistencies among literature reviews on miRNA dysregulation in T2D

miRNA	Literature review						
	Guay (2011) [32]	Guay (2012) [33]	Hamar (2012) [34]	Karolina (2012) [11]	McClelland (2014) [35]	Natarajan (2012) [36]	Shantikumar (2012) [14]
miR-103 (adipose)	N	–	D	–	U	–	N
miR-107 (adipose)	D	–	–	–	U	–	–
miR-132 (adipose)	–	–	U	–	–	–	D
miR-143 (adipose)	N	–	–	D	–	–	N
miR-144 (liver)	D	–	–	U	–	–	–
miR-192 (kidney)	–	–	U	N	N	N	–
miR-21 (kidney)	–	–	–	D	U	N	–
miR-29c (liver)	N	–	–	–	–	–	–
miR-375 (islets)	D	U	–	U	U	–	U

11–50% of reproducible results [29–31]. We also found that the findings from recent literature reviews on miRNAs were discrepant (Table 1). Therefore, this meta-analysis method would fill this gap to identify consistently dysregulated miRNAs in T2D.

2 Materials

1. Statistical software R (https://www.r-project.org) and RStudio (https://www.rstudio.com).
2. Installation of *metafor* package in R environment.
3. An example dataset with dysregulated miRNAs (Additional file `data.csv`).

2.1 Instructions

R could be downloaded and installed from https://www.r-project.org and RStudio could be downloaded from https://www.rstudio.com. In RStudio we can install *metator* package [37] (*see* **Note 1**).

```
Console ~/

R version 3.3.2 (2016-10-31) -- "Sincere Pumpkin Patch"
Copyright (C) 2016 The R Foundation for Statistical Computing
Platform: x86_64-w64-mingw32/x64 (64-bit)

R is free software and comes with ABSOLUTELY NO WARRANTY.
You are welcome to redistribute it under certain conditions.
Type 'license()' or 'licence()' for distribution details.

R is a collaborative project with many contributors.
Type 'contributors()' for more information and
'citation()' on how to cite R or R packages in publications.

Type 'demo()' for some demos, 'help()' for on-line help, or
'help.start()' for an HTML browser interface to help.
Type 'q()' to quit R.

[workspace loaded from ~/.RData]

> install.packages("metafor")
Installing package into 'C:/Users/lenovo/Documents/R/win-library/3.3'
(as 'lib' is unspecified)
trying URL 'https://cran.rstudio.com/bin/windows/contrib/3.3/metafor_1.9-9.zip'
Content type 'application/zip' length 2212763 bytes (2.1 MB)
downloaded 2.1 MB

package 'metafor' successfully unpacked and MD5 sums checked
```

Fig. 2 R code for *metafor* package installation. The words in red under R code indicate the package is being installed and the subsequent words in black indicate the package has been installed successfully

The process for package installation is shown in Fig. 2. The example data as part of a full dataset [7] is used in the statistical meta-analysis of this chapter.

3   Methods

In general, meta-analysis focuses on answering a well-defined question (*see* **Note 2**) [38]. The question of our interest, i.e., which miRNAs are consistently dysregulated, is to be addressed by meta-analysis, which includes a comprehensive search of relevant studies, an impartial selection according to appropriate criteria, unbiased assessment of study quality, transparent data extraction, and reproducible statistical analysis [38]. Here, we summarize a meta-analysis workflow to identify the dysregulated miRNAs in T2D (Fig. 3).

3.1   Identification

Since meta-analysis is conducted to gather and synthesize the evidence on a particular topic, the first step is to comprehensively search related studies from some important databases, such as PubMed, Web of Science, ScienceDirect, MINDLINE, ProQuest, and Embase. Here, PubMed, ScienceDirect, Embase, and Google Scholar were searched to identify relevant miRNA profiling studies

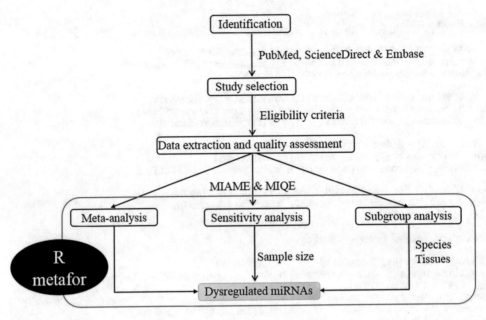

Fig. 3 A workflow for meta-analysis of dysregulated miRNAs

of T2D. An example search strategy for PubMed is provided as follows (*see* **Note 3**):

("miRNA," "diabetes," and "expression" in the title/abstract) or ("miRNA," "diabetes," and "profile" in the title/abstract) or ("miRNA," "diabetes," and "profiling" in the title/abstract) or ("microRNA," "diabetes," and "expression" in the title/abstract) or ("microRNA," "diabetes," and "profile" in the title/abstract) or ("microRNA," "diabetes," and "profiling" in the title/abstract).

3.2 Study Selection (Screening, Eligibility, and Inclusion)

After identification of relevant studies, study selection criteria are used to include or exclude studies. Eligible studies have to meet the inclusion criteria: (1) they are miRNA expression profiling studies on human patients or on animal models of T2D; (2) they compare diabetic and nondiabetic samples; (3) they use miRNA expression arrays; (4) they report cutoff criteria of differentially expressed miRNAs; and (5) they report sample sizes. In our exclusion criteria, miRNA profiling studies using saliva or urine samples are excluded because we focus on the miRNAs in blood. However, if we were studying miRNAs in oral cancer [39] and urinary tract cancer [40–42], saliva and urine samples would be important. In any case, a meta-analysis report should provide a flow diagram of study selection, which includes identification, screening, eligibility extraction, and inclusion steps. The PRISMA guideline [8] provides a four-stage flow diagram, which is a template downloadable for use. Figure 4 shows our example study selection process according to our selection criteria (*see* **Note 4**).

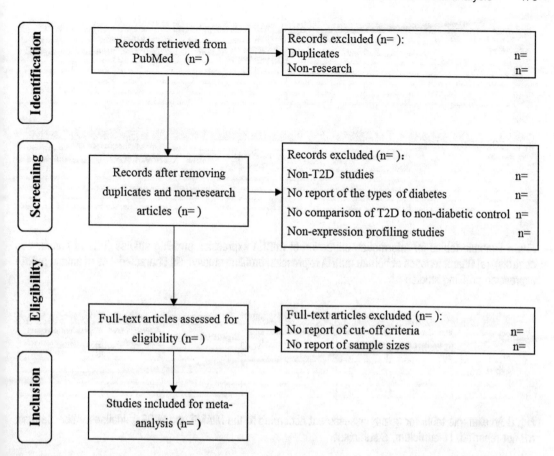

Fig. 4 Flow diagram of study selection. The process of study selection, including identification, screening, eligibility, and inclusion stages, is depicted in the flow diagram

3.3 Data Extraction and Quality Assessment

From the full text and supplementary information of each included expression profiling study, the following eligibility items (Fig. 5) are collected and recorded for subsequent analysis: first author, year of publication, location of study, selection and characteristics of recruited T2D patients or animal models of T2D, etc. Quality assessment of arrays is performed according to the Minimum Information About a Microarray Experiment (MIAME) guideline [9] and the Minimum Information for Publication of Quantitative Real-time PCR Experiments (MIQE) guideline [43] (*see* **Note 5**). Figure 6 shows an example table for quality assessment, and Fig. 7 shows the results of the quality assessment of the included studies.

3.4 Statistical Meta-analysis

Extracted data are transferred to the statistical software R [44] with the package *metafor* [37] for meta-analysis under a random-effects model. The outcomes are represented in terms of $\log_{10}$ odds ratios (logORs), based on the numbers of dysregulation events in both T2D and nondiabetic control samples (*see* **Note 6**), with their 95%

	A	B	C	D	E	F	G	H	I	J	K	L
1	First author (reference)	Year	T2D						Differentially expressed miRNAs			
2			Country	Period	Tissue	Clincal status	No. of samples (T2D/nondiabetic)	Platform	Cut-off criteria	Total	Upregulated	Downregulated
3												
4												
5												
6												

(A)

	A	B	C	D	E	F	G	H	I	J	K	L
1	First author (reference)	Year	Country	T2D					Differentially expressed miRNAs			
2				Traceable animal source	Tissue	Animal model	No. of samples (T2D/nondiabetic)	Platform	Cut-off criteria	Total	Upregulated	Downregulated
3												
4												
5												
6												

(B)

Fig. 5 Example tables for information extraction of miRNA expression profiling studies (T2D vs nondiabetic controls). (**a**) Characteristics of human miRNA expression profiling studies; (**b**) Characteristics of animal miRNA expression profiling studies

	A	B	C	D	E	F	G
1	Source of bias	Raw data of hybridisation	Actual data processing	Sample annotation and experimental variables	Experiment design	Annotation of array design	Experiment and data processing protocols
2	Study 1	NR	I	S	I	I	S
3	study n						
4							
5							

Fig. 6 An example table for quality assessment according to the MIAME and MIQE guidelines. Abbreviations: *NR* not reported, *I* insufficient, *S* sufficient

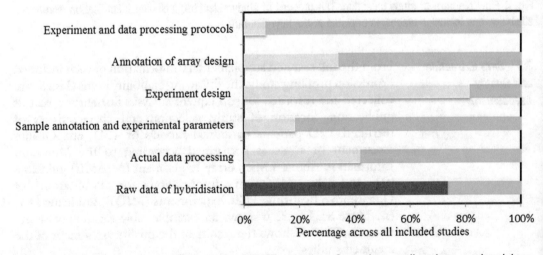

Fig. 7 Quality assessment according to the MIAME guideline. Green bars, yellow bars, and red bars, respectively, indicate the items that were sufficient in annotation, not sufficient in annotation and not reported

confidence intervals. Correction of *P* values (*see* **Note 7**) by such as Bonferroni method should be performed due to multiple testing. Adjusted *P* values less than 0.05 are considered statistically significant. R code for this meta-analysis is shown in Fig. 8.

```
#load metafor package
library(metafor)

#set current working directory
setwd("D:\\GoogleDownload\\book chapter")

#read data under current working directory
dat=read.csv("data.csv",header = TRUE)

#meta-analysis of miR-182 under the random effects model
res=rma(ai=event1, ci=event2, n1i=total1, n2i=total2, data=dat, subset=c(36:42),
        measure = "OR", method="REML")

#call the result
res

#adjust p value by Bonferroni corrections
p=p.adjust(res$pval,"bonferroni")

#call the adjusted p value
p
```

Fig. 8 R codes used for meta-analysis

3.5 Subgroup Analysis (See Note 8)

MiRNAs are differentially expressed among tissue types and species, with corresponding overall effects and heterogeneities. Subgroup analyses divide the extracted data of miRNA expression profiling according to tissue types (blood, muscle, pancreas, liver, etc.) and species (i.e., tissue specificity and species specificity). Technical details and full examples could be found in [7].

3.6 Sensitivity Analysis

Sensitivity analysis is performed on using stricter inclusion criteria such as sample sizes to test the robustness of findings. Sample size is a dominant factor affecting precision in determining the overall effects. Technical details and full examples could be found in [7].

4 Notes

1. RStudio is easier to use than ordinary R environment. RStudio will work only after proper installation of R.

2. When you have a question of interest suitable for conducting a meta-analysis, you should check whether there are existing meta-analyses, whether the existing meta-analyses can fully answer your question, and how your meta-analysis would make a difference in providing stronger evidence.

3. Detailed search strategy and search dates for databases should be documented for reproducibility and updating. You may follow the method to update the results.

4. Figure 3 shows the example results from a PubMed search, you should not only update it but also add the search results from other databases. The selection criteria are often based on the

	Outcome 1	Outcome 2	
Group 1	ai	bi	n1i
Group 2	ci	di	n2i

Fig. 9 A 2 × 2 table

study design, characteristics of participants, intervention (such as disease or healthy control, exposure or not) and outcome measures.

5. The profiling studies included in this example employ micro-arrays or PCR. For quality assessment, MIAME and MIQE would be appropriate. The choice of the quality assessment tools or scales is based on the design of included studies in specific fields. For example, randomized controlled trials should be evaluated according to the Cochrane Collaboration tool for risk of bias assessment tool while primary diagnostic accuracy studies should be evaluated according to the QUADAS-2 in medicine.

6. Meta-analyses in the health/medical sciences are often based on the data in 2 × 2 tables (Fig. 9):

where ai, bi, ci, and di denote the cell frequencies and n1i and n2i the row totals in the ith study. In our example, they are based on the numbers of dysregulation events in both T2D and nondiabetic control samples. log odds ratio is equal to the log of (ai*di)/(bi*ci). Suppose an miRNA is reported upregulation in a study, where the sample size is 6 both in type 2 diabetes and nondiabetic control groups, then the logOR is equal to the log of (6*6)/(0*0). A cell entry with zero value can be problematic especially for odds ratio. Adding a small (negligible) constant to the cells of the 2 × 2 tables is a common solution to this problem. For example, adding 0.1 to the cell entries with zero values, then the logOR will equal to 3.11. It should be noted that different software packages might deal with zero values differently.

7. P value correction methods include the Bonferroni (`bonferroni` in R) method in which P values are simply multiplied by the number of comparisons. Less conservative corrections include Holm (1979) (`holm`), Hochberg (1988) (`hochberg`), Hommel (1988) (`hommel`), Benjamini and Hochberg (1995) (`BH` or its alias `fdr`), and Benjamini and Yekutieli (2001) (`BY`) methods. Researchers could choose a correction method according to their study designs and purposes.

8. In general, subgroup analysis could be done on any characteristics of included studies to detect whether the study characteristics could explain the heterogeneities.

References

1. Koricheva J, Gurevitch J (2013) Place of meta-analysis among other methods of research synthesis. In: Koricheva J, Gurevitch J, Mengersen K (eds) Handbook of meta-analysis in ecology and evolution. Princeton University Press

2. Borenstein M, Hedges LV, Higgins JPT, Rothstein HR (2009) Introduction to meta-analysis. John Wiley & Sons, Ltd., Chichester. https://doi.org/10.1002/9780470743386

3. Evangelou E, Ioannidis JPA (2013) Meta-analysis methods for genome-wide association studies and beyond. Nat Rev Genet 14:379–389. https://doi.org/10.1038/nrg3472

4. Levinson DF (2005) Meta-analysis in psychiatric genetics. Curr Psychiatry Rep 7:143–151. https://doi.org/10.1007/s11920-005-0012-9

5. Borenstein M (2009) Effect sizes for continuous data. In: Cooper H, Hedges LV, Valentine JC (eds) The handbook of research synthesis and meta-analysis. Russell Sage Foundation

6. Tseng GC, Ghosh D, Feingold E (2012) Comprehensive literature review and statistical considerations for microarray meta-analysis. Nucleic Acids Res 40:3785–3799. https://doi.org/10.1093/nar/gkr1265

7. Zhu H, Leung SW (2015) Identification of microRNA biomarkers in type 2 diabetes: a meta-analysis of controlled profiling studies. Diabetologia 58:900–911. https://doi.org/10.1007/s00125-015-3510-2

8. Moher D, Liberati A, Tetzlaff J et al (2009) Preferred reporting items for systematic reviews and meta-analyses: the PRISMA statement (reprinted from annals of internal medicine). Phys Ther 89:873–880. https://doi.org/10.1371/journal.pmed.1000097

9. Minimum information about a microarray experiment – MIAME. http://www.mged.org/Workgroups/MIAME/miame_2.0.html

10. Kahn SE (2001) Clinical review 135: the importance of beta-cell failure in the development and progression of type 2 diabetes. J Clin Endocrinol Metab 86:4047–4058

11. Karolina DS, Armugam A, Sepramaniam S, Jeyaseelan K (2012) MiRNAs and diabetes mellitus. Expert Rev Endocrinol Metab 7:281–300. https://doi.org/10.1586/eem.12.21

12. Winer N, Sowers JR (2004) Epidemiology of diabetes. J Clin Pharmacol 44:397–405. https://doi.org/10.1177/0091270004263017

13. International Diabetes Federation (IDF) (2015) IDF Diabetes Atlas, 7th edn. idf.org. doi:https://doi.org/10.1289/image.ehp.v119.i03

14. Shantikumar S, Caporali A, Emanueli C (2012) Role of microRNAs in diabetes and its cardiovascular complications. Cardiovasc Res 93:583–593. https://doi.org/10.1093/cvr/cvr300

15. Rodriguez A, Griffiths-Jones S, Ashurst JL, Bradley A (2004) Identification of mammalian microRNA host genes and transcription units. Genome Res 14(10):1902. https://doi.org/10.1101/gr.2722704

16. Lee Y, Kim M, Han J et al (2004) MicroRNA genes are transcribed by RNA polymerase II. EMBO J 23:4051–4060. https://doi.org/10.1038/sj.emboj.7600385

17. He L, Hannon GJ (2004) MicroRNAs: small RNAs with a big role in gene regulation. Nat Rev Genet 5:522–531. https://doi.org/10.1038/nrg1379

18. Bartel DP (2004) MicroRNAs: genomics, biogenesis, mechanism, and function. Cell 116:281–297. https://doi.org/10.1016/S0092-8674(04)00045-5

19. Arroyo JD, Chevillet JR, Kroh EM et al (2011) Argonaute2 complexes carry a population of circulating microRNAs independent of vesicles in human plasma. Proc Natl Acad Sci U S A 108:5003–5008. https://doi.org/10.1073/pnas.1019055108

20. Vickers KC, Palmisano BT, Shoucri BM et al (2011) MicroRNAs are transported in plasma and delivered to recipient cells by high-density lipoproteins. Nat Cell Biol 13:423–433. https://doi.org/10.1038/ncb2210

21. Gibbings DJ, Ciaudo C, Erhardt M, Voinnet O (2009) Multivesicular bodies associate with components of miRNA effector complexes and modulate miRNA activity. Nat Cell Biol 11:1143–1149. https://doi.org/10.1038/ncb1929

22. Suárez Y, Sessa WC (2009) MicroRNAs as novel regulators of angiogenesis. Circ Res

104:442–454. https://doi.org/10.1161/CIRCRESAHA.108.191270

23. Carrington JC, Ambros V (2003) Role of microRNAs in plant and animal development. Science 301:336–338. https://doi.org/10.1126/science.1085242

24. Fabian MR, Sonenberg N, Filipowicz W (2010) Regulation of mRNA translation and stability by microRNAs. Annu Rev Biochem 79:351–379. https://doi.org/10.1146/annurev-biochem-060308-103103

25. Bagge A, Clausen TR, Larsen S et al (2012) MicroRNA-29a is up-regulated in beta-cells by glucose and decreases glucose-stimulated insulin secretion. Biochem Biophys Res Commun 426:266–272. https://doi.org/10.1016/j.bbrc.2012.08.082

26. Karolina DS, Tavintharan S, Armugam A et al (2012) Circulating miRNA profiles in patients with metabolic syndrome. J Clin Endocrinol Metab 97:E2271–E2276. https://doi.org/10.1210/jc.2012-1996

27. Locke JM, Harries LW (2012) MicroRNA expression profiling of human islets from individuals with and without type 2 diabetes: promises and pitfalls. Biochem Soc Trans 40:800–803. https://doi.org/10.1042/BST20120049

28. Liu J, Liu W, Ying H et al (2012) Analysis of microRNA expression profile induced by AICAR in mouse hepatocytes. Gene 512:364–372. https://doi.org/10.1016/j.gene.2012.09.118

29. Begley CG, Ellis LM (2012) Raise standards for preclinical cancer research. Nature 483:531–533. https://doi.org/10.1038/483531a

30. Prinz F, Schlange T, Asadullah K (2011) Believe it or not: how much can we rely on published data on potential drug targets? Nat Rev Drug Discov 10:712. https://doi.org/10.1038/nrd3439-c1

31. Mobley A, Linder SK, Braeuer R et al (2013) A survey on data reproducibility in cancer research provides insights into our limited ability to translate findings from the laboratory to the clinic. PLoS One 8:e63221. https://doi.org/10.1371/journal.pone.0063221

32. Guay C, Roggli E, Nesca V et al (2011) Diabetes mellitus, a microRNA-related disease? Transl Res 157:253–264. https://doi.org/10.1016/j.trsl.2011.01.009

33. Guay C, Jacovetti C, Nesca V (2012) Emerging roles of non-coding RNAs in pancreatic β-cell function and dysfunction. Diabetes Obes Metab 14:12–21

34. Hamar P (2012) Role of regulatory microRNAs in type 2 diabetes mellitus related inflammation. Nucleic Acids Ther 22:289–294

35. McClelland AD, Kantharidis P (2014) MicroRNA in the development of diabetic complications. Clin Sci (Lond) 126:95–110. https://doi.org/10.1042/CS20130079

36. Natarajan R, Putta S, Kato M (2012) MicroRNAs and diabetic complications. J Cardiovasc Transl Res 5:413–422

37. Viechtbauer W (2010) Conducting meta-analyses in R with the metafor package. J Stat Softw 36:1–48

38. Centre for Reviews and Dissemination (2009) Systematic reviews: CRDs guidance for undertaking reviews in health care. Cent Rev Dissemination, Univ York, 2008. https://doi.org/10.1017/CBO9781107415324.004

39. Park N, Zhou H, Elashoff D (2009) Salivary microRNA: discovery, characterization, and clinical utility for oral cancer detection. Clin Cancer Res 15:5473–5477

40. Hanke M, Hoefig K, Merz H et al (2010) A robust methodology to study urine microRNA as tumor marker: microRNA-126 and microRNA-182 are related to urinary bladder cancer. Urol Oncol 28:655–661. https://doi.org/10.1016/j.urolonc.2009.01.027

41. Weber JA, Baxter DH, Zhang S et al (2010) The microRNA spectrum in 12 body fluids. Clin Chem 56:1733–1741

42. Yamada Y, Enokida H, Kojima S et al (2011) MiR-96 and miR-183 detection in urine serve as potential tumor markers of urothelial carcinoma: correlation with stage and grade, and comparison with urinary cytology. Cancer Sci 102:522–529. https://doi.org/10.1111/j.1349-7006.2010.01816.x

43. Bustin S, Benes V, Garson J et al (2009) The MIQE guidelines: minimum information for publication of quantitative real-time PCR experiments. Clin Chem 55:611–622. https://doi.org/10.1373/clinchem.2008.112797

44. R Core Team (2015) R: A language and environment for statistical computing. R Found Stat Comput, Vienna, Austria 0:{ISBN} 3-900051-07-0. doi:ISBN 3-900051-07-0

INDEX

Mohini Gore and Umesh B. Jagtap (eds.), *Computational Drug Discovery and Design*, Methods in Molecular Biology, vol. 1762, https://doi.org/10.1007/978-1-4939-7756-7, © Springer Science+Business Media, LLC, part of Springer Nature 2018

Printed in the United States
By Bookmasters